# URINARY TRACT INFECTIONS

Edited by **Peter Tenke**

**Urinary Tract Infections**
Edited by Peter Tenke

**Published by InTech**
Janeza Trdine 9, 51000 Rijeka, Croatia



**Publishing Process Manager** Dragana Manestar

**Technical Editor** Teodora Smiljanic

**Cover Designer** InTech Design Team

Additional hard copies can be obtained from orders@intechopen.com

Urinary Tract Infections, Edited by Peter Tenke
p. cm.
ISBN 978-953-307-757-4

For EU product safety concerns:
IN TECH d.o.o., Prolaz Marije Krucifikse Kozulić 3, 51000 Rijeka, Croatia,
info@intechopen.com or visit our website at intechopen.com.

# Meet the editor

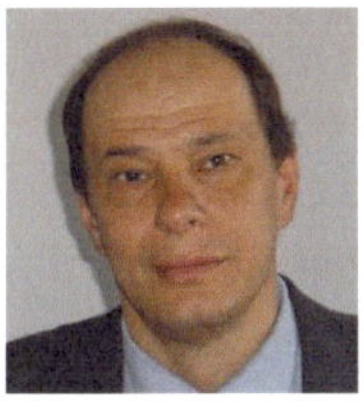

Dr. Peter Tenke was born in 1960 in Budapest. He graduated at the Semmelweis Medical University, Budapest in 1985, and become a licensed urologist in 1989. The main field of his scientific interest are infections in urology and uro-oncology. He received his PhD in 2005 (Foreign bodies in uro-infections), and since then, he is the head of the Department of Urology at South-Pest Hospital. He earned his Habilitation in 2008. Dr. Tenke is a member of the Hungarian and the European Association of Urology, and a Board Member of the European Society for Infection of Urology (ESIU) since 2005. He has delivered many lectures and seminars world-wide about urological infections, especially the role of catheters and foreign bodies. He is also a proud father of two beautiful children.

# Contents

# Preface

Urinary tract infections (UTIs) are among the most common bacterial infections worldwide, with enormous financial implications. About 50 % of women will experience at least one UTI episode during their lifetime, and there are about 7 million out of office visits and 1 million emergency department visits due to UTI in the USA alone, resulting in 100 000 hospital admissions annually. UTIs are also the leading cause of hospital-acquired infections, being responsible for 40% of all such cases, causing a substantial burden of expenses with significant consequences to morbidity and mortality. Therefore, the appropriate management of UTIs is a major medical and financial issue. The aim of this book is to give a summary about the different aspects of the diagnosis, management and prevention of urinary tract infections for all medical disciplines.

This book contains three main sections. In the first section the authors cover the different clinical manifestations of UTI, with special emphasis on some hard-to-treat diseases, such as recurrent UTIs, prostatitis or complicated upper UTIs. The authors also cover special conditions in respect to treatment, such as asymptomatic bacteriuria or pregnancy, and special patient groups, such as acute care settings or psychiatric patients.

The traditional treatment for UTIs is antibiotic therapy. Since the rate of bacterial resistance to antibiotics increases worldwide, the up-to-date knowledge about antibiotic resistance is an issue of growing importance. The second section deals with antibiotics and the available alternative strategies for the prevention and treatment of UTIs.

The third section deals with urinary tract infections in children, with emphasis on some special issues, such as the debates on the management of paediatric UTIs and acute lobar nephronia.

**Dr. Peter Tenke**
Department of Urology
Jahn Ferenc South Pest Hospital
Budapest,
Hungary

# Part 1

## Clinical Manifestations

# 1

# A Review of Uncomplicated Urinary Tract Infections

Tze Shien Lo[1,3] and Augusto Alonto[2,3]
[1]*Veterans Affairs Medical Center and*
[2]*Sanford Health Organization*
[3]*University of North Dakota School of Medicine & Health Sciences*
*Fargo, North Dakota,*
*United States of America*

## 1. Introduction

Urinary tract infections (UTIs) can be classified as either uncomplicated or complicated. Uncomplicated UTIs occur mostly in young women who are sexually active and who have normal genitourinary anatomy. These patients usually have had no previous risk factors otherwise, and no previous surgeries or manipulation of the genital tract. This chapter will discuss the epidemiology, pathogenesis, infecting organisms, clinical manifestations, diagnosis, treatment, and prevention of uncomplicated UTIs.

## 2. Epidemiology

UTIs are one of the most common infections caused by bacteria. UTIs account for more than 8 million doctor's visits each year in the U.S. These infections generate more than 3 million prescriptions, and costs an estimated $3.5 billion dollars annually to treat (University of Michigan Health System, 2010)

UTIs occur more frequently in women than in men, and will occur in roughly half of women during their lifetime. In men, decreased urinary flow from enlarged prostates increase the risk of infection. (University of Michigan Health System, 2010)

## 3. Pathogenesis

The urinary system includes the kidneys, ureters, bladder, and the urethra (Figure 1). This system removes body waste; specifically, urea, from the blood. Urea is carried in the bloodstream to the kidneys. The kidneys extract urea from the blood through filtering units called nephrons. Urea, along with other waste products and water, forms the urine. Urine then passes through the kidneys, to the ureters. From the ureters, urine flows into the bladder. The bladder collects urine and, intermittently, it passes out of the bladder into the urethra, which is a tube that excretes urine from the body.

Many different problems can occur within the urinary tract. Aging can decrease the action of muscles within the urinary system and decrease excretion of urine; therefore, urine may back up and an infection can develop. Injuries from trauma or surgery can also cause infection. In addition, other illnesses and medical conditions can predispose decreased emptying of urine, which can then predispose to infection. These illnesses include prostatic enlargement in elderly men, diabetes mellitus, nephrolithiasis (kidney stones), and other neurologic conditions that can also cause a neurogenic bladder. Manipulation and instrumentation such as insertion of urinary catheters can cause UTIs.

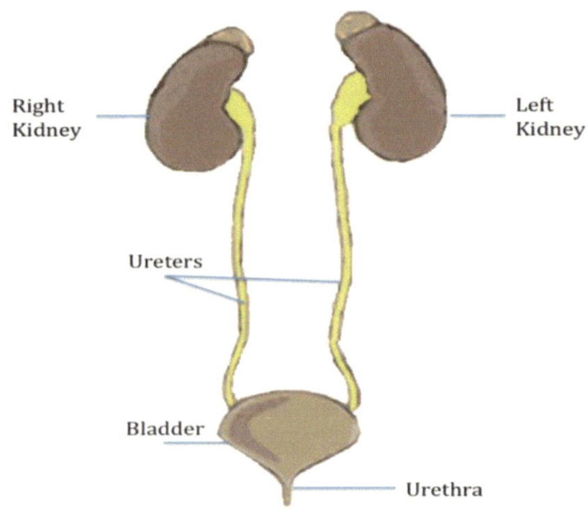


Fig. 1. Urinary System.

Usually, the urinary tract is able to eliminate harmful bacteria. High urine osmolarity and acidity inhibit the growth of most pathogens in the urine. However, these same characteristics can also decrease white blood cells' effectiveness in clearing infection. As such, these urinary characteristics, despite being a noxious environment for bacteria to thrive, can also lower resistance to infections by rendering white blood cells less effective. (Alonto, 2007)

Bacteria can enter the urinary tract through two main routes: ascending route and hematogenous route. The most common way to develop UTI is via the ascending route. Bacteria can enter the urinary tract through the urethra. From the urethra, bacteria can then ascend into the bladder, ureters, and kidneys. Infection of the kidneys is called pyelonephritis. (Alonto, 2007)

Hematogenous route of infection can occur in patients who have bacteremia from other foci of infection such as endocarditis. The pathogenic bacteria that enter the blood stream can then infect the renal parenchyma, causing pyelonephritis, and even renal abscesses.

UTIs are most commonly caused by bacteria that enter the bladder through the urethra. The genitourinary anatomy of women predisposes them to UTIs. Their urethras are shorter, and closer to the anus, providing easier access for fecal bacteria to enter the urethra. This is the major reason women experience infections significantly more frequently than men.

Many other conditions can increase the chances of developing UTIs. These conditions include menopause, diabetes, advanced age, kidney stones, pregnancy, and urinary tract instrumentation. In men, prostatic hypertrophy blocks the flow of urine and, because of this, there is also increased chance of developing UTIs in men with this condition.

Table 1 explains the most common terms used for urinary tract infections.

| | |
|---|---|
| Urinary tract infection | Microbial (bacterial, viral, fungal, etc.) infection that affects any part of the urinary tract |
| Lower urinary tract infection | Infection of either the bladder or the urethra. |
| Upper urinary tract infection | Although the upper urinary tract is composed of the kidneys and ureters, upper urinary tract infection generally affects the kidneys |
| Pyelonephritis | Infection affecting the kidneys |
| Cystitis | Infection affecting the bladder |
| Urethritis | Infection affecting the urethra. Common pathogens causing urethritis include *Chlamydia trachomatis* and *Neisseria gonorrhoeae* |
| Cervicitis | Infection affecting the cervix. Mostly due to pathogens causing sexually transmitted diseases such as *Chlamydia trachomatis* and *Neisseria gonorrhoeae* |
| Prostatitis | Infection of the prostate |
| Renal abscess | Infection of the renal parenchyma which forms purulent collection within or around the renal parenchyma |
| Bacteruria | Presence of bacteria in the urine. Does not necessarily indicate presence of infection. Does not need to be treated in most instances, if patient is asymptomatic. |
| Pyuria | Presence of white blood cells in the urine. Indicates inflammation, not necessarily from infection. |

Table 1. Terms Used for Specific Urinary Tract Infections.

## 4. Infecting organisms

Uropathogens have characteristics that enable them to be successful in causing infections of the urinary tract. Adhesins enable the attachment to host membranes. Capsular polysaccharides, hemolysins, cytotoxic necrotizing factor (CNF) protein, and aerobactins are other factors that enable uropathogens to invade the urinary tract. Table 2 lists common virulence factors associated with pathogens causing UTIs. (Brusch, 2010)

| Virulence Factors |
|---|
| Adherence |
| Calculi formation |
| Toxin production |
| Lipopolysaccharides |
| Capsular polysaccharide |
| Hemolysins |
| Biofilm |
| Aerobactins |

Table 2. Virulence Factors in Uropathogens.

The most common pathogen causing UTIs is *Escherichia coli* (*E. coli*), causing 70-95% of urinary tract infections. Other organisms that can be responsible for UTIs include Gram-positive cocci, such as *Staphylococcus saprophyticus* and *Enterococcus faecalis*. Other Gram-negative organisms responsible for causing UTIs include *Klebsiella* species and *Proteus* species. Hospitalized patients can develop complicated UTIs, and more common organisms isolated in these infections include Gram-negative organisms such as *Pseudomonas aeruginosa*, *Enterobacter* species, and *Acinetobacter* species; Gram-positive organisms including *Staphylococcus aureus*; and even yeast. Table 3 lists organisms that can be seen in urinary tract infections. (Brusch, 2010)

| | |
|---|---|
| **Pyelonephritis** | **Gram-positive Bacteria**<br>*Staphylococcus aureus*<br>*Staphylococcus saprophyticus*<br>**Gram-negative Bacteria**<br>*Escherichia coli*<br>*Klebsiella* species<br>*Proteus* species<br>*Pseudomonas aeruginosa*<br>*Enterobacter* species |
| **Cystitis** | **Gram-negative Bacteria**<br>*Escherichia coli*<br>*Klebsiella* species<br>*Proteus* species<br>**Gram-positive Bacteria**<br>*Staphylococcus saprophyticus*<br>*Enterooccus* species<br>*Staphylococcus aureus* |
| **Urethritis** | *Chlamydia trachomatis*<br>*Neisseria gonorrhoeae*<br>*Ureaplasma urealyticum* |

Table 3. Organisms Associated with Urinary Tract Infections.

## 5. Clinical manifestations

The clinical manifestations of UTIs can vary significantly, especially in the extremes of age. UTIs in children can present with different symptoms. Symptoms in children younger than 2 years of age tend to be nonspecific, and can include fever, vomiting, and failure to thrive.

In contrast, the elderly patient who has a UTI may be asymptomatic. When symptoms are present, they can include abdominal pain or mental status changes.

However, the classic symptoms of acute uncomplicated cystitis include dysuria, change in urinary frequency, urinary urgency, hematuria, and suprapubic pain. Fever is usually absent in those with lower UTIs.

In general, acute uncomplicated pyelonephritis classically presents with flank pain, abdominal pain, nausea, vomiting, fever, and costovertebral angle tenderness. Symptoms of cystitis may or may not be present in those with pyelonephritis. When present, these signs can occur 24-48 hours prior to appearance of symptoms of pyelonephritis. Some patients with acute pyelonephritis can present with sepsis.

## 6. Diagnosis

There are many different etiologies, both infectious and non-infectious, that can present with acute dysuria. The differential diagnosis of acute dysuria may include pyelonephritis, cystitis, urethritis, infectious vaginitis, atrophic vaginitis, and interstitial cystitis. A good history and physical examination usually gives the clinician enough information to make a correct diagnosis in most situations.

| | |
|---|---|
| Acute cystitis | |
| Acute pyelonephritis | |
| Urethritis | |
| | *Chlamydia trachomatis*<br>*Neisseria gonorrhoeae*<br>*Trichomonas vaginalis*<br>*Candida albicans*<br>*Herpes simplex virus*<br>Irritant urethritis |
| Vaginitis | |
| | *Candida albicans*<br>*Trichomonas vaginalis*<br>Bacterial vaginosis<br>Atrophic vaginitis |
| Interstitial cystitis | |

Table 4. Differential Diagnoses of Acute Cystitis.

The most valuable diagnostic test for UTI is a urine analysis. The preferred definition of pyuria is at least 10 leukocytes/mm$^3$ of midstream urine by counting changer. Using this definition, the majority of patients with bacteruria will have pyuria as well. Pyuria is present in almost all patients with acute cystitis. If pyuria is not seen, an alternative cause for the patient's symptoms will need to be considered. (Brusch, 2010)

Urine dipstick is a rapid screening test for detecting pyuria, as it can detect the presence of leukocyte esterase. The urine dipstick also detects nitrite, which signifies the presence of *Enterobacteriaceae,* bacteria which convert nitrite to nitrate. Although the nitrite test is a sensitive test for detecting *Enterobacteriaceae,* it may not detect other pathogens. (Brusch, 2010)

Urine in the bladder is sterile. However, because the urethra is usually contaminated with bacteria, collected urine specimens are frequently not sterile. A midstream, clean-voided urine, can separate contamination from urinary tract infection. Urine specimens from most patients with UTIs should have at least $10^5$ bacteria/mL. Patients without infection should have less than $10^4$ bacteria/mL. However, there are some patients with urinary infections that have fewer than $10^5$ bacteria/mL in urine. (Sobel & Kaye, 2005)

The Infectious Diseases Society of America consensus definition of cystitis for use in antibiotic treatment studies is $10^3$ bacteria/mL or more of an uropathogen, and for pyelonephritis $10^4$ bacteria/mL.

Acceptable methods for urine collection include midstream clean catch, catheterization, and suprapubic aspiration. (Sobel & Kaye, 2005)

## 7. Treatment

Because overuse and abuse of antimicrobial agents has led to rapidly evolving resistance of pathogens to this precious class of medications, appropriate administration of antibiotics to treat UTIs cannot be overemphasized. Appropriate use of antibiotics include correct indications, correct choice of antibiotic(s) (according to local resistance data or culture data), and timely administration of the agent(s) with appropriate dosage and treatment duration.

### 7.1 Asymptomatic bacteriuria (Alcaide & Lichtstein, 2004)

This condition is defined by the presence of more than $10^5$ bacteria/mL in the urine of a patient without urinary tract and/or constitutional symptoms. Antibiotic treatment for asymptomatic bacteriuria is not indicated unless the woman is pregnant or the patient is about to undergo a urologic procedure, e.g. cystoscopy. Prescribing antibiotics in patients with asymptomatic bacteriuria exposes them to potential adverse drug reactions, such as development of *C. difficile* infection and increased selective pressure leading to the development of antimicrobial resistance. Unfortunately, despite data not supporting the prescription of antibiotics to patients with asymptomatic bacteriuria, many clinicians administer antibiotics to this group of patients based on individual habit or convention rather than clinical evidence or guidelines.

### 7.2 Acute uncomplicated cystitis (AUC)

As described in the section "Infecting Organisms", the most common etiologic agent of AUC is *E. coli*. Other common pathogens are *S. saprophyticus, E. faecalis, Klebsiella* species and *Proteus* species. The selection of antibiotics should target the above common pathogens.
The following is a detailed description of commonly used antibiotics recommended for treating AUC (Mascaretti, 2003a; Dielubanza & Schaeffer, 2011; Gupta et al., 2011).

#### 7.2.1 Nitrofurantoin monohydrate/macrocrystals

Nitrofurantoin is reduced by bacterial flavoproteins to highly reactive intermediates which are active in damaging the DNA of susceptible bacteria. Most stains of *E. coli, S. saprophyticus* and *Enterococcus* species are sensitive to nitrofurantoin. However, most species of *Proteus* and *Klebsiella* are less susceptible to this drug.
Nitrofurantoin is indicated for the treatment of AUC only. Because it is eliminated without achieving antibacterial concentration in plasma or tissues, nitrofurantoin is not indicated for treating pyelonephritis. Because the rate of excretion of nitrofurantoin is linearly related to creatinine clearance, impaired renal function may decrease its efficacy and increase systemic toxicity of the drug (Petri, 2006).
Common side effects of nitrofurantoin are nausea, vomiting and diarrhea. However, the macrocrystal form appears to have lower gastrointestinal adverse reactions. Insidious irreversible interstitial pulmonary fibrosis can develop in elderly taking nitrofurantoin chronically. Therefore, patients who are taking this drug long term should undergo pulmonary function tests and chest radiography periodically.
Gupta et al. demonstrated that a 5-day course of nitrofurantoin is equivalent, clinically and microbiologically, to a 3-day course of trimethoprim-sulfamethoxazole (Gupta et al., 2007). The 2011 updated IDSA guidelines for uncomplicated urinary tract infection also recommended using nitrofurantoin monohydrate/macrocrystals 100 mg by mouth twice daily for 5 to 7 days (Gupta et al., 2011).

### 7.2.2 Trimethoprim/sulfamethoxazole (TMP/SMX)

TMP/SMX inhibits bacterial DNA, RNA and protein synthesis by interfering with folic acid synthesis. TMP/SMX's spectrum will cover *E. coli* and *S. saprophyticus*, the two most uropathogens in causing AUC. TMP/SMX has excellent tissue penetration, so it can be used to treat upper urinary tract infection, including uncomplicated pyelonephritis.
Skin rash and gastrointestinal adverse reactions; including nausea, vomiting, and anorexia are the common side effects of TMP/SMX. The dose should be reduced in patients with renal impairment.
TMP/SMX 160/800mg (double strength tablets) by mouth twice daily for 3 days is the recommended regimen for empirical treatment of AUC, provided the local community resistance prevalence of common uropathogens to TMP/SMX is less than 20%.

### 7.2.3 Fosfomycin trometamol

Fosfomycin inhibits bacterial cell wall synthesis by irreversibly inactivating the enzyme pyruvoyl transferase, an enzyme crucial in the synthesis of cell walls by bacteria. Fosfomycin exhibits a broad spectrum of activity against Gram positive and gram negative bacteria including *E. coli* and *P. mirabilis* (Mascaretti, 2003b).
Fosfomycin is well tolerated. Common side effects are headache, diarrhea and nausea.
In a multicenter clinical trial comparing single-dose fosfomycin with a 7-day course of nitrofurantoin for the treatment of AUC in female patients, Stein showed that bacteriologic and clinical cure rates of a single 3-g dose of fosfomycin and 7-day course of nitrofurantoin were comparable (Stein, 1999). Minasssian et al. from The United Kingdom also demonstrated that a single dose of 3g of fosfomycin trometamol had a comparable microbiological cure rate and was similar to a 5-day course of trimethoprim (Minassian et al., 1998). Fosfomycin is approved as a single dose of 3g powder mixed with water to treat AUC.

### 7.2.4 Fluoroquinolones

The fluoroquinolones inhibit relaxation of supercoiled DNA and cause breakage of DNA strands by inhibiting DNA gyrase and topoisomerase IV in susceptible bacteria.
The fluoroquinolones that are commonly used to treat AUC are ciprofloxacin and levofloxacin. Both offer excellent coverage for Gram positive and Gram negative bacteria including *Enterobacteriaceae*. Common side effects of ciprofloxacin and levofloxacin are headache, nausea, diarrhea, abdominal pain and constipation. A rare complication may be Achilles tendon rupture in elderly patients.
Arredondo-Garcia et al. conducted a randomized, multicenter, open-label, prospective study to compare the bacteriologic and clinical efficacy of oral ciprofloxacin 250mg twice daily for 3 days vs oral trimethoprim/sulfamethoxazole 160/800mg twice daily for 7 days vs oral norfloxacin 400mg twice daily for 7 days for treatment of AUC. The authors were able to show that a 3-day regimen of oral ciprofloxacin was clinically and bacteriologically at least as effective as a 7-day course of TMP-SMX and norfloxacin (Arredondo-Garcia et al., 2004). The empirical regimen of oral ciprofloxacin and oral levofloxacin for treating AUC is 250 mg twice daily for 3 days and 250 mg once a day for 3 days, respectively.

### 7.2.5 β-lactam agents

β-lactam agents that can be used to treat AUC include amoxicillin-clavulanate and oral second and third generation cephalosporins. Only amoxicillin-clavulanate will be described

in this chapter. Amoxicillin inhibits bacterial cell wall synthesis by binding to the penicillin-binding proteins. Clavulanate inhibits β-lactamases that inactivate amoxicillin.
Amoxicillin-clavulanate has a broad spectrum which covers Gram positive bacteria, including *S. saprophyticus*; and Gram negative bacteria, including *E. coli* and *P. mirabilis*. Most common side effects of amoxicillin-clavulanate are diarrhea, nausea, vomiting and skin rash. Serious side effects include *C. difficile* colitis and Stevens-Johnson syndrome.
In a randomized, single-blind treatment trial of 370 women with AUC with either a 3-day regimen of amoxicillin-clavulanate vs a 3-day regimen of oral ciprofloxacin, Hooton et al. demonstrated that the former was not as effective as the latter for the treatment of AUC (Hooton et al., 2005). Therefore, the recommended empirical regimen for treating AUC with amoxicillin-clavulanate is 500/125 mg by mouth three times a day for a range of 3 to 5 days.

### 7.3 Infectious Disease Society of America (IDSA) guidelines for treatment of uncomplicated urinary tract infections

The 2010 updated International Clinical Practice Guidelines for the treatment of acute uncomplicated cystitis (AUC) and pyelonephritis in women was published in the March 1, 2011 issue of Clinical Infectious Disease (Gupta et al., 2011). These guidelines were also endorsed by the European Society for Microbiology and Infectious Diseases. Table 5 summarizes the treatment guidelines for acute uncomplicated cystitis. Table 6 indicates the retail price of antibiotics used in treating AUC.

| AGENT | DOSE | DURATION |
|---|---|---|
| Nitrofurantoin monohydrate | 100 mg BID | 5 - 7 days |
| Nitrofurantoin macrocrystal | 100 mg BID | 5 - 7 days |
| Trimethoprim-sulfamethoxazole | 160/800 mg BID | 3 days |
| Fosfomycin trometamol | 3 g | Single dose sachet |
| Fluoroquinolones | Dose varies by agent | 3-day regimen |
| B-lactams | Dose varies by agent | 3-5 day regimen |

Table 5. Treatment guidelines for urinary tract infections published in 2010 by The Infectious Disease Society of America.

| Antibiotic | **Retail Price** |
|---|---|
| Nitrofurantoin monohydrate (100 mg twice daily ) | $13.50 (5 days)<br>$18.90 (7 days) |
| Nitrofurantoin macrocrystal (100 mg twice daily) | $19.00 (5 days)<br>$26.13 (7 days) |
| Trimethoprim-sulfamethoxazole (160/800 mg twice daily) | $4.00 (3 days) |
| Fosfomycin trometamol (3 g single-dose sachet) | $50.86 (1 day) |
| Ciprofloxacin (250 mg twice daily) | $17.70 (3 days) |
| Levofloxacin (25 mg once daily) | $36.00 (3 days) |
| Amoxicillin-clavulanate | $13.80 (3 days)<br>$23.00 (5 days) |

Prices derived from www.drugstore.com

Table 6. Retail price in the United States for commonly used antibiotics to treat AUC.

### 7.4 Treatment of uncomplicated pyelonephritis

The IDSA guidelines also recommend the following for management of acute uncomplicated pyelonephritis (Gupta et al., 2011).

- A urine culture and susceptibility test should always be performed, and initial empirical therapy should be tailored to the infecting uropathogen.
- Oral ciprofloxacin (500 mg twice daily) for 7 days, with or without an initial 400 mg dose of intravenous ciprofloxacin, is appropriate in patients not requiring hospitalization where the prevalence of resistance of community uropathogens to fluoroquinolones does not exceed 10%. If the prevalence of fluoroquinolone resistance is thought to exceed 10%, an initial 1-time intravenous dose of a long-acting parenteral antimicrobial, such as 1 g of ceftriaxone or a consolidated 24-h dose of an aminoglycoside is recommended.
- A once-daily oral fluoroquinolone, including ciprofloxacin (1000 mg extended release for 7 days) or levofloxacin (750mg for 5 days), is an appropriate choice for therapy in patients not requiring hospitalization where the prevalence of resistance of community uropathogens is not known to exceed 10%.
- Oral trimethoprim-sulfamethoxazole (TMP/SMX) (160/800 mg twice-daily for 14 days) is appropriate if the uropathogen is known to be susceptible. If TMP/SMX is used when the susceptibility is not known, an initial intravenous dose of a long-acting parenteral antimicrobial, such as 1 g of ceftriaxone or a consolidated 24-hour dose of an aminoglycoside is recommended.
- Oral β-lactam agents are less effective than other agents. If an oral β-lactam agent is used, an initial intravenous dose of a long-acting parenteral antimicrobial, such as 1g of ceftriaxone or a consolidated 24-hour dose of an aminoglycoside is recommended.
- Cases requiring hospitalization should initially be treated with an intravenous antimicrobial regimen; such as a fluoroquinolone, an aminoglycoside with or without ampicillin, an extended-spectrum cephalosporin, or extended–spectrum penicillin with or without an aminoglycoside, or a carbapenem. The choice among these agents should be based on local resistance data, and the regimen should be tailored on the basis of susceptibility results.

## 8. Prevention

The prevention of UTIs can be classified into two categories, non-antimicrobial and antimicrobial strategies.

### 8.1 Non antimicrobial strategy

A large population-based case-control study conducted by Fihn, et al. demonstrated that use of condoms coated with the spermicide nonoxynol-9 during intercourse was associated with a higher incidence of urinary tract infection caused by *E. coli* in young women (Fihn et al., 1996). Hooton et al. also demonstrated in a prospective study that recent use of a diaphragm with spermicide was one of the independent risk factors for symptomatic UTI (Hooton et al., 1996). Thus, sexually active women should be advised to avoid spermicide use during intercourse.

Postcoital voiding has been advocated as a positive behavioral modification to prevent UTI (Stamm, 2010). However, a population-based, prospective cohort study did not showed that postcoital voiding was associated with decreased incidents of acute cystitis after multivariable analysis (Jackson et al., 2004)

Other non-antimicrobial strategies to prevent acute UTI have been investigated. Cranberries and other berries containing proanthocyanidins was proven, in vitro, to prevent uropathogens such as *E. coli* from adhering to urinary epithelium ( Zafriri et al., 1989). Kontiokari et al. conducted an open, randomized controlled 12-month follow-up trial which showed that cranberry-lingonberry was more effective in reducing recurrence of UTI compared to lactobacillus GG drink or no intervention (Kontiokari et al., 2001). However, a recent double-blind, placebo-controlled study of the effects of cranberry on risk of recurring UTI study demonstrated that, among healthy college women with acute UTI, those drinking 8 oz of 27% cranberry juice twice daily, did not experience a decrease in the 6-month incidence of a second UTI, compared with those drinking a placebo (Barbosa-Cesnik et al., 2011).

Use of lactobacillus-containing probiotics has been proposed for the prevention of UTI. However, a review article by Barrons et al concluded that use of lactobacillus for the prevention of UTI remain inconclusive and controversial ( Barrons et al., 2008).

Although a randomized double-blind, placebo-controlled trial of a topically applied intravaginal estriol cream revealed that estriol was more effective in preventing recurrent UTI in postmenopausal women ( Raz & Stam, 1993), the use of low dose oral estrogen did not reduce frequency of UTI (Brown et al., 2001; Cardozo et al., 1998).

In recent years, there has been great enthusiasm for the development of a vaccine to prevent UTIs because of the increasing resistance of uropathogens against antimicrobials and concerns for adverse reactions from antimicrobials. A double-blind study involved 75 patients randomly assigned to either placebo or vaginal mucosal suppository vaccines. The vaccine suppositories contained 10 strains of heat-killed uropathogenic bacteria. The study demonstrated that vaginal suppository vaccines were effective in reducing recurrence of *E. coli* UTI compared to placebo (Hopkins, 2007). So far there is no licensed vaccine for prevention of UTIs available in the USA.

### 8.2 Antimicrobial strategies (Dielubanza & Schaeffer, 2011; Foster, 2008)

Antimicrobial prophylaxis is a more effective way to prevent recurrence of UTI. However, this strategy carries the potential of promoting resistance and development of adverse reactions.

Low-dose continuous antimicrobial prophylaxis nitrofurantoin (100 mg daily), cephalexin (250 mg daily), and TMP-SMX (daily or 3 times a week) have been used successfully as low-dose antimicrobial prophylaxis for women with frequent UTIs.

Other strategies that were found to be effective in preventing recurrent UTI are postcoital prophylaxis and self-start therapy. Postcoital prophylaxis is appropriate for women who tend to develop UTI after intercourse. A single dose of antibiotic is used following intercourse. Self-start therapy is for women who are unwilling to take antibiotic continuously for prevention of recurrent UTI. By this method, the patient diagnoses UTI herself with a urine dipstick or by recognizing incipient UTI symptoms and starts a 3-day course of antibiotics immediately.

## 9. References

Alonto, A. (2007). Urinary Tract Infections. In: *Textbook of Diagnostic Microbiology.* C. L. Mahon, D. Lehman & G. Manuselis (eds.), pp. 1010-1029. Sauders, 1-4160-2581-2, St. Louis, MO, USA.

Alcaide, M. and Lichtstein, D.M. (2004) How Best to Treat Urinary Tract Infections in Adults: A Rational Approach. *Consultant* (July 2004) pp. 1145-1151. In print and available at: www.ConsultantLive.com.

Arredondo-Garcia, J.L., Figueroa-Damian, R., Rosas, A., et al. (2004). Comparison of short-term treatment regimen of ciprofloxacin versus long-term treatment regimens of trimethoprim/sulfamethoxazole or norfloxacin for uncomplicated lower urinary tract infections: a randomized, multicentre, open-label, prospective study. *Journal of Antimicrobial and Chemotherapy* 54(4) (October 2004) pp. 840-3, 15347634. Epub 2004 Sep 3.

Barbosa-Cesnik, C., Brown, M.B., Buxton M., et al. (2011) Cranberry Juice Fails to Prevent Recurrent Urinary Tract Infection: Results From a Randomized Placebo-Controlled Trial. *Clinical Infectious Diseases* 52(1) (January 2011) pp. 23-30, 521-0001.

Barrons, R. and Tassone D. (2008) Use of Lactobacillus probiotics for bacterial genitourinary infections in women: a review. *Clinical Therapeutics* 30(3) (March 2008) pp. 453-68, 18405785.

Brown, JS, Vittinghoff E, Kanaya AM, et al. (2001). Urinary tract infections in postmenopausal women: effect of hormone therapy and risk factors. *Obstetrics and Gynecology* 98(6) (December 2001) pp. 1045-52, 11755552.

Brusch, J. (2010) *Urinary Tract Infection in Females* (Reference section) (M. S. Bronze, Ed.) Retrieved May 5, 2011, from Medscape: http://emedicine.medscape.com/article/233101 (overview and clinical sections).

Cardozo, L., Benness, C. and Abbott, D. (1998). Low dose oestrogen prophylaxis for recurrent urinary tract infections in elderly women. *British Journal of Obstetrics and Gynaecology* 105(4) (April 1998) pp. 403-407, 9609266.

Dielubanza, E.J. and Schaeffer A.J. (2011). Urinary Tract Infections in Women. *The Medical Clinics of North America* 95 pp. 27-41, 0025-7125.

Fihn S.D., Boyko, E.J., Normand, E.H., et al. (1996). Association between use of spermicide-coated condoms and *Escherichia coli* urinary tract infections in young women. *American Journal of Epidemiology* 144(5) (September 1996) pp. 512-520, 8781467.

Foster, RT. (2008). Uncomplicated Urinary Tract Infections. *Obstetrics and Gynecology Clinics of North America*. 35 (2008) pp. 235-248, 0889-8545/08.

Gupta, K, Hooton, TM, Roberts, PL, et al. (2007) Short-Course Nitrofurantoin for the Treatment of Acute Uncomplicated Cystitis in Women. *Arch Intern Med* 167(20) (November 2007) pp. 2207-2212, 17998493.

Gupta, K, Hooton, TM, Naber, KG, et al. (2011) International Clinical Practice Guidelines for the Treatment of Acute Uncomplicated Cystitis and Pyelonephritis in Women: A 2010 Update by the Infectious Diseases Society of America and the European Society for Microbiology and Infectious diseases. *Clinical Infectious Diseases*. 52(5) (March 2011) pp. 103-120, 1058-4838.

Hooton, T.M., Scholes, D., Hughes, J.P., et al. (1996) A prospective study of risk factors for symptomatic urinary tract infection in young women. *N Engl J Med* 335(7) (August 1996) pp. 468-74, 8672152.

Hooton, TM, Scholes, D, Gupta, K, et al. (2005) Amoxicillin-clavulanate vs ciprofloxacin for the treatment of uncomplicated cystitis in women: a randomized trial. *JAMA* 293(8) (February 2005) pp. 949-55, 15728165.

Hopkins, W.J., Elkahwaji, J., Beierle, L.M., et al. (2007) Vaginal mucosal vaccine for recurrent urinary tract infections in women: results of a phase 2 clinical trial. *Journal of Urology* 177(4) (April 2007) pp. 1349-53, 17382730.

Jackson, SL, Boyko, EJ, Scholes D, et al. (2004). Predictors of urinary tract infection after menopause: a prospective study. *The American Journal of Medicine;* 117(12) (December 2004) pp. 903-11, 15629728.

Kontiokari, T , Sundqvist, K., Nuutinen, M, et al. (2001) Randomized trial of cranberry-lingonberry juice and Lactobacillus GG drink for the prevention of urinary tract infections in women. *BMJ* 322(7302) (June 2001) pp. 1571, 11431298.

Mascaretti, OA. (2003a) Antibacterial agents that cause damage to DNA 5-nitrofurans. In: *Bacteria versus Antibacterial Agents. An integrated approach* pp. 315-317. American Society of Microbiology (ASM) Press. 1-55581-258-9. Washington DC.

Mascaretti, OA. (2003b) Antibacterial agents that cause damage to DNA 5-nitrofurans. In: *Bacteria versus Antibacterial Agents. An integrated approach* pp. 199-202. American Society of Microbiology (ASM) Press. 1-55581-258-9. Washington DC.

Minassian, MA, Lewis, DA, Chattopadhyay, D, et al. (1998) A comparison between single-dose fosfomycin trometamol (Monuril) and a 5-day course of trimethoprim in the treatment of uncomplicated lower urinary tract infection in women. *International Journal of Antimicrobial Agents* 10(1) (April 1998) pp. 39-47, 9624542.

Petri, W.A., Jr. (2006). Sulfonamides, Trimethoprime-Sulfamethoxazole, Quinolones, and Agents for Urinary Tract Infections. In: *Goodman and Gilman's The Pharmacological Basis of Therapeutics* (11th Edition), McGraw-Hill, 0-07-142280-3, New York, NY.

Raz, R. and Stamm, WE. (1992) A controlled trial of intravaginal estriol in postmenopausal women with recurrent urinary tract infections. *N Engl J Med* 329(11) (September 1993) pp. 753-6, 8350884.

Sobel, J. and Kaye D (2005). Urinary Tract Infections. In: *Principles and Practice of Infectious Diseases*, Elsevier, Inc., 0-443-06643-4 (pp. 875-901). Philadelphia, PA, USA.

Stamm WE. (2010). Urinary tract infections, pyelonephritis, and prostatitis. In: *Harrison's Infectious Diseases*. Dennis L. Kasper, Anthony S. Fauci (Eds). pp 272-282. McGraw Hill. 978-0-07-170293-5. New York, NY.

Stein, GE. (1999) Comparison of single-dose fosfomycin and a 7-day course of nitrofurantoin in female patients with uncomplicated urinary tract infection. *Clinical Therapeutics* 21(110) (November 1999) pp. 1864-1872, 10890258.

University of Michigan Health System. (2010, Nov. 12). *News Release*. Retrieved May 2, 2011, from Science Daily:
http://www.sciencedaily.com/releases/2010/11/101112141128.htm

Zafriri, D, Ofek, I, Adar, R, et al. (1989) Inhibitory activity of cranberry juice on adherence of type 1 and type P fimbriated Escherichia coli to eucaryotic cells. *Antimicrobial Agents and Chemotherapy* 33(1) (January 1989) pp. 92-98, 2653218.

www.Drugstore.com - Access Date: May 4, 2011 (drugstore.com, inc., 411 108th Ave NE, Suite 1400, Bellevue, WA 98004; Phone: 425-372-3200)

# 2

# Current Management Strategies for Uncomplicated and Complicated Cystitis

Niall F. Davis and Hugh D. Flood
*Department of Urology, Mid-Western Regional Hospital, Dooradoyle, Co. Limerick, Ireland*

## 1. Introduction

Acute cystitis is defined as a superficial infection of the bladder mucosa. Approximately 10% of females are diagnosed with cystitis on an annual basis and over 50% of females will have at least one episode of cystitis during their lifetime (Foxman 2002, Foxman et al. 2000). Typically, uncomplicated cystitis occurs in late adolescence and during the second and fourth decades in females with up to 30% of females 20 to 40 years of age having a history of cystitis (Hooton et al. 1996). Symptoms such as fever, chills and flank pain are absent as acute cystitis is not associated with involvement of the upper urinary tracts. Risk factors for acute cystitis include sexual intercourse, the use of spermicides and ascending bowel flora. Males with underlying structural and functional deficiencies of the genitourinary tract may also develop acute cystitis (Krieger et al. 1993). After the initial infection many patients tend to have recurrence with 25% to 50% of patients having another infection within 1 year. Recurrent episodes of cystitis are defined as symptomatic infections that follow the clinical resolution of a previous episode after treatment and their incidence is 3% to 5%.

Although the vast majority of patients presenting with cystitis respond promptly to appropriate therapy, early identification and treatment of patients with complicated cystitis remains a significant clinical challenge to physicians and urologists. Herein, we discuss appropriate management strategies for patients presenting with symptoms consistent with both uncomplicated and complicated cystitis. We also place particular emphasis on appropriate antimicrobial treatment regimens for cystitis and discuss emerging patterns of resistance among different uropathogens.

## 2. Acute uncomplicated cystitis

### 2.1 Clinical presentation

Typically, cystitis presents with symptoms that include dysuria, frequency, urgency and suprapubic pain. Occasionally, foul smelling urine and haematuria may develop (Fig. 1). The likelihood of cystitis in female patients presenting with these symptoms ranges from 50% to 90% (Bent et al. 2002, Wong et al. 1985). The likelihood cystitis is up to 90% in a female patient who has had cystitis and presents with symptoms suggestive of recurrence (Gupta et al. 2001a, Gupta et al. 2001b). As cystitis only affects the mucosal layers of the bladder fever and rigors do not develop. Differential diagnosis for females presenting with these symptoms should include vaginitis, sexually transmitted infections (STIs) and urethral pathology.

It is important to differentiate cystitis from other conditions where dysuria may also be present. Specific features within the history, physical examination and voided urine may differentiate between vaginitis, urethral infections caused by STIs and other miscellaneous conditions associated with dysuria. Characteristic features of vaginitis include irritative voiding with vaginal irritation and an insidious onset. Urinary symptoms such as frequency, suprapubic pain and haematuria are usually absent. The patient may also give a history of vaginal discharge and multiple sexual partners. Common causes of STIs are herpes simplex virus (HSV), gonorrhoea and chlamydia. Urethritis also causes subacute dysuria and is associated with a history of urethral discharge and multiple sexual partners. In male patients urethral discharge with inflammatory cells or pyuria is characteristic and common causes of urethritis in males include gonorrhoea, chlamydia, HSV and trichomoniasis. Culture and immunological analysis are indicated for diagnostic purposes

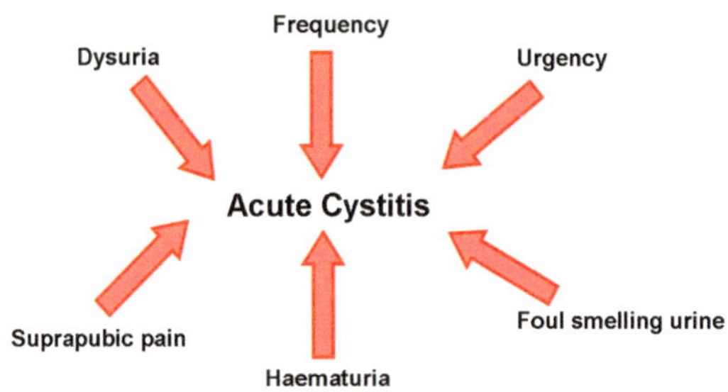


Fig. 1. Common presenting symptoms associated with acute cystitis. Typically, patients present with dysuria, frequency, urgency and suprapubic pain.

## 2.2 Risk factors

The most important risk factors for acute cystitis in female patients are previous episodes of cystitis and frequent or recent sexual activity as celibate females rarely present with cystitis (Scholes et al. 2000). The relative odds of acute cystitis during the first 48 hours after sexual intercourse are increased by 60 fold and spermicidal agents increase the risk of infection from E. coli or S. saprophyticus by 2 - 3 fold (Fihn et al. 1998, Nicolle et al. 1982, Strom et al. 1987). Females that frequently develop recurrent episodes of cystitis are more likely to have a maternal history of the condition and to have developed their first episode at an early age (Fihn 2003, Scholes et al. 2000). In healthy postmenopausal females sexual activity is a less important predictor of cystitis in comparison to younger females and oestrogen deficiency is believed to play a greater role (Boyko et al. 2002). Recurrent cystitis in postmenopausal females is more likely in patients with cystoceles, urinary incontinence and a previous history of genitourinary surgery (Raz et al. 2000). Female patients with diabetes mellitus are twice as likely to develop cystitis compared to non-diabetic females. The risk of acute cystitis also increases in elderly females residing in institutionalised settings with the risk of infection showing a direct correlation with increasing age and physical disability (Nicolle et al. 2005).

## 2.3 Laboratory diagnosis

A laboratory diagnosis of suspected acute cystitis is based on microscopic urinalysis that indicates the presence of pyuria, bacteriuria and haematuria. Pyuria on microscopy has a sensitivity of 95% and a specificity of 70% (Fihn 2003). The presence of bacteriuria has a sensitivity of 40% to 70% and a specificity of 85% to 90% depending on the number of bacteria identified (Hurlbut and Littenberg 1991). Dipstick analysis for bacteria (nitrite) or pyuria (leukocyte esterase) are convenient but remain less sensitive than microscopic assessment of the urine. The accuracy of the findings on a culture of midstream urine (MSU) depends on how a positive urine culture is defined. Traditionally, $10^5$ cfu/ml is applied to a voided urine sample. Although the specificity is high it is important to note that the sensitivity is only in the region of 50%. Lowering the threshold to $10^2$ cfu/mL in cases of young females with suspected cystitis raises the sensitivity without affecting the specificity (Nicolle et al. 2005, Stamm 1982). Therefore, urine culture remains the definitive diagnostic investigation for acute cystitis and the presence of $10^2$ cfu/mL or more of urine indicates active infection.

Admittedly, routine urine culture is not always necessary for diagnostic purposes (McIsaac et al. 2002). It is considered more cost-effective to manage and treat patients symptomatic of uncomplicated cystitis without an initial urine culture because antimicrobial therapy is often completed before culture results are made available. This theory was validated in one study that demonstrated pre-therapeutic urine cultures for UTIs increases cost by up to 40% but only decreases the duration of symptoms by 10%(Carlson and Mulley 1985). Therefore, in females with recent onset of symptoms suggestive of cystitis, without the features of a complicated UTI, a urinalysis that is positive for bacteriuria, pyuria, haematuria or a combination should provide sufficient evidence of a UTI and a urine culture may be omitted. Importantly, a urine culture should be obtained when symptoms and urine examination findings leave a diagnosis of cystitis in doubt. In addition, pretherapeutic urine cultures are also necessary for managing patients with a recent history of antimicrobial therapy. It has also been demonstrated that treating acute uncomplicated cystitis by telephone consultation is safe and effective in primary care settings (Barry et al. 2001, Fenwick et al. 2000, Saint et al. 1999). Importantly, inclusion criteria for these studies are females at low risk (i.e. without a prior history of UTI, without symptoms suggestive of vaginitis or cervicitis and less than 55 years of age). Females that do not meet these criteria should be seen in person and examined (Fenwick et al. 2000).

### 2.4 Causative microorganisms

E. coli is the responsible uropathogen in 75% to 90% of female patients diagnosed with acute cystitis and Staphylococcus saprophiticus acoounts for 10% to 20% of cases (Jordan et al. 1980, Latham et al. 1983, Ronald 2002). Less common organisms include Klebsiella, Proteus and Enterococci. E. coli and other Enterobacteriaceae are the most commonly diagnosed organisms in male patients.

### 2.5 Management

A 3 day course of oral trimethoprim- sulfamethoxazole (TMP-SMX) results in eradication of pathogens within 7 days after commencing treatment in approximately 94% of females (Warren et al. 1999). Single-dose treatment is less efficacious than the 3 day course with eradication rates approaching 87%; however single-dose treatment is associated with fewer side-effects (11% versus 18%) (Warren et al. 1999). TMP-SMX is effective and inexpensive for empirical therapy. Therefore, TMP-SMX is recommended in areas where the prevalence of resistance to these drugs among E. coli strains causing cystitis is less than 20%(Warren et al.

1999). When used alone, TMP is as efficacious as TMP-SMX and is associated with fewer side effects, probably because of the absence of the sulfa component. It can be prescribed to patients who are allergic to sulfa.

Interestingly, a number of more recent studies have demonstrated that resistance to TMP-SMX is increasing in many different countries (Bean et al. 2008, Daza et al. 2001, De Francesco et al. 2007, Ling et al. 2006, Sader et al. 2005) (Fig. 2). One study from Israel demonstrated that 29% of cultures grew TMP-SMX resistant organisms in patients with uncomplicated cystitis. In this study microbiological cure was achieved in 86% of patients with TMP-SMX susceptible microorganisms but in only 42% of those with TMP-SMX resistant organisms (Raz et al. 2002). Another prospective study from the United Kingdom (UK) demonstrated resistance to TMP in 13.9% of isolates and patients with resistant isolates had a longer median time to symptom resolution (7 versus 4 days; p=0.0002), more frequent revisits to their attending physician (39% versus 6% in the first week, p<0.0001), more subsequent antibiotics (36% versus 4% in the first week, p<0.0001) and higher rates of subsequent bacteria at 1 month (42% versus 20% with susceptible isolates) (McNulty et al. 2006). Recent studies from the United States have demonstrated TMP-SMX resistance rates of 15% to 23% in isolates from patients with acute uncomplicated cystitis (Colgan et al. 2008, Hames and Rice 2007). In a study from Japan 17% of isolates from patients with cystitis showed resistance to TMP-SMX and abandonment of TMP-SMX as first line therapy for acute uncomplicated cystitis is currently under consideration in this region (Yamamoto et al. 2009).

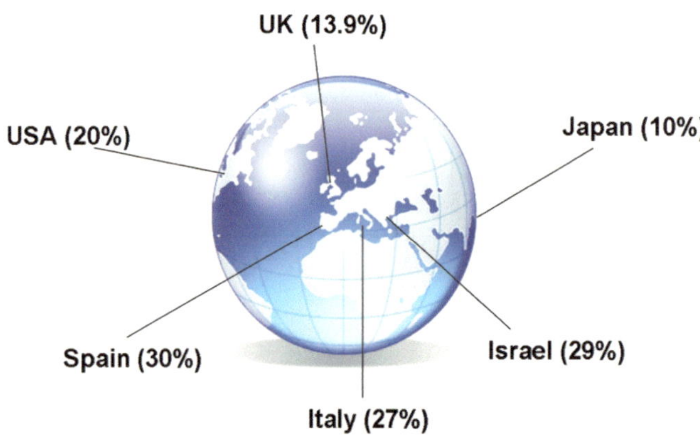


Fig. 2. Increasing rates of resistance for TMP-SMX treatment regimen for acute uncomplicated cystitis.

Resistant strains can be partially predicted from a history of recent antimicrobial usage. It has also been demonstrated that females who have been treated with TMP-SMX are 16 times less likely to be re-infected with an isolate resistant to this agent compared with females who have not take recent antimicrobial therapy (Brown et al. 2002). Furthermore, females that have taken other antimicrobial agents are two-fold more likely to be infected with a resistant isolate. Although the resistance rate to TMP-SMX is as high as 20% in some regions the bacteriologic eradication rate is approximately 80% and the clinical cure rate is approximately 85% (Manges et al. 2001, Wright et al. 1999). On account of these increasing resistance rates some authorities advocate the following criteria for prescribing TMP-SMX (Gupta et al. 2001b, Steinke et al. 1999):

- No known drug allergy
- No recent history of antibiotic usage
- Local prevalence to resistance is less than 15 - 20%

Although less than 5% of urine isolates are resistant to nitrofurantoin, it is considerably less active than TMP-SMX against aerobic Gram-negative rods other than E. coli. Furthermore, nitrofurantoin is more expensive than TMP-SMX. It is usually well tolerated, however it is frequently prescribed for 7 days and this may cause significant gastrointestinal upset. The macrocrystalline formulation is taken every 6 hours and the monohydrate macrocrystal is taken twice daily. The monohydrate formulation is associated with fewer side-effects. Nitrofurantoin is not associated with plasmid-mediated resistance and is a suitable choice for patients with recent exposure to other antimicrobial agents (Fihn 2003).

Fluoroquinolones offer excellent activity and are usually well tolerated (Henry et al. 2002). Their resistance is less than 5% in most regions (Hooton et al. 2004, Warren et al. 1999); however resistance rates are beginning to increase worldwide (although not as high as that of TMP-SMX) (Yamamoto et al. 2010) (Muratani and Matsumoto 2006). In the Mediterranean region up to one-third of strains that demonstrate reduced susceptibility to flouroquinolones and cause uncomplicated cystitis belong to two clonal groups: O15:H1 and O25:H4 (Cagnacci et al. 2008). This implies that strains belonging to these two clonal groups play a major role in determining the increasing rate of flouroquinolone resistant E. coli strains in the community. One study from Japan reported fluoroquinolone resistance in 8% of isolates from patients with acute uncomplicated cystitis (Yamamoto et al. 2009). Worryingly, resistance rates for E. coli isolated from acute uncomplicated cystitis to ciprofloxacin increased from 15.2% in 2002 to 23.4% in 2006 in South Korea (Yamamoto et al. 2010) (Fig. 3).

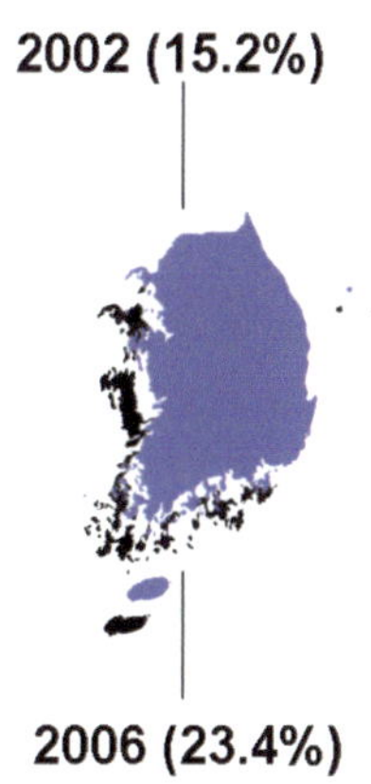


Fig. 3. Increasing rates of resistance for E. coli against ciprofloxacin in South Korea from 2002 to 2006.

The efficacy of ofloxacin is greater than TMP-SMX with recurrence rates of 8% to 9% 6 weeks after therapy has been completed (Hooton et al. 1991). Other fluoroqinolones have similar efficacy however they should be regarded as a second line treatment option due to their high cost and to preserve their sensitivity against uropathogens. Their use for uncomplicated cystitis should be limited to patients that are allergic to less expensive drugs, to patients with previous exposure to antimicrobial agents causing bacterial resistance and to regions where resistance to TMP-SMX is greater than 20%. When TMP-SMX is contraindicated a 3 day course of ciprofloxacin, levofloxacin, norfloxacin, lomefloxacin or gatifloxacin is an appropriate alternative. Importantly, fluoroquinolones are less active against S. saprophyticus and many Gram-negative uropathogens (Fihn 2003).

Fosfomycin tromethamine is taken as a single dose of powder from a sachet and is another option for treating uncomplicated cystitis. It is less effective than TMP-SMX and fluoroquinolones and should only be considered when more effective agents cannot be prescribed (Warren et al. 1999). Further limitations of fosfomycin tromethamine are its poor efficacy against S. saprophyticus and its expensive nature. The high *in vitro* resistance to ampicillin and sulfonamide and the high cost of amoxicillin/clavulanate and the cephalocrystalline sporins limit their usefulness in the setting of acute uncomplicated cystitis. More than 90% of females report the absence of acute urinary symptoms within 72 hours after commencement of antimicrobial therapy (Fihn et al. 1988). Phenazopyridine or Uristat can be prescribed in females with severe persistent dysuria. Although this compound is available over the counter there is concern that females with severe dysuria are not seeking medical care and are also at risk of side effects such as headache, gastrointestinal upset, rash and nephrotoxicity (Fihn 2003). Resistance rates of E. coli to antibiotic regimes are illustrated in Table 1.

| Antimicrobial Agent | Italy | Spain | USA | UK | China | Japan |
|---|---|---|---|---|---|---|
| Ampicillin | 49 | 65 | - | 54 | - | - |
| Amoxicillin/clavulanate | 8 | 37 | 12 | 12 | 29 | 2 |
| Piperacillin | 30 | - | - | - | - | - |
| Piperacillin/ tazobactam | 1 | 68 | - | - | 7 | - |
| Nitrofurantoin | 9 | 7 | 3 | 5 | - | 1 |
| TMP | - | - | - | 39 | - | - |
| TMP-SMX | 27 | 37 | 20 | - | - | 10 |
| Ciprofloxacin | 19 | 22 | 5 | 9 | 51 | 8 |
| Gentamicin | 6 | 10 | - | 5 | 39 | 2 |
| Cefalexin | - | - | - | 8 | - | - |
| Cephazolin | 7 | - | - | - | - | - |
| Cefpodoxime | - | - | 2 | 6 | - | 5 |
| Cefuroxime | - | 13 | 24 | - | - | - |
| Cefprozil | - | - | 3 | - | - | - |
| Cefotaxime | - | 4 | - | - | 14 | - |
| Ceftazidime | - | - | - | - | 3 | - |
| Ceftriaxone | 2 | - | - | - | - | - |
| Cefdinir | - | - | 2 | - | - | 5 |
| Cefoperazone | - | - | - | - | 17 | - |
| Cefperazone/sulbactam | - | - | - | - | 5 | - |
| Cefipime | - | 3 | - | - | 8 | - |

Table 1. Resistance rate of E. coli isolated from patients with community acquired infections (depicted as percentage) (Bean et al. 2008, Daza et al. 2001, De Francesco et al. 2007, Ling et al. 2006, Sader et al. 2005, Yamamoto et al.).

#### 2.5.1 Cranberry juice

Proanthocyanidins found in cranberry juice have been long advocated to play a preventative role against cystitis. It appears that proanthocyanidins inhibit the attachment of uropathogens to the surface of the uroepithlium. Randomised trials suggest that 200-750 ml of cranberry juice or cranberry-concentrate tablets reduce the risk of symptomatic recurrent infection by 12-20%(Avorn et al. 1994, Kontiokari et al. 2001, Stothers 2002). Interestingly, the amount of cranberry juice found within products marketed as cranberry juice is highly variable and ranges from 5-100%.

### 2.6 Duration of therapy

In female patients with uncomplicated cystitis 3 days of therapy is the preferred treatment regimen. One study that reviewed over 300 clinical trials of single-dose, 3-day or 7-day treatment with TMP-SMX, fluroquinolones and β-lactam antimicrobial agents found that 3-day therapy is more effective than single-dose therapy (Table 2). In addition, 3-day therapy with TMP-SMX, amoxicillin or cloxacillin is associated with cure rates that are comparable with longer courses of therapy and an incidence of adverse effects that are as low as single-dose therapy (Warren et al. 1999). Seven-day therapy is associated with a higher incidence of adverse effects and is only recommended in females with symptoms longer than 1 week, in male patients and in individual patients that have complicating risk factors

| Circumstance | Drug | Dosage | Frequency | Duration (Days) |
|---|---|---|---|---|
| Female | | | | |
| Healthy | Ciprofloxacin | 500mg | BD | 3 |
| | Levofloxacin | 500mg | QDS | 3 |
| | TMP-SMX | 1 double strength tablet (160 - 800mg) | BD | 3 |
| | Trimethoprim | 100mg | BD | 3 |
| | Nitrofurantoin | 100mg | BD | 3 |
| | Norfloxacin | 400mg | BD | 3 |
| Symptoms >7 days, recent UTI, Age >65 years, Diabetes, Diaphragm use | TMP-SMX | As Above | As Above | 7 |
| | Fluoroquinolone | | | 7 |
| Pregnancy | Amoxicillin | 250mg | TDS | 7 |
| | Cephalexin | 500mg | QDS | 7 |
| | Nitrofurantoin | As Above | As Above | 7 |
| Males | | | | |
| | Fluoroquinolone | As Above | As Above | 7 |
| | TMP-SMX | As Above | As Above | 7 |

Table 2. Current treatment regimens for acute uncomplicated cystitis.

### 2.7 Cost of therapy

The cost of treating acute uncomplicated cystitis involves the initial evaluation, the cost of the drug administered and the subsequent follow-up (Table 3). Good cost effectiveness is achieved with adequate efficacy against the most common uropathogen, E. coli. Intuitively, the lower the effectiveness against E. coli, the greater number of revisits, cases of progression to pyelonephritis and the higher the follow-up cost. Notably, antimicrobial cost is a poor predictor of cost-effectiveness as demonstrated in one study that compared the most expensive and least expensive drugs (fluroquinolones and TMP-SMX respectively). Results showed that both regimens are equally cost effective and that both of these drugs are also more cost effective against nitrofurantoin (Rosenberg 1999).

| Antimicrobial Agent | Approximate Retail Cost ($) | Side effects |
|---|---|---|
| Trimethoprim-sulfamethoxazole (TMP-SMX) | 1.83 | Anorexia. Nausea, vomiting, rash, urticaria, blood dyscrasias, hypersensitivity, hepatic necrosis |
| Trimethoprim | 4.33 | Diarrhoea, rash, glossitis, taste changes, blood dyscrasias, hypersensitivity |
| Norfloxacin | 25.21 | Dizziness, restlessness, headache, diarrhoea, nausea, rash, vaginitis, convulsions, psychosis, hypersensitivity, tendon rupture |
| Ciprofloxacin | 53.56 | Similar to norfloxacin |
| Levofloxacin | 43.92 | Similar to norfloxacin |
| Gatifloxicin | 21.61 | Similar to norfloxacin |
| Lomefloxacin | 35.96 | Similar to norfloxacin |
| Nitrofurantoin macrocrystals | 35.29 | Anorexia, nausea, vomiting, headache, pulmonary hypersensitivity, hepatotoxicity, haemolytic anaemia, peripheral neuropathy |
| Nitrofurantoin monohydrate macrocrystals | 29.96 | Similar to nitrofurantoin macrocrystals (gastrointestinal effects less common) |
| Fosfomycin tromethamine | 33.97 | Nausea, vomiting, vaginitis, rash, hypersensitivity |

Table 3. Cost of treatment regimens for acute uncomplicated cystitis (Rosenberg 1999).

### 2.8 Follow-up

In general, young female patients that are asymptomatic after antimicrobial therapies do not require a follow-up visit or repeat MSU. A follow up visit is recommended with MSU in older females and in all male patients with cystitis. Urological evaluation with ultrasound, computed tomography (CT) or cystoscopy is unnecessary in females and is also usually unnecessary in male patients that respond appropriately to antimicrobial therapy (Abarbanel et al. 2003, Lipsky 1989). However, one study demonstrated that up to 50% of males with UTIs have a significant urological abnormality. Finally, patients that do not respond to antimicrobial therapy should undergo appropriate microbiological evaluations (Andrews et al. 2002).

## 3. Asymptomatic bacteriuria

Asymptomatic bacteriuria can be defined as a microbiological diagnosis based on the isolation of a specified quantitative count of bacteria in a properly collected specimen of urine from a patient who is without symptoms or signs consistent with cystitis. Absence of symptoms is usually obvious in healthy patients, however an asymptomatic UTIs may be more difficult to diagnose in catheterised or neurologically compromised patients. A single catheterised urine specimen with a solitary isolate of $10^2$ cfu/mL is diagnostic of bacteriuria in catheterised male and female patients (Nicolle et al. 2005). Concomitant pyuria ranges from 30% in young females to 100% in catheterised patients (Hooton et al. 2000). Importantly, other co-factors like bladder calculi can induce mucosal inflammation in this patient cohort. Therefore, the presence of pyuria alone is insufficient for a diagnosis of bacteriuria.

The prevalence of asymptomatic bacteriuria among the general population varies with age, gender and the presence of abnormalities in the genitourinary tract (Nicolle et al. 2005) (Table 4). E. coli is the most common uropathogen isolated in patients with asymptomatic bacteriuria and it is usually a less virulent strain than in isolates from symptomatic patients (Svanborg and Godaly 1997). Enterobactericeae and Gram-positive uropathogens are more commonly isolated in patients with abnormalities of the genitourinary tract. Pseudomonas aeruginosa and Proteus are more prevalent among patients living in residential care.

| Patient Population | Prevalence (%) |
|---|---|
| Premenopausal females | 1.0 - 5.0 |
| Pregnant females | 1.9 - 9.5 |
| Postmenopausal females (age: 50-70) | 2.8 - 8.6 |
| Diabetic patients | |
| Males | 0.7 - 11 |
| Females | 9.0 - 27 |
| Elderly patients in the community | |
| Males | 3.6 - 19 |
| Females | 10.8 - 16 |
| Elderly patients in nursing homes | |
| Males | 14 -50 |
| Females | 25 - 50 |
| Patients with spinal cord injuries | |
| Self-intermittent catheterisation (SIC) | 23 - 89 |
| Sphincterotomy and condom catheter *in situ* | 57 |
| Patients undergoing haemodialysis | 28 |
| Indwelling catheter | |
| Short-term | 9 - 23 |
| Long-term | 100 |

Table 4. Prevalence of asymptomatic bacteria among different patient populations (Nicolle et al. 2005).

### 3.1 Management of asymptomatic bacteriura

In general, management of asymptomatic bacteriuria is governed by the patient cohort and their risk factors for adverse outcomes that may be prevented with appropriate antimicrobial treatment. In adult populations it has been shown that asymptomatic bacteriuria is not harmful and treatment of asymptomatic bacteriuria does not decrease the frequency of symptomatic UTIs or improve patient outcomes. Therefore, screening and treating asymptomatic bacteriuria is discouraged in populations other than in pregnant females and in patients undergoing urological procedures (Nicolle et al. 2005) (Table 5).

| Patient Cohort | Recommended | Not recommended |
|---|---|---|
| Premenopausal non pregnant females | | X |
| Pregnant females | X | |
| Diabetic females | | X |
| Elderly patients residing in the community | | X |
| Elderly patients residing in nursing homes | | X |
| Patients with spinal cord injuries | | X |
| Patient with indwelling catheters* | | X |
| Urological inteventions | X | |
| Immunocompromised patients | | X |

*Antimicrobial treatment of asymptomatic female patients with catheter-associated bacteriuira persisting >48 hours should be considered.

Table 5. Algorithm for screening and treating asymptomatic bacteriuria (Nicolle et al. 2005).

## 4. Complicated cystitis

Complicated cystitis may occur in patients with a compromised urinary tract or by a very resistant uropathogen. The clinical spectrum of complicated cystitis can range from mild cystitis to life-threatening infections of the kidney and urospesis (Table 6). Urine cultures are mandatory to identify the invading uropathogen and its antimicrobial susceptibility in this group of patients. The following are common host-factors that predispose to complicated cystitis:

- Functional and/or structural abnormalities of the urinary tract
- Recent instrumentation of the urinary tract
- Recent usage of antimicrobial therapy
- Diabetes mellitus
- Immunosuppression
- Pregnancy
- Hospital-acquired infections

Due to the wide range of host conditions and uropthogens that are associated with complicated cystitis appropriate guidelines for empirical therapy remain limited. Patients with mild to moderate illness can be treated on an outpatient basis with oral fluroquinolones. If the susceptibility pattern of the pathogen is known TMP-SMX may also be effective (Stamm and Hooton 1993).

| Pathogens | Mitigating Circumstances | Recommended Empirical Treatment |
|---|---|---|
| E. coli, Proteus species, Klebsiella species, Pseudomonas species | Mild-to-moderate illness, no nausea or vomiting-outpatient therapy | Oral* norfloxacin, ciprofloxacin or ofloxacin for 10-14 days |
| Serratia species, enterococci, staphylococci | Severe illness or urospesis-hospitalisation required | Parenteral** ampicillin and gentamicin, ciprofloxacin, levofloxacin, ceftriaxone, aztreonam, ticarcillin- clavulanate or imipenem-cilastin until fever has subsided; then oral trimethoprim-sulfamethoxazole, norfloxacin, ciprofloxacin or levofloxacin for 14-21 days |

* Oral regimens for pyelonephritis and complicated UTI are as follows: trimethoprim-sulfamethoxazole, 160 to 800 mg, BD; norfloxacin, 400mg, BD; ciprofloxacin, 500 mg, BD; levofloxacin, 500 mg, 500 mg/day.

** Parenteral regimens are as follows: ciprofloxacin, 400mg, BD; levofloxacin, 500mg/ day; gentamicin 1mg/kg TDS; ceftriaxone, 1-2 g/ day; ampicillin, 1 g QDS; imipenem-cilastin, 250-500 mg QDS; ticarcillin-clavulanate, 3.1 g QDS; and aztreonam 1 g TDS.

Table 6. Treatment strategies for complicated cystitis (Stamm and Hooton 1993).

For hospitalised patients intravenous ampicillin and gentamicin provides adequate coverage against most pathogens. Antimicrobial therapy can also be modified when sensitivity data are available. Therapy is usually continued for 10 to 14 days and switched from parenteral to oral whenever possible. Repeat urine culture should be performed 7 and 14 days after therapy to ensure adequate efficacy has been achieved (Fihn 2003).

### 4.1 Unresolving cystitis

Persistent infection suggests that initial antimicrobial therapy has been inadequate at eliminating bacterial growth and concomitant symptoms from the genitourinary tact. Repeat urinalysis and MSU are indicated if the symptoms of UTI do not resolve by the end of treatment or if symptoms begin to recur shortly after therapy. If the patient's symptoms are severe it is prudent to commence empirical therapy with a fluoroquinolone until the MSU results have been obtained.

Resistance to the antimicrobial agent selected to treat the infection is the most common cause for patients with persistent unresolving UTIs. The patient may have a recent history of antimicrobial therapy and colonisation of the bowel with resistant bacteria has subsequently developed. In addition, tetracycline, sulfonamides and β-lactams cause plasmid-mediated R factors that simultaneously carry resistance to multiple antimicrobial agents. The development of resistance in a previously susceptible population of bacteria is the second most common cause of resistant UTIs and this issue may arise in up to 5% of patients that are receiving antimicrobial therapy. Resistance to antimicrobial therapy is easily diagnosed as the culture taken on therapy shows that the previously susceptible population has been replaced by resistant bacteria of the same species. More resistant strains of bacteria usually emerge when the concentration of antimicrobial therapy in the urine is insufficient to eradicate all bacteria present. This phenomenon usually occurs in patients who are underdosed and in patients who are poorly compliant with their prescribed regimen. Rapid reintroduction of a new resistant species while the patient is undergoing antimicrobial therapy may also cause resistant UTI. Reinfection mimicking unresolved bacteriuria should increase the index of suspicion for an enterovesical fistula. The following list represents the more common causes of persistent unresolving cystitis

- Bacterial resistance to the antimicrobial agent selected for treatment.
- Development of resistance from previously susceptible bacteria
- Bacteriuira resulting from 2 different bacterial species with different susceptibilities
- Reinfection with a new, resistant species during initial therapy for the original susceptible organism
- Azotemia
- Analgesia abuse leading to papillary necrosis
- Staghorn calculi providing a nidus for resistant bacteria to attach

If the repeat urine culture (obtained from when the patient was on therapy) demonstrates that the initial bacterial species is still present and susceptible to the antimicrobial agent selected to treat the infection, it is likely that the unresolved infection is caused by an inability to deliver sufficient concentrations of antimicrobial agents into the urinary tracts or an excessive number of bacteria may be over-riding the activity of the antimicrobial agent.

In addition, antimicrobial levels are usually lower than the minimal inhibitory concentration required for eradicating the infecting organism in patients with uraemia. Severe defects in the medullary collecting system impair the kidney's concentrating ability and can dilute the antimicrobial agent, particularly in patients with papillary necrosis. Large masses of bacteria within the genitourinary tract are frequently seen with a large staghorn calculus. In this situation the urinary concentration of antimicrobial agent may be large, however it may be inadequate to sterilise the large volume of infected urine. This phenomenon may occur because susceptible bacteria cannot be inhibited once a specific critical density is reached. Rarely, patients with a variant of Munchausen's syndrome may present with unresolving cystitis. These patients tend to inoculate their bladders with uropathogens or wilfully avoid antimicrobial agents. Careful bacteriologic observations usually indicate the implausibility of the clinical picture.

### 4.2 Laboratory diagnosis

In cases of unresolving cystitis urinalysis and urine culture are required to investigate the uropathogen responsible for the persistent infective process. Renal function and imaging of the genitourinary tract should be performed if repeat culture demonstrates sensitivity of the uropathogen to the antimicrobial agent presecribed. This investigative regimen is employed to identify any abnormalities within the urinary tract. Empirical treatment of unresolving cystitis is based on the assumption that the infecting uropathogen is resistant. Fluoroquinolones provide sufficient antimicrobial coverage in most situations and should be prescribed for 7 days. Adjustments to this regime can be performed when bacterial susceptibilities have been made available. Finally, urine cultures should be repeated during and 7 days after therapy to ensure adequate eradication has been achieved.

### 4.3 Recurrent cystitis

Recurrent episodes are caused by re-emergence of bacteria from a site within the urinary tract (persistence) or from new infective uropathogens outside the urinary tract (reinfection) (Fig. 4). Bacterial persistence must be caused by the same uropathogen on each occasion and reinfections typically occur at varying intervals and are usually cause by different species of bacteria. It is important to differentiate between persistence and reinfections as management protocols differ. Patients with bacterial persistence can be cured of recurrent cystitis by indentifying and surgically removing/ correcting the focus of infection. Patients complaining of recurrent reinfection usually require long-term medical management as a structural defect is not usually present. Reinfections in males occasionally occur and are usually as a result of an underlying abnormality such as urethral stricture. In these situations surgical evaluation is warranted.

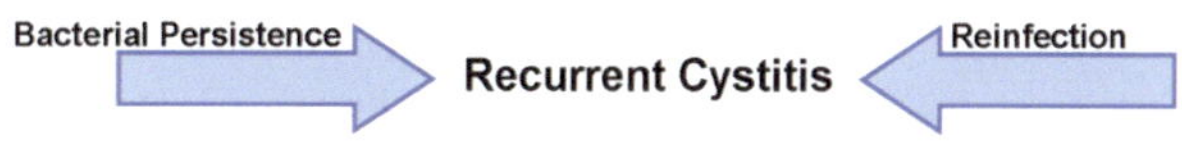


Fig. 4. Re-emergence of bacteria from within the urinary tract (persistence) or invasion of new bacteria (reinfection) is the most common causes of recurrent cystitis.

#### 4.3.1 Bacterial persistence

After the initial episode has resolved recurrence with the same organism arises from a site within the genitourinary tract. The site of bacterial persistence is usually excluded from high concentrations of the antimicrobial agent. It is generally accepted that there are 12 correctable urological abnormalities that may cause bacteria to persist within the genitourinary tract. These abnormalities are illustrated in Table 7 and may be difficult to diagnose. Some causes may require cystoscopic localisation of the infection (with ureteral catheters) to accurately define the focus of bacterial persistence.

- Infected stones
- Chronic bacterial prostatitis
- Unilateral infected atrophic kidneys
- Ectopic ureters and ureteral duplication
- Foreign bodies
- Urethral diverticula and infected periurethral glands
- Unilateral medullary sponge kidneys
- Non-refluxing, normal appearing, infected ureteral stumps after nephrectomy
- Infected urachal cyst
- Infected communicating cysts of the renal calyces
- Papillary necrosis
- Perivesical abscess with fistula to bladder

Table 7. Urological abnormalities causing bacterial persistence that may be amenable to surgical correction.

It is important to identify patients with bacterial persistence as they represent the only patient cohort with a surgically curable cause of recurrent UTIs. Radiological and endoscopic evaluation of the urinary tract is necessary with excreting urography/ CT and cystoscopic assessment providing the initial screening investigations. Diverticulum and nonrefluxing ureteral stumps can be diagnosed with retrograde urography. In patients in whom the focus of infection cannot be eradicated, long-term, low-dose antimicrobial suppression is necessary to prevent symptoms of infection. The antimicrobial drugs used for low-dose prophylaxis will also be effective for bacterial suppression if the persistent strain is susceptible. These include nitrofurantoin, TMP-SMX, cephalexin, and the fluoroquinolones

### 4.3.2 Recurrent infections

Females with recurrent infections and who are exposed to vaginal spermicides from either condoms or diaphragms should consider alternative methods of contraception or protection from sexually transmitted infections (STIs). Continuous and postcoital prophylaxis with low-dose antimicrobial agents is effective in treating recurrent cystitis and prophylactic treatment should not be commenced until active infection has been eradicated (Hooton 2001). Absence of infection can be confirmed by a negative urine culture 1-2 weeks after treatment has been discontinued.

Continuous prophylaxis is a potential option for females who have had 2 or more symptomatic infections over a 6 month period. Randomised, placebo-controlled trials have demonstrated that continuous prophylaxis with nitrofurantoin, trimethoprim (± sulfamethoxazole), ciprofloxacin or norfloxacin decreases recurrent episodes by 95% (i.e. from 2 to 3 episodes per patient/ year to 0.1 to 0.2 episodes per patient/ year) and may also prevent episodes of pyelonephritis (Hooton 2001). Notably, one agent is not recommended over another because studies to date have lacked sufficient statistical power. In general, antimicrobial prophylaxis is initiated on a trial basis for a 6 month period. If good outcomes are reported the agent may be continued for 2 to 5 years without the emergence of a resistant organism (Stamm et al. 1991). The rate of chronic adverse effects associated with antimicrobial agents ranges from 7% to 40% for trimethoprim containing regimens, from 0% to 40% for nitrofurantoin, from 7 to 21% for norfloxacin and up to 13% for ciprofloxacin (Chew and Fihn 1999). Gastrointestinal disturbances, rash and yeast vaginitis are the most common adverse effects encountered (Fig. 5).

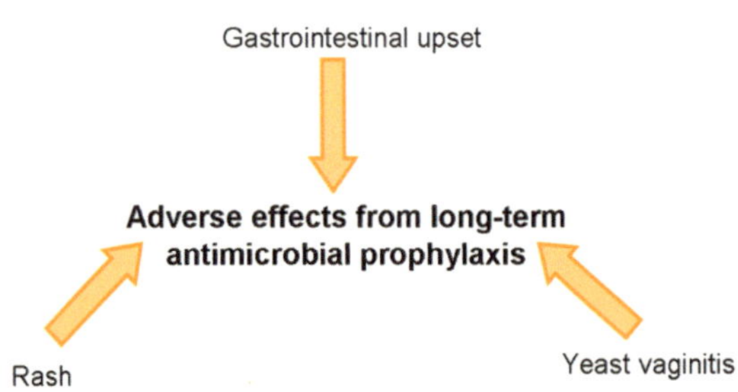


Fig. 5. Common adverse effects associated with long-term antimicrobial prophylaxis against recurrent episodes of cystitis.

Post-coital prophylaxis is an attractive option for female patients that describe a direct association between sexual intercourse and subsequent cystitis. A reduction in the frequency of recurrences has been demonstrated when nitrofurantoin, TMP-SMX or fluroquinolones have been administered post-coitus (Stapleton et al. 1990) (Table 8). Intermittent self-treatment as opposed to continuous treatment has also been recommended in some scenarios. Many females can accurately self-diagnose acute cystitis and may be instructed to commence a 3-day course of an antimicrobial agent at the onset of symptoms (Gupta et al. 2001a). However, females are advised to seek medical attention if symptoms persist 48-72 hours after completing the appropriate antimicrobial course. Interestingly, several studies have also demonstrated that postcoital voiding does not play a preventative role for recurrent cystitis. In addition, it appears that poor urinary hygiene does not predispose to recurrent cystitis (Scholes et al. 2000, Strom et al. 1987).

| Regimen | Infections per patient per year | Reference |
|---|---|---|
| Nitrofurantoin, 50 or 100 mg daily | 0.09 | (Bailey et al. 1971) |
| Nitrofurantoin, 50mg daily | 0.19 | |
| Placebo | 2.1 | |
| Sulfamethoxazole, 500mg daily | 2.5 | (Harding et al. 1982) |
| TMP-SMX, 40 and 200mg daily | 0.1 | |
| Methenamine mandelate, 2g daily + acorbic acid 2g | 1.6 | |
| Nitrofurantoin, 50mg daily | 0.32 | (Kasanen et al. 1978) |
| Methenamine hippurate, 1g daily | 0.39 | |
| Trimethoprim, 100mg daily | 0.13 | |
| TMP-SMX, 80 and 400 mg daily | 0.19 | |
| Cephalexin, 125 mg daily | 0.10 | (Gower 1975) |
| TMP-SMX, 40 and 200 mg daily | 0.00 | (Stamey et al. 1977) |
| Nitrofurantoin marcocrystals, 100mg daily | 0.74 | |
| TMP-SMX, 40 and 200 mg 3-times weekly | 0.1 | (Harding et al. 1979) |
| TMP-SMX, 40 and 200 mg daily | 0.15 | (Stamm et al. 1980) |
| Trimethoprim, 100 mg daily | 0.00 | |
| Nitrofurantoin marcocrystals, 100mg daily | 0.14 | |
| Placebo | 2.8 | |
| Nitrofurantoin, 50 mg twice daily | 0.19 | (Brumfitt et al. 1981) |
| Methenamine hippurate, 1g twice daily | 0.57 | |
| TMP-SMX, 40 and 200 mg 3-times weekly | 0.14 | (Harding et al. 1982) |
| Trimethoprim, 100 mg daily | 1.53 | (Brumfitt et al. 1983) |
| Methenamine hippurate, 1g daily | 1.38 | |
| Povidone-iodine wash, twice daily | 1.79 | |
| TMP-SMX, 40 and 200 mg daily | 0.2 | (Wong et al. 1985) |
| Self-administered cotrimoxazole, 4 x 80 and 400mg | 2.2 | |
| Cephalexin, 250 mg daily | 0.18 | (Martinez et al. 1985) |
| Trimethoprim, 100 mg daily | 1.0 | (Brumfitt et al. 1985) |
| Nitrofurantoin macrocrystals, 100 mg daily | 0.16 | |
| Nitrofurantoin, 200 mg daily | 0.00 | (Nicolle et al. 1989) |
| Norfloxacin, 200 mg daily | 0.00 | |
| Norfloxacin, 200 mg daily | 0.04 | (Raz and Boger 1991) |

Table 8. Low-dose prophylactic regimes for recurrent cystitis in females.

## 5. Conclusions

It is important for urologists to be familiar with appropriate management strategies for cystitis because of its highly prevalent nature in the community. Currently, recommended treatment regimens for uncomplicated cystitis include 3-day therapy with fluroquinolones or nitrofurantoin as resistance rates appear to be increasing when TMP-SMX is administered. Worryingly, recent studies have demonstrated an increasing number of isolates of fluoroquinolone-resistant pathogens and this merits concern for the future. Female patients that complain of frequent recurrences should be advised to avoid exposure to vaginal spermicides and prophylaxis or methods of self-administration may be considered. Imaging studies should be reserved for patients presenting with complicated episodes of cystitis. The increasing incidence of antimicrobial resistance in conjunction with the highly prevalent nature of cystitis suggests that prudent and appropriate use of antimicrobial agents is becoming increasingly important.

## 6. References

Abarbanel, J., Engelstein, D., Lask, D. and Livne, P. M. (2003) 'Urinary tract infection in men younger than 45 years of age: is there a need for urologic investigation?', *Urology,* 62(1), 27-9.

Andrews, S. J., Brooks, P. T., Hanbury, D. C., King, C. M., Prendergast, C. M., Boustead, G. B. and McNicholas, T. A. (2002) 'Ultrasonography and abdominal radiography versus intravenous urography in investigation of urinary tract infection in men: prospective incident cohort study', *BMJ,* 324(7335), 454-6.

Avorn, J., Monane, M., Gurwitz, J. H., Glynn, R. J., Choodnovskiy, I. and Lipsitz, L. A. (1994) 'Reduction of bacteriuria and pyuria after ingestion of cranberry juice', *JAMA,* 271(10), 751-4.

Bailey, A., Walker, A., Hadley, A. and James, D. G. (1971) 'Cephalexin. A new oral antibiotic', *Torax,* 20(1), 15-9.

Barry, H. C., Hickner, J., Ebell, M. H. and Ettenhofer, T. (2001) 'A randomized controlled trial of telephone management of suspected urinary tract infections in women', *J Fam Pract,* 50(7), 589-94.

Bean, D. C., Krahe, D. and Wareham, D. W. (2008) 'Antimicrobial resistance in community and nosocomial Escherichia coli urinary tract isolates, London 2005-2006', *Ann Clin Microbiol Antimicrob,* 7, 13.

Bent, S., Nallamothu, B. K., Simel, D. L., Fihn, S. D. and Saint, S. (2002) 'Does this woman have an acute uncomplicated urinary tract infection?', *JAMA,* 287(20), 2701-10.

Boyko, E. J., Fihn, S. D., Scholes, D., Chen, C. L., Normand, E. H. and Yarbro, P. (2002) 'Diabetes and the risk of acute urinary tract infection among postmenopausal women', *Diabetes Care,* 25(10), 1778-83.

Brown, P. D., Freeman, A. and Foxman, B. (2002) 'Prevalence and predictors of trimethoprim-sulfamethoxazole resistance among uropathogenic Escherichia coli isolates in Michigan', *Clin Infect Dis,* 34(8), 1061-6.

Brumfitt, W., Cooper, J. and Hamilton-Miller, J. M. (1981) 'Prevention of recurrent urinary infections in women: a comparative trial between nitrofurantoin and methenamine hippurate', *J Urol,* 126(1), 71-4.

Brumfitt, W., Hamilton-Miller, J. M., Gargan, R. A., Cooper, J. and Smith, G. W. (1983) 'Long-term prophylaxis of urinary infections in women: comparative trial of trimethoprim, methenamine hippurate and topical povidone-iodine', *J Urol,* 130(6), 1110-4.

Brumfitt, W., Smith, G. W., Hamilton-Miller, J. M. and Gargan, R. A. (1985) 'A clinical comparison between Macrodantin and trimethoprim for prophylaxis in women with recurrent urinary infections', *J Antimicrob Chemother,* 16(1), 111-20.

Cagnacci, S., Gualco, L., Debbia, E., Schito, G. C. and Marchese, A. (2008) 'European emergence of ciprofloxacin-resistant Escherichia coli clonal groups O25:H4-ST 131 and O15:K52:H1 causing community-acquired uncomplicated cystitis', *J Clin Microbiol,* 46(8), 2605-12.

Carlson, K. J. and Mulley, A. G. (1985) 'Management of acute dysuria. A decision-analysis model of alternative strategies', *Ann Intern Med,* 102(2), 244-9.

Chew, L. D. and Fihn, S. D. (1999) 'Recurrent cystitis in nonpregnant women', *West J Med,* 170(5), 274-7.

Colgan, R., Johnson, J. R., Kuskowski, M. and Gupta, K. (2008) 'Risk factors for trimethoprim-sulfamethoxazole resistance in patients with acute uncomplicated cystitis', *Antimicrob Agents Chemother,* 52(3), 846-51.

Daza, R., Gutierrez, J. and Piedrola, G. (2001) 'Antibiotic susceptibility of bacterial strains isolated from patients with community-acquired urinary tract infections', *Int J Antimicrob Agents,* 18(3), 211-5.

De Francesco, M. A., Ravizzola, G., Peroni, L., Negrini, R. and Manca, N. (2007) 'Urinary tract infections in Brescia, Italy: etiology of uropathogens and antimicrobial resistance of common uropathogens', *Med Sci Monit,* 13(6), BR136-44.

Fenwick, E. A., Briggs, A. H. and Hawke, C. I. (2000) 'Management of urinary tract infection in general practice: a cost-effectiveness analysis', *Br J Gen Pract,* 50(457), 635-9.

Fihn, S. D. (2003) 'Clinical practice. Acute uncomplicated urinary tract infection in women', *N Engl J Med,* 349(3), 259-66.

Fihn, S. D., Boyko, E. J., Chen, C. L., Normand, E. H., Yarbro, P. and Scholes, D. (1998) 'Use of spermicide-coated condoms and other risk factors for urinary tract infection caused by Staphylococcus saprophyticus', *Arch Intern Med,* 158(3), 281-7.

Fihn, S. D., Johnson, C., Roberts, P. L., Running, K. and Stamm, W. E. (1988) 'Trimethoprim-sulfamethoxazole for acute dysuria in women: a single-dose or 10-day course. A double-blind, randomized trial', *Ann Intern Med,* 108(3), 350-7.

Foxman, B. (2002) 'Epidemiology of urinary tract infections: incidence, morbidity, and economic costs', *Am J Med,* 113 Suppl 1A, 5S-13S.

Foxman, B., Barlow, R., D'Arcy, H., Gillespie, B. and Sobel, J. D. (2000) 'Urinary tract infection: self-reported incidence and associated costs', *Ann Epidemiol,* 10(8), 509-15.

Gower, P. E. (1975) 'The use of small doses of cephalexin (125 mg) in the management of recurrent urinary tract infection in women', *J Antimicrob Chemother,* 1(3 Suppl), 93-8.

Gupta, K., Hooton, T. M., Roberts, P. L. and Stamm, W. E. (2001a) 'Patient-initiated treatment of uncomplicated recurrent urinary tract infections in young women', *Ann Intern Med,* 135(1), 9-16.

Gupta, K., Hooton, T. M. and Stamm, W. E. (2001b) 'Increasing antimicrobial resistance and the management of uncomplicated community-acquired urinary tract infections', *Ann Intern Med,* 135(1), 41-50.

Hames, L. and Rice, C. E. (2007) 'Antimicrobial resistance of urinary tract isolates in acute uncomplicated cystitis among college-aged women: choosing a first-line therapy', *J Am Coll Health,* 56(2), 153-6.

Harding, G. K., Buckwold, F. J., Marrie, T. J., Thompson, L., Light, R. B. and Ronald, A. R. (1979) 'Prophylaxis of recurrent urinary tract infection in female patients. Efficacy of low-dose, thrice-weekly therapy with trimethoprim-sulfamethoxazole', *JAMA,* 242(18), 1975-7.

Harding, G. K., Ronald, A. R., Nicolle, L. E., Thomson, M. J. and Gray, G. J. (1982) 'Long-term antimicrobial prophylaxis for recurrent urinary tract infection in women', *Rev Infect Dis,* 4(2), 438-43.

Henry, D. C., Jr., Bettis, R. B., Riffer, E., Haverstock, D. C., Kowalsky, S. F., Manning, K., Hamed, K. A. and Church, D. A. (2002) 'Comparison of once-daily extended-release ciprofloxacin and conventional twice-daily ciprofloxacin for the treatment of uncomplicated urinary tract infection in women', *Clin Ther,* 24(12), 2088-104.

Hooton, T. M. (2001) 'Recurrent urinary tract infection in women', *Int J Antimicrob Agents,* 17(4), 259-68.

Hooton, T. M., Besser, R., Foxman, B., Fritsche, T. R. and Nicolle, L. E. (2004) 'Acute uncomplicated cystitis in an era of increasing antibiotic resistance: a proposed approach to empirical therapy', *Clin Infect Dis,* 39(1), 75-80.

Hooton, T. M., Johnson, C., Winter, C., Kuwamura, L., Rogers, M. E., Roberts, P. L. and Stamm, W. E. (1991) 'Single-dose and three-day regimens of ofloxacin versus trimethoprim-sulfamethoxazole for acute cystitis in women', *Antimicrob Agents Chemother,* 35(7), 1479-83.

Hooton, T. M., Scholes, D., Hughes, J. P., Winter, C., Roberts, P. L., Stapleton, A. E., Stergachis, A. and Stamm, W. E. (1996) 'A prospective study of risk factors for symptomatic urinary tract infection in young women', *N Engl J Med,* 335(7), 468-74.

Hooton, T. M., Scholes, D., Stapleton, A. E., Roberts, P. L., Winter, C., Gupta, K., Samadpour, M. and Stamm, W. E. (2000) 'A prospective study of asymptomatic bacteriuria in sexually active young women', *N Engl J Med,* 343(14), 992-7.

Hurlbut, T. A., 3rd and Littenberg, B. (1991) 'The diagnostic accuracy of rapid dipstick tests to predict urinary tract infection', *Am J Clin Pathol,* 96(5), 582-8.

Jordan, P. A., Iravani, A., Richard, G. A. and Baer, H. (1980) 'Urinary tract infection caused by Staphylococcus saprophyticus', *J Infect Dis,* 142(4), 510-5.

Kasanen, A., Anttila, M., Elfving, R., Kahela, P., Saarimaa, H., Sundquist, H., Tikkanen, R. and Toivanen, P. (1978) 'Trimethoprim. Pharmacology, antimicrobial activity and clinical use in urinary tract infections', *Ann Clin Res,* 10 Suppl 22, 1-39.

Kontiokari, T., Sundqvist, K., Nuutinen, M., Pokka, T., Koskela, M. and Uhari, M. (2001) 'Randomised trial of cranberry-lingonberry juice and Lactobacillus GG drink for the prevention of urinary tract infections in women', *BMJ,* 322(7302), 1571.

Krieger, J. N., Ross, S. O. and Simonsen, J. M. (1993) 'Urinary tract infections in healthy university men', *J Urol,* 149(5), 1046-8.

Latham, R. H., Running, K. and Stamm, W. E. (1983) 'Urinary tract infections in young adult women caused by Staphylococcus saprophyticus', *JAMA,* 250(22), 3063-6.

Ling, T. K., Xiong, J., Yu, Y., Lee, C. C., Ye, H. and Hawkey, P. M. (2006) 'Multicenter antimicrobial susceptibility survey of gram-negative bacteria isolated from patients with community-acquired infections in the People's Republic of China', *Antimicrob Agents Chemother,* 50(1), 374-8.

Lipsky, B. A. (1989) 'Urinary tract infections in men. Epidemiology, pathophysiology, diagnosis, and treatment', *Ann Intern Med,* 110(2), 138-50.

Manges, A. R., Johnson, J. R., Foxman, B., O'Bryan, T. T., Fullerton, K. E. and Riley, L. W. (2001) 'Widespread distribution of urinary tract infections caused by a multidrug-resistant Escherichia coli clonal group', *N Engl J Med,* 345(14), 1007-13.

Martinez, F. C., Kindrachuk, R. W., Thomas, E. and Stamey, T. A. (1985) 'Effect of prophylactic, low dose cephalexin on fecal and vaginal bacteria', *J Urol,* 133(6), 994-6.

McIsaac, W. J., Low, D. E., Biringer, A., Pimlott, N., Evans, M. and Glazier, R. (2002) 'The impact of empirical management of acute cystitis on unnecessary antibiotic use', *Arch Intern Med,* 162(5), 600-5.

McNulty, C. A., Richards, J., Livermore, D. M., Little, P., Charlett, A., Freeman, E., Harvey, I. and Thomas, M. (2006) 'Clinical relevance of laboratory-reported antibiotic resistance in acute uncomplicated urinary tract infection in primary care', *J Antimicrob Chemother,* 58(5), 1000-8.

Muratani, T. and Matsumoto, T. (2006) 'Urinary tract infection caused by fluoroquinolone- and cephem-resistant Enterobacteriaceae', *Int J Antimicrob Agents,* 28 Suppl 1, S10-3.

Nicolle, L. E., Bradley, S., Colgan, R., Rice, J. C., Schaeffer, A. and Hooton, T. M. (2005) 'Infectious Diseases Society of America guidelines for the diagnosis and treatment of asymptomatic bacteriuria in adults', *Clin Infect Dis,* 40(5), 643-54.

Nicolle, L. E., Harding, G. K., Preiksaitis, J. and Ronald, A. R. (1982) 'The association of urinary tract infection with sexual intercourse', *J Infect Dis,* 146(5), 579-83.

Nicolle, L. E., Harding, G. K., Thompson, M., Kennedy, J., Urias, B. and Ronald, A. R. (1989) 'Prospective, randomized, placebo-controlled trial of norfloxacin for the prophylaxis of recurrent urinary tract infection in women', *Antimicrob Agents Chemother,* 33(7), 1032-5.

Raz, R. and Boger, S. (1991) 'Long-term prophylaxis with norfloxacin versus nitrofurantoin in women with recurrent urinary tract infection', *Antimicrob Agents Chemother,* 35(6), 1241-2.

Raz, R., Chazan, B., Kennes, Y., Colodner, R., Rottensterich, E., Dan, M., Lavi, I. and Stamm, W. (2002) 'Empiric use of trimethoprim-sulfamethoxazole (TMP-SMX) in the treatment of women with uncomplicated urinary tract infections, in a geographical area with a high prevalence of TMP-SMX-resistant uropathogens', *Clin Infect Dis,* 34(9), 1165-9.

Raz, R., Gennesin, Y., Wasser, J., Stoler, Z., Rosenfeld, S., Rottensterich, E. and Stamm, W. E. (2000) 'Recurrent urinary tract infections in postmenopausal women', *Clin Infect Dis,* 30(1), 152-6.

Ronald, A. (2002) 'The etiology of urinary tract infection: traditional and emerging pathogens', *Am J Med,* 113 Suppl 1A, 14S-19S.

Rosenberg, M. (1999) 'Pharmacoeconomics of treating uncomplicated urinary tract infections', *Int J Antimicrob Agents,* 11(3-4), 247-51; discussion 261-4.

Sader, H. S., Biedenbach, D. J., Streit, J. M. and Jones, R. N. (2005) 'Cefdinir activity against contemporary North American isolates from community-acquired urinary tract infections', *Int J Antimicrob Agents,* 25(1), 89-92.

Saint, S., Scholes, D., Fihn, S. D., Farrell, R. G. and Stamm, W. E. (1999) 'The effectiveness of a clinical practice guideline for the management of presumed uncomplicated urinary tract infection in women', *Am J Med,* 106(6), 636-41.

Scholes, D., Hooton, T. M., Roberts, P. L., Stapleton, A. E., Gupta, K. and Stamm, W. E. (2000) 'Risk factors for recurrent urinary tract infection in young women', *J Infect Dis,* 182(4), 1177-82.

Stamey, T. A., Condy, M. and Mihara, G. (1977) 'Prophylactic efficacy of nitrofurantoin macrocrystals and trimethoprim-sulfamethoxazole in urinary infections. Biologic effects on the vaginal and rectal flora', *N Engl J Med,* 296(14), 780-3.

Stamm, W. E. (1982) 'Recent developments in the diagnosis and treatment of urinary tract infections', *West J Med,* 137(3), 213-20.

Stamm, W. E., Counts, G. W., Wagner, K. F., Martin, D., Gregory, D., McKevitt, M., Turck, M. and Holmes, K. K. (1980) 'Antimicrobial prophylaxis of recurrent urinary tract infections: a double-blind, placebo-controlled trial', *Ann Intern Med,* 92(6), 770-5.

Stamm, W. E. and Hooton, T. M. (1993) 'Management of urinary tract infections in adults', *N Engl J Med,* 329(18), 1328-34.

Stamm, W. E., McKevitt, M., Roberts, P. L. and White, N. J. (1991) 'Natural history of recurrent urinary tract infections in women', *Rev Infect Dis,* 13(1), 77-84.

Stapleton, A., Latham, R. H., Johnson, C. and Stamm, W. E. (1990) 'Postcoital antimicrobial prophylaxis for recurrent urinary tract infection. A randomized, double-blind, placebo-controlled trial', *JAMA,* 264(6), 703-6.

Steinke, D. T., Seaton, R. A., Phillips, G., MacDonald, T. M. and Davey, P. G. (1999) 'Factors associated with trimethoprim-resistant bacteria isolated from urine samples', *J Antimicrob Chemother,* 43(6), 841-3.

Stothers, L. (2002) 'A randomized trial to evaluate effectiveness and cost effectiveness of naturopathic cranberry products as prophylaxis against urinary tract infection in women', *Can J Urol,* 9(3), 1558-62.

Strom, B. L., Collins, M., West, S. L., Kreisberg, J. and Weller, S. (1987) 'Sexual activity, contraceptive use, and other risk factors for symptomatic and asymptomatic bacteriuria. A case-control study', *Ann Intern Med,* 107(6), 816-23.

Svanborg, C. and Godaly, G. (1997) 'Bacterial virulence in urinary tract infection', *Infect Dis Clin North Am,* 11(3), 513-29.

Warren, J. W., Abrutyn, E., Hebel, J. R., Johnson, J. R., Schaeffer, A. J. and Stamm, W. E. (1999) 'Guidelines for antimicrobial treatment of uncomplicated acute bacterial cystitis and acute pyelonephritis in women. Infectious Diseases Society of America (IDSA)', *Clin Infect Dis,* 29(4), 745-58.

Wong, E. S., McKevitt, M., Running, K., Counts, G. W., Turck, M. and Stamm, W. E. (1985) 'Management of recurrent urinary tract infections with patient-administered single-dose therapy', *Ann Intern Med,* 102(3), 302-7.

Wright, S. W., Wrenn, K. D. and Haynes, M. L. (1999) 'Trimethoprim-sulfamethoxazole resistance among urinary coliform isolates', *J Gen Intern Med,* 14(10), 606-9.

Yamamoto, S., Akiyama, K., Yoshimoto, T., Kanokogi, M., Yabumoto, H., Ihara, H., Ishikawa, E., Yoshioka, M., Kokura, K. and Shima, H. (2009) 'Clinical efficacy of oral administration of 200 mg gatifloxacin once daily for 3 days for the treatment of patients with uncomplicated cystitis', *J Infect Chemother,* 15(2), 104-7.

Yamamoto, S., Higuchi, Y. and Nojima, M. (2010) 'Current therapy of acute uncomplicated cystitis', *Int J Urol,* 17(5), 450-6.

3

# Urinary Tract Infections and Dysfunctional Voiding

Minardi Daniele, d'Anzeo Gianluca,
Conti Alessandro and Muzzonigro Giovanni
*Department of Clinical and Specialist Sciences - Urology, Polytechnic University of the Marches Region Medical School – A.O. Ospedali Riuniti, Ancona*
*Italy*

## 1. Introduction

Urinary tract infections are a common disease in the population. It has been estimated that half of all women are likely to suffer from at least one episode of UTIs in their life and one third will require an antibiotic treatment (Foxman, 2003).
Pathogen-related conditions (such as the presence of invasion or virulence factors) affect the severity of the infection and its resistance to antibiotic therapy, but also different host-related characteristics have been individuated, that play a role, in particular in the possibility of infection recurrence.
There are defence mechanisms that allow to counteract every attempt of the microorganisms to ascend the urinary tract. The basis of this defence is represented mainly by the semi-continuous stream of new (sterile) urine, coming from the upper urinary tract, that is stored only for a limited period of time in the bladder and afterwards completely eliminated. In this way the possibility of the microorganisms to proliferate is limited to a very narrow period of time and the immune system becomes able to eliminate efficiently the residual limited amount of colonies. Obstructing conditions causing incomplete bladder emptying after micturition set the patients at risk of infection development through overgrowth of ascending bacterial colonies.
The main causes of retention in women are listed in Table 1. Some of them are secondary to anatomic factors, while others depend on neurologic alterations affecting, in last consequence, the mechanisms of pelvic floor relaxation and detrusor contraction and their coordination. A particular category of voiding disturbances is represented by patients with alterations of detrusor-sphincter coordination in the absence of uropathy or neuropathic disorders. The individuals affected, mainly women, present frequently recurrent UTIs associated to a tendency to urinary retention.
In this chapter this disorder and its relation with infection recurrence are presented; the most common diagnostic procedures and their findings in the dysfunctional voiding and the possible treatment options are considered.

## 2. Pathophysiology of dysfunctional voiding

The normal micturition cycle can be divided in two phases: a storage phase, with passive filling by bladder relaxation and sphincter muscle contraction, and a voiding phase, with pelvic floor muscle relaxation and bladder contraction allowing micturition. In physiological conditions the two phases are well distinguished, and muscular groups aimed at filling and emptying switch alternatively from a relaxed to a contracted condition. This system is guaranteed by a correct voluntary and involuntary coordination of the nervous circuits and allows the individual to conduct a regular everyday life, without involuntary wetting or urine accumulation.

There are conditions in which, although the circuit is correctly functional and no anatomical obstructions are present, there is an impaired capacity of emptying the bladder. This situation, called dysfunctional voiding (DV), is often shown in particular in young healthy women, who go to the physician because of frequent episodes of recurrent UTIs.

DV is defined as an abnormality of bladder emptying in neurologically normal individuals in whom there is increased external sphincter activity during voluntary voiding (Carlson et al., 2001; Messelink et al., 2005).

It has been referred to by various terms, including pseudodyssynergia, external sphincter spasticity and non relaxing external urethral sphincter (Carlson et al., 2001). Its etiology is to date controversial, the clinical presentation varies and the precipitating event in autonomic somatic dyssynergia usually remains obscure (Yagci et al., 2005).

The prevalence of learned voiding dysfunction among adults is unknown, but it has been suggested that this disorder is more frequent than commonly recognized (Groutz et al., 2001): Jorgensen reported 0.5% prevalence rate among patients referred for urodynamic evaluation.

As far as it is known, DV seems to be the result of the combination of both inherited factors and behavioural conditions (Everaert et al., 2000). It is thought to be often acquired in the childhood, during toilet training when the children learn to control sphincteric activity, but can also appear in older ages, with higher frequency in the female sex. An inappropriate contraction of pelvic floor muscles, thereby tightening the urinary sphincter complex represents the key point of this mechanism. Activation of the pelvic floor muscles seems to start in consequence of the flow-rate exceeding a certain threshold and to cease spontaneously after it has fallen again below it.

This incoordination of bladder-sphincter function in children may represent a developmental abnormality (Allen & Bright, 1978), that can lead not only to lower urinary tract symptoms, but may cause structural and functional changes, including obstruction and consequent bladder trabeculations, residual urine and bacteriuria; detrusor hypertrophy and consequent vesico-ureteral reflux (VUR) or hydroureter/hydronephrosis may develop (Hinman, 1986; Groutz et al., 2001).

DV could represent the result of a learned behavior, evolving from attempt to suppress impending or active bladder contractions by inappropriately contracting the pelvic floor muscles, thereby tightening the urinary sphincter complex. The first step in the development of dysfunctional voiding could then reside in an underlying form of bladder overactivity, which the patient learns to control from the childhood through volitional contractions of the muscles of the pelvic floor. This leads to a condition of insufficient pelvic floor relaxation (or contractions) also in response to the physiological contractions during micturition. As the time goes by, this condition can evolve to a situation of high-pressure voiding, as in all obstruction sets. VUR, if not already present, can develop and, combined with the increased tendency to the development of recurrent UTIs, can further facilitate the occurrence of pyelonephritis and subsequent renal scarring (Chandra, 1995; Acar et al., 2009).

As a result, people affected from DV tend to develop chronic urinary retention, since high urethral pressures during micturition, due to incomplete sphincter relaxation, do not allow complete bladder emptying, and to develop, in the mid-long term, recurrent UTIs from an ascending way.

Also incontinence can develop during this process. This can be due to the accentuation of the primitive condition of detrusor overactivity, or, later, to the development of bladder underactivity, resulting in inability to empty and overflow incontinence (lazy bladder syndrome) (Norgaard et al., 1998).

An additional role for urethral instability in the pathogenesis of DV has been claimed, to explain the symptoms of urgency in DV. Sudden variations in the urethral pressure during bladder filling in people affected by DV were demonstrated, represented by pressure decreases with short periods of electromyography silence, intermittent urethral pressure increases with short perineal spasms, or urethral pressure decreases with silent electromyography, combined with different degrees of bladder instability (Vereecken & Proesmans, 2000).

Furthermore, some degree of external sphincter hypertrophia was noted in some studies conducted on females affected from dysfunctional voiding and a positive correlation between dysfunctional behaviors and sphincter volume postulated (Minardi et al., 2008). Its role in the pathogenesis is, anyway, still to be determined.

Behavioral or functional abnormalities which predispose to UTIs in women with normal urinary tract or only minor abnormalities are neglected in most recommended protocols for evaluation of urinary tract infections (McKenna & Herndon, 2000) .

The commonest cause of urinary retention in young women in dysfunctional voiding is a primary disorder of sphincter relaxation (Fowler's syndrome). It is defined as the combination of urinary retention, abnormal electromyographic activity of the urethral rhabdosphincter and polycystic ovaries (Fowler et al., 1988); it was further observed that this overactivity can lead to hypertrophic changes of the urethral rhabdosphincter (Wiseman et al., 2002). The full etiology of this condition remain to be elucidated but it has been hypothesized that the disorder is due to a hormonally sensitive channel alteration, which results in a sustained involuntary contraction of the striated urethral sphincter (Kavia et al., 2006). This in turn has an inhibitory effect on detrusor contractions as well as inhibiting sensations of the desire to void.

On light microscopy the urethral rhabdosphincter fiber diameter did not differ among patients with disorder of sphincter relaxation compared to normal patients, but electron microscopy showed excessive peripheral sarcoplasm with lipid and glycogen deposition, and sarcoplasmic accumulation of normal mitochondria, reflecting the increased energy requirement of an overactive urethral rhabdosphincter (Andrich et al., 2005).

EMG of the pubo-coccygeal muscles (together with recordings of other urodynamic variables) is helpful in revealing inappropriate EMG activity during micturition (Deindl et al., 1998).

Women perceive voiding dysfunction less commonly as an important urinary symptom. The most reported voiding symptom was poor urinary stream. Its prevalence with or without hesitancy ranged from 15% to 45%, intermittency (20% to 35%), incomplete emptying (30% to 50%), and abdominal straining (10%). These seem more severe in younger women than older women, except for poor stream which is common in older women (10% of women aged 19 to 29 years and 40% of women aged $\geq$ 80 years) (Al-Hayek & Abrams, 2004).

The association of dysfunctional voiding with recurrent UTIs is documented; dysfunctional voiding can disrupt the laminar urinary flow through the urethra, causing UTIs as bacteria are transferred back from the meatus to the bladder as a result of the "milk-back" phenomenon (Carlson et al., 2001; Yagci et al., 2005). It has been estimated that up to 42% with dysfunctional voiding suffer from recurrent UTIs episodes.
An extreme form of dysfunctional voiding is represented by Hinman-Allen syndrome, also called non-neurogenic neurogenic bladder syndrome (NNNBS). Hinman and Baumann and Allen described, independently, in the 70s, this condition in two series of children with severe functional dysfunction producing changes indistinguishable from an obstructive factor (Hinman & Baumann, 1973). Objective findings of NNNB syndrome are represented by severe obstructive uropathy, with elevated postvoid residual (PVR) urine volume, thickened, trabeculated bladder wall, recurrent UTIs, and acquired VUR and hydronephrosis. It often presents in the more complex form of dysfunctional elimination syndrome, including also the development of fecal disturbances and usually leads to very serious consequences including renal failure (Claudon et al., 2010).
Clinical criteria have been developed to help in distinguishing between NNNB syndrome and neurogenic bladder: in Hinman-Allis syndrome there is intact perineal sensation and anal tone, normal anatomy and function of the lower extremities are found, there is no evidence of skin lesions overlying the sacrum, normal lumbosacral spine at plain radiography, and normal spinal cord at MR imaging (Johnson et al., 1992). A relation between this abnormal bladder behavior in children, developed during their period of toilet training and a difficult familial-social condition (in particular the presence of a history of sexual harassment) has been reported in over 50% of the subjects affected (Ellsworth et al., 1995; Davila et al., 2003).

## 3. Diagnostic procedures

Some parameters have been developed, in order to classify a voiding disturbance as true Dysfunctional Voiding. There are clinical and laboratory requirements. Furthermore, a deep evaluation of all possible complicating factors need to be performed and the results must also be monitored after a treatment.

### 3.1 History taking, examination and questionnaires

A correct case history collection represents the first and most important step in the diagnostis of DV.
Voiding habits of patients presenting with symptoms of recurrent cystitis (pelvic pain or burning, frequent voiding, nocturia, blood in urine) must be carefully collected. A voiding diary can also be useful. In older patients also a pediatric history should be deeply collected, as far as possible.
Examination of the external genitalia, with particular care for eventual secretions can allow to exclude different etiologies, or address to particular infectious agents. Furthermore, in the female, a thorough inspection for vaginal wall prolapse should be always made, since they could account for obstructive symptoms, even in initial cases (Dancz & Ozel, 2011).
For pediatric patients also several questionnaires have been developed to assess voiding dysfunction (Tuygun et al., 2007). The most accepted is represented by the standardized dysfunctional voiding symptom score (DVSS) (Farhat et al., 2000). It consists of questions, the pediatric patient can easily understand and answer, while the parents are asked to

evaluate whether possible traumatic events have recently occurred that could justify the raise of the symptoms. The reliability of the test in predicting voiding dysfunction in the subsequent strumental iter was proven through different studies and could be successfully adapted to settings presenting cultural differences from western countries (Bartkowski & Doubrava, 2004; Calado et al., 2010).

A similar but more complex test, that can better fit to an adult population is represented by the Pelvic Floor Inventories Leiden (PelFIs), developed at the University of Leuven, aimed at the evaluation of a broader spectrum of different pelvic floor disorders. It consists of 83 items related to micturition, defecation and sexual dysfunction symptoms (Voorham-van der Zalm et al., 2008). It offers very good results in terms of validity and reliability. (Voorham-van der Zalm et al., 2011).

Although self assessment questionnaires represent a valid item in the evaluation of pelvic disorders, as reported in the literature, it is authors' belief that they cannot be considered as a substitute of the general clinical assessment on the basis of the personal judgement and experience of the physician, and a complete evaluation must be always be made after a (video)urodynamic , that is able not only to give a more correct and quantitative assessment of the disturbances felt by the patient, but also to discover mechanisms that could not be directly correlated with the symptoms and would therefore remain undiscovered, only based on patient's perceptions.

### 3.2 Urinalysis

In women presenting to their physician compelling of recurrent pelvic pain symptoms, chemical and cultural urine analysis represent the first line examination. The finding of high levels of nitrate in the urine, or the presence of leucocytes, is highly suggestive for the presence of urease producing bacteria. The importance of urinalysis in dysfunctional voiding relies on the need of stating the actual presence of recurrent UTIs; at the same time, it is necessary to prove the efficacy of an antibiotic therapy and to exclude the onset of an asymptomatic bacteruria.

### 3.3 Urodynamics

Functional assessment through urodynamics (UD) or with video-urodynamics (VUD) represents a second-level examination for UTIs assessment, but become mandatory in cases of treatment refractory recurrent UTIs. Some findings are typical of DV at the urodynamic evaluation. In these cases the contextual registration of needle EMG is very helpful (Minardi et al., 2008).

### 3.4 Ultrasound

Genito-urinary ultrasound (US) - in experts hands - represents an important tool in the evalutation of all cases of urinary tract dysfunctions, allowing a first examination of morphological changes, that are present in case of obstructed voiding, and a first assessment of the integrity of the urinary system. Advances in ultrasound equipment such as the development of vaginal probes allowing the use of higher frequency ultrasound have led to a dramatic increase in the resolution of images obtained and to date perineal US is held as an effective, well-tolerated and affordable diagnostic procedure (Sendag et al., 2003).

In the evaluation of the characteristics of the lower urinary tract US can also be used to evaluate the anatomy of the urethro-vesical junction and the mobility of the bladder neck for the study of stress urinary incontinence (Kolbl et al., 1988; Quinn et al., 1988; Khullar et al., 1996; Sarnelli et al., 2003).

Bladder neck mobility can be demonstrated by perineal or vaginal ultrasound and measured using the symphysis pubis as the immobile reference point; perineal ultrasonography allows visualization and measurement of the angle between the proximal mobile part and the distal fixed part of the urethra.

Under these aspects US offers several advantages over other imaging modalities: using US urethral sphincter volume and detrusor wall thickness could be investigated in women with urinary incontinence, urinary retention and detrusor instability (Kondo et al., 2001; Schafer et al., 2002; Oliveira et al., 2006); in patients with detrusor overactivity a positive correlation was observed between rhabdosphincter thickness and detrusor contraction pressure, and between rhabdosphincter thickness and urethral resistance, and mean maximum urethral closure pressure and sphincter volume (Major et al., 2002; Wiseman et al., 2002).

Sendag et al , applying perineal ultrasound, found that posterior urethro-vesical angle was significantly different both at rest and on straining in patients with stress incontinence, as well as the angle between the vertical axis and urethral axis and the descensus diameter (Sendag et al., 2003).

Perineal ultrasonography provides also serial non-invasive examinations for assessing the condition of the bladder wall; the normal bladder wall is 3 to 6 mm thick although it varies with intravesical volume; it may be thickened secondary to chronic infection, inflammation after surgery, or radiation; a decrease in bladder wall thickness may suggest clearing of an infection or inflammation; measurement of bladder wall thickness may be helpful for detecting detrusor overactivity (Schaer et al., 1995; Khullar et al., 1996; Yang & Huang, 2003; Minardi et al., 2007).

In their study, Khullar et al averaged the bladder wall thickness at the trigone, dome, and anterior bladder wall to develop criteria for detection of detrusor overactivity, others assumed that measurement of the bladder dome is sufficient to define bladder wall thickness, even if they did not find that women with detrusor overactivity had an appreciably thicker bladder wall than other study groups (Khullar et al., 1996; Yang & Huang, 2003).

US has also been shown to be a reproducible method of assessing urethral sphincter volume (Digesu et al., 2009).

Using 2D ultrasound, on axial US images the normal urethra has a characteristic target-like appearance and is seen as composed by four concentric rings of different echogenicity (Minardi et al., 2007).

In patients with detrusor overactivity a positive correlation was observed between rhabdosphincter thickness and detrusor contraction pressure, and between rhabdosphincter thickness and urethral resistance, as measured by maximal urethral closure pressure (Major et al., 2002).

Morphologic changes in the sphincter echo-texture can occur as result of a variety of factors; but while an intrinsic sphincter deficiency can easily be suggested on axial US images by loss of its normal characteristic target-like appearance, the coexistence of abnormal urethral rings and increased detrusor wall thickness might be due to functional compressive urethral obstruction from sphincter overactivity, both of idiopathic or neurological origin (Minardi et al., 2007).

Under this aspect the introduction of three-dimensional (3D) ultrasound has proven very useful to the morphologic assessment of the pelvic floor.

The advent of 3D images has improved the potential of US technique to measure volumes of structures. The advantages of 3D technology over two dimensions specifically include an ability to cross reference measurements so that the image measured is the best possible one obtainable and therefore in theory reduce the error of these measurements (Toozs-Hobson et al., 2001).

In fact, 3D measurements are produced from assessment of all three planes, each of which will have a biological variation. 3D ultrasound offers a potential advantage over 2D scanning of increased sensitivity, with a reduction in the error from conventional 2D imaging as the operator can constantly cross reference in all three major planes simultaneously and therefore ensure that any surface area being measured in the best possible reproduction. Since the scan may be manipulated in any plane, the image may be viewed from several perspective prior to the actual measurement (Toozs-Hobson et al., 2001). Technical developments enable rapid automated volume acquisition in real time, and currently available transducers designed for abdominal use are well suited for translabial/transperineal imaging (Dietz, 2004). Useful applications are represented by imaging of the urethra, the levator ani and paravaginal supports, prolapse and implants used in pelvic floor reconstruction and anti-incontinence surgery (Dietz, 2004).

Three-dimensional reconstruction of the female human urethral sphincter have shown the precise structure of the muscle layers (smooth and striated muscle fibers) and nerve fibers (myelinated and unmyelinated) and their relations with the urethra and vaginal wall. The proximal third consisted of a circular smooth muscle sphincter, the middle third consisted of two circular layers of smooth and striated muscle fibers and the distal third consisted of a circular layer of smooth muscle fibers surrounded by omega-shaped layer of striated muscle fibers (Karam et al., 2005).

In studies conducted on women with stress-urinary incontinence three-dimensional ultrasound has been shown to be a reproducible method of assessing urethral sphincter volume, where it has been shown to correlate with the area under the urethral pressure profile curve, suggesting a relationship between structural and functional anatomy (Toozs-Hobson et al., 2001; Athanasiou et al., 1999; Robinson et al., 2004).

Perineal ultrasound was used by our group to assess function and morphology of the urethral sphincter and of the detrusor muscle in the evaluation of dysfunctional voiding in female patients with recurrent urinary tract infections (UTIs) (Minardi et al., 2008).

The study population comprised women referred to our Department with more than a 3-year period of recurrent UTIs, and dysfunctional voiding. The diagnosis of dysfunctional voiding was made according to Carlson et al., where an increased external sphincter activity during voiding was recorded on multichannel video urodynamics (Carlson et al., 2001).

The sonographic examination (ESAOTE, model. Technos MP, Genova, Italy) was performed with the patients supine, using both the translabial approach (3.5 MHz sector probe) and the introital approach (6.5 MHz end fire endovaginal probe); the latter was used to allow proper location of the end extremity of the probe close to mid urethra and, due to its superior spatial resolution, to provide a more detailed depiction of minute structure when examining the echogenic texture of the urethra. Image orientation and display on the screen were standardized so that the transducer appears at the bottom, the left side is the ventral aspect of the patient and the upper is the cranial aspect, as described (Schaer et al., 1995; Minardi et al., 2007). The posterior urethro-vesical angle, the proximal pubo-urethral distance and the angle of urethral inclination were calculated, as described (Minardi et al., 2007). The thickness of the bladder detrusor wall was measured at the dome of the bladder.

Visualization of the four-rings different echo texture of the urethra was performed in the same scan plane. Urethral sphincter volume was assessed by measurements of 3 dimensions; they were first determined in the axial plane by measuring the transverse and anteroposterior dimension at the estimated point of widest transverse dimension; the longitudinal dimension was measured in the sagittal plane just off the midline; the ellipsoid volume formula was then applied as follows: volume = height x width x length x 0.52.
Urethral sphincter volume was measured using a 7.5 MHz transvaginal ultrasound probe, where volume was calculated using formula for the volume of a cylinder, as described (Kondo et al., 2001; Wiseman et al., 2002).
We observed that maximum urethral sphincter volume was significantly increased in patients with recurrent UTIs and dysfunctional voiding (2.87+0.41 $cm^3$) compared to patients with recurrent UTIs and normal perineal activity during voiding and to control patients (1.77+0.62 cm3 and 1.61+0.32 $cm^3$ respectively); abnormal findings at ultrasound included thickening of individual rings, haziness of contours and change in echogenic texture with loss of the characteristic four-rings appearance; these findings were observed only in patients with dysfunctional voiding (Minardi et al., 2008).
Detrusor wall thickness as assessed by suprapubic ultrasound ranged from 2.2 to 9.3 mm.; it was significantly thicker in patients with dysfunctional voiding (7.83+0.8 mm) compared to patients with recurrent UTIs and normal perineal activity during voiding and to control patients (3.81+1.1 mm. and 3.92+1.8 mm. respectively).
The ROC analysis showed that, to identify a patient with dysfunctional voiding, a sphincter volume threshold of 1.94 $mm^3$ has 100% sensitivity and 63.2% specificity; a detrusor thickness threshold of 4.95 mm has 100% sensitivity and 85.4% specificity; at these cut-off values, 56.9% of patients with dysfunctional voiding had both the two ultrasound parameters above the threshold level (Minardi et al., 2008).
In our study by the analysis of opening/maximum flow detrusor pressure and mean/maximum urethral closure pressure, patients with recurrent UTIs associated with dysfunctional voiding are obstructed; similarly, by the analysis of detrusor thickness and striated sphincter volume at ultrasound, we can diagnose obstruction. We have found positive correlations between opening/maximum flow detrusor pressure and urethral sphincter volume, between mean/maximum urethral closure pressure and urethral sphincter volume, and between detrusor thickness and urethral sphincter volume in patients with recurrent UTIs associated with dysfunctional voiding; the increased urethral sphincter volume, as a consequence of a dysfunctional voiding, can be the cause of a functional obstruction (Minardi et al., 2008). An increased urethral sphincter volume, as a consequence of a dysfunctional voiding, can be the cause of functional obstruction.
Based on our experience, dysfunctional voiding can be suspected by ultrasound in women with recurrent UTIs, when an increase of detrusor thickness and of striated sphincter volume is observed. Data derived from the ROC curves about cut-off values of urethral sphincter volume and detrusor thickness allow us to propose perineal ultrasound as a first line diagnostic approach in the evaluation of dysfunctional voiding in women with recurrent UTIs.
Therefore, we have suggested that a first line approach in female patients with recurrent UTIs can be done by flow electromyography, with recording of urine flow and perineal activity during voiding, and by perineal ultrasound, with the evaluation of detrusor wall thickness and of sphincter volume; these investigation in our experience are able to select

patients with dysfunctional voiding. According to results of our study, multichannel video urodynamics can therefore represent a second line diagnostic approach in selected patients.

## 4. Treatment options

DV treatment is particularly problematic: the aim is to restore a normal voiding pattern, to reduce excessive detrusor and pelvic floor activity, to improve voiding and storage symptoms and especially to reduce UTIs incidence. DV therapy combines pharmacological treatment, physical therapy and behavioral therapy.

DV treatment, with particular reference to UTIs, benefits, from a long time, of biofeedback, which has been employed for the first time in the 80's, on babies followed up for 3 years, with complete voiding pattern normalization (Hellstrom et al., 1987). Afterwards, many studies were focused on the linkage between DV and UTIs, trying to find therapeutic protocols which would be able to normalize voiding pattern and reduce UTIs recurrence and, from the other side, be simple to manage for the patient and, when in the pediatric age, for his family.

De Paepe et al. published in 1998 the first prospective clinical trial aimed to investigate the role of biofeedback modulation (BFM) in UTIs prevention in young girls (De Paepe et al., 1998). Girls of age under 14 were enrolled, with urodynamic-confirmed DV diagnosis. In the first phase of the treatment, patients were taught to take self-consciousness of perineal musculature and afterwards they started BFM. During this period, trimethoprim and anticholinergic drugs, in case of overactivity, were prescribed. The antibiotic treatment was stopped at the end of the BFM protocol and the patients were followed-up for 6 months. Considering an UTIs-free period of 6 months, at least the 83% of patients of age over 6 years were free from infections. Moreover, the Authors reported also a complete resolution of vescico-ureteral reflux in 5 of 6 cases. This study, which was of great importance because it shed light on the ability of BFM in reducing urinary infections, had several limitations, especially the absence of a control group (very important in this setting, because of the frequent spontaneous resolution of predisposing factors at this age, e.g reflux), and relatively short follow-up.

VUR is a determinant factor which is able to predispose DV patient to recurrent UTIs. In this regard, Kibar et al studied in deep the linkage between BFM treatment and frequency of VUR in children with DV (Kibar et al., 2007). Eighty-six patients of age over 5 years were enrolled in a BFM program; of these, 78 completed the protocol. At the end of 6 months follow-up, the Authors reported a significant improvement in all the considered parameters, both in symptoms (enuresis, incontinence, frequency, urgency) and urodynamics parameters. Moreover, the 29% of VUR improved, with a complete resolution in 63% of cases. Considering the frequency of spontaneous resolution of VUR in this age group, Authors concluded that BFM treatment could be considered as a good option alternative to watchful-waiting.

In the pathophysiology of recurrent UTIs in DV patient, post-void residual is of crucial importance. Kibar and coll focused their attention in a prospective randomized trial in which 94 kids with flowmetric and electromiographic profile compatible with DV, and a PVR higher than 20 ml were enrolled (Kibar et al., 2010). Patients were randomized in two groups, in the first one kids were informed with behavioral rules, in the other patients received also BFM. At the end of the treatment, there was a complete resolution of PVR in 64,5% in the group which received both treatments vs. th 34,4% in the first group. Moreover, Authors reported a reduction of UTIs in both groups.

BFM was applied not only in pediatric population, but also recently in adult female patients with recurrent UTIs and DV. In a prospective randomized clinical trial, we examined 142 women assigned to 4 treatment groups (Minardi et al., 2010) The first group underwent only uroflowmetry BFM, the second only BFM, the third both the two treatments and the fourth only antibiotic treatment when needed. During the treatment and at the end of the protocol, patients underwent periodic urine cultures and periodic evaluation of symptom scores and urodynamics parameters, trying to show variation in the subjective and objective domain. Only 86 subjects completed the protocol. Authors observed an improvement not only in the obstructive symptoms but also on irritative domain, as well as on urodynamic parameters, with results that remained stable until the end of follow-up period of 24 months. UTIs incidence was dramatically reduced in all the three group of treatment, but remained unchanged in the group that received only antibiotic therapy. The low compliance that emerged from this protocol, stresses the commitment, sometimes considerable, required to the patient in order to complete the protocol and to keep in touch with the hospital. This is of utmost importance because dropping out the protocol leads to a significant worsening of the results.

| | |
|---|---|
| **Neurologic causes** | Neurologic diseases (e.g. Multiple sclerosis, Lateral amyotrophic sclerosis, Parkinson disease) |
| | Spinal lesions/trauma |
| | Pharmacological treatments (e.g. TCA, antimuscarinic agents, alpha agonists, ganglion-blockers) |
| | Endocrine (e.g. Diabetes mellitus, hypotiroidismus) |
| **Non-neurologic causes** | Mechanic intrinsic bladder outlet obstruction (e.g.prostatic hyperplasia, bladder neck disease, urethral stenosis, bladder prolapse) |
| | Extrinsic obstruction (e.g pelvic masses, pelvic organs prolapse) |
| | Psychogenic (e.g. anxiety syndrome, hysteria) |
| | Inflammatory (e.g. urethritis, prostatitis, herpes) |
| | Myopathy (detrusor myopathy, myasthenia gravis) |
| | Iatrogenic (e.g. after pelvic surgery) |
| | Idiopathic causes |

Table 1. Most common causes of Urinary retention.

Anyway, some open questions remain, in particular on which parameters should be considered to establish the success of therapy and which prognostic factor the clinician can use in this setting. Nelson and coll evaluated the importance of urodynamic parameters in the evaluation of BFM treatment outcomes in DV patients (Nelson et al., 2004). This study confirmed the beneficial effect of BFM on the resolution of recurrent UTIs, but there was no correlation between the clinical improvement and urodynamic parameters improvement. In this study, which involved 81 pediatric patients followed up for more than 9 months after the end of BFM, there was no statistically significant difference in urodynamic parameters (in particular PVR and maximum flow) between those who had persistence of UTIs and those who benefit from this therapy.

In a retrospective study on 77 boys with DV, Drzewiecki and coll. showed that some parameters are able to predict the success of BFM therapy (Drzewiecki et al., 2009). The Authors noted that compliance and commitment during the treatment are both determinant factors, considering that at least 6 sessions are required for pediatric patients and that the probability of flow normalization after the third session are reduced to 5%.

At present, there is no evidence about this point in the adult population; so future randomized trials should also aim to identify predictive factors in order to tailor the treatment to any specific patient as much as possible.

## 5. References


Acar, B., Arikan, F. I., Germiyanoglu, C. & Dallar, Y. (2009). Influence of high bladder pressure on vesicoureteral reflux and its resolution. *Urol Int*, Vol. 82, No.1, (2009), pp. 77-80, ISSN 1423-0399 (Electronic) 0042-1138 (Linking)

Al-Hayek, S. & Abrams, P. (2004). Women's lower urinary tract function and dysfunction: definitions and epidemiology. *Minerva Ginecol*, Vol. 56, No.4, (August 2004), pp. 311-325, ISSN 0026-4784 (Print) 0026-4784 (Linking)

Allen, T. D. & Bright, T. C., 3rd (1978). Urodynamic patterns in children with dysfunctional voiding problems. *J Urol*, Vol. 119, No.2, (Febuary 1978), pp. 247-249, ISSN 0022-5347 (Print) 0022-5347 (Linking)

Andrich, D. E., Rickards, D., Landon, D. N., Fowler, C. J. & Mundy, A. R. (2005). Structural assessment of the urethral sphincter in women with urinary retention. *J Urol*, Vol. 173, No.4, (April 2005), pp. 1246-1251, ISSN 0022-5347 (Print) 0022-5347 (Linking)

Athanasiou, S., Khullar, V., Boos, K., Salvatore, S. & Cardozo, L. (1999). Imaging the urethral sphincter with three-dimensional ultrasound. *Obstet Gynecol*, Vol. 94, No.2, (August 1999), pp. 295-301, ISSN 0029-7844 (Print) 0029-7844 (Linking)

Bartkowski, D. P. & Doubrava, R. G. (2004). Ability of a normal dysfunctional voiding symptom score to predict uroflowmetry and external urinary sphincter electromyography patterns in children. *J Urol*, Vol. 172, No.5 Pt 1, (November 2004), pp. 1980-1985; discussion 1985, ISSN 0022-5347 (Print) 0022-5347 (Linking)

Calado, A. A., Araujo, E. M., Barroso, U., Jr., Netto, J. M., Filho, M. Z., Macedo, A., Jr., Bagli, D. & Farhat, W. (2010). Cross-cultural adaptation of the dysfunctional voiding score symptom (DVSS) questionnaire for Brazilian children. *Int Braz J Urol*, Vol. 36, No.4, (July-August 2010), pp. 458-463, ISSN 1677-6119 (Electronic) 1677-5538 (Linking)

Carlson, K. V., Rome, S. & Nitti, V. W. (2001). Dysfunctional voiding in women. *J Urol*, Vol. 165, No.1, (January 2001), pp. 143-147; discussion 147-148, ISSN 0022-5347 (Print) 0022-5347 (Linking)

Chandra, M. (1995). Reflux nephropathy, urinary tract infection, and voiding disorders. *Curr Opin Pediatr*, Vol. 7, No.2, (April 1995), pp. 164-170, ISSN 1040-8703 (Print) 1040-8703 (Linking)

Claudon, P., Fotso-Kamdem, A. & Aubert, D. (2010). [The non-neurogenic neurogenic bladder (Hinman's syndrome) in children: What are pronostic criteria based on a 31 cases multicentric study]. *Prog Urol*, Vol. 20, No.4, (April 2010), pp. 292-300, ISSN 1166-7087 (Print) 1166-7087 (Linking)

Dancz, C. E. & Ozel, B. (2011). Is there a pelvic organ prolapse threshold that predicts bladder outflow obstruction? *Int Urogynecol J Pelvic Floor Dysfunct*, (February 22 2011), ISSN 1433-3023 (Electronic) 0937-3462 (Linking)

Davila, G., Bernier, F., Franco, J. & Kopka, S. (2003). Bladder dysfunction in sexual abuse survivors. *J Urol*, Vol. 170, (August 2003), pp. 476-479, ISSN

De Paepe, H., Hoebeke, P., Renson, C., Van Laecke, E., Raes, A., Van Hoecke, E., Van Daele, J. & Vande Walle, J. (1998). Pelvic-floor therapy in girls with recurrent urinary tract infections and dysfunctional voiding. *British journal of urology*, Vol. 81 Suppl 3, (May 1998), pp. 109-113, ISSN 0007-1331 (Print) 0007-1331 (Linking)

Deindl, F. M., Vodusek, D. B., Bischoff, C., Hofmann, R. & Hartung, R. (1998). Dysfunctional voiding in women: which muscles are responsible? *Br J Urol*, Vol. 82, No.6, (December 1998), pp. 814-819, ISSN 0007-1331 (Print) 0007-1331 (Linking)

Dietz, H. P. (2004). Ultrasound imaging of the pelvic floor. Part II: three-dimensional or volume imaging. *Ultrasound Obstet Gynecol*, Vol. 23, No.6, (June 2004), pp. 615-625, I SSN 0960-7692 (Print) 0960-7692 (Linking)

Digesu, G. A., Robinson, D., Cardozo, L. & Khullar, V. (2009). Three-dimensional ultrasound of the urethral sphincter predicts continence surgery outcome. *Neurourol Urodyn*, Vol. 28, No.1, (2009), pp. 90-94, ISSN 1520-6777 (Electronic) 0733-2467 (Linking)

Drzewiecki, B. A., Kelly, P. R., Marinaccio, B., Borer, J. G., Estrada, C. R., Lee, R. S. & Bauer, S. B. (2009). Biofeedback training for lower urinary tract symptoms: factors affecting efficacy. *The Journal of urology*, Vol. 182, No.4 Suppl, (October 2009), pp. 2050-2055, ISSN 1527-3792 (Electronic) 0022-5347 (Linking)

Ellsworth, P., Merquerian, P. & Copening, M. (1995). Sexual abuse: another causative factor in dysfunctional voiding. *J Urol*, Vol. 153, (March 1995), pp. 773-776

Everaert, K., Van Laecke, E., De Muynck, M., Peeters, H. & Hoebeke, P. (2000). Urodynamic assessment of voiding dysfunction and dysfunctional voiding in girls and women. *Int Urogynecol J Pelvic Floor Dysfunct*, Vol. 11, No.4, (2000), pp. 254-264, ISSN 0937-3462 (Print) 0937-3462 (Linking)

Farhat, W., Bagli, D. J., Capolicchio, G., O'Reilly, S., Merguerian, P. A., Khoury, A. & McLorie, G. A. (2000). The dysfunctional voiding scoring system: quantitative standardization of dysfunctional voiding symptoms in children. *J Urol*, Vol. 164, No.3 Pt 2, (September 2000), pp. 1011-1015, I SSN 0022-5347 (Print) 0022-5347 (Linking)

Fowler, C. J., Christmas, T. J., Chapple, C. R., Parkhouse, H. F., Kirby, R. S. & Jacobs, H. S. (1988). Abnormal electromyographic activity of the urethral sphincter, voiding dysfunction, and polycystic ovaries: a new syndrome? *BMJ*, Vol. 297, No.6661, (December 3 1988), pp. 1436-1438, ISSN 0959-8138 (Print) 0959-535X (Linking)

Foxman, B. (2003). Epidemiology of urinary tract infections: incidence, morbidity, and economic costs. *Dis Mon*, Vol. 49, No.2, (February 2003), pp. 53-70, ISSN 0011-5029 (Print) 0011-5029 (Linking)

Groutz, A., Blaivas, J. G., Pies, C. & Sassone, A. M. (2001). Learned voiding dysfunction (non-neurogenic, neurogenic bladder) among adults. *Neurourol Urodyn*, Vol. 20, No.3, (2001), pp. 259-268, ISSN 0733-2467 (Print) 0733-2467 (Linking)

Hellstrom, A. L., Hjalmas, K. & Jodal, U. (1987). Rehabilitation of the dysfunctional bladder in children: method and 3-year followup. *The Journal of urology*, Vol. 138, No.4, (October 1987), pp. 847-849, I SSN 0022-5347 (Print) 0022-5347 (Linking)

Hinman, F. & Baumann, F. W. (1973). Vesical and ureteral damage from voiding dysfunction in boys without neurologic or obstructive disease. *J Urol*, Vol. 109, No.4, (April 1973), pp. 727-732, I SSN 0022-5347 (Print) 0022-5347 (Linking)

Hinman, F., Jr. (1986). Nonneurogenic neurogenic bladder (the Hinman syndrome)--15 years later. *J Urol*, Vol. 136, No.4, (October 1986), pp. 769-777, I SSN 0022-5347 (Print) 0022-5347 (Linking)

Johnson, J. F., 3rd, Hedden, R. J., Piccolello, M. L. & Wacksman, J. (1992). Distention of the posterior urethra: association with nonneurogenic neurogenic bladder (Hinman syndrome). *Radiology*, Vol. 185, No.1, (October 1992), pp. 113-117, I SSN 0033-8419 (Print) 0033-8419 (Linking)

Karam, I., Droupy, S., Abd-Alsamad, I., Uhl, J. F., Benoit, G. & Delmas, V. (2005). Innervation of the female human urethral sphincter: 3D reconstruction of immunohistochemical studies in the fetus. *Eur Urol*, Vol. 47, No.5, (May 2005), pp. 627-633; discussion 634, I SSN 0302-2838 (Print) 0302-2838 (Linking)

Kavia, R. B., Datta, S. N., Dasgupta, R., Elneil, S. & Fowler, C. J. (2006). Urinary retention in women: its causes and management. *BJU Int*, Vol. 97, No.2, (February 2006), pp. 281-287, I SSN 1464-4096 (Print) 1464-4096 (Linking)

Khullar, V., Cardozo, L. D., Salvatore, S. & Hill, S. (1996). Ultrasound: a noninvasive screening test for detrusor instability. *Br J Obstet Gynaecol*, Vol. 103, No.9, (September 1996), pp. 904-908, I SSN 0306-5456 (Print) 0306-5456 (Linking)

Kibar, Y., Ors, O., Demir, E., Kalman, S., Sakallioglu, O. & Dayanc, M. (2007). Results of biofeedback treatment on reflux resolution rates in children with dysfunctional voiding and vesicoureteral reflux. *Urology*, Vol. 70, No.3, (September 2007), pp. 563-566; discussion 566-567, I SSN 1527-9995 (Electronic) 0090-4295 (Linking)

Kibar, Y., Piskin, M., Irkilata, H. C., Aydur, E., Gok, F. & Dayanc, M. (2010). Management of abnormal postvoid residual urine in children with dysfunctional voiding. *Urology*, Vol. 75, No.6, (June 2010), pp. 1472-1475, I SSN 1527-9995 (Electronic) 0090-4295 (Linking)

Kolbl, H., Bernaschek, G. & Wolf, G. (1988). A comparative study of perineal ultrasound scanning and urethrocystography in patients with genuine stress incontinence. *Arch Gynecol Obstet*, Vol. 244, No.1, 1988), pp. 39-45, I SSN 0932-0067 (Print) 0932-0067 (Linking)

Kondo, Y., Homma, Y., Takahashi, S., Kitamura, T. & Kawabe, K. (2001). Transvaginal ultrasound of urethral sphincter at the mid urethra in continent and incontinent women. *J Urol*, Vol. 165, No.1, (Jan 2001), pp. 149-152, I SSN 0022-5347 (Print) 0022-5347 (Linking)

Major, H., Culligan, P. & Heit, M. (2002). Urethral sphincter morphology in women with detrusor instability. *Obstet Gynecol*, Vol. 99, No.1, (January 2002), pp. 63-68, I SSN 0029-7844 (Print) 0029-7844 (Linking)

McKenna, P. H. & Herndon, C. D. (2000). Voiding dysfunction associated with incontinence, vesicoureteral reflux and recurrent urinary tract infections. *Curr Opin Urol*,

Vol. 10, No.6, (November 2000), pp. 599-606, I SSN 0963-0643 (Print) 0963-0643 (Linking)

Messelink, B., Benson, T., Berghmans, B., Bo, K., Corcos, J., Fowler, C., Laycock, J., Lim, P. H., van Lunsen, R., a Nijeholt, G. L., Pemberton, J., Wang, A., Watier, A. & Van Kerrebroeck, P. (2005). Standardization of terminology of pelvic floor muscle function and dysfunction: report from the pelvic floor clinical assessment group of the International Continence Society. *Neurourol Urodyn*, Vol. 24, No.4, 2005), pp. 374-380, I SSN 0733-2467 (Print) 0733-2467 (Linking)

Minardi, D., d'Anzeo, G., Parri, G., Polito, M., Jr., Piergallina, M., El Asmar, Z., Marchetti, M. & Muzzonigro, G. (2010). The role of uroflowmetry biofeedback and biofeedback training of the pelvic floor muscles in the treatment of recurrent urinary tract infections in women with dysfunctional voiding: a randomized controlled prospective study. *Urology*, Vol. 75, No.6, (June 2010), pp. 1299-1304, I SSN 1527-9995 (Electronic) 0090-4295 (Linking)

Minardi, D., Parri, G., d'Anzeo, G., Fabiani, A., El Asmar, Z. & Muzzonigro, G. (2008). Perineal ultrasound evaluation of dysfunctional voiding in women with recurrent urinary tract infections. *J Urol*, Vol. 179, No.3, (March 2008), pp. 947-951, I SSN 1527-3792 (Electronic) 0022-5347 (Linking)

Minardi, D., Piloni, V., Amadi, A., El Asmar, Z., Milanese, G. & Muzzonigro, G. (2007). Correlation between urodynamics and perineal ultrasound in female patients with urinary incontinence. *Neurourol Urodyn*, Vol. 26, No.2, (2007), pp. 176-182; discussion 183-174, I SSN 0733-2467 (Print) 0733-2467 (Linking)

Nelson, J. D., Cooper, C. S., Boyt, M. A., Hawtrey, C. E. & Austin, J. C. (2004). Improved uroflow parameters and post-void residual following biofeedback therapy in pediatric patients with dysfunctional voiding does not correspond to outcome. *The Journal of urology*, Vol. 172, No.4 Pt 2, (October 2004), pp. 1653-1656; discussion 1656, I SSN 0022-5347 (Print) 0022-5347 (Linking)

Norgaard, J. P., van Gool, J. D., Hjalmas, K., Djurhuus, J. C. & Hellstrom, A. L. (1998). Standardization and definitions in lower urinary tract dysfunction in children. International Children's Continence Society. *Br J Urol*, Vol. 81 Suppl 3, (May 1998), pp. 1-16, I SSN 0007-1331 (Print) 0007-1331 (Linking)

Oliveira, F. R., Ramos, J. G. & Martins-Costa, S. (2006). Translabial ultrasonography in the assessment of urethral diameter and intrinsic urethral sphincter deficiency. *J Ultrasound Med*, Vol. 25, No.9, (September 2006), pp. 1153-1158; quiz 1159-1160, I SSN 0278-4297 (Print) 0278-4297 (Linking)

Quinn, M. J., Beynon, J., Mortensen, N. J. & Smith, P. J. (1988). Transvaginal endosonography: a new method to study the anatomy of the lower urinary tract in urinary stress incontinence. *Br J Urol*, Vol. 62, No.5, (November 1988), pp. 414-418, I SSN 0007-1331 (Print) 0007-1331 (Linking)

Robinson, D., Toozs-Hobson, P., Cardozo, L. & Digesu, A. (2004). Correlating structure and function: three-dimensional ultrasound of the urethral sphincter. *Ultrasound Obstet Gynecol*, Vol. 23, No.3, (March 2004), pp. 272-276, I SSN 0960-7692 (Print) 0960-7692 (Linking)

Sarnelli, G., Trovato, C., Imarisio, M., Talleri, D. & Braconi, A. (2003). Ultrasound assessment of the female perineum: technique, methods, indications and ultrasound anatomy. *Radiol Med*, Vol. 106, No.4, (October 2003), pp. 357-369, I SSN 0033-8362 (Print) 0033-8362 (Linking)

Schaer, G. N., Koechli, O. R., Schuessler, B. & Haller, U. (1995). Perineal ultrasound for evaluating the bladder neck in urinary stress incontinence. *Obstet Gynecol*, Vol. 85, No.2, (February 1995), pp. 220-224, I SSN 0029-7844 (Print) 0029-7844 (Linking)

Schafer, W., Abrams, P., Liao, L., Mattiasson, A., Pesce, F., Spangberg, A., Sterling, A. M., Zinner, N. R. & van Kerrebroeck, P. (2002). Good urodynamic practices: uroflowmetry, filling cystometry, and pressure-flow studies. *Neurourol Urodyn*, Vol. 21, No.3, 2002), pp. 261-274, I SSN 0733-2467 (Print) 0733-2467 (Linking)

Sendag, F., Vidinli, H., Kazandi, M., Itil, I. M., Askar, N., Vidinli, B. & Pourbagher, A. (2003). Role of perineal sonography in the evaluation of patients with stress urinary incontinence. *Aust N Z J Obstet Gynaecol*, Vol. 43, No.1, (February 2003), pp. 54-57, I SSN 0004-8666 (Print) 0004-8666 (Linking)

Toozs-Hobson, P., Khullar, V. & Cardozo, L. (2001). Three-dimensional ultrasound: a novel technique for investigating the urethral sphincter in the third trimester of pregnancy. *Ultrasound Obstet Gynecol*, Vol. 17, No.5, (May 2001), pp. 421-424, I SSN 0960-7692 (Print) 0960-7692 (Linking)

Tuygun, C., Sertcelik, N., Bakirtas, H., Cakici, H., Cetin, K. & Imamoglu, A. M. (2007). Usefulness of a new dysfunctional voiding and incontinence scoring system in predicting treatment effect in children with voiding dysfunction. *Urol Int*, Vol. 79, No.1, (2007), pp. 76-82, I SSN 0042-1138 (Print) 0042-1138 (Linking)

Vereecken, R. L. & Proesmans, W. (2000). Urethral instability as an important element of dysfunctional voiding. *J Urol*, Vol. 163, No.2, (February 2000), pp. 585-588, I SSN 0022-5347 (Print) 0022-5347 (Linking)

Voorham-van der Zalm, P. J., Berzuk, K., Shelly, B., Kamin, B., Putter, H., Lycklama, A. N. G. A., Pelger, R. C. & Stiggelbout, A. M. (2011). Validation of the pelvic floor inventories Leiden (PelFIs) in English. *Neurourol Urodyn*, Vol. 30, No.4, (April 2011), pp. 536-540, I SSN 1520-6777 (Electronic) 0733-2467 (Linking)

Voorham-van der Zalm, P. J., Stiggelbout, A. M., Aardoom, I., Deckers, S., Greve, I. G., Nijeholt, G. A. & Pelger, R. C. (2008). Development and validation of the pelvic floor inventories Leiden (PelFIs). *Neurourol Urodyn*, Vol. 27, No.4, (2008), pp. 301-305, I SSN 0733-2467 (Print) 0733-2467 (Linking)

Wiseman, O. J., Swinn, M. J., Brady, C. M. & Fowler, C. J. (2002). Maximum urethral closure pressure and sphincter volume in women with urinary retention. *J Urol*, Vol. 167, No.3, (March 2002), pp. 1348-1351; discussion 1351-1342, I SSN 0022-5347 (Print) 0022-5347 (Linking)

Yagci, S., Kibar, Y., Akay, O., Kilic, S., Erdemir, F., Gok, F. & Dayanc, M. (2005). The effect of biofeedback treatment on voiding and urodynamic parameters in children with voiding dysfunction. *J Urol*, Vol. 174, No.5, (November 2005), pp. 1994-1997; discussion 1997-1998, I SSN 0022-5347 (Print) 0022-5347 (Linking)

Yang, J. M. & Huang, W. C. (2003). Bladder wall thickness on ultrasonographic cystourethrography: affecting factors and their implications. *J Ultrasound Med*, Vol. 22, No.8, (August 2003), pp. 777-782, I SSN 0278-4297 (Print) 0278-4297 (Linking)

4

# Prostatitis: From Diagnosis to Treatment

Stylianos Kontos[1], Vasilis Migdalis[2],
Stefanos Kachrilas[1] and Athanasios G. Papatsoris[2]
[1]*Department of Urology, Nikaia General Hospital,*
[2]*2nd Department of Urology, School of Medicine, University of Athens, Sismanoglio Hospital, Athens;*
*Greece*

## 1. Introduction

Urinary tract infections (UTIs) are a significant source of morbidity and mortality, despite the widespread use of antibiotics. Prostatitis is a prevalent and debilitating disease, representing the most common urological diagnosis in men under the age of 50 years. Despite its prevalence and its drain on health care resources, our understanding of the etiology, diagnosis and treatment of prostatitis has not advanced to a widely accepted level.

Recently, a consensus has been reached on the definition and classification of prostatitis. Traditionally, prostatitis has been classified into the four clinical entities: i) Acute bacterial prostatitis (ABP), ii) Chronic bacterial prostatitis (CBP) iii) Non or abacterial prostatitis (NBP), iv) Prostatodynia. To improve the definition and understanding of prostatitis a new classification system has been proposed by the National Institute of Health (NIH). It includes: i) ABP, ii) CBP, represents the traditional forms of acute and chronic bacterial prostatitis, defined by the presence of both prostatic inflammation and uro-pathogenic bacteria in prostatic culture, iii) Chronic pelvic pain syndrome (CPPS) with the inflammatory and non-inflammatory type, which is characterized by prostatitis like symptoms in the absence of bacterial localization to the prostate iv) asymptomatic inflammatory prostatitis, which is characterized by pathogenic evidence of prostatic inflammation in patients without symptoms (includes patients who have prostatic inflammation diagnosed after prostatic biopsy) (Magri et al., 2010).

Risk factors that allow bacterial colonization and/or infection of the prostate with potentially pathogenic bacteria include intraprostatic ductal reflux; phimosis; specific blood groups; unprotected anal intercourse; UTI; acute epididymitis; indwelling urethral or condom catheters; and transurethral operations (especially in men who have infected urine) (Westesson & Shoskes, 2010).

In a study, nearly 9.7% of male respondents (aged 20 to 74 years) reported pain or discomfort in the perineum or with ejaculation or both, plus a total pain score (possible 0 to 21) of 4 or greater (Vaidyanathan & Mishra, 2008). This location and level of pain would be sufficient to lead most physicians to make a diagnosis of chronic prostatitis (CP). In this age group, 6.6% of men reported similar symptoms over the previous week with a pain score of 8 or greater, which would place them in the moderate or severe category (Vaidyanathan & Mishra, 2008).

The modern era of prostatitis management began in the 1960s with Meares and Stamey's description of the four-glass lower urinary tract segmented localization study. With this insight, prostatic massage as the mainstay of prostatitis therapy was abandoned, and antimicrobial therapy was rationalized for the percentage of patients with bacteria. Unfortunately, the vast majority of patients who were diagnosed with a nonbacterial cause continued to suffer the indignities of dismal urologic management (Wagenlehner & Naber, 2009).

## 2. Acute bacterial prostatitis (ABP)

### 2.1 Etiology & pathogenesis

ABP is a generalized infection of the prostate gland and is associated with both lower UTI and generalized sepsis. The most common cause of bacterial prostatitis is the Enterobacteriaceae family of gram-negative bacteria, which originate from the gastrointestinal flora. Aerobic gram-negative organisms principally cause ABP. The incidence of infection by various species and their antibiotic susceptibilities follow those of organisms that regularly infect the urine (Bruyere, 2010).

*E. coli* is implicated in 80% of infections. *Pseudomonada aeroginosa, Serratia, Klebsiella* and *Proteas* species account for 10-15% of the cases and enterococci for 10-15%. Bacteria reside deep in the ducts of the prostate gland and tend to form aggregates (also called bio-films); this appears to be a protective mechanism that allows bacteria to persist in the prostate gland even when the concomitant cystitis is treated with antibiotics (Bruyere, 2010).

The gram-positive bacteria become pathogenic only under special circumstances. Anaerobes infections are usually polymicrobial. Most infections occur in the peripheral zone, where the ducts drain horizontally into the urethra, facilitating reflux of urine as well as intraductal stasis. Glands of the central zone empty obliquely and completely into the prostatic urethra, preventing easy reflux and stagnation. Invasion by rectal bacteria, either directly or via lymphogenous spread, has also been suggested to cause prostatitis (Maglakelidze, 2009).

Investigators have demonstrated that urine and its metabolites (i.e. urate) are present in the prostatic secretion of patients with CP. Prostatic inflammation and subsequent symptoms may be simply due to a chemically induced inflammation secondary to the noxious substances in the urine that have refluxed into the prostatic duct (Bruyere, 2010).

### 2.2 Clinical features

ABP is marked by fever and chills; rectal, low back, and perineal pain; urinary urgency, frequency and dysouria. Prostatic swelling may result in acute urinary retention. Malaise, arthralgia, and myalgia are also common. Digital rectal examination reveals an exquisitely tender, enlarged gland that is irregularly firm and warm. The urine may be cloudy and malodorous because of concomitant UTI. Gross hematuria may be observed occasionally.

Physical examination is an important part of the evaluation of a patient with prostatitis, but it is usually not helpful in making a definitive diagnosis or further classifying prostatitis. It assists in ruling out other perineal, anal, neurologic, pelvic, or prostate pathologies and is an integral part of the lower urinary tract evaluation.

In ABP, the patient may be systemically toxic: flushed, febrile, tachycardic, tachypnoic, and even hypotensive. The patient usually has suprapubic discomfort due to a degree of urinary retention. Perineal pain and anal sphincter spasm may complicate the digital rectal examination. The prostate itself is usually described as warm, buggy, and exquisitely tender. In cases of ABP, prostatic massage is believed to be unnecessary and even harmful (Erlikh et al., 2009).

### 2.3 Diagnosis

ABP is often diagnosed on the basis of symptoms and physical examination. A complete blood count typically shows leukocytosis with a shift toward immature forms. Transurethral catheterization as well as prostatic massage should be avoided. Acute urinary retention requiring bladder drainage should be managed with a suprapubic tube. The voided urine usually shows pyuria and microscopic hematuria due to a UTI (Bruyere, 2010).

### 2.4 Management

Empiric treatment should not be delayed, and should be directed primarily against gram-negative rods and enterococci. Patients will often respond dramatically to agents that would otherwise diffuse poorly into prostatic tissue. The choice of antibiotic is ultimately guided by in vitro susceptibility tests. The flouroquinolones work very well as initial therapy, as does TMP-SMX. The recommended duration of antibiotic treatment is 4-6 weeks in order to prevent the development of complications such as prostatic abscess and chronic prostatitis. Supportive measures include antipyretics, analgesics, stool softeners, hydration and bed rest. Patients with significant co morbidities, sepsis, immunodeficiency and acute urinary retention need hospital admission. Any transurethral catheterization or instrumentation is contraindicated during the phase of acute infection. Acute urinary retention should be managed with suprapubic drainage until the patient is able to void spontaneously (Weidner et al., 2008).

### 2.5 Complications

Some patients may progress to chronic bacterial prostatitis, especially if attention is not focused on bacterial eradication. Prostatic abscess can develop in the setting of acute prostatitis. Immunocompromised patients, diabetics, those with indwelling urethral catheters, or those on chronic dialysis are at higher risk for this complication (Weidner et al., 2008).

## 3. Chronic bacterial prostatitis (CBP)

### 3.1 Etiology & pathogenesis

Chronic bacterial prostatitis is associated with recurrent lower UTIs secondary to focal uropathogenic bacteria residing in the prostate gland. Gram-negative bacteria and enterococci are usually the causative microorganisms in CBP. Mycoplasms, ureoplasms and chlamydial species are appreciable pathogens in BCP and most of them are also implicated in the chronic pelvic pain syndromes. Intraprostatic reflux, ductal anatomy, secretory dysfanction and alkaline prostatic secretions contribute to CBP.

Reflux of urine and possibly bacteria into the prostatic ducts has been postulated as one of the most important etiologic mechanisms involved in the pathogenesis of chronic bacterial and nonbacterial prostatic inflammation. Anatomically, the ductal drainage of the peripheral zone is more susceptible than other prostatic zones to intraprostatic ductal reflux (Wagenlehner et al., 2008). Investigators have measured high levels of urate and creatinine in EPS, which they postulated was caused by urine reflux into the prostatic ducts (Touma & Nickel, 2010). Furthermore, carbon particles have been found in the EPS macrophages and prostatic acini and ductal system after surgery in men with nonbacterial prostatitis.

Bacterial microcolonies may adhere to ductal and acinar walls and become impervious to antibiotics. Prostatic calculi also provide sanctuary for pathogens. A large proportion of men

with CBP have multiple prostatic calculi demonstraded on transrectal ultrasound. Prostatic calculi can serve as a source for bacterial persistence and recurent UTIs.
It is believed that the source of the pain is located at the pelvic area of the sacrum, coccyx, ischial tuberosity, pubic rami, and endopelvic fascia (Saini et al., 2008). These areas are immediately adjacent to the prostate and bladder and can be recognized by the demonstration of a hyperirritable spot (myofascial trigger point) that is painful on compression. It is hypothesized that the formation of myofascial trigger points in this area may be correlated with mechanical abnormalities in the hip and lower extremities, toilet straining, sexual abuse, repetitive trauma, constipation, heavy sports, trauma or unusual sexual activity, recurrent infections, and surgery (Sandhu, 2008).

### 3.2 Clinical features

The physical examination of a patient with category II CBP and category III CPPS is usually unremarkable. Careful examination and palpation of external genitalia, groin, perineum, coccyx, external anal sphincter, and internal pelvic side walls may pinpoint prominent areas of pain or discomfort (Magri et al., 2010). The digital rectal examination should be performed after the patient has produced pre- prostatic massage urine specimens. The prostate may be normal in size and consistency, and it has also been described as enlarged and boggy. The degree of elicited pain during prostatic palpation is variable and is unhelpful in differentiating a prostatitis syndrome. The prostate should be carefully checked for prostatic nodules before a vigorous prostatic massage is performed (Westesson and Shoskes, 2010).
Most patients report dysuria as well as urgency, frequency, and nocturia. Low back and perineal pain or discomfort may be present. The natural history is marked by disease relapse with occasional acute exacerbations, at which time fever, chills and malaise might manifest. Sometimes, the diagnosis is made in an asymptomatic patient in whom bacteriuria is found incidentally. There are no characteristic findings on digital rectal examination. The prostate frequently feels normal although tenderness, swelling, and firmness may be present. Secondary epididymitis is sometimes present. Hematuria, hematospermia and urethral discharge are usually rare (Jonsson & Hedelin, 2008).

### 3.3 Diagnosis

The 4-glass test is the standard in prostatitis diagnosis. This technique allows localization of bacteria by examining specimens from the urethra, midstream urine, and prostatic secretions. The examiner obtains the first voided 10 mL of urine (urethral specimen), a late midstream sample (bladder specimen), a specimen of prostatic secretions following prostatic massage, and the first voided 10 mL of urine following the massage. The specimens are labeled VB1, VB2, EPS, and VB3, respectively, and they are sent for bacterial identification and quantification using standard microbiologic methods. Two or more bacterial localization tests may then be required to identify the pathogenic bacteria. If no organisms can be cultured, and the prostatic fluid has increased leukocyte count (> 10 per HPF), a diagnosis of chronic pelvic pain syndrome (inflammatory type) can be made (Westesson & Shoskes, 2010). Despite sterilization in the urine, the pathogen often remains sheltered in the prostate because most antibiotics diffuse poorly into prostatic fluid. The prostate-specific antigen may be elevated.

### 3.4 Management

At least 3-4 months of treatment is generally recommended, although some studies have reported success with a 4-week course of a fluoroquinolone. Factors that promote antibiotic diffusion into the prostate include lipid solubility, weak binding to plasma proteins, and an uncharged state. Suppressive antibiotic therapy aimed at eliminating bacterial growth in the urine is often instituted. Most antibiotics are concentrated in the urine, allowing for reduced dosing while maintaining bactericidal efficacy. The most common daily suppressive regimens are nitrofurantoin (100 mg daily), TMP-SMX (200 mg daily), and ciprofloxacin (250 mg daily). Suppressive therapy can provide relief from symptoms for most men. Transurethral prostatectomy (TURP) has been described as an alternative treatment. Surgical therapy often provides the only chance at cure in relapsing cases. Studies of patients undergoing TURP for chronic bacterial prostatitis followed by 6-8 weeks of antibiotic therapy report varying success rates (30%-100%).

### 3.5 Complications

Recurrent UTIs are a major complication of CBP that may even result to infertility. Reports of successful treatment of prostatitis leading to improvement in semen parameters and pregnancy rates have been made. Although more difficult to quantify, CBP has a negative impact on the patient's quality of life.

## 4. Chronic pelvic pain syndrome (CPPS)

### 4.1 Etiology & pathogenesis

CPPS is the most common form of prostatitis and the most poorly understood. CPPS categories are divided into inflammatory (category IIIA) and noninflammatory (category IIIB) forms, based on the presence of leukocytes in the prostatic fluid. The inflammatory type was previously called "nonbacterial prostatitis" (associated with elevated prostatic immunoglobulin level); while the non-inflammatory type was called "prostatodynia" (not associated with increased immunoglobulins). Several studies have demonstrated chlamydial antigens in the prostatic fluid and anti-chlamydial antibodies in the serum of men with CPPS. In a study, transperineal prostate biopsy of men with CPPS failed to detect chlamydia by either immunofluorescence or culture (Wagenlehner et al., 2008). There seems to be an association between backflow of urine into the prostatic ducts and a subsequent chemically induced inflammatory prostatitis. Backflow of urine could lead to high concentrations of urinary urate and creatinine in the prostate fluid, resulting in a chemical prostatitis. Investigators have demonstrated a positive correlation between leukocyte count and urate concentration in the prostate fluid (Touma & Nickel, 2010).

Anatomic or neurophysiologic obstruction resulting in high-pressure dysfunctional flow patterns has been implicated in the pathogenesis of prostatitis. Urodynamic studies confirm that many patients, particularly those with prostatodynia, have obstructive flow rate patterns (e.g. decreased maximal flow rate). During video-urodynamic studies, many patients with prostatitis show incomplete funneling of the bladder neck as well as vesicourethral dysynergic patterns. Dysynergic voiding may lead to autonomic overstimulation of the perineal-pelvic neural system with subsequent development of a chronic neuropathic pain state. Alternatively, dysfunctional voiding may result in intraprostatic ductal reflux (Hedelin & Fall, 2008). Investigators have found an increased maximal urethral closure pressure and a decreased urinary flow rate in patients with CPPS compared with control patients (Strauss & Dimitrakov, 2010). They attributed the high maximal urethral closure pressure to increased adrenergic stimulation in the proximal urethra and bladder neck and proposed that this might cause intraprostatic reflux of urine. Based on these observations they suggested the use of the term "painful male urethral syndrome". Furthermore, spasm of the pelvic floor muscles alone or in combination with bladder neck dysfunction may contribute to chronic pelvic pain (Strauss & Dimitrakov, 2010).

### 4.2 Clinical features

Voiding dysfunction consisting of dysuria, slow stream, urgency, and frequency. Sexual dysfunction may also be reported. On digital rectal examination the prostate may be tender. During palpation patients may have tenderness of the pelvic floor muscles and a tight anal sphincter (Dellabella et al., 2009).

### 4.3 Diagnosis

The EPS in patients with inflammatory CPPS shows numerous leukocytes and lipid-laden macrophages. A 5-fold increase in leykocytes and an 8-fold increase in lipid-laden macrophages may be revealed in such patients in comparison control subjects. Urodynamic studies may disclose urethral hypertonia and diminished flow in the absence of striated sphincter dyssynergia (Vaidyanathan & Mishra, 2008).

### 4.4 Management

Patients may experience symptomatic improvement with antibiotics. This has prompted the recommendation of a trial of antibiotic therapy. If chlamydia is suspected, then tetracycline, minocycline, doxycycline or erythromycin should be administered. Antibiotic therapy should continue for several weeks. Alpha blockers may improve urination and symptoms. By decreasing adrenergic tone in the proximal urethra, alpha blockers alleviate urethral hypertonia and may prevent intraprostatic reflux of urine. Intraprostatic ductal reflux of urine increases the concentration of metabolites containing purine and pyrimidine bases in the prostatic ducts, resulting in inflammation (Sandhu, 2008).

High concentrations of urate in urine can be reduced with the use of allopurinol, a xanthine oxidase inhibitor. This may alleviate chemical irritation in the prostate caused by refluxed urine. Studies have demonstrated a significant effect of allopurinol on urate concentration in the prostatic fluid resulting in symptoms improvement (Maglakelidze 2009). Pelvic floor relaxation techniques, biofeedback, prostate massage, and muscle relaxants may reduce pelvic floor spasticity and chronic pelvic pain (Maglakelidze, 2009). Interestingly, a pollen extract (Cernilton) was recently assessed in a multicentre, prospective, randomised, double-blind, placebo-controlled phase 3 study (Wagenlehner, 2009). Participants were randomised to receive oral capsules of the pollen extract or placebo for 12 weeks. Compared to placebo, the pollen extract significantly improved total symptoms, pain, and QoL in patients with inflammatory CP/CPPS without severe side-effects.

Prostatic inflammation is associated with category III CPPS, while elevated cytokine levels are noted in the semen and EPS of patients with inflammatory CPPS. Non-steroidal anti-inflammatory drugs, steroids, and immunosuppressive medication theoretically may improve the symptoms. Surgical therapy with transrurethral microwave thermotherapy or neodynium:YAG laser has also been suggested (Hedelin & Fall, 2008).

### 4.5 Complications

CPPS may have a negative effect in fertility. Lower sperm counts and abnormal morphologic and motility parameters have been described in affected patients. These parameters may worsen with time. As with chronic bacterial prostatitis, the quality of life is adversely affected (Jonsson & Hedelin, 2008).

## 5. Epilogue

ABP can be efficiently treated with antibiotics that will eventually eradicate the bacteria. CBP treatment is based on long term antibiotic regimens. CP/CPPS management needs multimodal medication with antibiotics, alpha blockers, anti-inflammatory drugs and hormonal agents (Westesson & Shoskes, 2010).

Chronic nonbacterial prostatitis and prostatodynia (category III CPPS) constitute the vast majority of prostatitis cases and are difficult to manage. Performing a lower urinary tract evaluation (at least a two-glass premassage and postmassage screen) to rule out uro-pathogens, microscopy of postprostatic massage urine sediment (to differentiate inflammatory from non-inflammatory CPPS), and employment of the newly validated NIH-CPSI will allow optimal management (Strauss & Dimitrakov, 2010). Available treatments include: i) antibiotics that cover potential pathogens (including Chlamydia and Ureaplasma, at least in category IIIA); ii) alpha blockers (especially in patients with obstructive voiding symptoms); iii) anti-inflammatory agents; iv) muscle relaxants; v) pento-san polysulfate (in patients with bladder or interstitial cystitis-like symptoms); and vi) physical therapy (i.e. prostate, perineal, or pelvic floor massage, myofascial trigger point release, and biofeedback). For refractory symptoms, other treatment modalities include microwave hyperthermia or thermotherapy and TURP (Magri et al., 2010).

Asymptomatic inflammatory prostatitis (category IV) does not require symptomatic therapy. However, antibiotic medication may be indicated in patients who are scheduled to undergo endoscopic procedures, and in patients with concomitant inflammation and infertility (Murphy et al., 2009).

## 6. References


Bruyere, F. (2010)"Acute bacterial prostatitis in adult men." Prog Urol 20(11): 815-7.

Dellabella, M., Milanese, G., Sigala, S., d'Anzeo, G., Arrighi, N., Bodei, S., Muzzonigro, G. (2009). "The role of the prostatic stroma in chronic prostatitis/chronic pelvic pain syndrome." Inflamm Res 58(12): 829-36.

Erlikh, N., Miullerad, M., Khazanov, V. (2009). "Prostatic inflammation and chronic pelvic pain: diagnosis and treatment." Urologiia (1): 81-4.

Hedelin, H., Fall, M. (2008). "Controversies in chronic abacterial prostatitis/pelvic pain syndrome." Scand J Urol Nephrol 42(3): 198-204.

Jonsson, K., Hedelin, H. (2008). "Chronic abacterial prostatitis: Living with a troublesome disease affecting many aspects of life." Scand J Urol Nephrol 42(6): 545-50.

Maglakelidze, G. M. (2009). "The current approaches to chronic prostatitis problems." Georgian Med News(176): 21-6.

Magri, V., Perletti G., Bartoletti, R., Cai, T., Emelyanova, I., Mehik, A., Morgia, G., Skerk, V., Trinchieri, A., Wagenlehner, F.M., Naber, K.G. "Critical issues in chronic prostatitis. (2010)" Arch Ital Urol Androl 82(2): 75-82.

Mishra, V. C., Browne, J., Emberton, M. (2008). "Role of repeated prostatic massage in chronic prostatitis: a systematic review of the literature." Urology 72(4): 731-5.

Murphy, A. B., Macejko, A., Taylor, A., Nadler, R.B. (2009). "Chronic prostatitis: management strategies." Drugs 69(1): 71-84.

Saini, R., Gonzalez, R. R., Te, A.E. (2008). "Chronic pelvic pain syndrome and the overactive bladder: the inflammatory link." Curr Urol Rep 9(4): 314-9.

Sandhu, J. S. (2008). "Prostate cancer and chronic prostatitis." Curr Urol Rep 9(4): 328-32.

Strauss, A. C., Dimitrakov, J. D. (2010) "New treatments for chronic prostatitis/chronic pelvic pain syndrome." Nat Rev Urol 7(3): 127-35.

Touma, N. J., Nickel, J. C. (2010) "Prostatitis and chronic pelvic pain syndrome in men." Med Clin North Am 95(1): 75-86.

Vaidyanathan, R., Mishra, V. C. (2008). "Chronic prostatitis: Current concepts." Indian J Urol 24(1): 22-7.

Wagenlehner, F. M., Diemer, T., Naber, K. G., Weidner, W. (2008). "Chronic bacterial prostatitis (NIH type II): diagnosis, therapy and influence on the fertility status." Andrologia 40(2): 100-4.

Wagenlehner, F. M., Naber, K. G., Bschleipfer, T, Brähler, E, Weidner, W. (2009). "Prostatitis and male pelvic pain syndrome: diagnosis and treatment." Dtsch Arztebl Int 106(11): 175-83.

Wagenlehner, F.M., Schneider, H., Ludwig, M., Schnitker, J., Brähler, E., Weidner, W. (2009). "A pollen extract (Cernilton) in patients with inflammatory chronic prostatitis-chronic pelvic pain syndrome: a multicentre, randomised, prospective, double-blind, placebo-controlled phase 3 study." Eur Urol 56(3):544-51.

Weidner, W., Anderson, R. U. (2008). "Evaluation of acute and chronic bacterial prostatitis and diagnostic management of chronic prostatitis/chronic pelvic pain syndrome with special reference to infection/inflammation." Int J Antimicrob Agents 31 (Suppl 1): 91-5.

Weidner, W., Wagenlehner, F. M., Marconi, M., Pilatz, A., Pantke, K.H., Diemer, T. (2008). "Acute bacterial prostatitis and chronic prostatitis/chronic pelvic pain syndrome: andrological implications." Andrologia 40(2): 105-12.

Westesson, K. E., Shoskes, D. A. (2010)"Chronic prostatitis/chronic pelvic pain syndrome and pelvic floor spasm: can we diagnose and treat? " Curr Urol Rep 11(4): 261-4.

Wittschieber, D., Schenkenberg, S., Dietel, M., Erbersdobler, A. (2010)"The significance of chronic prostatitis for the etiopathology of prostate cancer." Urologe A 49(8): 947-51.

# 5

# Complicated Upper Urinary Tract Infection

Nasser Shakhssalim[1], Mohammad Samzadeh[2]
and Seyed Mohammad Ghahestani[3]
*[1]Assistant Professor of Urology, Urology and Nephrology Research Center (UNRC), Shahid Labbafinejad Medical Center, Shahid Beheshti University of Medical Sciences (SBUMS), Tehran,*
*[2]Resident of Urology, UNRC, Shahid Labbafinejad Medical Center,SBUMS, Tehran,*
*[3]Fellowship of Pediatric Urology*
*Tehran university of medical sciences(TUMS), Children Medical Center Hospital*
*I.R. Iran*

## 1. Introduction

A renal abscess is an accumulation of pus inside renal parenchyma. The presence of pus can be substantiated by means of imaging or percutaneous aspiration. When we say pus, we usually mean liquefaction while there is also another entity we can call a gaseous abscess resembling emphysematous pyelonephritis in imaging, but following a more benign course such as a localized renal abscess [1].

### 1.1 Pathophysiology

A host of organisms may cause a renal abscess. There seems to be a chronological shift of organisms from staphylococci to Gram negatives since 25 years ago with prevailing use of antibiotics.[2] Currently, the most common organisms are *E. coli, Klebsiella pneumoniae, Pseudomona aeruginosa* and *Staphylococcus aureus* [3]. Other unusual organisms are likely and clinical background should raise the suspicion e.g. *Salmonella parathyphi A* [4], *Salmonella typhimurium* [5], *Nocardia* [6], *Morganella morganii* [7], *Streptococcus group B* [8], *Serratia marcescens* [9]. In immunocompromised and AIDS patients, other opportunistic organisms like *Aspergillus fumigatus* [10] and *Mycobacterium avium complex* [11] may also be involved. Special clinical scenarios must raise suspicion toward specific organisms. Endophthalmitis accompanied by renal abscess has been reported with *Klebsiella pneumonia* and *Serratia marcescens* [9, 12]. In one case, *Salmonella virchow* phage type 1 renal abscess was reported in association with pelvis transitional cell carcinoma [13]. Renal abscess may also happen as a consequence of infective endocarditis metastasis [14].
Predisposing factors are diabetes mellitus, urolithiasis, immunosuppression [15] and vesicoureteral reflux [16-19]. Nevertheless, it may happen in previously healthy people [20, 21].

### 1.2 Clinical presentation

Although fever, nausea and vomiting, abdominal and flank pain are cited as usual clinical features [3], yet in some instances the symptoms may be insidious and nonspecific [19, 22]. Disguised clinical presentations must not be ignored since renal abscess with infectious

metastases to the lung has been mistaken with Wilm's tumor [22]. Acute peritonitis as first manifestation of a renal abscess has also been reported.[23]Endophthalmitis associated with renal abscess and *klebsiella pneumonia*[12, 23, 24] and *Serratia marcescens* [9] was mentioned. Renal abscess has also been reported in accompaniment with transitional cell carcinoma [25] and renal cell carcinoma [13, 25, 26] in the same kidney so a nonresolving mass must be approached with suspicion.
It looks that renal abscess has a high potential for infectious metastasis reasonably justified by high vascularity of the kidney; hence, a whole body physical exam must never be underrated.

### 1.3 Paraclinic findings

In a series of pediatric patients, urine culture was positive in 60% and blood culture was positive in only 2%.[3]. In another series, less than half of the patients had either an abnormal urinalysis or urine culture [17]. Thus, there is a high likelihood of negative urine and blood cultures. Leukocytosis is common [17]and elevated blood urea and creatinine have been linked with poorer prognosis [15].
Sonography is undoubtedly a very useful and accessible tool for detecting renal pathologies, but there are still some doubts on its reliability as the sole diagnostic tool for detecting and confirming a renal abscess. It seems wise to use sonography as a screening tool and then proceed to CT scan if any mass or nephromegaly is seen. The inclusion of nephromegaly as a criterion to perform a computerized tomography seems to increase the sensitivity of sonography [3]. Actually, we may see a hypoechoic or anechoic mass or nephromegaly. There may also be debris inside the mass moving in the position changes [27]. CT must also be performed in those patients with normal sonogram, but discordant clinical behavior (lack of response to antibiotics, infectious metastases, papillary necrosis, etc), or if there remains any doubt in diagnosis based on sonography.
CT is the most accurate modality for detecting a renal abscess [27]. An abscess usually appears as a well-defined low-density mass. An irregular and thick wall or pseudocapsule is better imaged after contrast enhancement [28, 29]. A separately defined entity called gaseous abscess can also be effectively diagnosed by CT. On CT, gas-forming renal abscesses appear as discrete gas pockets without purulent material within the renal parenchyma. The interesting point is that in this entity, despite emphysematous pyelonephritis gas persisted to exist in images several months after treatment [1]. In CT, gas has a HU number$\leq$ -150 but liquid $\pm$10 HU [27]. Although, Inidium 111 and Gallium isotope scans may have a role in diagnosis, but false negative results have been reported [30]. These scans may be particularly useful when the location of infectious intra abdominal process is still unknown.
In children with a history of febrile urinary infection, performing a MCUG must not be neglected. Not only this helps to detect vesicoureteral reflux, but also reveals many unsuspected bladder outlet and urethral pathologies. A DMSA scan 6 to 12 months later can show the extent of damage to renal parenchyma [3].

### 1.4 Management

The treatment of renal abscess has changed from open intervention to percutaneous drainage and intravenous antibiotic therapy. In a retrospective but critical analytic study, abscesses less than 3cm in diameter responded well to antibiotic therapy, those between 3 and 5 cm responded 92% to single percutaneous treatment (using either sonography or CT guidance), and in abscesses above 5cm responded to multiple drainages (alternatively a temporary indwelling pigtail) and antibiotic treatment.[31]. Percutaneous treatment seems as effective as open surgical drainage [31, 32]. The presence of immunocompromised state must push us one step forward to a more aggressive approach. The choice of antibiotic in cases of percutaneous drainage can best be based on aspirate culture results. In non-drained cases, positive urine culture can guide the treatment that an empirical regimen covering both Gram-negative enteric bacteria and staphylococci can be used otherwise. In small abscesses which do not respond to antibiotics in a timely manner, a percutaneous drainage can be both curative and diagnostic.

Three to six weeks of parenteral and oral antibiotic may be necessary [3], but the duration of antibiotic treatment and time of switching to oral treatment must be based on clinical response and sonographic follow up. As previously cited, concomitance with renal malignancies have been reported thus lack of adequate response to treatment must raise a suspicion.

## 2. Perinephric abscess

### 2.1 Introduction

Perinephric abscess refers to accumulation of pus inside Gerota's fascia. There may also be gas bubbles especially in diabetics due to glucose fermentation [33] and this should not be mistaken with separate entity of emphysematous pyelonephritis.

The incidence ranges from 1 to 10 cases for every 10,000 hospital admissions. Men and women are affected with equal frequency. [33] In a population based cohort retrospective study in an eleven-year follow-up period [34] the incidence rates for the diabetics and the control subjects were 4.6 and 1.1/10000 person-years, respectively, representing an adjusted hazard ratio of 3.81 (95% confidence interval 3·44-4·23). Therefore, diabetes mellitus in an immunocompromised setting stands as a major predisposing factor.

### 2.2 Pathophysiology

Most of perinephric abscesses are caused by ascending enteric Gram-negative bacteria.[35]. In a study of 26 cases, 67% of cultures yielded enteric Gram-negative bacteria[36], however, metastatic staphylococcal infections still happen [33].This entity may also follow the chronological shift of causative organism of renal abscess. A host of other unusual bacteria have also been reported. Among those, *Shigella flexneri* [37], *Stenotrophomonas maltophilia* [38], *Nocardia* [39] group B *streptococcus* [40], *Candida glabrata* [41], *Aspergillus fumigates* [42], *Listeria monocytogenes* [43], coagulase-negative *Staphylococcus* [44], *Salmonella* [45], *Torulopsis glabrata* [46, 47], *Bacteroides fragilis* [48] and *Trichomonas vaginalis* [49] have been reported to cause perinephric abscess in non-transplant patients. *Mycoplasma hominis* [50], *Streptococcus agalactiae* [51], Nocardia[52], and Gardnerella vaginalis[53] have been reported to cause perinephric abscess in patients with kidney graft. In a review of kidney transplant patients with perinephric abscess, staphylococci with a prevalence of 36%, and aerobic Gram-negative rods with a prevalence of 32% were the most common pathogens. Also of note were the presence of anaerobes (28%) and candida albicans (4%) [54].

There are also predisposing conditions strongly related with development of perinephric abscess. In a study on 23 patients, the predisposing conditions were identified as follows: diabetes mellitus in 65.2% , history of nephrolithiasis in 43.47%, and the history of urological

surgery in 17.38% [55]. In some older series (1977) diabetes had a smaller role, and the main role was attributed to nephrolithiasis (76%)[36].
Some special conditions have been described in accompaniment or as a cause of perinephric abscess: urinary extravasation associated with renal colic [56], colon carcinoma [57],renal cell carcinoma [58], extracorporeal shockwave lithotripsy [59-61], splenic abscess [62, 63], and ruptured retrocecal appendicitis [64, 65]. One must not ignore these conditions in the management of a perinephric abscess.

### 2.3 Clinical presentation

It may either present as an insidious disease or an acute process. Ascending infections have been described to follow an insidious course, but metastatic staphylococcal abscesses may show a dramatic course [33]. Yeast abscesses have been described to follow a chronic course with nonspecific symptoms that the usual culprits are *Candida* and *Torulopsis* species [66]. A patient with perinephric abscess has been presented with just a chronic diarrhea and weight loss [67]. Therefore, in most cases a high level of suspicion is necessary to proceed to appropriate imaging modalities. Unusual presentations as acute peritonitis [68, 69], acute pancreatitis [70], and fulminant hepatic failure [71] have been described too. A subcutaneous abscess in the loin may root in a perinephric abscess [72]. Nephrobronchial fistula may happen in the context of an unknown perinephric abscess; hence, if a patient presents perirenal suppurative process with the chest x-ray findings consistent with pleural effusion or pulmonary infiltrates, perinephric abscess have to be considered in differential diagnosis along with malignancy [73].

### 2.4 Paraclinic findings

Aspirate cultures are undoubtedly the best guide for antibiotic treatment. Laboratory findings have also been correlated with prognosis and outcome.
In a retrospective study recruiting 23 patients, hemoglobin levels and white blood cells counts were associated with the loss of the renal unit, thrombocytopenia was linked with septic shock, and hyponatremia with mortality [55].
In this study, a hemoglobin concentration greater than 10.5 g/dl and a white blood cell count lower than 15 x 10(3) / microL were associated with nephrectomy, and a platelet count lower than 140 x 10(3) / microL with septic shock. General mortality was 8.69%, and 78.3% of patients required nephrectomy. Patients who died had fever, anemia, a white blood cell count greater than 16 x 10(3) / microL, platelet count lower than 130 x 10(3) / microL, and hyponatremia of 125 mEq/L or lower at hospital admittance, and all of them had septic shock that required nephrectomy.
Sonography alone may have a substantial risk of incorrect or missed diagnosis. In a study, perinephric abscesses which were not seen in ultrasonography were those associated with pyonephrosis, abscesses smaller than 6 cm and gas-forming abscesses [74]. Although sonography has an important role as a non-ionizing accessible tool of first investigation, it could be misleading in some cases. One should not hesitate performing a CT scan in cases of urinary tract infection with an unusual course or resistant to antibiotic treatment with normal sonography. In another study, sonography failed to show abscesses smaller than 2-3 Cm.
CT scan has also the advantage of detecting concomitant pathologies cited before. As nephrolithiasis has been cited as a major predisposer, the investigation must be completed both with and without contrast for optimal results. Gallium-67 scintigraphy appears to be useful in detecting perinephric abscess in patients with polycystic kidney disease undergoing chronic hemodialysis [75].

### 2.5 Management

Antibiotic treatment must be guided by urine, blood or aspirate culture. Before the culture results get ready, a regimen covering both Gram-negative enteric bacteria and staphylococci is usually adopted. However, the mainstay of treating a perinephric abscess is drainage [33]. A percutaneous approach is preferred in most cases unless in multilocular, very large abscesses with extremely viscous purulent material in which open drainage is necessary. Laparoscopic treatment has been reported [76], but evidently it has not been introduced as a standard method yet.

Controlling diabetes mellitus or any underlying condition is mandatory. A urinary obstruction must be dealt with by either a percutaneous stent, or double J stent, or open intervention. In blood dyscrasias recombinant human granulocyte colony-stimulating factor may be helpful [77]. Unusual causative or accompanying conditions cited before must be cautiously addressed. Hematuria is uncommon in cases of perinephric abscess. When hematuria is present in a patient with perinephric abscess further evaluation is necessary to rule out an associated malignant process [58].

## 3. Spectrum of infected hydronephrosis and pyonephrosis

### 3.1 Introduction

Infected hydronephrosis denotes bacterial infection in a hydronephrotic kidney. Pyonephrosis occurs when suppurative destruction of parenchyma has begun. By definition, both conditions occur in obstructed kidneys. The level of obstruction varies from a calyceal infundibulum (pyocalyx) to bladder outlet (pyocystitis/pyonephrosis).

### 3.2 Pathophysiology

The same organisms responsible for acute pyelonephritis may infect a hydronephrotic kidney and ultimately lead to pyonephrosis. *Staphylococcus aureus, Mycobacterium tuberculosis, Candida albicans* and *Anaerobes* are other putative organisms [78-80]. The etiology of obstruction may also vary and must be differentiated on the context of patient's age and medical history. One must consider that in many cases there may be a disparity between voided urine culture and pelvis urine culture aspirated by needle or nephrostomy; hence, the best antibiotic regimen must cover both organisms after the aspirate from pelvis is obtained [81].

### 3.3 Clinical presentation

A patient with these conditions have usually fever and chills, loin pain(in almost all), CVA tenderness, lower urinary tract symptoms(48%), and palpable renal mass (58%)[82]. In a study, an initial body temperature of above 38.5 degrees Celsius ($P=0.0004$) and an elevated BMI ($P=0.002$) were connotative as predictors of urosepsis. [83] However, occasionally the symptoms may be vague or even totally absent [84].The author draws your attention to a case of pyocalyx which may only have a lost calyx in EXU without clinical symptoms of infection where an inappropriate ESWL to treat a stone may cause sepsis and eventual death (unpublished data).

### 3.4 Paraclinic findings

As previously stated, blood culture, voided urine, and pelvis aspirate guides the antibiotic treatment. CRP and ESR were used to differentiate between the infected hydronephrosis and pyonephrosis with a cut-off at 3mg/dl for CRP and 100 mm/hr for ESR as useful adjuncts for sonographic studies [85]. Cr and blood biochemistry leads to treatment in cases

of bilateral obstruction or functional solitary kidneys. The role and presence of predisposers like diabetes or immunocompromised states not formerly known must not be overlooked and should be evaluated with appropriate investigations.
In patients with clinical suspicion of renal infection, sonography has an accuracy of up to 96%.[86]. Sonography can distinguish internal echoes inside the pelvicalyceal system or areas of decreased echogenicity inside parenchyma. As previously said, combining sonography findings with CRP and ESR may further increase the accuracy of differentiating between infected hydronephrosis and pyonephrosis.
MRI with diffusion-weighted images (MRI Dw) and Apparent Diffusion Coefficient (ADC) are helpful to distinguish between infected hydronephrosis and pyonephrosis[87].The extremely low ADC of the renal pelvis of the pyonephrotic kidney accounts for its signal hyperintensity on diffusion-weighted images as well as signal hypointensity on ADC maps. However, the decision to use MRI must be based on the fact that whether or not it could change the treatment strategy. Other modalities may be used to discover the etiology of obstruction e.g. a spiral non-contrast CT may be the best tool to detect an obstructive ureteral stone.
One must avoid using a retrograde pyelography as it increases the internal pressure of an obstructed infected system and may cause urosepsis. Therefore, t should only be done after the infection has been eradicated. In addition to relieving the obstruction in the acute phase, percutaneous nephrostomy provides the opportunity of antegrade pyelography afterwards. Hence, one can have a near physiologic dynamic image while maintaining a safety valve.

### 3.5 Management

Starting antibiotic treatment and relieving obstruction in an obstructed infected kidney are urgent. One starts antibiotic empirically covering Gram-negatives, anaerobes, and staphylococci, and then tailors the regimen according to the aspirate culture. Percutaneous nephrostomy has proved to be an ideal option for obstruction relief in multiple case series including a prospective study while gaining a reliable culture and providing access for subsequent imaging[88-91]. A considerable disparity has been found between the results of the pelvis aspirate and the voided urine culture.[81]Nevertheless, the choice of the method for relieving obstruction must be astutely individualized. In a pelvic kidney with overlying bowel, percutaneous nephrostomy is no longer the ideal first line option and a retrograde stent may be preferred if proved feasible. In a child with duplex system and upper moiety pyonephrosis, upper moiety cutaneous pyelostomy may be performed. For an irreversibly non-functional kidney with a thin parenchyme, a primary nephrectomy may be curative. In many cases, a strict differentiation between infected hydronephrosis and pyonephrosis does not seem to radically change the treatment strategy.

## 4. Acute focal bacterial nephritis (AFBN) or lobar nephronia

### 4.1 Introduction

Acute focal bacterial nephritis (AFBN) or acute lobar nephronia represents as an acute localized non-liquefactive infection of the kidney caused by bacterial infection [92]. This stipulates that the mass should not contain drainable pus. Actually, it is a precursor step to a frank renal abscess before liquefaction. In a study by Klar et al. (1993), of 210 pediatric patients admitted to hospital with manifestations of urinary tract infection, 13 had AFBN.

Evolution to renal abscess happened in 25%, but all responded well to antibiotic therapy [93]. However, it looks that incidence rate may vary according to the ease of access to medical facilities and cultural background that may alter the interval between the commencement of manifestations of the acute pyelonephritis and the time that antibiotic therapy is instituted.

### 4.2 Pathophysiology

The same process that causes acute pyelonephritis may evolve into AFBN and eventually abscess. In children, both hematogenous [94] and ascending routes [16] have been suspected. Congenital urologic abnormalities especially vesicoureteral reflux has been linked with AFBN. Unusual and fastidious organisms e.g. brucellosis especially in endemic areas must be kept in mind [95]. Diabetes mellitus is a major predisposing factor in all complicated urinary tract infections [96].

### 4.3 Clinical presentation

Clinical manifestations are similar to acute pyelonephritis, but probably in a more severe and durable form. Fever, chills and costovertebral angle tenderness along with signs and symptoms of SIRS(Systemic Inflammatory Response Syndrome) could happen [92]. However, atypical and imitating clinical pictures may happen as nephrectomy with a misdiagnosis of renal tumoral mass has been reported; hence, the condition has also been referred to as renal inflammatory pseudotumor [97].

### 4.4 Paraclinic findings

One expects an active urinalysis and a positive urine culture in many cases, but the point is that in some patients these laboratory findings are absent and a high level of suspicion must be put on such cases [94, 98].

The value of sonography in diagnosis of AFBN has been somewhat controversial. Some consider an average accuracy [99] or even low accuracy [100] in sonography that fails to show half and even over the half of the cases. Another study attributes a high accuracy for sonographic findings of nephromegaly and focal mass in a pediatric group of patients with a specificity of 86% and a sensitivity of up to 95%.[101]. The author thinks one must also consider the chronological evolution of sonographic technology between 1988[99], 1989[100] and 2004([101]. Newer sonographic apparatus may well be relied upon in revealing renal pathologies.

Reported sonographic appearances of AFBN are varied, but are typically described as being echopoor [102], yet at least in one study in 17 patients, the abnormal areas were echogenic in 12 of them, echopoor in three, and of mixed echogenicity in two [102]. In sonographic follow-up, the inflammatory mass may diminish and disappear in 4 weeks. [92].

The most valuable modality for detection of AFBN is computerized tomography [103] used as reference standard to assess other modalities [29]. AFBN in CT is typically hypodense [99] and may help to differentiate them with renal tumors that are most commonly hyperdense. Different patterns could be seen in CT that they have been linked with prognosis and severity of the disease. In a retrospective study, the CT appearance of AFBN was categorized into three groups: Group I: wedge-shaped lesions (focal or diffuse); Group II: focal mass-like lesions; and Group III: diffuse (multifocal) mass-like lesions.

The clinical features in Group I patients displayed many similarities with those in uncomplicated acute pyelonephritis (APN) responding to antibiotic therapy promptly. Patients in Group II were successfully treated with antibiotics, but had a protracted clinical course with a slower clinical improvement than Group I. Evolution to renal abscess happened, though uncommonly. In comparison, 33% of the patients in Group III died despite antibiotic therapy[104].

We must not neglect to detect associated anomalies of urinary tract especially vesicoureteral reflux. In children, doing a MCUG is mandatory. In adults, decision to perform a MCUG must be made on the basis of whether VUR can do any further harm or the need for additional intervention.

### 4.5 Management

The mainstay of treatment in AFBN is antibiotics. There is a well-designed RCT to determine the best duration of treatment [105]. In this study, a three-week antibiotic course was clearly superior to a two-week course. The treatment began with parenteral form, and then, switched to oral form 2 to 3 days after defervescence. Antibiotic must be directed against Gram-negative organisms and staphylococci while the culture results are not ready, or in the cases that urine and blood cultures are negative and clinical suspicion is high [94].

As previously stated, patients with diffuse mass-like lesions on CT may have a grave prognosis as 30% of them may die of the disease [104]. Therefore, one could infer that in such cases a more vigorous approach including surgery has to be considered.

## 5. Chronic pyelonephritis

### 5.1 Introduction

Chronic pyelonephritis is the result of an underlying renal or urinary tract disease with the subsequent repeated renal infection that ends in scarring, atrophy of the kidney, and eventual renal insufficiency [106]. Besides the history of UTIs, complicating defects such as major anatomic anomalies, urinary tract obstruction, nephrolithiasis, renal dysplasia, analgesic abuse , or most commonly, vesicoureteral reflux (VUR) in young children could be detected in patients with end-stage renal disease and chronic pyelonephritis. Nonetheless, it has never been found that renal insufficiency has been caused by non-obstructive uncomplicated UTI alone [107, 108].

There is a gender susceptibility in chronic pyelonephritis as it is twice more common in females than in males; there is also a higher occurrence in infants and young children (younger than 2 years old) than in older children and adults. Although the greatest risk of renal scarring has been reported in young children, additional renal scars could be the result of repeated infections. [109] There is a three-time higher possibility of VUR and chronic pyelonephritis in white children than in African-American children [110]. VUR could be accompanied by UTIs in 30-45% of children. Moreover, in siblings of patients with chronic pyelonephritis, VUR prevalence rate could reach up to around 35% [111, 112].

Chronic renal infection can worsen renal impairment significantly in patients with underlying functional or structural urinary tract abnormalities; hence, diagnosis, localization, and treatment of chronic renal infection are crucial to be found by appropriate studies. The diagnosis is made by radiologic or pathologic examination rather than mere clinical presentation.

In women and in contrary to a 2% to 5% prevalence of bacteriuria, pyelonephritis without complications by obstruction or urinary tract malformation does not result in end-stage renal disease [111].

## 5.2 Pathology

In chronic pyelonephritis, the affected kidney in gross is often diffusely shrunk, scarred, and pitted. The scars could be described as Y-shaped, flat, broad-based depressions with red-brown granular bases. Usually, there is a polar scarring with underlying calyceal distortion and blunting with thin parenchyma that the cortico-medullary demarcation is lost [113].
There are microscopic changes that are usually patchy together with an interstitial infiltrate of lymphocytes, plasma cells, and occasional polymorphonuclear cells. Some portions of the parenchyma are probably replaced by fibrosis and although glomeruli may be preserved, periglomerular fibrosis is commonly observed. In parts of the involved areas, glomeruli could be completely fibrosed along with atrophied tubules. At times, leukocytes and hyaline casts are present in the tubules that the latter may resemble the thyroid colloid where the description renal thyroidization is originated [114]. On the whole, the changes are nonspecific that could be seen in toxic exposures, post-obstructive atrophy, hematologic disorders, post irradiation nephritis, ischemic renal disease, and nephrosclerosis too [113].

## 5.3 Clinical presentation

Chronic pyelonephritis is usually asymptomatic in many individuals until it produces renal insufficiency and then the symptoms are similar to those of any other form of chronic renal failure, but they may have a history of frequent UTIs. A strong correlation between renal scarring and recurrent UTIs exists in children [115]. Although the developing kidney appears to be very susceptible to damage, and this susceptibility appears to be age dependent, in adult kidneys, renal scarring induced by UTIs is rare.
If it is believed that a patient's chronic pyelonephritis is an end result of many episodes of acute pyelonephritis, a history of intermittent symptoms of fever, lethargy, flank pain, and dysuria could be extracted. Moreover, there is a poor correlation between urinary findings and the presence of renal infection. Bacteriuria and pyuria as the hallmarks of UTI, are not predictive of renal infection since patients with significant renal infection may have sterile urine if the infection is outside of the collecting system or in case of an obstructed ureter draining the kidney [107].
Chronic pyelonephritis often progress asymptomatically and the diagnosis is usually incidental during the radiologic investigation to evaluate for the complications associated with renal insufficiency, such as hypertension, visual impairments, headaches, fatigue, and polyuria.
Leukocytes or proteinuria may be detected in urinalysis in these patients, but it is likely to be normal. The severity of renal impairment could be reflected by serum creatinine levels. If there is an active infection, urine cultures might be positive.
Differential diagnosis for chronic pyelonephritis includes chronic renal failure, hypertension, nephrolithiasis, pyonephrosis, perinephric abscess, acute pyelonephritis, uremia, tuberculosis, and some tumor-like lesions in the kidney, namely, xanthogranulomatous pyelonephritis, malacoplakia, and lymphoma [116].
Chronic pyelonephritis might cause morbidity and mortality by causing following conditions:(1) focal glomerulosclerosis, (2) proteinuria, (3) progressive renal scarring, (4) hypertension, (5) end-stage renal disease and (6) xanthogranulomatous pyelonephritis

(XPN) [112]. The rate of XPN occurrence is 8.2% in such patients and it reaches up to 25% in patients with pyonephrosis [117].

### 5.4 Paraclinic findings

Asymmetry and irregularity of the kidney outlines or a small and atrophic kidney on the affected side could be easily detected in intravenous pyelogram or CT scan. The characteristic signs include focal coarse renal scarring, atrophy and cortical thinning, hypertrophy of residual normal tissue (which may mimic a mass lesion) with blunting and dilation (clubbing) of one or more underlying calyces [118, 119].

In children with gross reflux, voiding cystourethrogram (VCUG) findings may reveal urine reflux into the renal pelvis and ureteral dilatation [112].

Ultrasonography could be used as an alternative that it similarly demonstrates these findings. The best imaging modality to look for renal scarring is DMSA [120]. By providing high-resolution images of the renal cortex, it allows for both qualitative and quantitative characterization of renal injury and impairment. Areas of scarring can be seen as photopenic areas usually at poles [120, 121].

Once the radiologic changes of chronic pyelonephritis have been established, it is important to consider that the repeat of imaging is unlikely to come up with further findings[121].

### 5.5 Management

Since the damage caused by chronic pyelonephritis is irreversible, the management of the radiographic evidence of pyelonephritis should be focused on treating the existing infection, preventing future infections, and monitoring and preserving renal function.

Restricting dietary protein intake can decrease progressive renal injury. The course of renal failure progression could be decelerated through regular checking of blood pressure and aggressive blood pressure control. ACE inhibitors are considered to be particularly beneficial in this setting.

Careful antimicrobial susceptibility tests and the selection of the non-nephrotoxic drugs that yield high urine concentrations must be the basis for the treatment of existing infection. Since there is a possible reduction in renal concentrating ability in pyelonephritis, it may impair excretion and concentration of the antimicrobial drug needed to achieve acceptable bactericidal levels in urine. In order to boost the chance of cure and to avoid recurrence, further progression, and renal damage, the duration of the antimicrobial therapy is recommended to be prolonged along with continuous prophylactic antibiotic regimes [122].

There is either an underlying renal (papillary) lesion or a urologic condition such as obstruction or calculus available that increases the susceptibility to the renal damage, thus appropriate nephrologic and urologic evaluation, treatment and prevention should be undertaken to identify and possibly correct these abnormalities.

Nephrectomy could become necessary in case of hypertension or pain for having a large stone burden in a nonfunctioning kidney.

## 6. Emphysematous pyelonephritis

### 6.1 Introduction

Emphysematous pyelonephritis (EPN) is defined as a rare, yet an acute severe necrotizing infection that involves renal parenchyma and its surrounding tissues causing the presence of gas in the renal parenchyma, collecting system or perinephric tissue [123, 124].

Kelly and MacCullum reported the first case of disease in 1898 [125], and then, Schultz and Klorfein introduced the term emphysematous pyelonephritis in 1962 [126].
It is considered as a rare disease as only 600 cases have been reported from 1966 to date [127]. According to some authors EPN is suggested when gas is detected within the renal parenchyma or perinephric space, yet it has been defined by several others as gas within the collecting system, parenchyma, perirenal space, or in any of these areas [128].
Gas could be found not only in the site of inflammation in the sub-capsular, perinephric, and pararenal spaces that in some cases, but gas was also detected even in the scrotal sac and spermatic cord [129].
Emphysematous pyelitis is a separate condition and refers to the presence of gas in the collecting systems only and could be secondary to instrumentation of the urinary tract. With proper medical management emphysematous pyelitis has an excellent prognosis; however, EPN requires special attention due to its life-threatening nature either with medical or surgical management.
Gas could be found in other conditions such as urinary endoscopic procedures, genitourinary trauma, communicating fistulas with the gastrointestinal tract, and produced by bacteria within the urinary tract [123].
The most common associated factor in EPN is diabetes mellitus that an uncontrolled DM is present in 95% of the cases [131] and the next common cause is urinary tract obstruction [127, 130] that urinary calculi are usually found to be the cause of obstruction [128].
A glucose-fermenting bacterial infection, impaired host immunity, decreased tissue perfusion, neurogenic bladder, alcoholism, drug abuse, urinary tract obstruction in non-diabetics and anatomic anomaly are considered to be the other reported risk factors in EPN [123, 130, 131].
With the female to male ratio of 4:1 in most studies, it is clear there is a greater tendency of the disease toward women [127, 131] that the reason for the higher incidence in females seems to originate from increased susceptibility to UTI. A urinary tract obstruction raises the risk of developing secondary EPN to as high as 25–40% [123]. Despite its worldwide spread, it seems to be geographically more common in Asia [127].

### 6.2 Pathogenesis

The mechanism of gas production is the fermentation of the glucose and lactate to carbon dioxide causing necrotizing infection in an appropriate tissue environment and it usually occurs in the presence of the organisms such as *E. coli*, *Klebsiella* spp., *Proteus* spp., *gram-negative facultative anaerobic* organisms. *E. coli* is found to be the causative agent in almost 70% of the reported cases isolated in urine or pus cultures [132]. There is a presence of bacteriemia in over 50% of the patients with the same organisms as those in urine or pus culture [130].
In addition to the aforesaid organisms, *Proteus mirabilis, Klebsiella pneumonia,* Group D *Streptococcus,* coagulase-negative *Staphylococcus,* and *Candida albicans* have been reported as the causative agent for EPN too [132].
In pathology, abscess formation, foci of micro- and macro-infarctions, vascular thrombosis, numerous gas-filled spaces and areas of necrosis surrounded by acute and chronic inflammatory cells implying septic infarction could be identified in kidney [130, 133].

### 6.3 Clinical presentation

Most patients are in their forties and fifties [127, 133-135]. The symptoms and signs are similar to pyelonephritis and include dysuria, fever, rigorous nausea, vomiting, and flank pain [127,129, 132].

The other clinical manifestations to be potentially considered are acute renal dysfunction, acid-base disturbances on blood gases, hyperglycemia, thrombocytopenia and impaired consciousness [129,130, 135]. There may be a rapid progress into septic shock that could even be the presenting feature in patients with severe emphysematous pyelonephritis [130, 132]. Of the most common physical signs, loin tenderness and in some cases crepitus around the renal area and the scrotum may also be felt [129,130, 132]. In laboratory tests, leucocytosis could be found in 70-80% of the cases that thrombocytopenia was seen in 15-20% of the patients [129, 135]. Since most patients suffer from diabetes mellitus, high blood glucose level is a common finding.

Among other positive findings in EPN, acute renal failure, microscopic or macroscopic hematuria, and severe proteinuria could be counted too [130].

In EPN prognosis, many identified factors affect mortality including a systolic blood pressure of less than 90 mmHg, disturbance of consciousness and an increase in serum creatinine level, thrombocytopenia (OR 22.68, 95% CI 4.4- 16.32) and bilateral EPN (OR 5.36, 95% CI 1.41 - 20.33) that both are attributable to dire prognosis. Antibiotic therapy alone has been associated with a higher risk of mortality (OR 2.85, 95% CI 1.19- 6.81) and it is in comparison to the additional interventions of percutaneous drainage (PCD) of the abscess or nephrectomy [127, 131]. Based on Wan *et al.* 's classification, EPN Type I, as seen below, has a ominous prognosis and it is due to the fact that a more fulminating clinical course and more extensive parenchymal damage exist [133].

Reportedly, although diabetes mellitus is a common risk factor for EPN, but surprisingly it does not culminate in an increased mortality [odds ratio (OR) 0.32, 95% CI 0.05-1.99] [133, 136]. There are also no increased risk of higher mortality in EPN with nephrolithiasis, etiologic factors such as *E. coli* or *K. pneumonia* [137, 138], age 50 years, female sex, history of UTIs, alcoholism, bacteremia, proteinuria (presence of urine protein greater than 3 gm/l on at least 2 occasions during admission), retinopathy, and macrohematuria (presence of urine red blood cells of over than 100 per high power field) [131].

### 6.4 Paraclinic findings

As the clinical and the laboratory findings will only point to sepsis of renal origin, emphysematous pyelonephritis is a radiological diagnosis mostly.

In support of the diagnosis, a plain radiograph is indicative of an abnormal gas shadow in the renal bed that an ultrasonography or CT will confirm the presence of intra renal gas to diagnose EPN. CT is considered to have the highest accuracy of 100%, hence, it is proven to be the most reliable diagnostic tool in EP diagnosis [129]. By identifying parenchymal destruction characteristics, it demonstrates the extent of EPN too [130,133, 135]. Since ultrasound diagnosis is very much dependent on the operator, it is not sufficiently specific when gas-containing lesions are to be characterized. Calculi or bowel gas are the origin of mistakes as gas appears as echogenic foci.

The accuracy of ultrasonography and plain radiograph of the abdomen is around 69 and 65%, respectively, and it necessitates exploiting abdominal CT for the sake of early diagnosis and further management of EPN [127].

By analysis based on CT findings, EPN has been classified into two types by Wan et al. in 1996. [127, 133] According to this classification in type I, there is a renal necrosis with either total absence of fluid content or the presence of a streaky/mottled gas pattern whereas there is a presence of renal or perirenal fluid along with a loculated gas pattern or the presence of gas in the collecting system in type II (Figure 1). Owing to more extensive parenchymal necrosis and more fulminating clinical course, type I EPN is associated with worse prognosis [133].

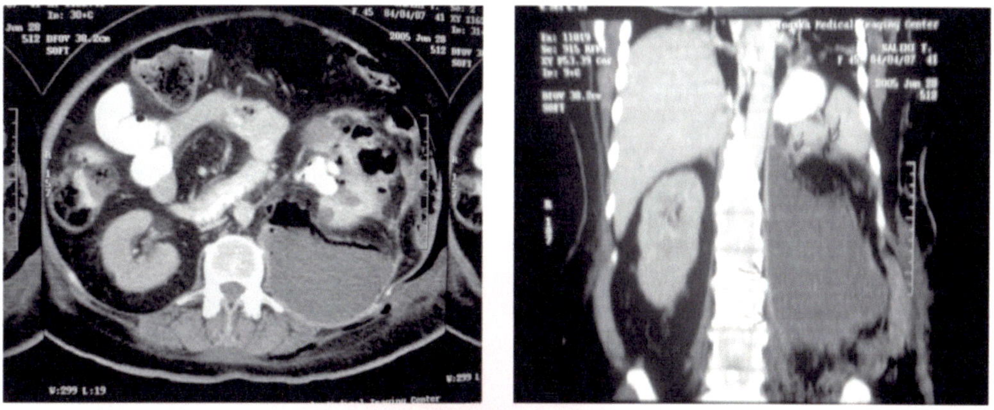

Fig. 1. CT scan showing a large collection with air-fluid level in left retroperitoneal cavity.(transverse and coronal view). ( Courtesy of Simforoosh N., Sharifiaghdas F., Parvin M.,et al. The book "Urology Cases in Practice". Labbafinejad Medical Center, Tehran, Iran.)

In a publication in 2000, Huang and Tseng introduced a new classification based on the CT findings described in more details and with more subcategories that was different to the one mentioned above [130]. Their classification can be summed up as: (1) Class1: the presence of gas in the collecting system only; (2) Class 2: the presence of gas in the renal parenchyma without extension to extrarenal space; (3) Class 3A: extension of gas or abscess to perinephric space; Class 3B: extension of gas or abscess to pararenal space; and (4) Class 4: bilateral EPN or solitary kidney with EPN.
The purpose of such detailed classification by Huang and Tseng was to show the correlation between the EPN classification and its management.
Nonetheless, the described classification by Wan *et al.* has been evaluated for the risk factors and the management of EPN in two published meta-analyses.

### 6.5 Management

In those patients under the treatment for pyelonephritis, the radiological diagnosis of Emphysematous Pyelonephritis could be overlooked unless appropriate imaging is taken.
In order to confirm the diagnosis in this group of patients, also in individuals with failure in responding to the standard line of therapy for pyelonephritis, an urgent CT scan should be taken.[134]
The preliminary treatment is a medical management(MM) by providing basic resuscitation measures of oxygen, intravenous fluids, acid base balance correction and proper antibiotics along with good glycemic control. It is also necessary to sustain systolic blood pressure at above 100 mmHg through fluid resuscitation or inotropic support if a need arises.
In case of observing deterioration in the clinical condition and the laboratory results, these patients should be looked after more vigorously as multi-organ support is possibly required.
The initial antibiotic therapy should be aimed at eliminating Gram-negative bacteria as the most common causative organisms. To fulfill this, Aminogycosides, α-lactamase inhibitors,

cephalosporins and quinolones could be administered guided by the local hospital policy. For the initial stage of treatment, a combination of aminoglycoside with any of the other three groups can be used. The choice of antibiotics could be changed for the type and number of organisms along with their individual sensitivities accordingly once the culture report is ready.

Emergency nephrectomy and/or open surgical drainage along with antibiotic therapy was the accepted treatment of EPN until the late 1980s that had a mortality rate of up to 40–50% [123, 139].

As introduced by Hudson et al., fluoroscopy guided percutaneous drainage (PCD) has been an option for treating EPN. [140] In a number of case studies later, patients have been successfully treated with a significant reduction in mortality rates in case of an early PCD in combination with medical management [129, 132]. PCD has also been found to be helpful in preserving the function of the affected kidney in about 70% of cases [127]. In patients who have been found to have localized areas of gas and in those with existing functioning renal tissue, early PCD should be performed.

Since more than one catheter can be used to drain all, hence, loculations, abscess or multiple abscesses are not contraindications for PCD [127, 141]. The first target of the PCD should be the abscess that is technically accessible easier and could significantly reduce the pressure on the viable renal tissue. As there is a better success rate if compared with ultrasonography, ideally the insertion of a pigtail drain of at least 14 Fr should be guided under CT [134].

Unless follow-up CT shows resolution of the EPN features, the drainage tubes should stay in place, and if needed, flushed with antibiotic solutions.

A gradual shift toward a nephron-sparing approach with early PCD has been noticed during the last decade with or without elective nephrectomy at a later stage. The various treatment strategies could be summarized as MM alone, early PCD plus MM, MM plus emergency nephrectomy, and PCD plus MM plus emergency nephrectomy [127] (Figure 2).

Chen *et al.* have recommended follow-up CT in 4 to 7 days as beneficial to look for non-communicating air/fluid collections in patients with early PCD plus MM [141]. This could also be found helpful in planning a nephrectomy for non-responders to PCD plus medical management.

MM with PCD has found to be the most successful management method (30–100%) in two meta-analysis of the management strategies which has also been linked with the lowest mortality rate at 13.5% ( *P* 0.001) [127]. Nonetheless, subsequent nephrectomy could be required in a small proportion of patients managed with MM and PCD and the reported mortality stands at 6.6% that is significantly lower than medical management only approach (50%), or emergency nephrectomy (25%) alone (p _0.001) [127, 131].

MM alone or combined with PCD can lead to a good outcome in Class 1 and 2 EPN based on the Huang and Tseng classification. The survival rate with MM plus PCD is 85% in patients with fewer than two risk factors in Class 3 and 4 EPN, however, MM plus PCD was unsuccessful in 92% of cases in those patients with more than two risk factors. In comparison with the Class 1 and 2 EPN, the number of non-responders in this group who require nephrectomy is higher [130, 132].

After PCD, the respective failure and mortality rates of 71% and 29% rate in Class 3A, and 30% and 19% in Class 3B have been described by Huang and Tseng [130].

A meta-analysis has revealed that in patients who underwent an early PCD, elective nephrectomy is required only in 13% of them [127]. These patients either do not respond well clinically to MM plus PCD, or on nuclear imaging they are found to have a nonfunctioning kidney.

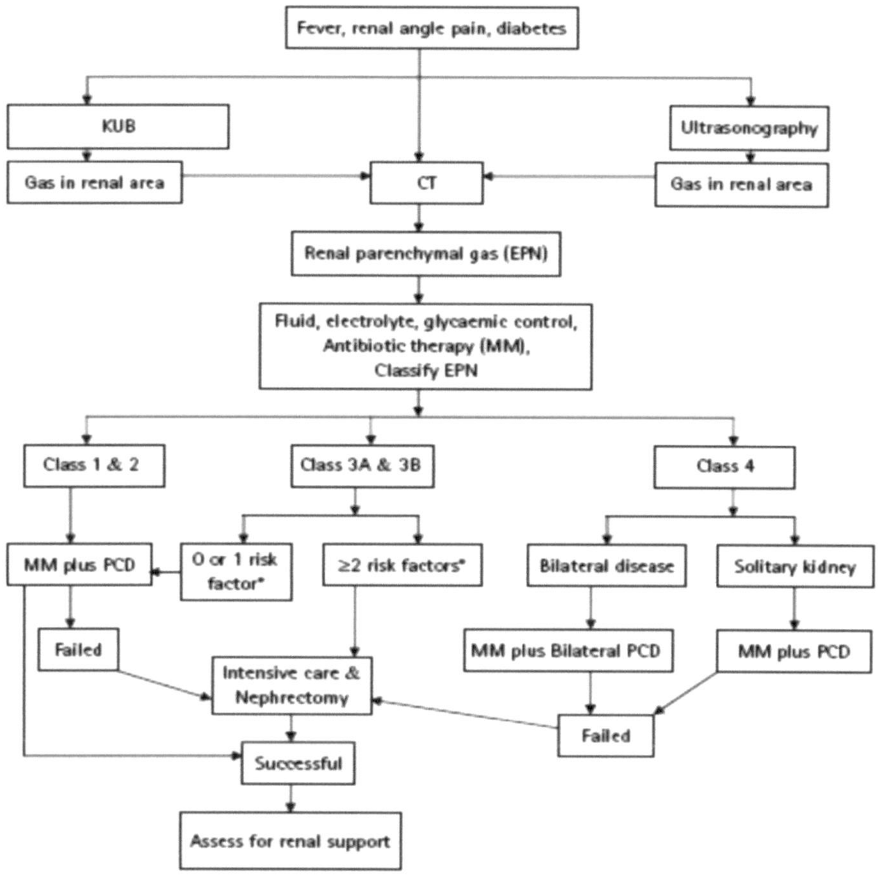


*Risk factors: diabetes, thrombocytopenia, acute renal failure, altered level of consciousness, shock.

Fig. 2. EPN Management algorithm that is based on clinico-radiological classification by Huang & Tseng [130]. KUB, plain abdominal film of kidney, ureter and bladder.

In these patients, nephrectomy can be either simple, or radical, or laparoscopic [124, 142]. The mortality rate could be as low as 10% if simple nephrectomy can be carried out [124, 138]. Laparoscopic nephrectomy has been performed successfully in these patients with the advantage of a shortened recovery period and hospital stay [142].

Renal support measures in the form of dialysis might be required in patients with EPN that it seems the availability of renal support reduces the mortality rate as concluded in a recent study [132].

The best management strategy should be chosen based on an individualized case by case approach until prospective randomized studies come up with a definite conclusion. The degree and extent of parenchymal loss together with the coexisting renal disease determine the long-term outcome for renal function and the need for further support.

# 7. Xanthogranulomatous pyelonephritis

## 7.1 Introduction

In medical literature, xanthogranulomatous pyelonephritis (XPN) is described as a rare, severe, chronic renal infection typically resulting in diffuse renal destruction. There is a unilateral involvement in most cases that ends in a nonfunctioning, enlarged kidney associated with obstructive uropathy as a result of nephrolithiasis [143]. The most common pathology that is attributed to the disease is the simultaneous obstruction of the ipsilateral renal unit, most commonly due to an underlying stone disease with concomitant urinary tract infection [143]. In 1916, Schlagenhaufer presented the first descriptions of the distinctive gross and macroscopic features of XPN; however, the term *xanthogranulomatous pyelonephritis* was introduced by Oberling in 1935 [144].

The characteristic of xanthogranulomatous pyelonephritis is the renal parenchyma destruction and its replacement by a chronic inflammatory infiltrate and lipid-laden macrophages called xanthoma cells [145] that in turn results in an enlarged kidney that is either poorly functional or non-functional.

Although the disease can be observed at any age, the majority of cases occur in middle-aged women. As it can affect the neonates, there is a possibility of prenatal origin as well [146]. XPN has been known to imitate virtually every other inflammatory disease of the kidney and on radiographic examination it is usually mistaken for renal cell carcinoma[147]. Moreover, because of the confusing microscopic similarities between xanthogranulomatous and clear cell adenocarcinoma of kidney on frozen section, it has ended in radical nephrectomy [145, 147, 148].

## 7.2 Pathogenesis

With regards to the pathogenesis, the primary factors involved in xanthogranulomatous pyelonephritis are nephrolithiasis, obstruction, and infection [149]. In up to 83% of the patients in various series, they have been found to have nephrolithiasis that staghorn type has comprised approximately one third to half of the renal stones [147, 150-152]. To a lower extent, there have also been reports of urinary tract obstruction as a result of UPJ obstruction, severe VUR and tumors (e.g. renal cell carcinoma, ureteral carcinoma, bladder carcinoma)[150, 153]. Also there is a greater risk of developing the disease in diabetics [154].

There has been a clinical and experimental postulation that primary obstruction with or without subsequent bacterial infection can lead to the tissue damage with the release of lipid material initiating the XPN. The lipid material is collected by macrophages. Then, these macrophages (xanthoma cells) are spread in sheets around parenchymal abscesses and calyces and are intermixed with lymphocytes, giant cells, and plasma cells. As spontaneous bacteriemia has been reported rarely, the bacteria seem to be of low virulence [143, 155].

Venous occlusion and hemorrhage, abnormal lipid metabolism, lymphatic blockage, failure of antimicrobial therapy in UTI, altered immunologic competence, and renal ischemia are the other factors possibly interrelated [156, 157].

The fact that XPN is treated successfully by nephrectomy, also the lack of other evidence for the systemic immune deficiency, has led to the assumption that immunological defect is unlikely. The reported malnutrition in these patients seems to be attributable to the effect of the XPN rather than its cause. Nonetheless, the cycle of events in the XPN pathogenesis is unclear [158].

In the studies so far, no single factor has found to be instrumental in the pathogenesis of this disease. Instead, insufficient host acute inflammatory response within an obstructed, ischemic, or necrotic kidney seems to be the culprit.

### 7.3 Pathology

Grossly, kidney involvement in xanthogranulomatous pyelonephritis could be diffuse (80%), or segmental as well as surrounding tissues.

The involved kidney is usually described as enlarged, with normal outline and the indication of nephrolithiasis, peripelvic fibrosis and dilated calyces filled with purulent material; however, the pelvis that is surrounded by fibrosis usually prevents pelvic dilation. Papillary necrosis leads to destruction of the papillae [143].

Typically, orange-yellow nodules of inflamed parenchymal tissue near the areas of tissue necrosis suppuration could be observed. Besides small localized abscess is a common finding. The renal cortex is thin and the xanthogranulomatous tissue usually replaces it. The renal capsule often thickens, and the inflammatory process expansion into the perinephric or paranephric space is common [143, 149, 156].

In microscopic examination, yellowish nodules that line the calyces and surround the parenchymal abscesses with dark sheets of lipid-laden macrophages or xanthoma cells (foamy histiocytes with small, dark nuclei and clear cytoplasm) could be noted (Figure 3). There is a mixture of the macrophages with a variety of inflammatory cells such as lymphocytes, plasma cells, neutrophils, and multinucleated giant cells. This seems necessary to mention that the presence of xanthogranulomatous cells is unspecific to xanthogranulomatous pyelonephritis and they may be found anywhere inflammation or obstruction exits [143, 156].

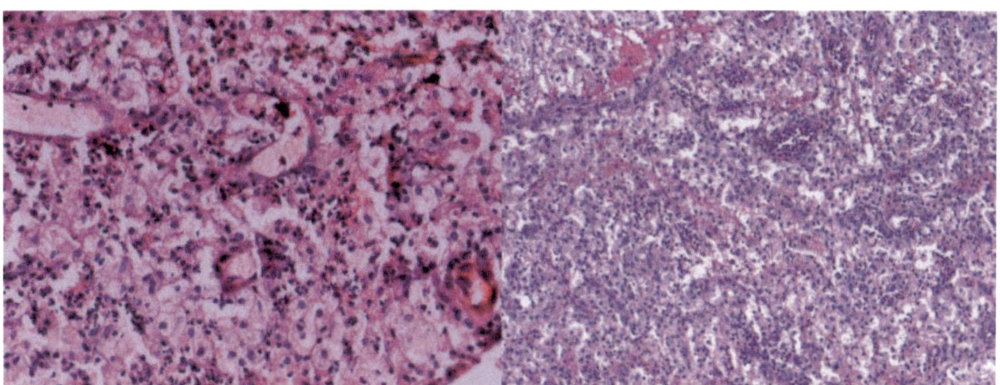

Fig. 3. Xanthogranulomatous pyelonephritis. Prominent foamy histocyes admixed with mononuclear cells.( Courtesy of Simforoosh N., Sharifiaghdas F., Parvin M.,et al. The book "Urology Cases in Practice". Labbafinejad Medical Center, Tehran, Iran.)

### 7.4 Clinical presentation

In patients with UTIs and a unilateral enlarged nonfunctioning or poorly functioning kidney with a stone or a mass lesion indistinguishable from malignant tumor, xanthogranulomatous pyelonephritis should be considered in the differential diagnosis. Since it has been termed "the great imitator" indicates the difficulty to characterize its clinical and radiologic features. As a result, in most cases the precise diagnosis is made at the time of histopathology after nephrectomy.

The disease presentation is nonspecific and its clinical demonstration varies markedly. The usual findings in most patients include flank pain, fever, and constitutional symptoms of fatigue, malaise, weight loss, and anorexia. Among those, a tender flank mass is the most common physical finding.

In up to 50% of patients, there are abnormal liver function tests with occasional hepatomegaly.

XGP inflammation could be extended into the perirenal or pararenal space, lymph nodes, ipsilateral Psoas muscle, colon, spleen, diaphragm, abdominal wall, and skin. This process is similar in pediatric patients and adults with similar clinical and pathologic findings. The classic triad is unilateral renal enlargement with little or no function and a large calculus in the renal pelvis without pelvic dilation in fifty to eighty percent of patients. A positive medical history for UTIs and urologic instrumentation could often be extracted. [152, 154, 155, 158, 159].

Although xanthogranulomatous pyelonephritis with its unknown etiology can occur at any age; however, the peak age for its incidence is in the fifth to the seventh decade that predominantly affects women with no preference of involving either kidney [158].

### 7.5 Paraclinic findings

In the literature review for the xanthogranulomatous pyelonephritis it can be realized that *Proteus* is the most common organism involved followed by E. coli [151, 158].The stone formation and subsequent chronic obstruction and irritation could be attributable to *Proteus* organisms [147]. Polymicrobial infections have found to be the responsible organisms in 33% of a series of 36 cases that included some anaerobics.

No microbial growth could be detected in the urine of one-third of the patients. It seems that the reason is either the preventive effect of the urinary tract obstruction not allowing the contaminated urine to reach the bladder, or it is because of the antibiotic treatment prior to the patient's admission [151]. In some cases, only the cultures of the tissue obtained during the operation could reveal the organism. The common findings in urinalysis are pyuria and proteinuria; nonetheless, urine culture is sterile in 35 % of patients. Blood tests are usually indicative of anemia and leukocytosis that hepatic dysfunction could be found in as high as 50% of the patients [159]. Azotemia or serious renal failure is uncommon due to the almost always unilateral involvement in xanthogranulomatous pyelonephritis [149].

In sonography, a global enlargement of the kidney is usually found. Instead of the normal renal parenchyma, many hypoechoic fluid-filled masses are detected that are debris-filled dilated calyces or foci of parenchymal destruction. In focal involvement, a solid mass is present in the involved segment of the kidney with an associated calculus in the collecting system or ureter. As to the differential diagnosis, renal cell carcinoma and other solid renal lesions must be considered [160].

A renal mass due to a localized renal enlargement could be presented. Less common findings in excretory urography are delayed function and possibly a massive hydronephrosis. Although smaller calcifications within the mass are not uncommon, however, they are not very specific.

The point of obstruction could be shown by retrograde pyelography that it also reveals the dilation of the renal pelvis and calyces. In contrast studies, extensive parenchymal damage could be demonstrated as an ulcerated pyelocalyceal system with multiple irregular filling defects.

The most valuable radiologic means in evaluating patients with xanthogranulomatous pyelonephritis is probably CT scanning (Figure 4). By using this radiologic technique, an enlarged nonfunctioning kidney with decreased contrast enhancement, dilated calyces, and the evidence of obstruction often by a renal stone could be demonstrated [161, 162]. At times, a large reniform mass with the renal pelvis closely encircling a central calcification, but without pelvic dilatation, could be demonstrated [160, 163]. In the scans, multiple water-density masses that are representative of dilated calyces and abscess cavities filled with varied amounts of pus and debris could be observed instead of normal renal parenchyma. On enhanced scans, however, the abundant vascularity within the granulation tissue could make the walls of these cavities demonstrate a prominent blush. In contrast to the tumors and other inflammatory lesions, the cavities themselves, do not enhance in the scans.

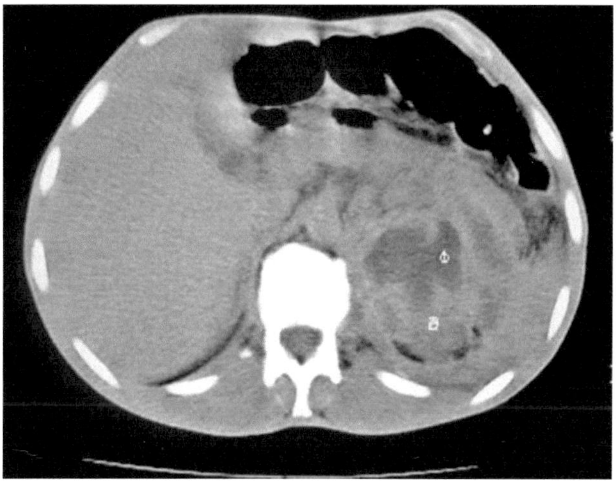

Fig. 4. CT scan :a multifocal mass in left kidney(transverse view). ( Courtesy of Simforoosh N., Sharifiaghdas F., Parvin M.,et al. The book "Urology Cases in Practice". Labbafinejad Medical Center, Tehran, Iran.)

In properly evaluating the involvements of the perirenal and pararenal tissues, CT scan is very helpful that could reveal extension of the inflammatory process into structures nearby, or abdominal wall [154, 161].

In order to confirm and quantify the differential lack of function in the involved kidney, $^{99m}Tc$-DMSA radionuclide renal scanning is exploited [149].

MRI has not excelled CT in assessing renal inflammation yet, however, it has the advantage of outlining extra renal extension of inflammation. On T1 and T2-weighted images, lesions of xanthogranulomatous pyelonephritis could emerge as cystic foci of intermediate intensity and hyper intensity signal, respectively [164].

Xanthogranulomatous pyelonephritis and renal cell carcinoma cannot usually be differentiated in the radiologic studies despite the distinctive radiologic signs. The decisive diagnosis is usually made pathologically, mostly after nephrectomy. In the last decade, however, a combination of increasingly sensitive radiologic investigations and suspicious clinical signs has made the preoperative diagnosis possible.

### 7.6 Differential diagnosis

In segmental xanthogranulomatous pyelonephritis with no calculus, the diagnosis may be difficult. In a small contracted kidney, the radiographic findings are nonspecific and non-diagnostic for XPN [161, 163].

The usual differential diagnoses for xanthogranulomatous pyelonephritis are Wilms tumor, renal cell carcinoma, renal abscess, infected renal cystic disease, tuberculosis, malakoplakia, and transitional renal cell carcinoma. There have also been the reports of cases associated with renal carcinoma [148, 155].

Differentiation between xanthogranulomatous pyelonephritis presented with massive pelvic dilation and pyonephrosis is not possible. In renal parenchymal malacoplakia, there may be renal enlargement and multiple inflammatory masses instead of the normal renal parenchyma, however, calculi are usually absent. Renal lymphoma could be presented by multiple hypoechoic masses in the kidney enclosing the contracted, non-dilated pelvis. Nevertheless, the clinical signs for lymphoma are clear and calculi are absent and the renal involvement is usually bilateral [160].

### 7.7 Management

The correct diagnosis is the first issue to tackle in the correct treatment of xanthogranulomatous pyelonephritis. XPN used to be diagnosed mostly postoperatively in the past [147]. With today's accurate modern CT technology, diagnosis nears 90% preoperatively [152, 158].

To stabilize the patient preoperatively, antimicrobial therapy is necessary that the renal function could be occasionally restored by eradicating the infection through long-term antimicrobial therapy[165].

In a study by Tasi et al., an adult case was reported who had bilateral diffuse XPN with no fever and was successfully managed by supportive care without renal replacement therapy. The subsequent eighteen-month follow-up was proven to be uneventful with relatively stable renal function (serum creatinine 10.6 mg/dl). Therefore, it seems fever could be used as an indicator for nephrectomy [166]. Nonetheless due to the limited reported cases, the significance of pyrexia should be investigated further for its importance to be fully recognized.

If the renal involvement is either diffuse or indistinguishable from a renal tumor preoperatively, nephrectomy is carried out. Nonetheless, for the localized xanthogranulomatous pyelonephritis, diagnosed preoperatively or at exploration, partial nephrectomy is preferred [147, 157].

To make the diagnosis solely on the basis of frozen section could be difficult as the lipid-laden macrophages associated with xanthogranulomatous pyelonephritis are very similar to clear cell adenocarcinoma. There also seems to be relations between the cells in xanthogranulomatous pyelonephritis and renal cell carcinoma, papillary transitional cell carcinoma of the pelvis or bladder, and infiltrating squamous cell carcinoma of the pelvis [148, 157]. As a result, nephrectomy should be performed if malignant renal tumor cannot be ruled out. In case of an encounter with enlarged lymph nodes, the nodes should be dissected to exclude coexisting renal cell carcinoma[148].

If there is a diffuse and extensive disease that extends to the retroperitoneum, nephrectomy accompanied by the removal of the perinephric fat and the dissection of granulomatous tissue from the diaphragm, great vessels, and bowel may be required.

If nephrectomy is not performed and incision and drainage is carried out instead, the patient may continue suffering from a prolonged incapacitating illness that could advance toward cutaneous fistula and in such cases an even more difficult nephrectomy will then be necessary [147].
Laparoscopic nephrectomy has been concluded as a reasonable approach to the treatment of xanthogranulomatous pyelonephritis in some literature reviews, but the fact is that most XPN cases were managed through open surgery and the conversion rate was high in those few cases that laparoscopic approach had been tried [159, 167].

## 8. Malacoplakia

### 8.1 Introduction

The Greek word "Malacoplakia" literally means soft plaque and the term is used for any unusual inflammatory disease that was originally described to affect the bladder, however, it has been found later that it could affect the genitourinary and gastrointestinal tracts, skin, lungs, bones, and mesenteric lymph nodes. Originally, this chronic inflammatory lesion was described by Michaelis and Gutmann in 1902. In 1903, it was characterized by von Hansemann as soft, yellow-brown plaques with large polygonal shaped macrophages and foamy eosinophilic cytoplasm (von Hansemann cells) that the pathognomonic PAS-positive granules are called Michaelis-Gutmann bodies [168]
Malacoplakia does not have exact known pathogenesis; however, it probably results from abnormal macrophage function against a bacterial infection, mostly *E. coli.*

### 8.2 Pathogenesis

Although the true pathogenesis is unknown, but there are several popular theories available. Of some 93 patients who had cultures of urine, diseased tissue, or blood, 89.4% were found to have coliform infections [168]. Of the total number of patients in this review, some 40% of the patients had an immunodeficiency syndrome, autoimmune disease, carcinoma, or another systemic disorder. In malacoplakia, this association of coliform infections and patients' compromised health status is well recognized.
The distinguishable Michaelis-Gutmann bodies are believed to originate from the phagolysosomes containing incompletely destroyed bacteria with abnormal deposition of calcium and iron [168]. As many authors agree there is a decreased intra cellular cGMP/cAMP ratio that seems to diminish capacity of macrophages for bacterial lysis. Hence, in Malacoplakia the assumption exists that the underlying cellular defect is the impaired intracellular killing of bacteria [169, 170]. The most frequent bacteria associated with malacoplakia are coliforms that in 75% of cases is E. coli [169].

### 8.3 Pathology

To diagnose the disease, biopsy should be carried out that the lesion has the characteristic large histiocytes, known as *von Hansemann cells,* and pathognomonic small basophilic, extracytoplasmic, or intracytoplasmic calculospherules called Michaelis-Gutmann bodies. Electron microscopy has been able to demonstrate the intact coliform bacteria and bacterial fragments within phagolysosomes of the foamy-appearing malacoplakic histiocytes [168]. It has been emphasized that Michaelis-Gutmann bodies though pathognomonic for the disease, may not be observed in early malacoplakia; hence, they are not necessary for the diagnosis [168, 171].

Large amounts of immunoreactive $\alpha_1$-antitrypsin have been detected in macrophages in malacoplakia involving the kidney and bladder [172]. In other pathologic processes that macrophages closely look alike the ones in malacoplakia, but without Michaelis-Gutmann bodies, they do not contain $\alpha_1$-antitrypsin that is with the exception for a few macrophages in tuberculosis and xanthogranulomatous pyelonephritis. In malacoplakia, hence, $\alpha_1$-antitrypsin immunohistochemical staining could be a useful test for an early and accurate differential diagnosis.

### 8.4 Clinical presentation

The majority of patients are females who are over the age of 50 with a recurrent urinary tract infection history. For the malacoplakia in the urinary tract, the female to male ratio is 4:1; however, this ratio does not stand for other body tissues [168, 169]. The affected patients who are mostly debilitated, are immunosuppressed, with other chronic diseases and they are similar to those patients on long-term steroid administration and individuals with acquired immunodeficiency syndrome, lymphoma, and diabetes mellitus [168].

Malacoplakia could appear through various clinical presentations that is appropriate to the location of the disease-associated plaques and can involve any portion of the urinary tract, nonetheless, the bladder is the most commonly involved site and it is followed by the renal parenchyma, ureters, and renal pelvis [168, 169].

The symptoms for the bladder malacoplakia that is more common than the other types of urinary tract involvement are bladder irritability and hematuria. In cystoscopy, mucosal plaques or nodules could be detected. With the progress of these lesions, they may become fungating, firm, sessile masses that result in filling defects of the bladder, ureter, or pelvis on excretory urograms. The disease process may cause distal ureter to be strictured or stenotic with subsequent renal obstruction or nonfunction [173].

In malacoplakia, the common renal parenchymal disease may be presented with flank pain or tenderness, palpable mass, pyuria, hematuria, and fever [173] accompanied by the history of urinary tract infections. Due to the usual enlargement of the affected kidney, it is commonly misdiagnosed as renal abscesses or malignant growths, particularly if there is concomitant lung involvement that can mimic metastatic disease [174]. In rare cases, malacoplakia has been reported as bilateral hydronephrosis and ureteral involvement [173, 175]. It can also cause renal vein thrombosis, inferior vena cava thrombosis, or progressive renal failure. Malacoplakia should be considered in the differential diagnosis of acute renal failure if it directly involves the renal parenchyma, also in those rare cases of bilateral renal disease that the end-stage renal failure has been resulted [173, 176].

The renal malacoplakia may extend beyond the kidney and it may also be potentially fatal due to post-infectious glomerulonephritis secondary to bacterial presence in the renal parenchyma, and unlike bladder involvements, is a progressive and destructive parenchymal disease [177, 178].

With the advancement of the medical science, renal parenchymal disease is no longer considered as a frequently fatal disease in the new millennium; however, the morbidity rate still remains high and progress toward renal failure will ensue in a considerable number of patients with time [176].

### 8.5 Paraclinic findings

*Urine cytology:* It could possibly reveal the presence of cells with Michaelis- Gutmann bodies in the urine sample tested [179].

Depending on the degree of internal necrosis, ultrasonography and CT may demonstrate a solid or cystic structure. Ultrasonography, CT, and arteriography are helpful means to establish the multifocal nature.

The most common sonographic finding in renal parenchymal malacoplakia is diffuse enlargement of the affected kidneys, and to a lower extent, hypoechoic lesions, distortion of parenchymal echoes, and increased echogenicity of the parenchyma could be observed too [180, 181].

The most common CT findings include nephromegaly and parenchymal inhomogeneity. The density of the foci of malacoplakia is less than the surrounding enhanced parenchyma. Nevertheless, there have been images available mimicking malignant renal infiltration presenting by masses with increased focal uptake, heterogenecity of focal necrosis, abscesses and multiple retroperitoneal lymph node of significant size with hypodense necrotic center [179, 182]. CT has also the best capability to demonstrate the extension beyond the kidney occurring either in multifocal or uniform malacoplakia [182].

The typical presentation of the multifocal malacoplakia on excretory urography is enlarged kidneys with multiple filling defects and it is on the contrary to the unifocal lesion that appears as a non-calcified mass indistinguishable from other inflammatory or neoplastic lesions. Moreover, renal calcification, lithiasis, and hydronephrosis do not exist [183].

In a typical arteriography, a hypovascular mass without peripheral neovascularity could be observed [183].

### 8.6 Differential diagnosis

Histopathologic analysis could establish the diagnosis; yet the diagnostic value of the cytologic analysis of fine-needle aspirates has also been demonstrated. Since malacoplakia has no characteristic clinical or radiologic sign, thus, biopsy is crucial both to confirm the diagnosis and to help exclude other possible pathologies [184].

In case of observing one or more renal masses, malacoplakia should be suspected, particularly in females with recurrent UTIs with *E. coli,* altered immune response syndromes, or cystoscopic evidence of malacoplakia or filling defects in the collecting system. In a renal transplant patient with these radiographic findings and persistent UTI who has received appropriate antimicrobial therapy, malacoplakia should also be suspected. The differential diagnoses to consider are renal cystic disease, neoplasia, and renal inflammatory disease [184]. To exclude cystic disease in general, careful sonographic and CT evaluations could be carried out. In the course of the disease, late renal involvement with metastatic disease or lymphomas usually occurs that is well documented. Most often, multifocal renal cell carcinoma is seen in the context of von Hippel-Lindau disease together with its other clinical manifestations. Similar to malacoplakia, signs and symptoms of UTI are usually available in the patients with xanthogranulomatous pyelonephritis and the involved kidney is enlarged; however, renal calculi and obstruction are common. Multiple renal abscesses are often the result of hematogenous dissemination originated by cardiac disease.

### 8.7 Management

To stabilize the disease process and to manage malacoplakia, the control of the UTIs should be the target of the treatment [168].

An antibiotic with an excellent cell membrane penetration is the cornerstone of treatment that fluoroquinolones are effective in up to 80 -90% of cases and since their debut in the

early 90's, they have been the greatest support in the literature to manage the disease [176, 185]. They have been the first choice of treatment due to the easy passage through the macrophage and histiocyte cell wall providing high concentrations there [179, 186].
Despite the use of various long-term antimicrobial agents such as many antituberculosis agents, however, the sulfonamides, rifampin, doxycycline, and TMP are found to be particularly useful owing to their intracellular bactericidal activity [179, 185].
In the patients that receive immunosuppressive therapy for any reason, the suspension of their medications is advisable during the treatment period.
As phagocytic dysfunction is supposedly the reason behind the malacoplakia, the use of ascorbic acid (Vitamin C) and cholinergic agents such as bethanechol in conjunction with antimicrobial therapy have been reported with good results in the restoration of phagocytic function [168, 179]. It is believed that the aforesaid agents work through increasing intracellular cyclic guanosine monophosphate levels (cGMP) that its biologic defect seemingly leads to macrophage dysfunction and its availability restores lysosomal function that in turn enhances phagocytosis.
If the disease progresses in spite of antimicrobial treatment, surgical intervention could be indicated that for the treatment of symptomatic unilateral renal lesions, nephrectomy is usually performed. As to the often very aggressive nature of the retroperitoneal involvement, it could be fatal [176, 179].
Prognosis seems appropriate to the extent of the disease in the long-term. In bilateral parenchymal renal malacoplakia or in the transplanted kidney the survival is usually limited to 6 months [179, 186]. On the opposite, the long-term survival after nephrectomy in the unilateral disease is good that in a literature review in 2003, the survival rate was found to be over 90% in such patients. Nonetheless due to the possible long-term relapse, these patients must always undergo close evaluation periodically [176].

## 9. References


[1] Best, C.D., et al., Clinical and radiological findings in patients with gas forming renal abscess treated conservatively. J Urol, 1999. 162(4): p. 1273-6.

[2] Rinder, M.R., Renal abscess: an illustrative case and review of the literature. Md Med J, 1996. 45(10): p. 839-43.

[3] Cheng, C.H., et al., Renal abscess in children: a 10-year clinical and radiologic experience in a tertiary medical center. Pediatr Infect Dis J, 2008. 27(11): p. 1025-7.

[4] D'Cruz, S., et al., Isolation of Salmonella paratyphi A from renal abscess. Indian J Pathol Microbiol, 2009. 52(1): p. 117-9.

[5] Dravid, M. and B.N. Joshi, Renal abscess due to Salmonella typhimurium. Indian J Pediatr, 1990. 57(4): p. 586-8.

[6] Valbuena Alvarez, R., et al., [Acute systemic nocardiosis. Renal abscess]. Arch Esp Urol, 1996. 49(5): p. 529-31.

[7] Osanai, S., et al., Renal abscess with Morganella morganii complicating leukemoid reaction. Intern Med, 2008. 47(1): p. 51-5.

[8] Woods, C.R. and M.S. Edwards, Renal abscess caused by group B Streptococcus. Clin Infect Dis, 1994. 18(4): p. 662-3.

[9] Lin, M.F., et al., Serratia marcescens renal abscess with endophthalmitis: a case report. J Microbiol Immunol Infect, 1998. 31(4): p. 245-8.

[10] Metta, H., et al., Renal abscess due to Aspergillus fumigatus as the only sign of disseminated aspergillosis in a patient with AIDS. Rev Iberoam Micol, 2010. 27(3): p. 136-9.
[11] Colebunders, R., et al., Renal abscess due to Mycobacterium avium complex in a human immunodeficiency virus-positive patient. Int J Infect Dis, 2002. 6(3): p. 238-9.
[12] Chen, K.J., et al., Endogenous Klebsiella pneumoniae endophthalmitis with renal abscess: Report of two cases. Int J Infect Dis, 2010. 14(5): p. e429-32.
[13] Olson, E.S., et al., A case report of renal abscess caused by Salmonella virchow phage type 1 associated with a papillary renal cell carcinoma. J Infect, 1999. 38(1): p. 56-7.
[14] Shoji, S., et al., [Renal infarction with renal abscess onset due to infective endocarditis: a case report]. Hinyokika Kiyo, 2008. 54(3): p. 221-3.
[15] Chang, S.W., et al., Klebsiella pneumoniae renal abscess. Zhonghua Yi Xue Za Zhi (Taipei), 2000. 63(10): p. 721-8.
[16] Shimizu, M., et al., Evolution of acute focal bacterial nephritis into a renal abscess. Pediatr Nephrol, 2005. 20(1): p. 93-5.
[17] Steele, B.T., C. Petrou, and J. de Maria, Renal abscess in children. Urology, 1990. 36(4): p. 325-8.
[18] Sugao, H., H. Takiuchi, and T. Sakurai, Acute focal bacterial nephritis and renal abscess associated with vesicoureteral reflux. Report of a case. Urol Int, 1988. 43(4): p. 253-6.
[19] Wang, Y.T., et al., Renal abscess in children: a clinical retrospective study. Acta Paediatr Taiwan, 2003. 44(4): p. 197-201.
[20] Pieretti, R.V., R. Pieretti-Vanmarcke, and A. Pieretti, Renal abscess in previously healthy girl. Urology, 2009. 73(2): p. 297-8.
[21] Ybarra, M.E., L. D'Ambrosio, and A. Fioravanti, [Renal abscess]. Arch Argent Pediatr, 2011. 109(2): p. 173-174.
[22] Constantine, S. and J. Kaye, Metastatic renal abscess mimicking Wilms' tumour. Pediatr Radiol, 2004. 34(11): p. 924-6.
[23] Sule, A.Z., Undiagnosed renal abscess presenting as acute bacterial peritonitis: case report. East Afr Med J, 2001. 78(9): p. 500-1.
[24] Deryckere, A., et al., [Endogenous Klebsiella pneumoniae endophthalmitis secondary to a renal abscess: a case report]. J Fr Ophtalmol, 2009. 32(4): p. 280-3.
[25] Gillitzer, R., et al., Transitional cell carcinoma of the renal pelvis presenting as a renal abscess. Urology, 2002. 60(1): p. 165.
[26] Perimenis, P., Pyonephrosis and renal abscess associated with kidney tumours. Br J Urol, 1991. 68(5): p. 463-5.
[27] Kawashima, A., C.M. Sandler, and S.M. Goldman, Imaging in acute renal infection. BJU Int, 2000. 86 Suppl 1: p. 70-9.
[28] Hoddick, W., et al., CT and sonography of severe renal and perirenal infections. AJR Am J Roentgenol, 1983. 140(3): p. 517-20.
[29] Soulen, M.C., E.K. Fishman, and S.M. Goldman, Sequelae of acute renal infections: CT evaluation. Radiology, 1989. 173(2): p. 423-6.
[30] Kumar, R., et al., Indium-111 leukocyte scanning. False-negative study in a renal abscess. Clin Nucl Med, 1986. 11(4): p. 274-5.
[31] Siegel, J.F., A. Smith, and R. Moldwin, Minimally invasive treatment of renal abscess. J Urol, 1996. 155(1): p. 52-5.
[32] Hung, C.H., et al., Immediate percutaneous drainage compared with surgical drainage of renal abscess. Int Urol Nephrol, 2007. 39(1): p. 51-5.

[33] Gardiner, R.A., R.A. Gwynne, and S.A. Roberts, Perinephric abscess. BJU Int, 2011. 107 Suppl 3: p. 20-3.
[34] Ko, M.C., et al., Incidence of renal and perinephric abscess in diabetic patients: a population-based national study. Epidemiol Infect, 2011. 139(2): p. 229-35.
[35] Hutchison, F.N. and G.A. Kaysen, Perinephric abscess: the missed diagnosis. Med Clin North Am, 1988. 72(5): p. 993-1014.
[36] Truesdale, B.H., S.N. Rous, and R.P. Nelson, Perinephric abscess: a review of 26 cases. J Urol, 1977. 118(6): p. 910-1.
[37] Al-Soub, H., et al., Shigella flexneri perinephric abscess and bacteremia. Ann Saudi Med, 2005. 25(5): p. 419-21.
[38] Vaidyanathan, S., et al., Superinfection of perinephric abscess by Stenotrophomonas maltophilia in a tetraplegic patient. Spinal Cord, 2005. 43(6): p. 394-5.
[39] D'Cruz, S., et al., Isolated nocardial subcapsular and perinephric abscess. Indian J Pathol Microbiol, 2004. 47(1): p. 24-6.
[40] Baumgardner, D.J., Perinephric abscess caused by group B streptococcus. Am Fam Physician, 2004. 69(12): p. 2764, 2766.
[41] Khemakhem, B., et al., [Candida glabrata perinephric abscess. A case report]. Ann Med Interne (Paris), 2001. 152(2): p. 134-6.
[42] Rajesh, G.D., et al., Perinephric abscess due to Aspergillus fumigatus. Indian J Pediatr, 2000. 67(7): p. 545-6.
[43] Gomber, S., et al., Perinephric abscess (presenting as abdominal pain) due to Listeria monocytogenes. Ann Trop Paediatr, 1998. 18(1): p. 61-2.
[44] Chitnavis, V. and C.R. Magnussen, Perinephric abscess due to a coagulase-negative Staphylococcus: case report and review of the literature. J Urol, 1993. 149(6): p. 1530-1.
[45] Rigg, K.M. and J.R. Sainsbury, Salmonella perinephric abscess. Br J Hosp Med, 1986. 36(4): p. 284-5.
[46] Khauli, R.B., S. Kalash, and J.D. Young, Jr., Torulopsis glabrata perinephric abscess. J Urol, 1983. 130(5): p. 968-70.
[47] Thompson, W.C. and J.W. Brock, 3rd, Torulopsis glabrata perinephric abscess: a case report. J Urol, 1983. 130(3): p. 529-30.
[48] Wunderlich, H.F., et al., Bacteroides fragilis perinephric abscess. J Urol, 1980. 123(4): p. 601-2.
[49] Suriyanon, V., K.E. Nelson, and V. Choomsai na Ayudhya, Trichomonas vaginalis in a perinephric abscess. A case report. Am J Trop Med Hyg, 1975. 24(5): p. 776-80.
[50] Camara, B., et al., Perihepatitis and perinephric abscess due to Mycoplasma hominis in a kidney transplant patient. Exp Clin Transplant, 2007. 5(2): p. 708-9.
[51] Santoro-Lopes, G., M. Halpern, and R.T. Goncalves, Perinephric abscess caused by Streptococcus agalactiae after renal transplantation. J Infect, 2005. 51(3): p. e145-7.
[52] Shohaib, S., Nocardial psoas and perinephric abscess in a renal transplant treated by surgery and antibiotics. Nephrol Dial Transplant, 1994. 9(8): p. 1209-10.
[53] Finkelhor, R.S., et al., Gardnerella vaginalis perinephric abscess in a transplanted kidney. N Engl J Med, 1981. 304(14): p. 846.
[54] Edelstein, H.E., R.E. McCabe, and E. Lieberman, Perinephric abscess in renal transplant recipients: report of seven cases and review. Rev Infect Dis, 1989. 11(4): p. 569-77.
[55] Maldonado-Alcaraz, E., et al., [Perinephric abscess: associated factors and mortality]. Arch Esp Urol, 2008. 61(1): p. 7-12.

[56] Harrow, B.R., Spontaneous urinary extravasation associated with renal colic causing a perinephric abscess. Am J Roentgenol Radium Ther Nucl Med, 1966. 98(1): p. 47-53.
[57] Feldman, M.A., R.E. Cotton, and W.M. Gray, Carcinoma of the colon presenting as left perinephric abscess. Br J Surg, 1968. 55(1): p. 21-6.
[58] Chintapalli, K., et al., Perinephric abscess with renal cell carcinoma. Urol Radiol, 1981. 3(2): p. 113-5.
[59] Karamalegos, A.Z., A.C. Diokno, and D.F. Moylan, Formation of perinephric abscess following extracorporeal shock-wave lithotripsy. Urology, 1989. 34(5): p. 277-80.
[60] Kochakarn, W. and K. Ratana-Olarn, Late perinephric abscess formation after extracorporeal shock wave lithotripsy. Br J Urol, 1991. 68(3): p. 323-4.
[61] Pautler, S.E., J.F. Vallely, and J.D. Denstedt, Perinephric abscess following extracorporeal shockwave lithotripsy. Can J Urol, 1998. 5(4): p. 623-626.
[62] Reese, J.H., R.U. Anderson, and G. Friedland, Splenic abscess arising by direct extension from a perinephric abscess. Urol Radiol, 1990. 12(2): p. 91-3.
[63] Reiber, K. and I. Leventhal, Splenic abscess as complication of perinephric abscess. Urology, 1987. 30(3): p. 269-71.
[64] Kao, C.T., et al., Right perinephric abscess: a rare presentation of ruptured retrocecal appendicitis. Pediatr Nephrol, 2002. 17(3): p. 177-80.
[65] Wani, N.A., et al., Perinephric abscess caused by ruptured retrocecal appendix: MDCT demonstration. Urol Ann, 2010. 2(1): p. 29-31.
[66] High, K.P. and V.J. Quagliarello, Yeast perinephric abscess: report of a case and review. Clin Infect Dis, 1992. 15(1): p. 128-33.
[67] McLellan, R.A., M.A. Fischer, and P. Belitsky, Perinephric abscess presenting as chronic diarrhea. Can J Urol, 2000. 7(2): p. 983-5.
[68] Khan, A., M.Z. Hotiana, and S. Khan, Perinephric abscess presenting as acute peritonitis. Trop Doct, 1993. 23(1): p. 32.
[69] Runyon, B.A., Bacterial peritonitis secondary to a perinephric abscess. Case report and differentiation from spontaneous bacterial peritonitis. Am J Med, 1986. 80(5): p. 997-8.
[70] Curran, A.J., et al., Perinephric abscess as a presentation of pancreatitis. Br J Urol, 1993. 71(1): p. 97-8.
[71] Teelucksingh, S., et al., Perinephric abscess mimicking fulminant hepatic failure. West Indian Med J, 1994. 43(2): p. 66-7.
[72] Tsukagoshi, D., et al., Perinephric abscess secondary to a staghorn calculus presenting as a subcutaneous abscess. CJEM, 2006. 8(4): p. 285-8.
[73] Hampel, N., T.A. Sidor, and L. Persky, Nephrobronchial fistula. Complication of perinephric abscess secondary to ureteral obstruction and pyonephrosis. Urology, 1980. 16(6): p. 608-10.
[74] Stojadinovic, M., S. Micic, and D. Milovanovic, Ultrasonographic and computed tomography findings in renal suppurations: performance indicators and risks for diagnostic failure. Urol Int, 2008. 80(4): p. 389-97.
[75] Sweet, R. and W.F. Keane, Perinephric abscess in patients with polycystic kidney disease undergoing chronic hemodialysis. Nephron, 1979. 23(5): p. 237-40.
[76] Bickel, A., I. Waxman, and A. Eitan, Laparoscopic treatment of a perinephric abscess. Surg Endosc, 1995. 9(4): p. 437-8.
[77] Tamura, K., et al., Successful treatment for perinephric abscess with recombinant human granulocyte colony-stimulating factor following nephrectomy in a patient of myelodysplastic syndrome: a case report. Biotherapy, 1990. 2(3): p. 223-6.

[78] Brook, I., Urinary tract and genito-urinary suppurative infections due to anaerobic bacteria. Int J Urol, 2004. 11(3): p. 133-41.
[79] Chijioke, A., Current concepts on pathogenesis of renal tuberculosis. West Afr J Med, 2001. 20(2): p. 107-10.
[80] Sharma, S., A. Mohta, and P. Sharma, Neonatal pyonephrosis--a case report. Int Urol Nephrol, 2004. 36(3): p. 313-5.
[81] Watson, R.A., et al., Percutaneous nephrostomy as adjunct management in advanced upper urinary tract infection. Urology, 1999. 54(2): p. 234-9.
[82] Watt, I. and J. Roylance, Pyonephrosis. Clin Radiol, 1976. 27(4): p. 513-19.
[83] Christoph, F., et al., How septic is urosepsis? Clinical course of infected hydronephrosis and therapeutic strategies. World J Urol, 2005. 23(4): p. 243-7.
[84] Kirk, D., Silent pyonephrosis as a cause of chronic ill-health. Lancet, 1982. 1(8274): p. 705-7.
[85] Wu, T.T., et al., The role of C-reactive protein and erythrocyte sedimentation rate in the diagnosis of infected hydronephrosis and pyonephrosis. J Urol, 1994. 152(1): p. 26-8.
[86] Subramanyam, B.R., et al., Sonography of pyonephrosis: a prospective study. AJR Am J Roentgenol, 1983. 140(5): p. 991-3.
[87] Chan, J.H., et al., MR diffusion-weighted imaging of kidney: differentiation between hydronephrosis and pyonephrosis. Clin Imaging, 2001. 25(2): p. 110-3.
[88] Baumgarten, D.A. and B.R. Baumgartner, Imaging and radiologic management of upper urinary tract infections. Urol Clin North Am, 1997. 24(3): p. 545-69.
[89] Chisena, S., [Echoguided percutaneous nephrostomy]. Arch Ital Urol Androl, 1998. 70(3): p. 133-6.
[90] Lledo Garcia, E., et al., [Initial treatment of pyonephrosis using percutaneous nephrostomy. Value of the technique]. Arch Esp Urol, 1993. 46(8): p. 711-8.
[91] Yoder, I.C., K.K. Lindfors, and R.C. Pfister, Diagnosis and treatment of pyonephrosis. Radiol Clin North Am, 1984. 22(2): p. 407-14.
[92] Li, Y. and Y. Zhang, Diagnosis and treatment of acute focal bacterial nephritis. Chin Med J (Engl), 1996. 109(2): p. 168-72.
[93] Klar, A., et al., Focal bacterial nephritis (lobar nephronia) in children. J Pediatr, 1996. 128(6): p. 850-3.
[94] Frosch, M., et al., [Acute focal bacterial nephritis in childhood]. Monatsschr Kinderheilkd, 1987. 135(12): p. 842-6.
[95] Loberant, N., et al., Acute focal bacterial nephritis in childhood brucellosis. Pediatr Radiol, 1995. 25 Suppl 1: p. S62-4.
[96] Patterson, J.E. and V.T. Andriole, Bacterial urinary tract infections in diabetes. Infect Dis Clin North Am, 1997. 11(3): p. 735-50.
[97] Qin, J.Y., [Acute focal bacterial nephritis: report of 7 cases]. Zhonghua Wai Ke Za Zhi, 1990. 28(7): p. 405-6, 445.
[98] Shinoda, G., et al., [A pediatric case of acute focal bacterial nephritis; comparison with the reports in Japanese child cases]. Kansenshogaku Zasshi, 2001. 75(11): p. 981-8.
[99] You, K., et al., [Focal infectious lesions of the renal parenchyma. Comparative contribution of echography and x-ray computed tomography]. J Radiol, 1988. 69(8-9): p. 509-16.
[100] Soulen, M.C., et al., Bacterial renal infection: role of CT. Radiology, 1989. 171(3): p. 703-7.

[101] Cheng, C.H., et al., Effective ultrasonographic predictor for the diagnosis of acute lobar nephronia. Pediatr Infect Dis J, 2004. 23(1): p. 11-4.
[102] Farmer, K.D., L.R. Gellett, and P.A. Dubbins, The sonographic appearance of acute focal pyelonephritis 8 years experience. Clin Radiol, 2002. 57(6): p. 483-7.
[103] Granados Molina, A., et al., [Acute lobar nephronia: Diagnosis, treatment and prognosis]. An Pediatr (Barc), 2007. 66(1): p. 84-6.
[104] Huang, J.J., et al., Acute bacterial nephritis: a clinicoradiologic correlation based on computed tomography. Am J Med, 1992. 93(3): p. 289-98.
[105] Cheng, C.H., Y.K. Tsau, and T.Y. Lin, Effective duration of antimicrobial therapy for the treatment of acute lobar nephronia. Pediatrics, 2006. 117(1): p. e84-9.
[106] Eke, N. and R.C. Echem, Chronic pyonephrosis associated with renal neovascularisation. Afr J Med Med Sci, 2004. 33(3): p. 267-9.
[107] Huland, H. and R. Busch, Chronic pyelonephritis as a cause of end stage renal disease. J Urol, 1982. 127(4): p. 642-3.
[108] Guarino, N., et al., Natural history of vesicoureteral reflux associated with kidney anomalies. Urology, 2005. 65(6): p. 1208-11.
[109] Pylkkanen, J., J. Vilska, and O. Koskimies, The value of level diagnosis of childhood urinary tract infection in predicting renal injury. Acta Paediatr Scand, 1981. 70(6): p. 879-83.
[110] Chand, D.H., et al., Incidence and severity of vesicoureteral reflux in children related to age, gender, race and diagnosis. J Urol, 2003. 170(4 Pt 2): p. 1548-50.
[111] Kohler, J.R., et al., Long-term effects of reflux nephropathy on blood pressure and renal function in adults. Nephron Clin Pract, 2003. 93(1): p. C35-46.
[112] Kohler, J., et al., Vesicoureteral reflux diagnosed in adulthood. Incidence of urinary tract infections, hypertension, proteinuria, back pain and renal calculi. Nephrol Dial Transplant, 1997. 12(12): p. 2580-7.
[113] Roberts, J.A., Mechanisms of renal damage in chronic pyelonephritis (reflux nephropathy). Curr Top Pathol, 1995. 88: p. 265-87.
[114] Braude, A.I., Current concepts of pyelonephritis. Medicine (Baltimore), 1973. 52(4): p. 257-64.
[115] Wennerstrom, M., et al., Primary and acquired renal scarring in boys and girls with urinary tract infection. J Pediatr, 2000. 136(1): p. 30-4.
[116] Tsuji, T., et al., Chronic pyelonephritis presenting as multiple tumor-like renal lesions. Intern Med, 2007. 46(12): p. 879-82.
[117] Alan, C., S. Ataus, and B. Tunc, Xanthogranulamatous pyelonephritis with psoas abscess: 2 cases and review of the literature. Int Urol Nephrol, 2004. 36(4): p. 489-93.
[118] Kawashima, A. and A.J. LeRoy, Radiologic evaluation of patients with renal infections. Infect Dis Clin North Am, 2003. 17(2): p. 433-56.
[119] Papadopoulos, G.I., et al., Chronic pyelonephritis presenting as a renal sinus tumor with retroperitoneal extension: a case report. J Med Case Reports, 2009. 3: p. 9054.
[120] Stoller, M.L. and B.A. Kogan, Sensitivity of 99mtechnetium-dimercaptosuccinic acid for the diagnosis of chronic pyelonephritis: clinical and theoretical considerations. J Urol, 1986. 135(5): p. 977-80.
[121] Craig, W.D., B.J. Wagner, and M.D. Travis, Pyelonephritis: radiologic-pathologic review. Radiographics, 2008. 28(1): p. 255-77; quiz 327-8.
[122] Chishti, A.S., et al., A guideline for the inpatient care of children with pyelonephritis. Ann Saudi Med, 2010. 30(5): p. 341-9.
[123] Michaeli, J., et al., Emphysematous pyelonephritis. J Urol, 1984. 131(2): p. 203-8.

[124] Pontin, A.R., et al., Emphysematous pyelonephritis in diabetic patients. Br J Urol, 1995. 75(1): p. 71-4.
[125] Kelly, H.A., XI. A Preliminary Report upon the Examination of the Bladder and Catheterization of the Ureters in Men. Ann Surg, 1898. 27(1): p. 71-3.
[126] Schultz, E.H., Jr. and E.H. Klorfein, Emphysematous pyelonephritis. J Urol, 1962. 87: p. 762-6.
[127] Somani, B.K., et al., Is percutaneous drainage the new gold standard in the management of emphysematous pyelonephritis? Evidence from a systematic review. J Urol, 2008. 179(5): p. 1844-9.
[128] Shokeir, A.A., et al., Emphysematous pyelonephritis: a 15-year experience with 20 cases. Urology, 1997. 49(3): p. 343-6.
[129] Narlawar, R.S., et al., Imaging features and guided drainage in emphysematous pyelonephritis: a study of 11 cases. Clin Radiol, 2004. 59(2): p. 192-7.
[130] Huang, J.J. and C.C. Tseng, Emphysematous pyelonephritis: clinicoradiological classification, management, prognosis, and pathogenesis. Arch Intern Med, 2000. 160(6): p. 797-805.
[131] Falagas, M.E., et al., Risk factors for mortality in patients with emphysematous pyelonephritis: a meta-analysis. J Urol, 2007. 178(3 Pt 1): p. 880-5; quiz 1129.
[132] Khaira, A., et al., Retrospective analysis of clinical profile prognostic factors and outcomes of 19 patients of emphysematous pyelonephritis. Int Urol Nephrol, 2009. 41(4): p. 959-66.
[133] Wan, Y.L., et al., Acute gas-producing bacterial renal infection: correlation between imaging findings and clinical outcome. Radiology, 1996. 198(2): p. 433-8.
[134] Ubee, S.S., L. McGlynn, and M. Fordham, Emphysematous pyelonephritis. BJU Int, 2010.
[135] Tang, H.J., et al., Clinical characteristics of emphysematous pyelonephritis. J Microbiol Immunol Infect, 2001. 34(2): p. 125-30.
[136] Abdul-Halim, H., et al., Severe emphysematous pyelonephritis in diabetic patients: diagnosis and aspects of surgical management. Urol Int, 2005. 75(2): p. 123-8.
[137] Kuo, Y.T., et al., Emphysematous pyelonephritis: imaging diagnosis and follow-up. Kaohsiung J Med Sci, 1999. 15(3): p. 159-70.
[138] Wan, Y.L., et al., Predictors of outcome in emphysematous pyelonephritis. J Urol, 1998. 159(2): p. 369-73.
[139] Ahlering, T.E., et al., Emphysematous pyelonephritis: a 5-year experience with 13 patients. J Urol, 1985. 134(6): p. 1086-8.
[140] Hudson, M.A., et al., Emphysematous pyelonephritis: successful management by percutaneous drainage. J Urol, 1986. 136(4): p. 884-6.
[141] Chen, M.T., et al., Percutaneous drainage in the treatment of emphysematous pyelonephritis: 10-year experience. J Urol, 1997. 157(5): p. 1569-73.
[142] Bauman, N., et al., Laparoscopic nephrectomy for emphysematous pyelonephritis. Can J Urol, 2005. 12(4): p. 2764-8.
[143] Parsons, M.A., et al., Xanthogranulomatous pyelonephritis: a pathological, clinical and aetiological analysis of 87 cases. Diagn Histopathol, 1983. 6(3-4): p. 203-19.
[144] Izzidien, A.Y., et al., Xanthogranulomatous pyelonephritis in childhood. J Pediatr Surg, 1980. 15(5): p. 686-9.
[145] Sugie, S., et al., Fine-needle aspiration cytology of xanthogranulomatous pyelonephritis. Urology, 1991. 37(4): p. 376-9.

[146] Youngson, G.G. and E.S. Gray, Neonatal xanthogranulomatous pyelonephritis. Br J Urol, 1990. 65(5): p. 541-2.
[147] Malek, R.S. and J.S. Elder, Xanthogranulomatous pyelonephritis: a critical analysis of 26 cases and of the literature. J Urol, 1978. 119(5): p. 589-93.
[148] Schoborg, T.W., et al., Xanthogranulomatous pyelonephritis associated with renal carcinoma. J Urol, 1980. 124(1): p. 125-27.
[149] Gregg, C.R., T.E. Rogers, and R.S. Munford, Xanthogranulomatous pyelonephritis. Curr Clin Top Infect Dis, 1999. 19: p. 287-304.
[150] Levy, M., R. Baumal, and A.A. Eddy, Xanthogranulomatous pyelonephritis in children. Etiology, pathogenesis, clinical and radiologic features, and management. Clin Pediatr (Phila), 1994. 33(6): p. 360-6.
[151] Chuang, C.K., et al., Xanthogranulomatous pyelonephritis: experience in 36 cases. J Urol, 1992. 147(2): p. 333-6.
[152] Nataluk, E.A., D.L. McCullough, and E.O. Scharling, Xanthogranulomatous pyelonephritis, the gatekeeper's dilemma: a contemporary look at an old problem. Urology, 1995. 45(3): p. 377-80.
[153] Grainger, R.G., A.J. Longstaff, and M.A. Parsons, Xanthogranulomatous pyelonephritis: a reappraisal. Lancet, 1982. 1(8286): p. 1398-401.
[154] Eastham, J., T. Ahlering, and E. Skinner, Xanthogranulomatous pyelonephritis: clinical findings and surgical considerations. Urology, 1994. 43(3): p. 295-9.
[155] Zugor, V., G.E. Schott, and A.P. Labanaris, Xanthogranulomatous pyelonephritis in childhood: a critical analysis of 10 cases and of the literature. Urology, 2007. 70(1): p. 157-60.
[156] McDonald, G.S., Xanthogranulomatous pyelonephritis. J Pathol, 1981. 133(3): p. 203-13.
[157] Tolia, B.M., et al., Xanthogranulomatous pyelonephritis: detailed analysis of 29 cases and a brief discussion of atypical presentations. J Urol, 1981. 126(4): p. 437-42.
[158] Gupta, S., C.E. Araya, and V.R. Dharnidharka, Xanthogranulomatous pyelonephritis in pediatric patients: case report and review of literature. J Pediatr Urol, 2010. 6(4): p. 355-8.
[159] Korkes, F., et al., Xanthogranulomatous pyelonephritis: clinical experience with 41 cases. Urology, 2008. 71(2): p. 178-80.
[160] Hartman, D.S., et al., Xanthogranulomatous pyelonephritis: sonographic--pathologic correlation of 16 cases. J Ultrasound Med, 1984. 3(11): p. 481-8.
[161] Demertzis, J. and C.O. Menias, State of the art: imaging of renal infections. Emerg Radiol, 2007. 14(1): p. 13-22.
[162] Hertle, L., et al., Computed tomography in xanthogranulomatous pyelonephritis. Eur Urol, 1984. 10(6): p. 385-8.
[163] Goldman, S.M., et al., CT of xanthogranulomatous pyelonephritis: radiologic-pathologic correlation. AJR Am J Roentgenol, 1984. 142(5): p. 963-9.
[164] Soler, R., et al., Focal xanthogranulomatous pyelonephritis in a teenager: MR and CT findings. Eur J Radiol, 1997. 24(1): p. 77-9.
[165] Brown, P.S., Jr., M. Dodson, and P.S. Weintrub, Xanthogranulomatous pyelonephritis: report of nonsurgical management of a case and review of the literature. Clin Infect Dis, 1996. 22(2): p. 308-14.
[166] Tsai, K.H., et al., Bilateral xanthogranulomatous pyelonephritis. J Chin Med Assoc, 2008. 71(6): p. 310-4.
[167] Tobias-Machado, M., et al., Laparoscopic nephrectomy in inflammatory renal disease: proposal for a staged approach. Int Braz J Urol, 2005. 31(1): p. 22-8.

[168] Stanton, M.J. and W. Maxted, Malacoplakia: a study of the literature and current concepts of pathogenesis, diagnosis and treatment. J Urol, 1981. 125(2): p. 139-46.
[169] Dobyan, D.C., L.D. Truong, and G. Eknoyan, Renal malacoplakia reappraised. Am J Kidney Dis, 1993. 22(2): p. 243-52.
[170] van Crevel, R., et al., Functional and morphological monocyte abnormalities in a patient with malakoplakia. Am J Med, 1998. 105(1): p. 74-7.
[171] Esparza, A.R., et al., Renal parenchymal malakoplakia. Histologic spectrum and its relationship to megalocytic interstitial nephritis and xanthogranulomatous pyelonephritis. Am J Surg Pathol, 1989. 13(3): p. 225-36.
[172] Callea, F., B. Van Damme, and V.J. Desmet, Alpha-1-antitrypsin in malakoplakia. Virchows Arch A Pathol Anat Histol, 1982. 395(1): p. 1-9.
[173] Sanchez, L.M., S.I. Sanchez, and J.L. Bailey, Malacoplakia presenting with obstructive nephropathy with bilateral ureter involvement. Nat Rev Nephrol, 2009. 5(7): p. 418-22.
[174] Ozkurkcugil, C., et al., A case of renal parenchymal malacoplakia with bilateral pulmonary lesions. Br J Urol, 1996. 77(1): p. 159-60.
[175] Koroku, M., et al., [Malacoplakia in the ureter and bladder]. Hinyokika Kiyo, 2005. 51(3): p. 183-5.
[176] Tam, V.K., et al., Renal parenchymal malacoplakia: a rare cause of ARF with a review of recent literature. Am J Kidney Dis, 2003. 41(6): p. E13-7.
[177] Yang, A.H., et al., Post-infectious glomerulonephritis in a patient with vesicorenal malacoplakia--coincidence or causal relationship? Nephrol Dial Transplant, 2000. 15(7): p. 1060-2.
[178] Sheerin, N.S., K.F. Bhatacharia, and M.C. Webb, Positron emission tomography in a patient with renal malacoplakia. Am J Kidney Dis, 2003. 42(3): p. E36-9.
[179] Velasquez Lopez, J.G., A. Velez Hoyos, and J.F. Uribe Arcila, [Malakoplakia in urology: six cases report and review of the literature]. Actas Urol Esp, 2006. 30(6): p. 610-8.
[180] Venkatesh, S.K., N. Mehrotra, and R.B. Gujral, Sonographic findings in renal parenchymal malacoplakia. J Clin Ultrasound, 2000. 28(7): p. 353-7.
[181] Mitchell, M.A., et al., Bilateral renal parenchymal malacoplakia presenting as fever of unknown origin: case report and review. Clin Infect Dis, 1994. 18(5): p. 704-18.
[182] Houston, T.K., 2nd, et al., Gallium-67-citrate scanning of renal parenchymal malacoplakia. J Nucl Med, 1998. 39(8): p. 1454-7.
[183] Trillo, A., W.B. Lorentz, and N.O. Whitley, Malakoplakia of kidney simulating renal neoplasm. Urology, 1977. 10(5): p. 472-7.
[184] Evans, N.L., J. French, and M.B. Rose, Renal malacoplakia: an important consideration in the differential diagnosis of renal masses in the presence of Escherichia coli infection. Br J Radiol, 1998. 71(850): p. 1083-5.
[185] Dohle, G.R., J. Zwartendijk, and J.H. Van Krieken, Urogenital malacoplakia treated with fluoroquinolones. J Urol, 1993. 150(5 Pt 1): p. 1518-20.
[186] Dasgupta, P., et al., Malacoplakia: von Hansemann's disease. BJU Int, 1999. 84(4): p. 464-9.

6

# Asymptomatic Bacteriuria: Significance for Different Patient Population

Thomas Nelius, Stephanie Filleur and Jonathan S. Nelson
*Texas Tech University Health Sciences Center*
*Departments of Urology and Microbiology*
*Lubbock*
*USA*

## 1. Introduction

Infections of the urinary tract (UTI) are one of the most common infections for which antibiotics are prescribed. Asymptomatic bacteriuria, or asymptomatic urinary infection, is a common condition (Nicolle, 2003). *Based on the microbiological definition, urinary tract infections are characterized by the presence of ≥$10^5$ colony-forming units per ml (CFUs/mL) of a single bacterial species or multiple organisms in two consecutive urine specimens, properly collected from a person with symptoms or signs of a UTI* (Rubin et al., 1992). However, the presence of a significant quantity of bacteria in the urine of an asymptomatic patient is known as asymptomatic bacteriuria. Quantitative criteria to establish the diagnosis of significant bacteriuria in an asymptomatic person are: 1. at least $10^5$ CFUs/mL of urine in a voided midstream, so called clean-catch specimen; and 2. at least 100 CFUs per mL of urine obtained by bladder catheterization. Despite several decades of research, there is still a considerable amount of controversy about the adequate management of bacteriuria. A common dilemma in clinical medicine is whether or not to treat asymptomatic bacteriuria. It is now recognized that certain patient characteristics can led to the development of symptomatic infections based on an asymptomatic bacteriuria. For several clinical scenarios, the antibiotic treatment of asymptomatic bacteriuria has been shown to improve patient outcomes. Based on clinical trials conducted over the last few decades, better recommendations for the management of bacteriuria in different patient population could be established. The Infectious Diseases Society of America (IDSA) established guidelines for the screening and treatment of asymptomatic bacteriuria (Nicolle et al., 2005). The optimal management depends significantly on specific patient characteristics, co-morbidities, and risk factors. Recent studies could prove that for certain patient populations, screening and treatment is beneficial or may be beneficial. However, for other clinical scenarios, screening and treatment for asymptomatic bacteriuria has not proven to be beneficial and therefore is highly controversial. Importantly, overtreatment of asymptomatic bacteriuria is a quality, safety, and cost issue. Recent studies have revealed a substantial gap between clinical practice, published guidelines, and recommendations (need reference). Treating physicians need to be aware that because of an increasing antimicrobial resistance, it is important to treat patients only if there is clear evidence of potential benefits. Therefore, in this chapter we review the most recent literature and provide up-to-date information for treating physicians on how to diagnose and when to treat asymptomatic bacteriuria.

### 1.1 Historical aspects

The use of quantitative urine cultures for the microbiological diagnosis of UTI was suggested and validated more than 50 years ago (Kass, 1957, 1962). If bacteria were isolated in quantitative counts of $\geq 10^5$ colony-forming units (CFU)/mL in a voided urine specimen from asymptomatic patients, the condition was described as asymptomatic bacteriuria. Interestingly, in this patient population the isolated organisms were always the same in paired specimens obtained by urinary catheterization. Quantitative counts of $\leq 10^5$ colony-forming units (CFU)/mL in a voided urine specimen usually resulted in a negative paired catheterized specimens. Therefore, $\leq 10^5$ colony-forming units (CFU)/mL in voided specimens were considered as contamination. The general acceptance and widespread use of this technique identified several clinically asymptomatic patient populations with an increased prevalence of positive urine cultures (Kunin, 1966). Specifically, pregnant women, patients with urogenital abnormalities, and patients with indwelling urethral catheters demonstrated a higher incidence of asymptomatic bacteriuria (Kunin, 1966). Antibiotic treatment of asymptomatic bacteriuria in pregnant women resulted in a significantly reduced incidence of pyelonephritis (Kass, 1962), which is considered an important concern in pregnancy. The obvious benefits of eradicating bacteriuria in asymptomatic pregnant women were interpreted to be generally applicable. Therefore, other patient populations with asymptomatic bacteriuria were also treated ordinarily (Kass, 1962). This treatment strategy was not based on clinical studies or facts, rather on the assumption that asymptomatic bacteriuria was consistently harmful in all populations and necessitated antibiotic treatment (Nicolle, 2006). Both basic and clinical research conducted over the last few decades, including long-term cohort studies and prospective randomized comparative trials in defined populations with asymptomatic bacteriuria, have improved the understanding of this clinical condition and addressed appropriate management (Nicolle, 2006).

## 2. Material and methods

To identify all relevant materials, comprehensive literature searches were performed via the data sources: MEDLINE, EMBASE, CINAHL and OVID using the key words: asymptomatic bacteriuria, pyuria, urinary tract infection, urine culture, UTI, antibiotic treatment. Relevant articles and references between 1962 and 2010 were reviewed and analyzed for data on the association between asymptomatic bacteriuria and antibiotic treatment. Reference lists from relevant review articles were also searched. Only articles published as formal papers in peer-reviewed journals were selected for inclusion if they reported outcomes of interest including potential benefits of antibiotic treatment for asymptomatic bacteriuria. The data base searches resulted in 1400 articles, of which 356 of 1400 pertained directly to asymptomatic bacteriuria and antibiotic treatment. The entirety of these articles was reviewed, forming the basis for the current review.

## 3. Results

### 3.1 Causes and pathogenesis of asymptomatic bacteriuria

The normal upper and lower urinary tract is considered sterile, except for the distal end of the urethra. Colonization with bacteria or development of an asymptomatic bacteriuria occurs due to ascension of bacteria into the urinary bladder or into the upper urinary tract, including the kidneys. Typically, the bacteria isolated from patients with asymptomatic bacteriuria are part of the normal colonizing flora of the periurethral area, vagina, or bowel. The most common organism isolated from patients with asymptomatic bacteriuria is almost uniformly Escherichia coli (Bennett et al., 1995, Hooton et al., 2000, Kunin et al., 1964, Leblanc &McGanity, 1964, Nicolle et al., 1983, Nicolle et al., 1987, Zhanel et al., 1995), with only two exceptions. In elderly institutionalized men, common organisms include Pseudomonas mirabilis, Providencia spp, and Pseudomonas aeruginosa. In patients with spinal cord injuries, only Klebsiella pneumonia and Streptococcus spp are more common (Bennett et al., 1995, Nicolle et al., 1983). However, a large variety of different bacteria can be isolated, including Citrobacter spp, Enterococcus spp, coagulase-negative staphylococcus species, and others (Bennett et al., 1995, Hooton et al., 2000, Kunin et al., 1964, Nicolle et al., 1983, Nicolle et al., 1987, Zhanel et al., 1995). The mechanisms causing asymptomatic bacteriuria are still not fully understood. Characterization and comparison of Escherichia coli strains from patients with asymptomatic bacteriuria and acute uncomplicated urinary infection/acute nonobstructive pyelonephritis revealed a lower frequency of genetic markers or phenotypic expression of potential virulence factors (Geerlings et al., 2001, Stenqvist et al., 1987, Svanborg &Godaly, 1997). The expression of virulence factors seems to be a key event determining symptoms or persistence (Andersson et al., 1991). Interestingly, several authors reported a local response even in the absence of clinical symptoms. A local response includes mainly pyuria (Bachman et al., 1993, Hooton et al., 2000, Kincaid-Smith &Bullen, 1965, Kunin et al., 1964, Nicolle, 1997, 2001, Zhanel et al., 1995), although other local inflammatory or immune markers, including cytokines and urinary immunoglobulins, may also be present (Nicolle, 1997, Svanborg &Godaly, 1997).

### 3.2 Diagnostic

#### 3.2.1 Urine culture

To establish the diagnosis of bacteriuria, a urine specimen for culture is necessary. There is a general agreement for men and women in the definition of the diagnostic approach in order to make the diagnosis bacteriuria (Evans et al., 1978, Gleckman et al., 1979, Hooton et al., 2000, Kunin, 1966, Lipsky et al., 1987, Ouslander et al., 1987, Rubin et al., 1992).

For men, a quantitative count of a potential uropathogen of $\geq 10^5$ CFU/mL in a single voided midstream clean-catch specimen or at least 100 CFUs per mL of urine from a catheterized specimen are reliable for identification of bacteriuria (Gleckman et al., 1979, Lipsky, 1989, Lipsky et al., 1987, Saint &Chenoweth, 2003, Warren et al., 1982). Exception exists for elderly men with external condom catheters. For this patient population, a quantitative count of $\geq 10^5$ CFU/mL is necessary for the diagnosis. The results were obtained by comparison with bacterial counts of concurrent catheterized specimens (Nicolle et al., 1988, Ouslander et al., 1987). Quantitative counts $\leq 10^5$ CFU/mL are consistent of bacterial colonization with periurethral organisms or contamination from the condom catheter itself.

For women, a quantitative count of a potential uropathogen of $\geq 10^5$ CFU/mL in at least two consecutive voided midstream clean-catch specimen or at least 100 CFUs per mL of urine from a catheterized specimen are reliable for identification of bacteriuria and the recommended standard (Kunin, 1966, Nicolle, 2003, Nicolle et al., 2005, Rubin et al., 1992). Identification of bacteriuria in women based on a single voided specimen has been reported to be 80% specific, and 95% specific for two specimens (Kunin et al., 1964, Rubin et al., 1992). The fact that there is an 80% concordance rate between the first and the second voided urine specimen is often related to a transient bacteriuria, a condition common in young women (Hooton et al., 2000).

According to the IDSA guideline, the criteria for identification of bacteriuria in specimens obtained from catheterized patients are similar for women and men. (Saint &Chenoweth, 2003). However, some authors defined bacteriuria differently in their studies, ranging from identification in a single voided urine (Geerlings et al., 2000, Hooton et al., 2000) to those requiring persistent bacteriuria from two or more specimens (Evans et al., 1978).

### 3.2.2 Nonculture urine tests

Nonculture urine tests are widely used in primary care settings to evaluate urinary symptoms or as a screening test. The sensitivity and specificity of nonculture urine tests are insufficient to diagnose bacteriuria in asymptomatic patients. Nonculture urine tests are the so called dipstick tests and are designed to identify leukocyte esterase and nitrite in the urine specimen. A urine dipstick leukocyte esterase test showing pyuria has a sensitivity of 75 to 96 percent and specificity of 94 to 98 percent (Sobel, 2005). However, the test is not specific enough and may also be positive with other inflammatory conditions of the genitourinary tract (e.g., vaginitis). Frequently, patient with asymptomatic bacteriuria do not have pyuria. The urine dipstick nitrite test has several limitations, and therefore has a high false-negative rate. Importantly, the test is unable to diagnose bacteriuria with non-nitrite–producing pathogens (Kunin &DeGroot, 1975). Both a delay between urine sample collection and testing, and insufficient time since the last void for bacteria to produce sufficient amount of nitrites to appear at detectable levels contribute to the high false-negative rate (Goossens et al., 1985, Kunin &DeGroot, 1975, McNair et al., 2000). A higher specificity can be achieved by combining the leukocyte esterase and nitrite tests results, but the quantitative urine culture remains the optimal screening test. A microscopic urine analysis is a useful additional test for the identification of bacteriuria (Colgan et al., 2006).

## 3.3 Epidemiology

Although asymptomatic bacteriuria is a common condition, its prevalence differs significantly between certain patient population. The prevalence depends on age, sex, sexual activity, pregnancy, the presence of genitourinary abnormalities, indwelling urinary catheters, and co-morbidities including diabetes mellitus and immunosuppressive conditions (Bakke &Digranes, 1991, Chaudhry et al., 1993, Nicolle, 1997, 2003, Waites et al., 1993, Zhanel et al., 1991). It more often affects women than men (Colgan et al., 2006). Studies could show that the type of organisms isolated from patients with asymptomatic bacteriuria is influenced by certain patient characteristics: e.g. a healthy person will most likely harbor E. coli, while a nursing home resident with a catheter is more likely to have a multi-drug-resistant polymicrobic flora (e.g., P. aeruginosa). Enterococcus species and gram-negative bacilli are common in men. In order to describe the prevalence for certain subgroups, a modified classification from Nicolle was used (Nicolle, 2003).

## 3.4 Prevalence and treatment outcomes for certain patient population

### 3.4.1 Healthy, young populations

**Pediatric Population**

The prevalence of asymptomatic bacteriuria in full-term infants and in premature infants is less than 1% and 3%, respectively (Edelmann et al., 1973). If bacteriuria is present in neonates and infants, congenital malformations, especially vesicoureteral reflux, need to be rule out (Whitworth, 1981). Even an asymptomatic bacteriuria can cause renal scars and subsequently renal insufficiency and hypertension later in life. Antibiotic therapy maybe recommended under these circumstances. In preschool aged children, the prevalence is approximately 0.8% for girls and is insignificant for boys, and is almost never identified beyond the newborn period (Siegel et al., 1980). Its prevalence subsequently increases slightly with age (Siegel et al., 1980). In school-age girls, the prevalence is around 2%-5% (Kunin, 1985). Two randomized controlled trials did not report significant differences in outcome when treating asymptomatic bacteriuria in girls with antibiotics or not (Lindberg, 1975, Savage et al., 1975). Others could show that girls with asymptomatic bacteriuria do experience more frequent symptomatic urinary infection compared with those without bacteriuria (Emans et al., 1979, Gillenwater et al., 1979). Antibiotic treatment in this clinical setting showed only little benefit (Sequelae of covert bacteriuria in schoolgirls. A four-year follow-up study, 1978, Covert bacteriuria in schoolgirls in Newcastle upon Tyne: a 5-year follow-up. Newcastle Covert Bacteriuria Research Group, 1981, Gillenwater et al., 1979, Lindberg et al., 1978, Siegel et al., 1980, Welch et al., 1976, Wettergren et al., 1990). Noteworthy, spontaneous resolutions are common, as well recontaminations and persistence for many years (Hansson et al., 1989, Kunin, 1985). More importantly, initiated antibiotic treatment in these conditions resulted subsequently in a higher incidence of symptomatic urinary infection in the *post-treatment* period (Hansson et al., 1989). Therefore, screening for or treatment of asymptomatic bacteriuria in healthy children is not recommended (Kemper &Avner, 1992, Lindberg et al., 1978, Wettergren et al., 1990).

**Non-pregnant premenopausal, women**

The prevalence of asymptomatic bacteriuria in young, healthy, premenopausal, non-pregnant women was reported between 0.7% and 5.2% (Bengtsson et al., 1998, Kunin &McCormack, 1968). It increases with age and sexual activity (Kunin &McCormack, 1968). Even without urological abnormalities, it is a common finding and shows a correlation with the use of a diaphragm or spermicide for birth control (Hooton et al., 2000, Peddie et al., 1986). A number of studies demonstrate that approximately 30% of women with asymptomatic bacteriuria will develop symptomatic episodes within 1 year (Asscher et al., 1969, Gaymans et al., 1976), however none of the studies show any benefit from treating (Alwall, 1978, Freedman, 1975, Gleckman, 1976, Tencer, 1988). In this patient population asymptomatic bacteriuria is not associated with any long-term adverse outcomes. Noteworthy, antimicrobial therapy given in this setting is rather associated with an increased frequency of symptomatic infection in the immediate *post-antibiotic* period (Foxman et al., 2001, Smith et al., 1997). Therefore, screening for and treatment of asymptomatic bacteriuria are not recommended for healthy, premenopausal, non-pregnant women. Moreover, eradication of bacteriuria by antibiotic courses is difficult, time consuming, costly, and potentially hazardous (Raz, 2003).

**Pregnant women**

The prevalence of asymptomatic bacteriuria during pregnancy ranges between 2% to 7% and is similar to non-pregnant women of the same age (Little, 1966, Plauche et al., 1981). Physiological changes during pregnancy, including dilatation of the ureters and renal pelvis, allow bacteria in the bladder to reach the kidneys and produce pyelonephritis (Shortliffe, 1986). 20% to 30% of bacteriuric pregnant women develop an acute pyelonephritis during pregnancy if untreated, in contrast to only 1-3% of pregnant women who received antibiotics (Golan et al., 1989, Kasviki-Charvati et al., 1982). It is well documented that acute pyelonephritis in late pregnancy is associated with prematurity (Gilstrap et al., 1981, McGrady et al., 1985, Mittendorf et al., 1992). Asymptomatic bacteriuria in pregnancy has also been associated with low-birth-weight infants and the possibility of perinatal death (Platt, 1987, Romero et al., 1989, Schieve et al., 1994, Wadland &Plante, 1989). Treatment of bacteriuria in pregnancy resulted in a 90% risk reduction, and also decreases premature delivery (see Table 4) (Gratacos et al., 1994). Therefore, screening for and antibiotic treatment of asymptomatic bacteriuria in pregnant women are beneficial (Nicolle, 2003).

**Healthy young men**

Only limited data are reported on the association between asymptomatic bacteriuria and young men. According to the literature, it is uncommon in healthy young adult men (Lipsky, 1989). The reported prevalence ranges between 0% and 1.5% (Freedman, 1975, Wilson et al., 1986). No significant differences were reported for heterosexual and homosexual men (Wilson et al., 1986). One clinical study reporting 1.5% prevalence of asymptomatic bacteriuria in young men could show that after careful questioning, all bacteriuric men had lower urinary tract symptoms, including dysuria (Wilson et al., 1986). Taking into consideration the limited reported results, asymptomatic bacteriuria is not a relevant clinical issue in young healthy men, and therefore, screening for asymptomatic bacteriuria is not recommended.

### 3.4.2 Elderly populations

**Community and institutionalized residents**

The prevalence of asymptomatic bacteriuria in the elderly populations is common and differs significantly between community residents and residents in long-term care facilities (Nicolle, 1997, 2003, 2006). The prevalence ranges between 6% to 50% in women, and 6% to 34% in men for community residents and increases with age (Boscia et al., 1986, Kunin &McCormack, 1968). An even higher prevalence was reported for elderly institutionalized residents (25% to 50% in women, and 15% to 40% in men) (Nicolle, 1997, 2003, 2006). Decreased estrogen effect on the genitourinary mucosa, urinary incontinence, prior urologic events including genitourinary surgery, urologic abnormalities such as cystoceles, as well as recurrent symptomatic infection in elderly women contribute to asymptomatic bacteriuria (Raz et al., 2000). For men, prostatic hypertrophy with bladder outlet obstruction was reported to be the major predisposing factor for the development of asymptomatic bacteriuria. Also the use of an external condom catheter to manage incontinence in men increases its prevalence (Ouslander et al., 1987). Several studies, including prospective, randomized studies, did not find any benefits when treating asymptomatic bacteriuria in this patient population. Specifically, no decrease in symptomatic episodes (Boscia et al., 1987, Nicolle et al., 1983, Nicolle et al., 1987) and no differences in morbidity and mortality were seen (Abrutyn et al., 1994, Nicolle et al., 1983, Nicolle et al., 1987, Ouslander et al., 1995). Noteworthy, residents treated for asymptomatic bacteriuria were reported to have an increased reinfection rate with resistant organisms and side effects from antibiotic treatment (Nicolle et al., 1987). Therefore, screening for or treatment of asymptomatic bacteriuria in elderly residents in the community and or institutionalized residents is not recommended (Nicolle, 2001, Pels et al., 1989).

### 3.4.3 Patients with chronic medical conditions

**Diabetes mellitus**

Several studies reported a prevalence of bacteriuria in diabetic women of 7% to 13% (Brauner et al., 1993, Geerlings et al., 2000, Zhanel et al., 1995), which is approximately a 3-fold higher prevalence than in non-diabetic women (Zhanel et al., 1991). Diabetic men do not show higher prevalence rates than non-diabetics (Zhanel et al., 1990, Zhanel et al., 1991). The reasons for the high prevalence in women are still not well understood. A main factor for asymptomatic bacteriuria might be the development of an autonomic neuropathy leading to impaired bladder voiding (Patterson &Andriole, 1997). The duration of diabetes mellitus and the presence of long-term diabetic complications such as nephropathy, retinopathy, peripheral vascular disease, and neuropathy were reported to be associated with asymptomatic bacteriuria (Vejlsgaard, 1966, Zhanel et al., 1995). There is evidence, that symptomatic urinary infection may be potentially more severe in diabetic than non-diabetic patients (Patterson &Andriole, 1997). Both, the severity of symptomatic infection and the higher prevalence of bacteriuria in diabetic women has led to the assumption that treatment of asymptomatic bacteriuria in this patient population might be beneficial (Screening for asymptomatic bacteriuria, hematuria and proteinuria. The U.S. Preventive Services Task Force, 1990). Several studies, including long term and/or prospective do not suggest that asymptomatic bacteriuria is harmful in diabetic women (Geerlings et al., 2001, Semetkowska-Jurkiewicz et al., 1995). Moreover, treatment did not show any significant benefits in terms of improved glucose control or delayed development of long-term complications of diabetes mellitus (Geerlings et al., 2001, Semetkowska-Jurkiewicz et al., 1995). Antimicrobial treatment of bacteriuria did not decrease the frequency or severity of symptomatic urinary infection. However, greater antimicrobial exposure and a higher frequency of adverse drug effects with antimicrobial therapy and a high rate of recurrent asymptomatic bacteriuria were observed following therapy (Harding et al., 2002). In summary, screening for and treatment of asymptomatic bacteriuria in diabetic women with asymptomatic bacteriuria and normal renal tracts should not be recommended.

**Patients with spinal cord-injuries**

The neurologic bladder dysfunction is the key event in the development of asymptomatic bacteriuria in this patient population (Erickson et al., 1982, Sanderson &Weissler, 1990, Schlager et al., 1995, Sotolongo &Koleilat, 1990). The prevalence of asymptomatic bacteriuria remains high independently of the method of bladder emptying (see Table 6-need ref). The preservation of a low pressure urinary tract decreased morbidity and mortality secondary to urosepsis and renal failure dramatically in this patient population (Hackler et al., 1989). However, symptomatic urinary tract infections are still a significant issue (DeVivo et al., 1985, Ditunno &Formal, 1994). Clinical studies, including prospective cohort studies and placebo-controlled trials show no decrease in symptomatic infection with antibiotic therapy for asymptomatic bacteriuria (Mohler et al., 1987) and no progression to renal failure with asymptomatic bacteriuria were observed, as long as a low urinary bladder pressure was maintained (Sotolongo &Koleilat, 1990). Therefore, screening for or treatment of asymptomatic bacteriuria in spinal cord injury populations is currently not recommended (Cardenas &Hooton, 1995, Ditunno &Formal, 1994).

**Kidney transplant patients**

Asymptomatic bacteriuria is a very common event after kidney transplantation, especially during the immediate post-transplantation period. Often the differentiation between asymptomatic bacteriuria and infection is difficult because of the presence of immunosuppressive medications, which can suppress symptoms and signs of infections. Ramsey et al. diagnosed 65 bladder infections in 35 of 65 transplant recipients during 14.7 months follow-up. In this study, 91% of the patients were asymptomatic and 57% of the infections occurred within 1 month, and approximately 80% by 6 months (Ramsey et al., 1979). In another study by Prat et al., 185 of 299 kidney transplant patients had at least one episode of infection with 96% of the episodes asymptomatic (Prat et al., 1985). Patients with persistent infection and urologic complications often experienced sepsis and graft loss. However, graft survival was not associated with the presence or absence of bacteriuria in patients without urologic complications (Griffin &Salaman, 1979, Ramsey et al., 1979). The frequency of both asymptomatic and symptomatic urinary infection in renal graft recipients has declined due to improved early post-transplantation management including routine perioperative antibiotics, short-term urethral catheterization, and use of long-term prophylactic antibiotics to prevent all post-transplant infections (Fox et al., 1990, Hoy et al., 1985). Fiorante et al. reported no differences in renal allograft prognosis between those who do not develop asymptomatic bacteriuria and those who do develop asymptomatic bacteriuria and are systematically treated. Systematic treatment of asymptomatic bacteriuria however, may reduce the incidence pyelonephritis (Fiorante et al.). Similar results were reported by others (Lyerova et al., 2001, Takai et al., 1998). Therefore, evidence to support screening recommendations in the post-transplant period is still deficient. According to the Immunocompromised Host Society Consensus Conference, periodic monitoring for urinary infection in post-transplant might beneficial, but a specific frequency of screening or clear recommendations for therapy if bacteriuria is identified were not given (Snydman, 2001).

**Other immunocompromised patients**

Other than kidney transplantation, no convincing data has been reported so far on the relationship between asymptomatic bacteriuria and organ transplantation, including bone marrow transplantation. For this reason, post-transplant screening and treatment for asymptomatic bacteriuria is highly controversial for this patient population (Guidelines for preventing opportunistic infections among hematopoietic stem cell transplant recipients, 2000, Snydman, 2001). Chemotherapy-induced granulocytopenia during the treatment of a variety of malignancies possibly represents a risk factor for patients with asymptomatic bacteriuria to develop urinary tract infections (Gurwith et al., 1979). Another immunosuppressive condition with a higher prevalence of asymptomatic bacteriuria is the infection with HIV (Awolude et al., 2011). Several studies suggest a correlation between low CD4+ counts and the presence of asymptomatic bacteriuria (Awolude et al., 2011, De Pinho et al., 1994, Hoepelman et al., 1992). No articles were identified addressing the use of antibiotic treatment for this patient population. The reason for the higher prevalence of asymptomatic bacteriuria and low CD4 counts is not well understood. Based on the lack of data in this clinical setting, routine screening and treatment of patients with HIV and asymptomatic bacteriuria cannot be recommended.

### 3.4.4 Patients with urological or gynaecological devices

**Catheterized patients**

Clear differences were reported in the literature on the relationship of asymptomatic bacteriuria and short-and long term transurethral bladder catheterization. No reports for suprapubic tubes were found in the peer-reviewed literature. The prevalence of asymptomatic bacteriuria correlates with several influencing factors, including the type and duration of bladder catheterization, qualification of the health-care personnel and the catheter system and care (MacFarlane, 1984).

**Patients with temporary transurethral or suprapubic indwelling catheters**

Single bladder catheterization is associated with less than 1% risk of developing asymptomatic bacteriuria for patients in an ambulatory setting (Garibaldi et al., 1974). The development of asymptomatic bacteriuria even after placement of short-term transurethral catheters is significant. Short term is defined as less than 30 days of bladder catheterization. The prevalence of asymptomatic bacteriuria increases on a daily basis by 2%-7% (Tambyah &Maki, 2000). A prevalence of nearly 100% was reported for elderly patients with an indwelling transurethral catheter and an open urine collecting bag system (Uehling et al., 1985), and 20% for patients with a closed urine collection system (MacFarlane, 1984). Early clinical studies could not demonstrate any benefits when treating patients with short-term indwelling catheters with antibiotics and asymptomatic bacteriuria (Butler &Kunin, 1968). A common dilemma is that approximately 80% of all patients with transurethral catheters are treated with antibiotics for other reasons, therefore it is difficult to define the significance of asymptomatic bacteriuria for this patient population (Johnson et al., 1990, Riley et al., 1995). It is noteworthy that the development of asymptomatic bacteriuria in patients with a permanent catheter is practically inevitable. According to Nicolle (Nicolle, 2003) screening and treatment of bacteriuria for patients with short-term indwelling catheters is recommended only for patients with certain risk factors, such as a pregnant woman or those undergoing an invasive urologic procedure.

**Patients with permanant transurethral or suprapubic indwelling catheters**

Long term or chronic indwelling catheters are defined as more than 30 days of bladder catheterization. For this patient population bacteriuria is universal. The main reason for the development of bacteriuria under these circumstances is the presence of a biofilm, a material composed of bacteria and extracellular bacterial substances in combination with certain urinary components including Tamm-Horsfall protein, magnesium, and calcium (Donlan &Costerton, 2002). Several studies suggest that patients with a chronic indwelling catheter have a higher morbidity from symptomatic urinary infection compared to patients without a catheter (Orr et al., 1996, Warren et al., 1987). Therefore, several prospective randomized studies were conducted to define the role of antibiotic treatment for this clinical scenario. Antibiotic treatment did not reduce the frequency of fever in treated patients compared to untreated patients with asymptomatic bacteriuria. A higher percentage of resistant organisms were encountered in the treatment group after antibiotic treatment and that antibiotic treatment rarely eliminated the bacteriuria (Alling et al., 1975, Warren et al., 1982). Therefore, patients with long-term indwelling catheters should not be screened and treated with antibiotic therapy for asymptomatic bacteriuria. None of the published studies could demonstrate any benefits of antibiotic treatment, but did demonstrate potential harm for the patient. However, antibiotic treatment might be considered for patients at high risk for certain complications, for instance infection of prosthetic devices (Raz, 2003).

**Other indwelling devices**

The mainstay in the treatment of ureteral obstruction is the use of ureteral stents. Similar to transurethral *catheters,* these devices are subject to biofilm development and asymptomatic bacteriuria (Riedl et al., 1999). Often it is difficult to differentiate between asymptomatic bacteriuria and bladder infection, as patients frequently report dysuria, frequency and urgency as a reaction to the indwelling ureteral stent. Studies have shown that prophylactic antibiotic treatment did not reduce bacterial colonization or prevent stent obstruction (Riedl et al., 1999). The evidence for screening and treatment in this setting is sparse and therefore not recommended. Fallahian et al. describe the use of intrauterine devices as a risk factor for urinary tract infections. For patients with asymptomatic bacteriuria, an intrauterine device therefore might not be the method of choice, and other contraceptive methods should be preferred (Fallahian et al., 2005).

### 3.4.5 Patients undergoing surgical intervention

**Urological surgery**

Patients with asymptomatic bacteriuria undergoing any surgical procedures or manipulations of the genitourinary tract are nearly uniformly at risk to develop complications. Surgery or trauma causes mucosal injuries allowing bacteria to penetrate the tissue causing local infection, or to invade the blood circulation resulting in bacteremia and/or sepsis. If left untreated, asymptomatic bacteriuria prior to the surgery resulted in bacteremia in 25%-80% of the patients (Olson &Cookson, 2000). Other authors could demonstrate that antibiotic treatment prior to the surgery can prevent bacteremia and sepsis (Grabe, 2001, Olson &Cookson, 2000). Olson et al. recommend antibiotic treatment only immediately before the procedure, since earlier initiation can result in reinfection with resistant bacterial strains (Olson &Cookson, 2000). Grabe suggests treatment of asymptomatic bacteriuria before urodynamic studies, ureteral stent placements, ureteroscopic procedures and transurethral resection of the prostate (Grabe, 2001). However, no general consensus exists for which urologic intervention requires preoperative treatment of asymptomatic bacteriuria (Grabe, 2001).

**Ileal Conduit and Orthotopic Neobladder**

The treatment of asymptomatic bacteriuria in patients with ileal conduit and orthotopic neobladder is controversial (Zhanel et al., 1990). Guinan et al. described the bacterial milieu in patients with ileal conduit (Guinan et al., 1972). The terminal ileum is in nearly 100% of the patients sterile. After creation of an ileal conduit the mucosa is rapidly colonized. The most common organisms are Proteus, Pseudomonas and E. coli. Aggressive treatment is recommended for patients with pyelonephritis or systemic signs of illness (Guinan et al., 1972).

**Other surgical interventions**

A small number of studies have evaluated the risk of deep joint infection after joint replacement surgery associated with the preoperative presence of asymptomatic bacteriuria. A retrospective analysis of 277 patients undergoing 364 total joint replacements showed that 35 patients had evidence of preoperative or perioperative asymptomatic bacteriuria. Joint infections were observed in 3 patients (1.1%) 9, 19, and 45 months. None of the joint infections were related to perioperative asymptomatic bacteriuria (Ritter &Fechtman, 1987). Glynn and Sheehan reported in a retrospective analysis that 55 of 299 patients admitted for hip or knee arthroplasty had asymptomatic bacteriuria and 2 patients were symptomatic upon admission (Glynn &Sheehan, 1984). Routine perioperative antibiotic treatment initiated pre or postoperatively was sufficient to prevent infection of the implant. Deep joint infection was not seen in any patients at 3-month follow-up, prompting the authors to conclude that asymptomatic bacteriuria is common and should not be a cause for postponement of surgery and that treatment with antibiotics can be implemented at any time perioperatively. In conclusion, asymptomatic bacteriuria may be a reservoir for bacterial contamination of the wound, or may identify a patient at increased risk of infection at any site, including implants, without having a causal relationship (Nelson et al., 1983). Present guidelines recommend to identify and treat any infection remote to the surgical site before an elective operation. It is only an assumption that this recommendation also includes asymptomatic bacteriuria (Mangram et al., 1999). However, screening and treatment of asymptomatic bacteriuria before any surgical procedures other certain urological procedures is currently not recommended. Coincidentally, the perioperative antibiotic prophylaxis given for most procedures is sufficient to suppress or eradicate asymptomatic bacteriuria and prevent symptomatic infections in the vast majority of cases.

## 4. Discussion

Asymptomatic bacteriuria is a common clinical finding in several different patient populations. A higher prevalence exists in patients with morphological or functional defects of the genitourinary tract and with indwelling urological devices. However, healthy individuals may also have asymptomatic bacteriuria. The central question for physicians and health care professionals is whether or not to treat asymptomatic bacteriuria. Continuous improvement has been made over the last few decades in documenting the epidemiology of asymptomatic bacteriuria. Patient populations with a high prevalence are well described. However, the natural history and guidelines for management are still controversial. Sufficient evidence exists to recommend screening and treatment for some patient populations with a high prevalence of asymptomatic bacteriuria, while for other populations no such recommendations exist.

| **Screening and treatment proven to be beneficial** |
|---|
| Pregnancy |
| Prior to traumatic genitourinary procedures |
| **Screening and treatment may beneficial** |
| Renal transplant recipient, first 6 months post-transplant |
| Immunocompromised patients (e.g. malignancy-chemotherapy) |
| Infected kidney stones |
| Vesicoureteral reflux in young children |
| Women with persistent catheter-acquired bacteriuria after catheter removal |

Table 1. Potential benefits of screening and treatment for asymptomatic bacteriuria.

This dilemma is based on the lack of good evidence from clinical trials investigating direct management strategies. Antibiotic treatment is only recommended if it has been shown to improve patient outcome.

Sufficient evidence exists to screen and treat asymptomatic bacteriuria in pregnant women and patients undergoing traumatic urological interventions (table 1). *Young children with vesicoureteral reflux, renal transplant recipients, transplant recipients during the first 6 months post-transplant, immunocompromised patients (e.g. malignancy-chemotherapy), and women with*

*persistent catheter-acquired bacteriuria after catheter removal might benefit from screening and treatment. However, the evidence is not strong enough to recommend it* (table 1).
Screening for asymptomatic bacteruria is highly controversial in the patient populations listed in table 2. Treating asymptomatic bacteriuria in these patient populations has not been found to improve outcomes. In fact, antibiotic treatment in these patient populations may be associated with significant adverse effects. Possible side effects reported in the literature include the development of symptomatic infections, re-infection with organisms of increased antimicrobial resistance, and side effects directly related to the antibiotics (Nicolle, 2003). Overtreatment of asymptomatic bacteriuria is a substantial quality, safety, and cost issue.

| Screening and treatment controversial or not beneficial |
|---|
| Healthy infants |
| Healthy women or men |
| Elderly men and women in the community or in long-term care facilities |
| Women with diabetes |
| Patients with HIV infection |
| Patients with short-term and /or chronic-indwelling indwelling urethral catheters* |
| Patients using intermittent catheterization |
| Patients with neurologic impairment of bladder emptying |
| Patients with chronic urologic or gynecological devices |

* not recommended for patient care; may be appropriate to screen for bacteriuria for nosocomial infection surveillance or outbreak control.

Table 2. No proven benefits of screening and treatment for asymptomatic bacteriuria.

Therefore, it is crucial to treat patients with asymptomatic bacteriuria only if there is evidence of potential benefits. Urine cultures are commonly ordered as part of a routine work-up in hospitalized patients, despite lower urinary tract symptoms. More importantly, patients with asymptomatic bacteriuria are frequently treated under these circumstances, accounting for a substantial burden of inappropriate antibiotic use in hospitals (Silver et al., 2009). Similar findings have been reported for patients in long-term care facilities for the elderly (Walker et al., 2000). Many research questions, however, still remain to be addressed in future clinical trials. The potential benefits of treatment need to be weighed against no treatment in order to maximize patient safety.

## 5. Acknowledgment

We would like to thank the library staff from Texas Tech University Health Sciences Center, Lubbock for their extraordinary support and assistance. On a special note, we would like to thank Carrie Gassett who showed great interest and support in our project.

## 6. References

Abrutyn, E et al. (1994). Does asymptomatic bacteriuria predict mortality and does antimicrobial treatment reduce mortality in elderly ambulatory women? *Annals of Internal Medicine*, Vol. 120, No. 10, (May 15 1994), pp. 827-833, ISSN 0003-4819

Alling, B et al. (1975). Effect of consecutive antibacterial therapy on bacteriuria in hospitalized geriatric patients. *Scandinavian journal of infectious diseases*, Vol. 7, No. 3, 1975), pp. 201-207, ISSN 0036-5548

Alwall, N. (1978). On controversial and open questions about the course and complications of non-obstructive urinary tract infection in adult women. Follow-up for up to 80 months of 707 participants in a population study and evaluation of a clinical series of 36 selected women with a history of urinary tract infection for up to 40 years. *Acta medica Scandinavica*, Vol. 203, No. 5, 1978), pp. 369-377, ISSN 0001-6101

Andersson, P et al. (1991). Persistence of Escherichia coli bacteriuria is not determined by bacterial adherence. *Infection and Immunity*, Vol. 59, No. 9, (Sep 1991), pp. 2915-2921, ISSN 0019-9567

Asscher, A W et al. (1969). Asymptomatic significant bacteriuria in the non-pregnant woman. II. Response to treatment and follow-up. *British Medical Journal*, Vol. 1, No. 5647, (Mar 29 1969), pp. 804-806, ISSN 0007-1447

Awolude, O A et al. (2011). Asymptomatic bacteriuria among HIV positive pregnant women. *Virulence*, Vol. 1, No. 3, (May-Jun 2011), pp. 130-133, ISSN 2150-5608

Bachman, J W et al. (1993). A study of various tests to detect asymptomatic urinary tract infections in an obstetric population. *Jama: The Journal of American Medical Association*, Vol. 270, No. 16, (Oct 27 1993), pp. 1971-1974, ISSN 0098-7484

Bakke, A &Digranes, A. (1991). Bacteriuria in patients treated with clean intermittent catheterization. *Scandinavian journal of infectious diseases*, Vol. 23, No. 5, 1991), pp. 577-582, ISSN 0036-5548

Bengtsson, C et al. (1998). Bacteriuria in a population sample of women: 24-year follow-up study. Results from the prospective population-based study of women in Gothenburg, Sweden. *Scandinavian Journal of Urology and Nephrology*, Vol. 32, No. 4, (Jul 1998), pp. 284-289, ISSN 0036-5599

Bennett, C J;Young, M N &Darrington, H. (1995). Differences in urinary tract infections in male and female spinal cord injury patients on intermittent catheterization. *Paraplegia*, Vol. 33, No. 2, (Feb 1995), pp. 69-72, ISSN 0031-1758

Boscia, J A et al. (1986). Epidemiology of bacteriuria in an elderly ambulatory population. *The American Journal of Medicine*, Vol. 80, No. 2, (Feb 1986), pp. 208-214, ISSN 0002-9343

Boscia, J A et al. (1987). Therapy vs no therapy for bacteriuria in elderly ambulatory nonhospitalized women. *Jama: The Journal of American Medical Association*, Vol. 257, No. 8, (Feb 27 1987), pp. 1067-1071, ISSN 0098-7484

Brauner, A et al. (1993). Bacteriuria, bacterial virulence and host factors in diabetic patients. *Diabet Medicine: a Journal of the British Medical Association*, Vol. 10, No. 6, (Jul 1993), pp. 550-554, ISSN 0742-3071

Butler, H K &Kunin, C M. (1968). Evaluation of specific systemic antimicrobial therapy in patients while on closed catheter drainage. *Journal of Urology*, Vol. 100, No. 4, (Oct 1968), pp. 567-572, ISSN 0022-5347

Cardenas, D D &Hooton, T M. (1995). Urinary tract infection in persons with spinal cord injury. *Archives of Physical Medicine and Rehabilitation*, Vol. 76, No. 3, (Mar 1995), pp. 272-280, ISSN 0003-9993

Chaudhry, A;Stone, W J &Breyer, J A. (1993). Occurrence of pyuria and bacteriuria in asymptomatic hemodialysis patients. *American Journal of Kidney Diseases*, Vol. 21, No. 2, (Feb 1993), pp. 180-183, ISSN 0272-6386

Colgan, R et al. (2006). Asymptomatic bacteriuria in adults. *American Family Physician*, Vol. 74, No. 6, (Sep 15 2006), pp. 985-990, ISSN 0002-838X

Covert bacteriuria in schoolgirls in Newcastle upon Tyne: a 5-year follow-up. Newcastle Covert Bacteriuria Research Group. (1981). *Archives of Disease in Childhood*, Vol. 56, No. 8, (Aug 1981), pp. 585-592, ISSN 1468-2044

De Pinho, A M et al. (1994). Urinary tract infection in men with AIDS. *Genitourinary Medicine*, Vol. 70, No. 1, (Feb 1994), pp. 30-34, ISSN 0266-4348

DeVivo, M J et al. (1985). The risk of bladder calculi in patients with spinal cord injuries. *Archives of International Medicine*, Vol. 145, No. 3, (Mar 1985), pp. 428-430, ISSN 0003-9926

Ditunno, J F, Jr. &Formal, C S. (1994). Chronic spinal cord injury. *New England Journal of Medicine*, Vol. 330, No. 8, (Feb 24 1994), pp. 550-556, ISSN 0028-4793

Donlan, R M &Costerton, J W. (2002). Biofilms: survival mechanisms of clinically relevant microorganisms. *Clinical Microbiology Reviews*, Vol. 15, No. 2, (Apr 2002), pp. 167-193, ISSN 0893-8512

Edelmann, C M, Jr. et al. (1973). The prevalence of bacteriuria in full-term and premature newborn infants. *The Journal of Pediatrics*, Vol. 82, No. 1, (Jan 1973), pp. 125-132, ISSN 0022-3476

Emans, S J;Grace, E &Masland, R P, Jr. (1979). Asymptomatic bacteriuria in adolescent girls: I. Epidemiology. *Pediatrics*, Vol. 64, No. 4, (Oct 1979), pp. 433-437, ISSN 0031-4005

Erickson, R P et al. (1982). Bacteriuria during follow-up in patients with spinal cord injury: I. Rates of bacteriuria in various bladder-emptying methods. *Archives of Physical Medicine and Rehabilitation*, Vol. 63, No. 9, (Sep 1982), pp. 409-412, ISSN 0003-9993

Evans, D A et al. (1978). Bacteriuria in a population-based cohort of women. *Journal of Infectious Diseases*, Vol. 138, No. 6, (Dec 1978), pp. 768-773, ISSN 0022-1899

Fallahian, M;Mashhady, E &Amiri, Z. (2005). Asymptomatic bacteriuria in users of intrauterine devices. *Urology Journal*, Vol. 2, No. 3, (Summer 2005), pp. 157-159, ISSN 1735-1308

Fiorante, S et al. Systematic screening and treatment of asymptomatic bacteriuria in renal transplant recipients. *Kidney International*, Vol. 78, No. 8, (Oct) pp. 774-781, ISSN 1523-1755

Fox, B C et al. (1990). A prospective, randomized, double-blind study of trimethoprim-sulfamethoxazole for prophylaxis of infection in renal transplantation: clinical efficacy, absorption of trimethoprim-sulfamethoxazole, effects on the microflora, and the cost-benefit of prophylaxis. *American Journal of Medicine*, Vol. 89, No. 3, (Sep 1990), pp. 255-274, ISSN 0002-9343

Foxman, B et al. (2001). Urinary tract infection among women aged 40 to 65: behavioral and sexual risk factors. *Journal of Clinical Epidemiology*, Vol. 54, No. 7, (Jul 2001), pp. 710-718, ISSN 0895-4356

Freedman, L R. (1975). Natural history of urinary infection in adults. *Kidney International. Supplement*, Vol. 4, No. (Aug 1975), pp. S96-100, ISSN 0098-6577

Garibaldi, R A et al. (1974). Factors predisposing to bacteriuria during indwelling urethral catheterization. *New England Journal of Medicine*, Vol. 291, No. 5, (Aug 1 1974), pp. 215-219, ISSN 0028-4793

Gaymans, R et al. (1976). Aprospective study of urinary-tract infections in a Dutch general practice. *Lancet*, Vol. 2, No. 7987, (Sep 25 1976), pp. 674-677, ISSN 0140-6736

Geerlings, S E et al. (2000). Is a second urine specimen necessary for the diagnosis of asymptomatic bacteriuria? *Clinical Infectious Diseases*, Vol. 31, No. 3, (Sep 2000), pp. E3-4, ISSN 1058-4838

Geerlings, S E et al. (2001). Virulence factors of Escherichia coli isolated from urine of diabetic women with asymptomatic bacteriuria: correlation with clinical characteristics. *Antonie Van Leeuwenhoek*, Vol. 80, No. 2, (Oct 2001), pp. 119-127, ISSN 0003-6072

Geerlings, S E et al. (2001). Consequences of asymptomatic bacteriuria in women with diabetes mellitus. *Archives of Internal Medicine*, Vol. 161, No. 11, (Jun 11 2001), pp. 1421-1427, ISSN 0003-9926

Geerlings, S E et al. (2000). Asymptomatic bacteriuria may be considered a complication in women with diabetes. Diabetes Mellitus Women Asymptomatic Bacteriuria Utrecht Study Group. *Diabetes Care*, Vol. 23, No. 6, (Jun 2000), pp. 744-749, ISSN 0149-5992

Gillenwater, J Y;Harrison, R B &Kunin, C M. (1979). Natural history of bacteriuria in schoolgirls. A long-term case-control study. *New England Journal of Medicine*, Vol. 301, No. 8, (Aug 23 1979), pp. 396-399, ISSN 0028-4793

Gilstrap, L C et al. (1981). Renal infection and pregnancy outcome. *American Journal of Obstetrics and Gynecology*, Vol. 141, No. 6, (Nov 15 1981), pp. 709-716, ISSN 0002-9378

Gleckman, R. (1976). The controversy of treatment of asymptomatic bacteriuria in non-pregnant women--resolved. *Journal of Urology*, Vol. 116, No. 6, (Dec 1976), pp. 776-777, ISSN 0022-5347

Gleckman, R et al. (1979). Reliability of a single urine culture in establishing diagnosis of asymptomatic bacteriuria in adult males. *Journal of Clinical Microbiology*, Vol. 9, No. 5, (May 1979), pp. 596-597, ISSN 0095-1137

Glynn, M K &Sheehan, J M. (1984). The significance of asymptomatic bacteriuria in patients undergoing hip/knee arthroplasty. *Clinical Orthopedics and Relatated Research*, Vol. No. 185, (May 1984), pp. 151-154, ISSN 0009-921X

Golan, A et al. (1989). Asymptomatic bacteriuria in normal and high-risk pregnancy. *European Journal of Obstetrics, Gynecology, and Reproductive Biology*, Vol. 33, No. 2, (Nov 1989), pp. 101-108, ISSN 0301-2115

Goossens, H et al. (1985). Prevalence of asymptomatic bacteriuria and comparison between different screening methods for its detection in infants. *European Journal of Epidemiology*, Vol. 1, No. 4, (Dec 1985), pp. 301-304, ISSN 0393-2990

Grabe, M. (2001). Perioperative antibiotic prophylaxis in urology. *Current Opinions in Urology*, Vol. 11, No. 1, (Jan 2001), pp. 81-85, ISSN 0963-0643

Gratacos, E et al. (1994). Screening and treatment of asymptomatic bacteriuria in pregnancy prevent pyelonephritis. *Journal of Infectious Diseases*, Vol. 169, No. 6, (Jun 1994), pp. 1390-1392, ISSN 0022-1899

Griffin, P J &Salaman, J R. (1979). Urinary tract infections after renal transplantation: do they matter? *British Medical Journal*, Vol. 1, No. 6165, (Mar 17 1979), pp. 710-711, ISSN 0007-1447

Guidelines for preventing opportunistic infections among hematopoietic stem cell transplant recipients. (2000). *Morbidity and Mortality Weekly Report, Recommendations and Reports*, Vol. 49, No. RR-10, (Oct 2000), pp. 1-125, CE121-127, ISSN 1057-5987

Guinan, P D et al. (1972). The bacteriology of ileal conduit urine in man. *Surgery, Gynecology, & Obstetrics*, Vol. 134, No. 1, (Jan 1972), pp. 78-82, ISSN 0039-6087

Gurwith, M J et al. (1979). A prospective controlled investigation of prophylactic trimethoprim/sulfamethoxazole in hospitalized granulocytopenic patients. *American Journal of Medicine*, Vol. 66, No. 2, (Feb 1979), pp. 248-256, ISSN 0002-9343

Hackler, R H;Hall, M K &Zampieri, T A. (1989). Bladder hypocompliance in the spinal cord injury population. *Journal of Urology*, Vol. 141, No. 6, (Jun 1989), pp. 1390-1393, ISSN 0022-5347

Hansson, S et al. (1989). Untreated asymptomatic bacteriuria in girls: I--Stability of urinary isolates. *British Medical Journal*, Vol. 298, No. 6677, (Apr 1 1989), pp. 853-855, ISSN 0959-8138

Hansson, S et al. (1989). Untreated asymptomatic bacteriuria in girls: II--Effect of phenoxymethylpenicillin and erythromycin given for intercurrent infections. *British Medical Journal*, Vol. 298, No. 6677, (Apr 1 1989), pp. 856-859, ISSN 0959-8138

Harding, G K et al. (2002). Antimicrobial treatment in diabetic women with asymptomatic bacteriuria. *New England Journal of Medicine*, Vol. 347, No. 20, (Nov 14 2002), pp. 1576-1583, ISSN 1533-4406

Hoepelman, A I et al. (1992). Bacteriuria in men infected with HIV-1 is related to their immune status (CD4+ cell count). *Aids*, Vol. 6, No. 2, (Feb 1992), pp. 179-184, ISSN 0269-9370

Hooton, T M et al. (2000). A prospective study of asymptomatic bacteriuria in sexually active young women. *New England Journal of Medicine*, Vol. 343, No. 14, (Oct 5 2000), pp. 992-997, ISSN 0028-4793

Hoy, W E et al. (1985). Altered patterns of posttransplant urinary tract infections associated with perioperative antibiotics and curtailed catheterization. *American Journal of Kidney Diseases*, Vol. 6, No. 4, (Oct 1985), pp. 212-216, ISSN 0272-6386

Johnson, J R et al. (1990). Prevention of catheter-associated urinary tract infection with a silver oxide-coated urinary catheter: clinical and microbiologic correlates. *Journal of Infectious Diseases*, Vol. 162, No. 5, (Nov 1990), pp. 1145-1150, ISSN 0022-1899

Kass, E H. (1957). Bacteriuria and the diagnosis of infections of the urinary tract; with observations on the use of methionine as a urinary antiseptic. *AMA Archives of Internal Medicine*, Vol. 100, No. 5, (Nov 1957), pp. 709-714, ISSN 0888-2479

Kass, E H. (1962). Pyelonephritis and bacteriuria. A major problem in preventive medicine. *Annals of Internal Medicine*, Vol. 56, No. (Jan 1962), pp. 46-53, ISSN 0003-4819

Kasviki-Charvati, P et al. (1982). Turnover of bacteriuria in old age. *Age and Ageing*, Vol. 11, No. 3, (Aug 1982), pp. 169-174, ISSN 0002-0729

Kemper, K J &Avner, E D. (1992). The case against screening urinalyses for asymptomatic bacteriuria in children. *American Journal of Diseases of Children*, Vol. 146, No. 3, (Mar 1992), pp. 343-346, ISSN 0002-922X

Kincaid-Smith, P &Bullen, M. (1965). Bacteriuria in Pregnancy. *Lancet*, Vol. 1, No. 7382, (Feb 20 1965), pp. 395-399, ISSN 0140-6736
Kunin, C M. (1966). Asymptomatic bacteriuria. *Annual Review of Medicine*, Vol. 17, No. 1966), pp. 383-406, ISSN 0066-4219
Kunin, C M. (1985). Does kidney infection cause renal failure? *Annual Review of Medicine*, Vol. 36, No. 1985), pp. 165-176, ISSN 0066-4219
Kunin, C M &DeGroot, J E. (1975). Self-screening for significant bacteriuria. Evaluation of dip-strip combination nitrite/culture test. *Jama: The Journal of American Medical Association*, Vol. 231, No. 13, (Mar 31 1975), pp. 1349-1353, ISSN 0098-7484
Kunin, C M;Deutscher, R &Paquin, A, Jr. (1964). Urinary Tract Infection in School Children: an Epidemiologic, Clinical and Laboratory Study. *Medicine (Baltimore)*, Vol. 43, No. (Mar 1964), pp. 91-130, ISSN 0025-7974
Kunin, C M &McCormack, R C. (1968). An epidemiologic study of bacteriuria and blood pressure among nuns and working women. *New England Journal Medicine*, Vol. 278, No. 12, (Mar 21 1968), pp. 635-642, ISSN 0028-4793
Leblanc, A L &McGanity, W J. (1964). The Impact of Bacteriuria in Pregnancy; a Survey of 1300 Pregnant Patients. *Texas Reports on Biology and Medicine*, Vol. 22, No. 1964), pp. 336-347, ISSN 0040-4675
Lindberg, U. (1975). Asymptomatic bacteriuria in school girls. V. The clinical course and response to treatment. *Acta paediatrica Scandinavica*, Vol. 64, No. 5, (Sep 1975), pp. 718-724, 0001-656X (Print) 0001-656X (Linking)
Lindberg, U et al. (1978). Asymptomatic bacteriuria in schoolgirls. VIII. Clinical course during a 3-year follow-up. *The Journal of Pediatrics*, Vol. 92, No. 2, (Feb 1978), pp. 194-199, ISSN 0022-3476
Lipsky, B A. (1989). Urinary tract infections in men. Epidemiology, pathophysiology, diagnosis, and treatment. *Annals of Internal Medicine*, Vol. 110, No. 2, (Jan 15 1989), pp. 138-150, ISSN 0003-4819
Lipsky, B A et al. (1987). Diagnosis of bacteriuria in men: specimen collection and culture interpretation. *Journal of Infectious Diseases*, Vol. 155, No. 5, (May 1987), pp. 847-854, ISSN 0022-1899
Little, P J. (1966). The incidence of urinary infection in 5000 pregnant women. *Lancet*, Vol. 2, No. 7470, (Oct 29 1966), pp. 925-928, ISSN 0140-6736
Lyerova, L et al. (2001). Urinary tract infection in patients with urological complications after renal transplantation with respect to long-term function and allograft survival. *Annals of Transplant*, Vol. 6, No. 2, 2001), pp. 19-20, ISSN 1425-9524
MacFarlane, D E. (1984). Catheter-associated urinary tract infections. Part I: Epidemiology, pathogenesis and bacteriology. *West Indian Medical Journal*, Vol. 33, No. 3, (Sep 1984), pp. 146-150, ISSN 0043-3144
Mangram, A J et al. (1999). Guideline for prevention of surgical site infection, 1999. Hospital Infection Control Practices Advisory Committee. *Infection Control and Hospital Epidemiology*, Vol. 20, No. 4, (Apr 1999), pp. 250-278; quiz 279-280, ISSN 0899-823X
McGrady, G A;Daling, J R &Peterson, D R. (1985). Maternal urinary tract infection and adverse fetal outcomes. *American Journal of Epidemiology*, Vol. 121, No. 3, (Mar 1985), pp. 377-381, ISSN 0002-9262
McNair, R D et al. (2000). Evaluation of the centrifuged and Gram-stained smear, urinalysis, and reagent strip testing to detect asymptomatic bacteriuria in obstetric patients.

*American Journal of Obstetrics and Gynecology*, Vol. 182, No. 5, (May 2000), pp. 1076-1079, ISSN 0002-9378

Mittendorf, R;Williams, M A &Kass, E H. (1992). Prevention of preterm delivery and low birth weight associated with asymptomatic bacteriuria. *Clinical Infectious Diseases*, Vol. 14, No. 4, (Apr 1992), pp. 927-932, ISSN 1058-4838

Mohler, J L;Cowen, D L &Flanigan, R C. (1987). Suppression and treatment of urinary tract infection in patients with an intermittently catheterized neurogenic bladder. *Journal of Urology*, Vol. 138, No. 2, (Aug 1987), pp. 336-340, ISSN 0022-5347

Nelson, C L et al. (1983). One day versus seven days of preventive antibiotic therapy in orthopedic surgery. *Clinical Orthopedics and Related Research*, Vol. No. 176, (Jun 1983), pp. 258-263, ISSN 0009-921X

Nicolle, L E. (1997). Asymptomatic bacteriuria in the elderly. *Infectious Disease Clinics of North America*, Vol. 11, No. 3, (Sep 1997), pp. 647-662, ISSN 0891-5520

Nicolle, L E. (2006). Asymptomatic bacteriuria: review and discussion of the IDSA guidelines. *International Journal of Antimicrobial Agents*, Vol. 28 Suppl 1, No. (Aug 2006), pp. S42-48, ISSN 0924-8579

Nicolle, L E. (2003). Asymptomatic bacteriuria: when to screen and when to treat. *Infectious Disease Clinics of North America*, Vol. 17, No. 2, (Jun 2003), pp. 367-394, ISSN 0891-5520

Nicolle, L E. (2001). Urinary tract infections in long-term-care facilities. *Infection Control and Hospital Epidemiology*, Vol. 22, No. 3, (Mar 2001), pp. 167-175, ISSN 0899-823X

Nicolle, L E. (2001). Urinary tract pathogens in complicated infection and in elderly individuals. *Journal of Infectious Diseases*, Vol. 183 Suppl 1, No. (Mar 1 2001), pp. S5-8, ISSN 0022-1899

Nicolle, L E et al. (1983). Bacteriuria in elderly institutionalized men. *New England Journal of Medicine*, Vol. 309, No. 23, (Dec 8 1983), pp. 1420-1425, ISSN 0028-4793

Nicolle, L E et al. (2005). Infectious Diseases Society of America guidelines for the diagnosis and treatment of asymptomatic bacteriuria in adults. *Clinical Infectious Diseases*, Vol. 40, No. 5, (Mar 1 2005), pp. 643-654, ISSN 1537-6591

Nicolle, L E et al. (1988). Urine specimen collection with external devices for diagnosis of bacteriuria in elderly incontinent men. *Journal of Clinical Microbiology*, Vol. 26, No. 6, (Jun 1988), pp. 1115-1119, ISSN 0095-1137

Nicolle, L E;Mayhew, W J &Bryan, L. (1987). Prospective randomized comparison of therapy and no therapy for asymptomatic bacteriuria in institutionalized elderly women. *American Journal of Medicine*, Vol. 83, No. 1, (Jul 1987), pp. 27-33, ISSN 0002-9343

Olson, E S &Cookson, B D. (2000). Do antimicrobials have a role in preventing septicaemia following instrumentation of the urinary tract? *The Journal of Hospital Infection*, Vol. 45, No. 2, (Jun 2000), pp. 85-97, ISSN 0195-6701

Orr, P H et al. (1996). Febrile urinary infection in the institutionalized elderly. *American Journal of Medicine*, Vol. 100, No. 1, (Jan 1996), pp. 71-77, ISSN 0002-9343

Ouslander, J G;Greengold, B &Chen, S. (1987). External catheter use and urinary tract infections among incontinent male nursing home patients. *Journal of the American Geriatrics Society*, Vol. 35, No. 12, (Dec 1987), pp. 1063-1070, ISSN 0002-8614

Ouslander, J G et al. (1987). An accurate method to obtain urine for culture in men with external catheters. *Archives of Internal Medicine*, Vol. 147, No. 2, (Feb 1987), pp. 286-288, ISSN 0003-9926

Ouslander, J G et al. (1995). Does eradicating bacteriuria affect the severity of chronic urinary incontinence in nursing home residents? *Annals of Internal Medicine*, Vol. 122, No. 10, (May 15 1995), pp. 749-754, ISSN 0003-4819

Patterson, J E &Andriole, V T. (1997). Bacterial urinary tract infections in diabetes. *Infectious Disease Clinics of North America*, Vol. 11, No. 3, (Sep 1997), pp. 735-750, ISSN 0891-5520

Peddie, B A et al. (1986). Association between diaphragm use and asymptomatic bacteriuria. *Australian and New Zealand Journal of Obstetrics & Gynaecology*, Vol. 26, No. 3, (Aug 1986), pp. 225-227, ISSN 0004-8666

Pels, R J et al. (1989). Dipstick urinalysis screening of asymptomatic adults for urinary tract disorders. II. Bacteriuria. *Jama: The Journal of American Medical Association*, Vol. 262, No. 9, (Sep 1 1989), pp. 1221-1224, ISSN 0098-7484

Platt, R. (1987). Adverse consequences of asymptomatic urinary tract infections in adults. *American Journal of Medicine*, Vol. 82, No. 6B, (Jun 26 1987), pp. 47-52, ISSN 0002-9343

Plauche, W C;Janney, F A &Curole, D N. (1981). Screening for asymptomatic bacteriuria in pregnant patients: three office screening systems versus quantitative culture. *Southern Medical Journal*, Vol. 74, No. 10, (Oct 1981), pp. 1227-1229, ISSN 0038-4348

Prat, V et al. (1985). Urinary tract infection in renal transplant patients. *Infection*, Vol. 13, No. 5, (Sep-Oct 1985), pp. 207-210, ISSN 0300-8126

Ramsey, D E;Finch, W T &Birtch, A G. (1979). Urinary tract infections in kidney transplant recipients. *Archives of Surgery*, Vol. 114, No. 9, (Sep 1979), pp. 1022-1025, ISSN 0004-0010

Raz, R. (2003). Asymptomatic bacteriuria. Clinical significance and management. *International Journal of Antimicrobial Agents*, Vol. 22 Suppl 2, No. (Oct 2003), pp. 45-47, ISSN 0924-8579

Raz, R et al. (2000). Recurrent urinary tract infections in postmenopausal women. *Clinical Infectious Diseases*, Vol. 30, No. 1, (Jan 2000), pp. 152-156, ISSN 1058-4838

Riedl, C R et al. (1999). Bacterial colonization of ureteral stents. *European Urology*, Vol. 36, No. 1, 1999), pp. 53-59, ISSN 0302-2838

Riley, D K et al. (1995). A large randomized clinical trial of a silver-impregnated urinary catheter: lack of efficacy and staphylococcal superinfection. *American Journal of Medicine*, Vol. 98, No. 4, (Apr 1995), pp. 349-356, ISSN 0002-9343

Ritter, M A &Fechtman, R W. (1987). Urinary tract sequelae: possible influence on joint infections following total joint replacement. *Orthopedics*, Vol. 10, No. 3, (Mar 1987), pp. 467-469, ISSN 0147-7447

Romero, R et al. (1989). Meta-analysis of the relationship between asymptomatic bacteriuria and preterm delivery/low birth weight. *Obstetrics & Gynecology*, Vol. 73, No. 4, (Apr 1989), pp. 576-582, ISSN 0029-7844

Rubin, R H et al. (1992). Evaluation of new anti-infective drugs for the treatment of urinary tract infection. Infectious Diseases Society of America and the Food and Drug Administration. *Clinical Infectious Diseases*, Vol. 15 Suppl 1, No. (Nov 1992), pp. S216-227, ISSN 1058-4838

Saint, S &Chenoweth, C E. (2003). Biofilms and catheter-associated urinary tract infections. *Infectious Disease Clinics of North America*, Vol. 17, No. 2, (Jun 2003), pp. 411-432, ISSN 0891-5520

Sanderson, P J &Weissler, S. (1990). A comparison of the effect of chlorhexidine antisepsis, soap and antibiotics on bacteriuria, perineal colonization and environmental contamination in spinally injured patients. *Journal of Hospital Infections*, Vol. 15, No. 3, (Apr 1990), pp. 235-243, ISSN 0195-6701

Savage, D C et al. (1975). Controlled trial of therapy in covert bacteriuria of childhood. *Lancet*, Vol. 1, No. 7903, (Feb 15 1975), pp. 358-361, ISSN 0140-6736

Schieve, L A et al. (1994). Urinary tract infection during pregnancy: its association with maternal morbidity and perinatal outcome. *American Journal of Public Health*, Vol. 84, No. 3, (Mar 1994), pp. 405-410, ISSN 0090-0036

Schlager, T A et al. (1995). Bacteriuria in children with neurogenic bladder treated with intermittent catheterization: natural history. *Journal of Pediatrics*, Vol. 126, No. 3, (Mar 1995), pp. 490-496, ISSN 0022-3476

Screening for asymptomatic bacteriuria, hematuria and proteinuria. The U.S. Preventive Services Task Force. (1990). *American Family Physician*, Vol. 42, No. 2, (Aug 1990), pp. 389-395, ISSN 0002-838X

Semetkowska-Jurkiewicz, E et al. (1995). The clinical course of untreated asymptomatic bacteriuria in diabetic patients--14-year follow-up. *Materia Medica Polona*, Vol. 27, No. 3, (Jul-Sep 1995), pp. 91-95, ISSN 0025-5246

Sequelae of covert bacteriuria in schoolgirls. A four-year follow-up study. (1978). *Lancet*, Vol. 1, No. 8070, (Apr 29 1978), pp. 889-893, ISSN 0140-6736

Shortliffe, L M. (1986). Asymptomatic bacteriuria: should it be treated? *Urology*, Vol. 27, No. 2 Suppl, (Feb 1986), pp. 19-25, ISSN 0090-4295

Siegel, S R et al. (1980). Urinary infection in infants and preschool children. Five-year follow-up. *American Journal of Diseases in Childrern*, Vol. 134, No. 4, (Apr 1980), pp. 369-372, ISSN 0002-922X

Silver, S A;Baillie, L &Simor, A E. (2009). Positive urine cultures: A major cause of inappropriate antimicrobial use in hospitals? *Canadian Journal of Infectious Diseases & Medical Microbiology*, Vol. 20, No. 4, (Winter 2009), pp. 107-111, ISSN 1918-1493

Smith, H S et al. (1997). Antecedent antimicrobial use increases the risk of uncomplicated cystitis in young women. *Clinical Infectious Diseases*, Vol. 25, No. 1, (Jul 1997), pp. 63-68, ISSN 1058-4838

Snydman, D R. (2001). Posttransplant microbiological surveillance. *Clinical Infectious Diseases*, Vol. 33 Suppl 1, No. (Jul 1 2001), pp. S22-25, ISSN 1058-4838

Sobel, J, Kaye, D. (2005). Urinary tract infections. *Principles and Practice of Infectious Diasease*, (6th edition), Elsvier Churchill Livingstone, ISBN 0443066434, Philadelphia, PA

Sotolongo, J R, Jr. &Koleilat, N. (1990). Significance of asymptomatic bacteriuria in spinal cord injury patients on condom catheter. *Journal of Urology*, Vol. 143, No. 5, (May 1990), pp. 979-980, ISSN 0022-5347

Stenqvist, K et al. (1987). Virulence factors of Escherichia coli in urinary isolates from pregnant women. *Journal of Infectious Diseases*, Vol. 156, No. 6, (Dec 1987), pp. 870-877, ISSN 0022-1899

Svanborg, C &Godaly, G. (1997). Bacterial virulence in urinary tract infection. *Infectious Disease Clinics of North America*, Vol. 11, No. 3, (Sep 1997), pp. 513-529, ISSN 0891-5520

Takai, K et al. (1998). Urinary tract infections following renal transplantation. *Clinical Transplantation*, Vol. 12, No. 1, (Feb 1998), pp. 19-23, ISSN 0902-0063

Tambyah, P A &Maki, D G. (2000). Catheter-associated urinary tract infection is rarely symptomatic: a prospective study of 1,497 catheterized patients. *Archives of Internal Medicine*, Vol. 160, No. 5, (Mar 13 2000), pp. 678-682, ISSN 0003-9926

Tencer, J. (1988). Asymptomatic bacteriuria--a long-term study. *Scandinavian Journal of Urology and Nephrology*, Vol. 22, No. 1, (1988), pp. 31-34, ISSN 0036-5599

Uehling, D T et al. (1985). Impact of an intermittent catheterization program on children with myelomeningocele. *Pediatrics*, Vol. 76, No. 6, (Dec 1985), pp. 892-895, ISSN 0031-4005

Vejlsgaard, R. (1966). Studies on urinary infection in diabetics. II. Significant bacteriuria in relation to long-term diabetic manifestations. *Acta medica Scandinavica*, Vol. 179, No. 2, (Feb 1966), pp. 183-188, ISSN 0001-6101

Wadland, W C &Plante, D A. (1989). Screening for asymptomatic bacteriuria in pregnancy. A decision and cost analysis. *Journal of Family Practice*, Vol. 29, No. 4, (Oct 1989), pp. 372-376, ISSN 0094-3509

Waites, K B;Canupp, K C &DeVivo, M J. (1993). Epidemiology and risk factors for urinary tract infection following spinal cord injury. *Archives of Physical Medicine & Rehabilitation*, Vol. 74, No. 7, (Jul 1993), pp. 691-695, ISSN 0003-9993

Walker, S et al. (2000). Why are antibiotics prescribed for asymptomatic bacteriuria in institutionalized elderly people? A qualitative study of physicians' and nurses' perceptions. *Canadian Medical Association Journal*, Vol. 163, No. 3, (Aug 8 2000), pp. 273-277, ISSN 0820-3946

Warren, J W et al. (1982). Cephalexin for susceptible bacteriuria in afebrile, long-term catheterized patients. *Jama: Journal of American Medical Association*, Vol. 248, No. 4, (Jul 23 1982), pp. 454-458, ISSN 0098-7484

Warren, J W et al. (1987). Fever, bacteremia, and death as complications of bacteriuria in women with long-term urethral catheters. *Journal of Infectious Diseases*, Vol. 155, No. 6, (Jun 1987), pp. 1151-1158, ISSN 0022-1899

Warren, J W et al. (1982). A prospective microbiologic study of bacteriuria in patients with chronic indwelling urethral catheters. *Journal of Infectious Diseases*, Vol. 146, No. 6, (Dec 1982), pp. 719-723, ISSN 0022-1899

Welch, T R et al. (1976). Recurrent urinary tract infection in girls. Group with lower tract findings and a benign course. *Archives of Diseases of Children*, Vol. 51, No. 2, (Feb 1976), pp. 114-119, ISSN 1468-2044

Wettergren, B et al. (1990). Six year follow up of infants with bacteriuria on screening. *British Medical Journal*, Vol. 301, No. 6756, (Oct 13 1990), pp. 845-848, ISSN 0959-8138

Whitworth, J A. (1981). Management of asymptomatic bacteriuria. *Australian and New Zealand journal of medicine*, Vol. 11, No. 3, (Jun 1981), pp. 321-328, ISSN 0004-8291

Wilson, A P et al. (1986). Prevalence of urinary tract infection in homosexual and heterosexual men. *Genitourinary Medicine*, Vol. 62, No. 3, (Jun 1986), pp. 189-190, ISSN 0266-4348

Zhanel, G G;Harding, G K &Guay, D R. (1990). Asymptomatic bacteriuria. Which patients should be treated? *Archives of Internal Medicine*, Vol. 150, No. 7, (Jul 1990), pp. 1389-1396, ISSN 0003-9926

Zhanel, G G;Harding, G K &Nicolle, L E. (1991). Asymptomatic bacteriuria in patients with diabetes mellitus. *Reviews of Infectious Diseases*, Vol. 13, No. 1, (Jan-Feb 1991), pp. 150-154, ISSN 0162-0886

Zhanel, G G;Nicolle, L E &Harding, G K. (1995). Prevalence of asymptomatic bacteriuria and associated host factors in women with diabetes mellitus. The Manitoba Diabetic Urinary Infection Study Group. *Clinical Infectious Diseases*, Vol. 21, No. 2, (Aug 1995), pp. 316-322, ISSN 1058-4838

# 7

# Urinary Tract Infections During Pregnancy

Anick Bérard[1,2], Fabiano Santos[1,2], Ema Ferreira[1,2] and Sylvie Perreault[1]
[1]*Faculty of Pharmacy, University of Montreal, Montreal, Quebec*
[2]*Research Center, CHU Sainte-Justine, Montreal, Quebec, Canada*

## 1. Introduction

Urinary tract infections (UTIs) are one of the most common medical complications of pregnancy (Mittal & Wing, 2005). It is estimated that one in three women of childbearing age will have a UTI (Duarte et al., 2008). Because of the normal physiologic changes induced by gestation, pregnant women are especially susceptible to these infections.

UTIs are characterized by the presence of infectious agents in the genito-urinary tract that cannot be explained by contamination. These agents have the potential to invade the tissues of the urinary tract and adjacent structures. The microbiological profile is well known and pathogens such as *Escherichia coli* have been present in the vast majority of cases (Sheffield & Cunningham, 2005). The infection may be limited to the growth of bacteria in the urine (which frequently don't produce symptoms) or it can result in several syndromes associated with an inflammatory response to the bacterial invasion. Actually, the term UTI represent a wide variety of conditions, including asymptomatic forms of UTIs, urethritis, cystitis, acute pyelonephritis and pyelonephritis with bacteremia or sepsis (Joseph DiPiro et al., 2011).

There are several classification methods for these infections. In this chapter, we will refer to UTIs as follows:

- Asymptomatic bacteriuria is defined as the presence of more than $10^8$ colonies/L of urine, without the symptoms of an acute UTI (Schnarr & Smaill, 2008);
- lower tract infection and upper tract infections, according to the anatomical site of contamination (Joseph DiPiro et al., 2011) ;
- Lower UTIs: The anatomical site of the infection can be the bladder (cystitis) and/or the urethra (urethritis) (Joseph DiPiro et al., 2011);
- Upper UTIs: The kidneys are the anatomical site of the infection (pyelonephritis associated with inflammation of the renal parenchyma, calices and pelvis) (Wagenlehner et al., 2009);
- Uncomplicated UTIs: infections occurring in individuals who lack structural or functional abnormalities of the urinary tract that interfere with the normal flow of urine or voiding mechanism (Joseph DiPiro et al., 2011);
- Complicated urinary tract infections: infections occurring in individuals with predisposing lesions of the urinary tract that interferes with the normal flow of urine and urinary tract defences. Common causes of predisposing lesions are birth defects,

kidney stones, catheters, or obstruction (Masson et al., 2009). An UTI during pregnancy is considered complicated.

During gestation, untreated UTIs can lead to several pregnancy complications, such as low birth weight infants, premature delivery, and occasionally, stillbirth. Prompt and efficacious treatment of symptomatic UTIs is warranted in pregnant women. Nevertheless, there is still some controversy regarding the screening and treatment of asymptomatic forms during gestation (Lin and Brown 2010; Lumbiganon et al., 2010; Schmiemann et al., 2010).

Given the prevalence and the potential impacts of UTIs on the health of the mother and her child, the objective of this chapter is to cover the most important clinical aspects of the epidemiology, etiology, physiopathology, pregnancy outcomes, and the treatment risks and benefits associated with UTIs during pregnancy.

## 2. Epidemiology

It is estimated that 2 to 10% of pregnant woman suffer from any form of UTIs (Lee et al., 2008). These infections complicate up to 20% of pregnancies and are responsible for the majority of antepartum admissions to the maternal–fetal medicine units (Sheffield & Cunningham, 2005).

The prevalence of asymptomatic forms of UTIs has remained constant across countries, and most of the recent observational studies report similar rates, ranging from 2 to 10% - similar to that of nonpregnant women (Duarte et al., 2008; Bahadi et al., 2010). Acute cystitis is prevalent in 1 to 4% of pregnant women (Wagenlehner et al., 2009).

Despite the relatively low prevalence of pyelonephritis during pregnancy (0.5 to 2%), it is estimated that 20% to 40% of pregnant women with asymptomatic bacteriuria will develop this condition later in gestation (Jolley & Wing, 2010). A study showed that if UTI is left untreated, 30% of mothers will develop acute pyelonephritis compared with 1.8% of non-bacteriuric controls[2]. Many studies have reported that pyelonephritis is more common during the second half of pregnancy, with an incidence peak during the last two trimesters of pregnancy (Gilstrap et al., 1981; Hill et al., 2005; Sharma & Thapa, 2007). Acute pyelonephritis may lead to adverse outcomes for the baby and the mother, such as premature delivery, low birth weight infants, preeclampsia, hypertension, renal failure and fetal death (Hill et al., 2005).

The prevalence of UTI in pregnancy is closely related to socioeconomic factors (Turck et al., 1962). Predictors of UTIs' asymptomatic forms include: welfare status, increasing maternal age, multiparity, risky sexual behavior, history of childhood UTIs and history of recurrent UTIs. It has been reported that indigent women have a five-fold greater incidence of bacteriuria than non-indigent populations (Turck et al., 1962; Golan et al., 1989). The prevalence is also markedly increased if women present certain pre-existing medical conditions, such as diabetes mellitus, sickle cell disease, immuno-deficiency states, urinary tract anatomic anomalies, spinal cord injuries and psychiatric illnesses (Ovalle et al., 1989). Nevertheless, there is some controversy on the effects of these host factors as predictors of UTIs (Fatima & Ishrat, 2006). UTI before pregnancy is a predictor for the diagnosis of asymptomatic bacteriuria at the first prenatal visit (Tugrul et al., 2005). Risk factors for developing cystitis and pyelonephritis in pregnancy include those stated before, as well as a history of *Clamidia trachomatis* infection, illicit drug use, and having less than 12 years of education (Verani et al., 2010).

It was suggested that UTIs screening and testing algorithms should be designed, incorporating identified risk factors in order to lower overall costs and to improve maternal and infant outcomes (Chng & Hall, 1982; Pastore et al., 1999). To date, no such algorithm has been prospectively evaluated (Schnarr & Smaill, 2008).

## 3. Etiology and physiopathology

### 3.1 Microbiology

In normal physiological circumstances, the genito-urinary tract is sterile. The microorganisms causing UTIs usually originate from the gastro-intestinal flora of the host. For example, during pregnancy bacteriuria can occur when bacteria from a fecal source gains access to the bladder by ascending the relatively short female urethra (Patterson & Andriole, 1997). Patogens causing bacteriuria are similar in both pregnant and nonpregnant women (Schnarr & Smaill, 2008). Although virtually every organism can be associated with UTIs, certain organisms predominate as a result of specific virulence and host susceptibility factors (Joseph DiPiro et al., 2011).

The most common agent implicated in uncomplicated UTIs is *Escherichia coli*, which accounts for 85% of non-hospital setting infections (Harris & Gilstrap, 1981; Millar & Cox, 1997; Sharma & Thapa, 2007). Other microorganisms such as *Staphylococcus saprophyticus* (5% to 15% of cases) (Mittal & Wing, 2005), *Gardnerella vaginalis, Chlamydia trachomatis, Klebsiella pneumoniae, Proteus spp., Pseudomonas aeruginosa, Enterococcus spp.* (5% to 10%), *Ureaplasma urealyticum* and lactobacilli have also been associated with UTIs. Although the clinical significance of these organisms on UTIs during pregnancy was not yet appreciated, a few small studies have reported improved outcomes following therapy against these agents (Gilbert et al., 1986; Cohen et al., 1990). The consensus is that during gestation, most UTIs are caused by a single organism. Nevertheless, organisms isolated from pregnant women with complicated UTIs are more varied and generally are more resistant to treatment than those found in uncomplicated infections. Anaerobic and other fastidious microorganisms have been identified in the urine of a large percentage of pregnant women, but the role played by these organisms on adverse perinatal outcomes is unknown (Gilbert et al., 1986). There is evidence that some bacterial strains can replicate inside the cells, explaining the difficulties in treating some cases, given that these strains are protected from the action of anti-infective drugs (Rosen et al., 2007). At present, there is no evidence showing advantages in routinely examining the urine for these uncommon organisms.

### 3.2 Physiopathology

For many years, pregnancy was seen as a period that naturally predisposes to all forms of UTIs. This was explained by the fact that genito-urinary anatomical and physiological changes induced by gestation predispose women with asymptomatic bacteriuria to develop symptomatic UTIs, leading to the impression that the number of UTIs was higher during this period of life (Nowicki, 2002). Nowadays, it is known that gestation itself is not the only responsible for the increased risk of UTIs. Throughout pregnancy, UTIs often persist, owing to re-infection (Foxman & Brown, 2003).

During gestation the urethra is colonized by bacteria originated from the gastro-intestinal and perineal flora (Naveen & Mathai, 2005). Other factors that can predispose urethral colonization include the use of some methods of contraception before pregnancy, such as spermicides and diaphragms (Fihn, 2003; Foxman & Brown, 2003). Although there is evidence that bladder infections follow colonization of the urethra, the mode of ascent of the microorganisms is not completely elucidated. After reaching the bladder, the organisms quickly multiply and can ascend the ureters to the kidneys. This sequence of events is more likely to occur if reflux of urine into the ureters and kidneys is present.

Bacterial colonization is facilitated as early as the renal pelvis and ureters begin to dilate (eighth week of gestation), and the bladder is displaced superiorly and anteriorly inside the intra-abdominal cavity (Jeyabalan & Lain, 2007). Mechanical compression caused by the enlarging uterus is the principle cause of this dilatation, but smooth muscle relaxation induced by progesterone may also play a role. The main consequences of these changes are the decrease in peristalsis of the ureters, followed by an increase in bladder capacity and urinary stasis. It is known that the decreased renal capacity to concentrate urine during pregnancy reduces the antibacterial activity of this fluid, leading it to excrete smaller amounts of potassium and higher amounts of glucose, amino acids and hormone degradation products. These biochemical alterations turn the urine into an alkaline solution, thus providing a suitable environment for bacterial growth (Dafnis & Sabatini, 1992). Additionally, the increase in the estrogen induced by gestation, contribute to the adhesion of certain *E. coli* strains to the type 1 uroepithelial cells (Roos et al., 2006).

Host protective factors such as the low glucose concentration of the urine, stability of the vaginal lactobacilli population, the influence of estrogens, the activity of Tamm-Horsfall protein, the presence of urinary mucus or slime (called glycosaminoglycan) and the immunologic defense mechanisms, makes the normal urinary tract generally resistant to invasion and efficient in rapidly eliminating microorganisms that reach the bladder (Parsons et al., 1978; Joseph DiPiro et al., 2011).

Specific subsets of *E. coli* clones identified with O, K and H antigens were shown to have increased propensity to cause UTIs (Kaper, 2005; Naveen & Mathai, 2005). An important virulence factor of bacteria is their ability to adhere to urinary epithelial cells, resulting in colonization of the urinary tract, bladder infections, and pyelonephritis. Uropathogenic *E. coli* have such virulence factors, known as fimbrias or *pilli*. These are adherence proteins (adhesins) expressed on the bacterial wall surface that promote binding to the epithelium of the vagina and urethra, thus increasing *E. coli* ability to cause UTIs (Sandberg et al., 1988). Adhesins include type 1, S and P fimbriae, and adhesins like Dr (Kaper, 2005). This property was recognized decades ago, and it is what differentiates uropathogenic *E. coli* from the gastro-intestinal commensal forms (Eden et al., 1976).

The type 1 fimbriae are prevalent and are probably involved in colonization of lower urinary tract (Naveen & Mathai, 2005). The role of P fimbriae in upper UTI is well documented (Wullt et al., 2002). These are present in 20% of faecal *E. coli*, 60% of cystitis causing, and 80% of *E. coli* isolated in pyelonehritis (Kaper, 2005). Attachment of P fimbriae to urinary tract epithelium is also associated with increased host inflammatory response (Wullt et al., 2002). Other factors that increase *E. coli* virulence include production of haemolysin, serum resistance and release of aerobactin (Wullt et al., 2002). Haemolysin provides *E. coli* a possible selective advantage by releasing iron from lysed erythrocytes and thus, enhancing pathogenicity by destroying phagocytic and epithelial cells (Naveen & Mathai, 2005).

Animal models and human data suggest that *E. coli* can remain hidden in large bacterial reservoirs within the host and can be reactivated to cause infection in the future, when there is some local decrease in the normal activity of the host defense factors (Mulvey et al., 2001;

Epp et al., 2010). Midstream urine samples from women with acute uncomplicated cystitis also showed evidence of intracellular bacterial communities of uropathogenic *E. coli* (Rosen et al., 2007). These communities are relatively protected from host immune response mechanisms and antibiotic therapy. They may be reactivated, causing recurrent UTI (Rosen et al., 2007).

There is some controversy concerning the role played by the physiological changes occuring during pregnancy which could be the main factor predisposing pregnant women to UTIs (Nowicki et al., 2011). Some authors claim that the biological complexity and molecular epidemiology of UTI suggest that mechanical obstruction can only partially explain the risk of developing gestational UTI (Nowicki, 2002). It is argued that if gestation alone predisposes to UTIs, urine stasis and obstruction should favour infection in the presence of avirulent random gram-negative and gram-positive species. Instead, 90% of gestational UTIs are associated with uropathogenic virulent *E. coli* strains, which (in contrast) are seldom isolated in the non-pregnant patients with urinary tract obstructive problems. To date, this issue remains controversial.

## 4. Clinical presentation and diagnosis

### 4.1 Clinical presentation

Given that UTIs correspond to the growth and multiplication of bacteria within the urinary tract, the resulting lesions can result in different degrees of severity. These infections can be grouped into four different clinical entities, according to the anatomical location of injury, maintaining relations between them (see Introduction section).

In 1962, Kass brought attention and concern to asymptomatic bacteriuria, noting that this form of infection was one of the most important predisposing factors for pyelonephritis in pregnant women (Kass, 1962). Since then, there was a step forward to recognize the importance of early diagnosis of this form of infection in early pregnancy, avoiding the complications of pyelonephritis (MacLean, 2001; Smaill, 2007). Asymptomatic bacteriuria is characterized by bacterial colonization of the urine, and if it shows no clinical symptoms, microbiological laboratory tests are needed to support its diagnosis (MacLean, 2001). Asymptomatic bacteriuria is defined by two consecutive clean-catch urine cultures with more than $10^8$ colonies/L of urine, with a single type of bacteria (Shand et al., 1970). It is believed that the vast majority of pregnant women that developing UTIs' symptomatic forms during gestation have asymptomatic bacteriuria at the time of conception. It was observed that 30% of women with asymptomatic bacteriuria developed symptomatic UTI during gestation (Gratacos et al., 1994).

Urethritis is characterized by urethral colonization resulting in dysuria and polyuria. Approximately 50% of pregnant women suffering from this complication do not have significant asymptomatic bacteriuria, and in 30% of them, urine cultures are negative. From a practical standpoint, only 20% of symptomatic patients have urine culture with more than $10^8$ colonies/L of urine. Another important detail is that some etiological agents involved in urethritis are germs commonly found in the vaginal cavity and that cause genital infections - some cannot be detected in routine urine cultures, such as *Chlamydia trachomatis* and *Mycoplasma hominis* (Nicolle, 2006). However, the potential invasiveness of these bacteria in the urinary tract is low.

Cystitis is the infection of the bladder, occurring in about 1 to 1.5% of pregnancies. Common clinical manifestations are dysuria, polyuria, suprapubic discomfort, and in some cases, hematuria (Le et al., 2004). Although dysuria and polyuria may suggest UTIs, these symptoms may concomitantly be present in pregnant women with other conditions, such as bacterial vaginosis (Duarte et al., 2008). In addition, hemorrhagic cystitis during pregnancy can be confounded with bleeding issued from a process that could be bacterial, viral, fungal, immune (allergic) and radiotherapy. Cystitis is associated with preterm delivery and should be treated as soon as detected (Fakhoury et al., 1994).

Pyelonephritis is the most severe form of UTI in pregnant women and may affect up to 2% of this population. Its occurrence is directly associated with the prevalence of asymptomatic bacteriuria among pregnant women (Gilstrap et al., 1981; Nowicki, 2002). This condition can occur with or without symptoms of cystitis. Overall, pyelonephritis is associated with worse maternal and prenatal prognosis (Schieve et al., 1994). Clinical signs and symptoms of pyelonephritis include flank pain (unilateral or bilateral) or abdominal pain, fever, anorexia, nausea and vomiting often associated with variable degrees of dehydration, chills, headache, and tachypinea. Respiratory failure and sepsis can be present in severe forms. Fever is elevated in the acute forms (Rosen et al., 2007). When considering the clinical diagnosis of UTIs during pregnancy, it is useful to remember that some symptoms of infection are difficult to characterize because they can be normally present during gestation, such as polyuria. In addition, asymptomatic bacteriuria does not present any clinical manifestation. However, patient history and risk factors can identify women at higher risk of UTI (Pastore et al., 1999; Nowicki, 2002; Fatima & Ishrat, 2006; Roos et al., 2006).

### 4.2 Diagnosis

Given the increased incidence of symptomatic UTI during pregnancy and its association with maternal and perinatal complications, screening of asymptomatic bacteriuria during pregnancy is requested with two urine samples obtained at different times. Testing a single sample may provide false-positive result in up to 40% of cases (MacLean, 2001). This measure can allow early start treatment and reduces the rate of progression to symptomatic infection and it's potentially harmfull consequences (Gratacos et al., 1994; Smaill, 2007).

Current laboratory tests for the diagnosis of UTI are based on the color changes of chemical reactants according to urine composition (dipstick analysis). Two of these are important for their rapidity and low costs: the test of nitrite and the test of leukocyte esterasis. The nitrite test is based on the ability of certain bacteria to reduce the urinary nitrate to nitrite. This test has 50% sensitivity and specificity of 97%, and can result in false positives when used on urine contaminated by normal vaginal bacteria or highly concentrated urine, given that the test follows colorimetric principles. The leukocyte esterase test has low sensitivity and specificity (25%) and can also result in false positives. Both tests have low sensitivity and therefore not suitable as screening tests for diagnosis, unless they are used in combination with other tests (McNair et al., 2000).

Microscopic urinalysis is the examination of one drop of centrifuged and uncoloured fresh urine, with dry objective (400 times magnification). The observation of any bacteria per field correlates with a urine culture of at least $10^8$ colonies/L of urine. Despite being a low cost test, its low sensitivity limits it to be indicated in the screening of asymptomatic bacteriuria (McNair et al., 2000). Current evidence seems to indicate that the microscopic analysis of a Gram-colored urine sample is a more suitable and rapid test for UTI screening. It consists in the microscopic observation of the urine bacteria Gram stain, improving the accuracy of microscopic urinalysis (Duarte et al., 2008).

Several alternative laboratory methods can be used for the diagnosis of UTIs with varying sensitivities and specificities. Therefore, the association of these tests can be necessary to confirm the positive results of a urinalysis. Moreover, for their meaningfull interpretation, it become imperative to use correct techniques for collecting the urine sample (aseptic perineal urine midstream, immediate transportation and refrigeration at 4 °C for, no later than 24 hours) (Nicolle, 2006).

Among the abnormalities likely to be detected in a urinalysis, we can find pyuria, hematuria, proteinuria and cylinders in the urinary sediment. These findings can indicate UTI, but actually they are just signs of inflammation and may also be present in other conditions. It should be remembered that a normal urinalysis result does not exclude the diagnosis of UTI, hence, not being ideal for screening of asymptomatic bacteriuria during pregnancy. However, in symptomatic patients, the result of this test is accepted for the initiation of therapy until the results of urine microbiologic culture are known (Nicolle, 2006; Duarte et al., 2008).

The urine microbiologic culture is considered the gold standard for laboratory diagnosis of UTI. It is the most accurate method to identify and quantify bacteria in the urine with high sensibility (MacLean, 2001). Its drawbacks are the relatively higher costs, the long time needed to achieve the number of bacterial colonies necessary for a sensitive result and the need for professionals and laboratories qualified for its elaboration (Rosen et al., 2007). The correct interpretation of a urine culture is crucial for therapeutic success. In asymptomatic cases, the finding of more than $10^8$ colonies/L of urine suggests infection. Values between $10^7$ and $10^8$ correspond to infection in 50% of cases. If the urine is collected by bladder catheterization, the finding of values above $10^6$ indicates infection; if the urine is issued by suprapubic aspiration, infection is diagnosed with any number of bacteria. In symptomatic cases, urine cultures are considered positive with up to $10^5$ bacteria/mL of urine (Nicolle, 2006).

Other important complementary tests include total and differential blood cells count, and dosage of metabolites such as urea and creatinine. These tests help to identify the severity of the infection, reflected in the hematologic and renal function parameters. However, they are not essential for the monitoring of patients with uncomplicated UTIs. Ultrasound of kidneys and urinary tract can be considered an important complementary examination. In addition of being rapid, inexpensive, easily accessible and totally safe for both mother and fetus, they can help to identify predisposing factors for adverse pregnancy outcomes, such as urinary calculus and pathological dilatation of the renal collecting system (Duarte et al., 2008).

## 5. UTIs and pregnancy outcomes

Several studies have associated UTIs during gestation with the risk of adverse perinatal and maternal outcomes. Some other studies failed to prove such associations (Gilstrap et al., 1981; Reddy & Campbell, 1985; Chen et al., 2010). Inconsistencies in the results of these studies could be due to selection bias, low statistical power and inadequate control for potential confounders. As stated before, the general consensus is that UTIs can lead to complications, such as low-birth-weight infants, premature delivery, and, occasionally, stillbirth (Lee et al., 2008).

### 5.1 UTIs and maternal outcomes

The maternal complications of UTI are a result of the tissue damage caused by bacterial endotoxins, especially in pyelonephritis (Neal, 2008). The most dramatic maternal complication associated with UTIs is bacteremia and septic shock, induced by resistant pyelonephritis (Mittal & Wing, 2005). Endotoxin-mediated damage includes diminished peripheral vascular resistance and changes in cardiovascular output. With the release of *E. coli* endotoxin active component of (lipid A) into the maternal circulation, a cascade response of pro-inflammatory cytokines, histamine, and bradykinins is precipitated, which may lead to the more serious complications (septic shock, disseminated intravascular coagulation, respiratory insufficiency, and adult respiratory distress syndrome (Galajdova, 2010)). This syndrome is defined as a disease of acute onset with bilateral infiltrates on chest radiograph and hypoxemia without evidence of pulmonary hypertension (Graves, 2002), and complicates 1% to 8% of cases of pyelonephritis in pregnancy (Wing, 1998). Women who have septic shock require admission to intensive care, immediate fluid resuscitation, and antimicrobial therapy. Although patients generally respond well to oxygen therapy, worsening dyspnea, tachypnea, and hypoxemia may signify progress to adult respiratory distress syndrome (Graves, 2002). Respiratory failure and pulmonary edema can result from an increased permeability of the alveolar-capillary membrane. This condition can be worsened by the use of hyperhydration and tocolytics, often administered for inhibition of preterm labor (Duarte et al., 2008). Although bacteremia is detected in 15-20% of women with severe pyelonephritis, few of them develop clinical manifestations of septic shock.

Other maternal complications that have been associated with UTIs during pregnancy are hypertension and preeclampsia (Conde-Agudelo et al., 2008; Rustveld et al., 2008), anemia (Fede, 1983), chorioamnionitis and endometritis (Schieve et al., 1994; Delzell & Lefevre, 2000). The causal nature of these associations is questionable, because it is not always clear whether an episode of UTI preceded the particular outcome of interest, especially in what concerns maternal hypertension and anemia (Schieve et al., 1994).

The relationship between UTIs during pregnancy and preeclampsia is consistent throughout studies performed over the last years, and is present in diverse settings worldwide (Conde-Agudelo et al., 2008). Several mechanisms have been proposed to explain how maternal infection might be involved in the etiology of preeclampsia or its manifestations. These include direct effects of the infectious agents on the arterial walls, including endothelial injury or dysfunction, acute atherosis, and local inflammation that might cause relative uteroplacental ischemia (von Dadelszen & Magee, 2002). Furthermore, some authors have hypothesized that the infection might be involved in both the initiation of the pre-eclampsia process (by increasing the risk of acute uteroplacental atherosis) and/or its potentiation (by amplifying the maternal systemic inflammatory response) (Herrera et al., 2001). Nevertheless, these hypotheses are issued from animal data and some other authors argue that the association between UTIs and preeclampsia may not be real and may be due to confounding. For example, abnormal changes associated with chronic pyelonephritis and papillary necrosis has been observed in almost half of women with bacteriuria during pregnancy (Whalley et al., 1965). These underlying diseases and the impairment of renal function they cause could, thus, account for the higher risk of preeclampsia among women with bacteriuria (Conde-Agudelo et al., 2008). More data is needed to determine whether the relationship between maternal UTIs and preeclampsia is causal.

Local complications, such as urinary obstruction, perinephric abscess and cellulitis are rare and when present, are associated with lithiasis or treatment-resistant microorganisms (Le et al., 2004; Neal, 2008).

### 5.2 UTIs and perinatal outcomes

The association between perinatal outcomes and UTIs has been studied for many years (Mittal & Wing 2005; Duarte et al., 2008). From a global health perspective, UTI is one of the most important and potentially preventable causes of early preterm birth (Simmons et al., 2010). Intrauterine infections are thought to be responsible for up to 50% of extreme preterm births of less than 28 weeks of gestation, where both neonatal mortality and morbidity are high (Simmons et al., 2010). Observational studies show an association between maternal UTIs and preterm birth and low birth weight (Gravett et al., 2010). Most of these studies are conducted in lower and middle income countries. Therefore, there is a great deal of heterogeneity between studies regarding the association between these infections and the risk of preterm birth (Beck et al., 2010). Among other recognized perinatal complications of UTI, we highlight premature rupture of membranes, intrauterine growth restriction, cerebral palsy/mental retardation and perinatal death (Romero et al., 1989; Polivka et al., 1997; McDermott et al., 2000; Duarte et al., 2008). Some cases of periventricular leukomalacia and fetal septicemia have been recently reported as a result of transplacental transfer of cytokines originated from maternal UTIs (Spinillo et al., 1998; Oda et al., 2008). Pregnancies complicated by UTIs are also associated with increased fetal mortality (McDermott et al., 2001).

It was estimated that 27% of preterm deliveries are associated with pre-existing UTIs (Turiani, 2009). In the same study, the investigators found that women with pyelonephritis had prevalence for low birth weight infants of 15% (defined as birth weight less than 2500 grams). Same findings were reported in a large cohort study conducted in the USA. In this study, UTIs were also associated with the risk of small-for-gestational-age newborns (Schieve et al., 1994). Evidence issued from microbiological analysis of the genito-urinary tract of women with premature labor or preterm rupture of membranes, show that UTI is the most important risk factor for perinatal morbidity and fetal death (Turiani, 2009). Data from 52 cases of neonatal sepsis showed that UTIs were present in 63% of cases (Ananthakrishnan & Gunasekaran, 2009). All the aforementioned adverse pregnancy outcomes are important predictors of neonatal mortality.

Data on the treatment of UTI and its effect on pregnancy outcomes corroborate the observation that these infections, if left untreated, are associated with low birth weight. In one study, the risk of preterm delivery in women who had asymptomatic UTI was two times greater than in unaffected women. With adequate treatment, the risk of low birth weight infants was 44% lower when compared to the untreated group (Gilstrap et al., 1981; Romero et al., 1989). These findings were confirmed in a recent Cochrane review which demonstrated the decreased incidence of pyelonephritis and low birth weight infants when asymptomatic UTI was treated (Smaill & Vazquez, 2007).

The increased incidence of preterm labor and delivery associated with UTIs can be explained by the inflammatory response induced by citokines and prostaglandins mediators. Another way in which preterm labor can be triggered is through the colonization of amniotic fluid by uropathogens originated from UTIs. These bacteria produce phospholipases A and C, that act as precursors of pro-contractile prostaglandins E2 and F2a, consequently triggering preterm labor (Duarte et al., 2008; Bhutta et al., 2010). There are several mechanisms suggested to explain the high rates of premature rupture of membranes in pregnant women with UTI. One of them is that UTIs induces the release of metalloproteinases by macrophages, via cytokines which degrade the membranes, predisposing them to rupture, in a similar way as do collagenasis and phospholipasis issued from bacteria (Sayres, 2010) (Wax et al., 2010).

There has also been a hypothesis suggesting that UTI during pregnancy is associated with child developmental delay and mental retardation (Broman, 1987). One study has found a 30% increase in the risk for cognitive delay in children whose mothers had UTI during pregnancy, when compared to children whose mothers were not infected (McDermott et al., 2001). Furthermore, when comparing untreated women with treated women, the risk of having infants with cognitive delay was 22% higher. These results support the association between UTI in pregnancy and cognitive delay and emphasize the importance of the rapid diagnosis and treatment. However, the multifactorial nature of these outcomes makes the determination of etiology difficult, and no firm consensus has been reached on this subject (Mittal & Wing 2005).

Given the burden of UTI during pregnancy, with regards to adverse maternal and pregnancy outcomes, these infections must be adequately diagnosed and efficient treatment must be initiated. Screening and treatment of assympomatic UTI during pregnancy is recommended by the U.S. Preventive Services Task Force (USPSTF, 2010). Given the evidence indicating that detection and treatment of asymptomatic bacteriuria with antibiotics significantly reduces the incidence of maternal UTIs and low birth weight, the USPSTF concludes that during pregnancy, there is high certainty that the net benefit of screening for asymptomatic bacteriuria is substantial. Nevertheless, in men and non-pregnant women, there is moderate certainty that the harms of screening for asymptomatic bacteriuria outweighs the benefits (Lin & Brown, 2010). The USPSTF discloses that the urine culture is the standard criterion for detecting asymptomatic bacteriuria. Nevertheless, as previously discussed, it is recognized that this test is expensive for routine screening in populations with a low prevalence of the condition. However, no currently available tests have a high enough sensitivity and negative predictive value (Lin & Fajardo, 2008). The screening tests used commonly in primary care (dipstick analysis and direct microscopy) have poor positive and negative predictive value for detecting bacteriuria in asymptomatic persons (Bandyopadhyay et al., 2005, 2010). Pregnant women with asymptomatic bacteriuria should receive antibiotic therapy directed at the cultured organism and follow-up monitoring. The screening intervals must be between 12 to 16 weeks' gestation or at the first pre-natal visit, if later, although there is no consensus in the literature as to the optimal timing and screening frequency for asymptomatic bacteriuria (McIsaac et al., 2005; Tugrul et al., 2005; Schnarr & Smaill, 2008).

## 6. Treatment of UTIs during pregnancy

Data from observational studies showed that the prevalence of anti-infective use during pregnancy is 24.5% (Santos et al., 2010a). Once the clinical diagnosis of UTI is established, treatment is mandatory even when no confirmation of the UTI etiological agent by the microbiologic culture test is available. As a consequence, the initial antibiotic therapy has the drawback of being empirical, and a variety of different antimicrobial agents can be used for the treatment of bacteriuria (Gilstrap & Ramin, 2001). Therefore, a periodic assessment of the sensitivity pattern of etiological agents against anti-infective drugs commonly used to treat UTIs must be done. This measure becomes extremely important given the growing number of bacterial resistant to the antibiotics that are deemed safe during pregnancy (Duarte et al., 2008). It is important to remember that therapy must be safe for both mother and fetus. Nearly all anti-infective drugs are able to cross the placenta, and therefore agents that may be harmful to the developing fetus should be avoided. Antibiotics that have been associated with teratogenic effects are quinolones, trimethropime/sulfamethoxazole, chloramphenicol, and tetracycline (Macejko & Schaeffer, 2007).

Quinolones has been associated to the development of arthropathy when given directly to immature animals and is not usually recommended for routine use during pregnancy. This adverse effect has not been described in humans (Gilstrap & Ramin, 2001; Macejko & Schaeffer, 2007; Lee et al., 2008). Tetracycline has been associated with yellow-brown discoloration of the deciduous teeth, when used after the 16th week of gestation, and gentamicin could potentially cause eighth nerve damage in the fetus (Dashe & Gilstrap, 1997; Schnarr & Smaill, 2008).

Given that pregnant women are not enrolled in randomised clinical trials assessing safety, there is no clear consensus on the choice of antibiotics and the duration of treatment during gestation. As a consequence, practice is more likely guided by national patterns of prescription and local bacterial resistance profiles (Schnarr & Smaill, 2008). Antibiotics commonly used for the treatment of UTIs during pregnancy have not been found to be associated with an increased risk of birth defects. Beta lactams antibiotics, such as penicillins and cephalosporins, are deemed safe during pregnancy and are commonly prescribed for the treatment of UTIs during the gestational period (Lee et al., 2008; Schnarr & Smaill, 2008; Guinto et al., 2010, Santos et al., 2010a). Despite the fact that no drug of this class has any apparent teratogenic properties, beta-lactams are sometimes associated with allergic and anaphylactic reactions. In addition, high bacterial resistance rates limit the use of some agents, such as amoxicillin or ampicillin (Dashe & Gilstrap, 1997; Guinto et al., 2010).

Safety of nitrofurantoin in pregnancy has already been demonstrated (Ben David et al., 1995). Nitrofurantoin only achieves therapeutic levels in the urine, so it cannot be used to treat pyelonephritis. This drug is not active against *Proteus* spp (Christensen, 2000; Sahm et al., 2001). There is a theoretical risk of nitrofurantoin-induced hemolytic anemia in the fetusor newborn, particularly in those with glucose-6-phosphate dehydrogenase (G6PD) deficiency (Smaill & Vazquez, 2007; Guinto et al., 2010).

Trimethoprim is a folic acid antagonist and its use during the first trimester has been associated with neural tube and cardiovascular defects in the newborn (Milo et al., 2005). Sulfonamides could theoretically displace bilirubin from albumin-binding sites and could cause severe jaundice leading to kernicterus. Practical evidence of this risk, however, is sparse (Smaill, 2000). Furtheremore, a recent study showed an association between exposure to sulphonamides during the last two trimesters of pregnancy and the risk of small for gestational age newborns (Santos et al., 2010b).

Follow-up of women with asymptomatic bacteriuria is important because approximately one third of them will experience a recurrent infection during pregnancy. For women with frequent recurrent episodes of bacteriuria or symptomatic UTIs, prophylactic continuous antibiotic treatment should be considered. However, the protracted use of antibiotics, especially ampicillin and cephalosporins, may interfere with the normal gastrointestinal flora. Prolonged use of these antibiotics may be associated with chronic vulvovaginitis secondary to overgrowth of *Candida albicans* (Gilstrap & Ramin 2001).

Table 1 summarizes most common therapeutic regimens currently proposed for the treatment of UTIs during pregnancy, according to the type of UTIs (Bruel et al., 2000; Milo et al., 2005; Mittal & Wing, 2005; Cimolai & Cimolai, 2007; Rosen et al., 2007; Duarte et al., 2008; Guinto et al., 2010).

| Urinary tract infection | Treatment regimen | Treatment options | Comments |
|---|---|---|---|
| Assymptomatic bacteriuria | Current standard of practice is to treat pregnant patients who have asymptomatic bacteriuria with at least 3 to 7 days of an oral anti-infective agent (Rubin et al., 1992; Connolly & Thorp, 1999; Christensen, 2000; Gilstrap & Ramin, 2001; Ovalle & Levancini, 2001). | Cephalexin 250-500 mg, po, qid<br>Nitrofurantoin 100 mg, po, qid or Nitrofurantoin (monohydrate/macro-crystals) 100 mg, po, bid, 7 days<br>Amoxicillin 500 mg, po, tid<br>Norfloxacin 400 mg, po, bid<br>Cefuroxim 250 mg, po, tid<br>SXT (320/1600 mg) po, once a day (avoid use during first trimester) | Single-dose and three days regimens have been used, but showed lack of efficacy. Some authors do not recommend during gestation (Rubin et al., 1992; Smaill & Vazquez, 2007). SXT was associated with a theoretical increased risk of neural tube defects and it may lead to neonatal kernicterus (Schnarr & Smaill, 2008). Nitrofurantoin was associated with theoretical risk of fetal hemolytic anemia when mother has G6PD deficiency (Smaill & Vazquez, 2007). Given the increased rates of bacterial resistance to ampicillin and cephalexin, one must verify hospital susceptibilities before prescribing b-lactam monotherapy (Mittal & Wing, 2005; Joseph DiPiro et al., 2011). |
| Urethritis and cystitis | Given that the pathogens associated with urethritis and cystitis are the same as those causing asymptomatic bacteriuria, the treatment of cystitis in pregnancy is the same as the treatment for asymptomatic bacteriuria, longer courses of therapy are usually recommended (7-10 days) (Gilstrap & Ramin, 2001). | Cefuroxim 250 mg, po, tid<br>Nitrofurantoin 100 mg, po, qid or Nitrofurantoin (monohydrate/macro-crystals) 100 mg, po, bid<br>Amoxicillin 500 mg, po, tid<br>SXT (320/1600 mg) po, once a day (avoid use during first trimester) | These agents are FDA class B category (Mittal & Wing, 2005). |

| Urinary tract infection | Treatment regimen | Treatment options | Comments |
|---|---|---|---|
| Pyelonephritis | Initial treatment must be parentheral (Vazquez & Villar, 2003; Duarte et al., 2008). First-line therapy often includes a first-generation cephalosporin. In an inpatient setting, parenteral antimicrobial therapy usually is continued until the patient is afebrile for 48 hours (Wing, 1998). The patient is switched to oral antimicrobial therapy for 2 weeks (total). | Ampicillin 2 grams, IV, q6h (+) Gentamicin 1.5-1.7/mg/kg, IV, q6 h<br>Gentamicin 1.5-1.7/mg/kg, IV, q8h<br>Ampicillin-sulbactam 3 grams, IV, q6 h<br>Ceftriaxone 1 gram, IV/IM, q24 h<br>Cefuroxime 0.75–1.5 grams, IV, q8 h<br>Cefazolin 2 grams, IV, q6–8 h<br>Mezlocillin 3 grams, IV, q6 h<br>Piperacillin 4 grams IV q8 h<br>Ticarcillin/clavulanate 3.1 grams, IV, q6h | Ampicillin monotherapy showed high incidence of resistant bacteria, and therefore, usually is used in conjunction with gentamicin (Dunlow & Duff, 1990).<br>To avoid exacerbation of the renal insufficiency that commonly accompanies pyelonephritis, drug serum levels should be monitored when using aminoglycosides, such as gentamicin (Wing, 1998). |

Table 1. Most common therapeutic regimens currently proposed for the treatment of UTIs during pregnancy (Abbreviations: po: by mouth; q: every; bid: twice a day; tid: three times a day; qid: four times a day; SXT: Trimethoprim/Sulfamethoxazole; IM: intramuscularly; IV: intravenously).

## 7. Conclusion

Urinary tract infection is a prevalent complication of pregnancy that can worsen maternal and perinatal prognosis. Untreated asymptomatic forms can progress to pyelonephritis, which is associated with preterm delivery, low birth weight infants and stillbirth. In addition to the increased incidence of UTIs during gestation, health care professionals must be aware that the choice of available anti-infective drugs are restricted, given the risk of certain of them for the fetus, and the potential for bacterial resistance. Most of the drugs used for the treatment of UTIs during pregnancy are not associated with an increased risk of birth defects. Early diagnosis followed by immediate and adequate therapy is essential during gestation, avoiding compromising maternal and neonatal health.

## 8. Acknowledgment

Dr. Anick Bérard is the recipient of a career award from the *Fonds de la Recherche en Santé du Québec* (FRSQ) and is on the endowment Research Chair of the Famille Louis-Boivin on

Medications, Pregnancy and Lactation at the Faculty of Pharmacy of the University of Montreal. Fabiano Santos is the recipient of the Sainte-Justine Hospital Foundation and the Foundation of Stars scholarship and of the Robert Dugal scholarship (Health Research Foundation and Faculty of Pharmacy of the University of Montreal). The authors have no conflict of interest to declare.

## 9. References

A U.S. Preventive Services Task Force. (2010) Screening for asymptomatic bacteriuria in adults: reaffirmation recommendation statement. Am Fam Physician, 81, 505.

Ananthakrishnan, S. & Gunasekaran, D. (2009) Etiology and risk factors for early onset neonatal sepsis. Indian J Med Microbiol, 27, 279.

Bahadi, A., El Kabbaj, D., Elfazazi, H., Abbi, R., Hafidi, M.R., Hassani, M.M., Moussaoui, R., Elouennass, M., Dehayni, M. & Oualim, Z. (2010) Urinary tract infection in pregnancy. Saudi J Kidney Dis Transpl, 21, 342-344.

Bandyopadhyay, S., Thakur, J.S., Ray, P. & Kumar, R. (2005) High prevalence of bacteriuria in pregnancy and its screening methods in north India. J Indian Med Assoc, 103, 259-262, 266.

Beck, S., Wojdyla, D., Say, L., Betran, A.P., Merialdi, M., Requejo, J.H., Rubens, C., Menon, R. & Van Look, P.F. (2010) The worldwide incidence of preterm birth: a systematic review of maternal mortality and morbidity. Bull World Health Organ, 88, 31-38.

Ben David, S., Einarson, T., Ben David, Y., Nulman, I., Pastuszak, A. & Koren, G. (1995) The safety of nitrofurantoin during the first trimester of pregnancy: meta-analysis. Fundam Clin Pharmacol, 9, 503-507.

Bhutta, Z.A., Lassi, Z.S., Blanc, A. & Donnay, F. (2010) Linkages among reproductive health, maternal health, and perinatal outcomes. Semin Perinatol, 34, 434-445.

Broman, S.H. (1987) Prenatal risk factors for mental retardation in young children. Public Health Rep, 102, 55-57.

Bruel, H., Guillemant, V., Saladin-Thiron, C., Chabrolle, J.P., Lahary, A. & Poinsot, J. (2000) [Hemolytic anemia in a newborn after maternal treatment with nitrofurantoin at the end of pregnancy]. Arch Pediatr, 7, 745-747.

Chen, Y.K., Chen, S.F., Li, H.C. & Lin, H.C. (2010) No increased risk of adverse pregnancy outcomes in women with urinary tract infections: a nationwide population-based study. Acta Obstet Gynecol Scand, 89, 882-888.

Chng, P.K. & Hall, M.H. (1982) Antenatal prediction of urinary tract infection in pregnancy. Br J Obstet Gynaecol, 89, 8-11.

Christensen, B. (2000) Which antibiotics are appropriate for treating bacteriuria in pregnancy? J Antimicrob Chemother, 46 Suppl 1, 29-34; discussion 63-25.

Cimolai, N. & Cimolai, T. (2007) Nitrofurantoin and pregnancy. CMAJ, 176, 1860-1861.

Cohen, I., Veille, J.C. & Calkins, B.M. (1990) Improved pregnancy outcome following successful treatment of chlamydial infection. JAMA, 263, 3160-3163.

Conde-Agudelo, A., Villar, J. & Lindheimer, M. (2008) Maternal infection and risk of preeclampsia: systematic review and metaanalysis. Am J Obstet Gynecol, 198, 7-22.

Connolly, A. & Thorp, J.M., Jr. (1999) Urinary tract infections in pregnancy. Urol Clin North Am, 26, 779-787.

Dafnis, E. & Sabatini, S. (1992) The effect of pregnancy on renal function: physiology and pathophysiology. Am J Med Sci, 303, 184-205.

Dashe, J.S. & Gilstrap, L.C., 3rd (1997) Antibiotic use in pregnancy. Obstet Gynecol Clin North Am, 24, 617-629.

Delzell, J.E., Jr. & Lefevre, M.L. (2000) Urinary tract infections during pregnancy. Am Fam Physician, 61, 713-721.

Duarte, G., Marcolin, A.C., Quintana, S.M. & Cavalli, R.C. (2008) [Urinary tract infection in pregnancy]. Rev Bras Ginecol Obstet, 30, 93-100.

Dunlow, S. & Duff, P. (1990) Prevalence of antibiotic-resistant uropathogens in obstetric patients with acute pyelonephritis. Obstet Gynecol, 76, 241-244.

Eden, C.S., Hanson, L.A., Jodal, U., Lindberg, U. & Akerlund, A.S. (1976) Variable adherence to normal human urinary-tract epithelial cells of Escherichia coli strains associated with various forms of urinary-tract infection. Lancet, 1, 490-492.

Epp, A., Larochelle, A., Lovatsis, D., Walter, J.E., Easton, W., Farrell, S.A., Girouard, L., Gupta, C., Harvey, M.A., Robert, M., Ross, S., Schachter, J., Schulz, J.A., Wilkie, D., Ehman, W., Domb, S., Gagnon, A., Hughes, O., Konkin, J., Lynch, J., Marshall, C., Society of, O. & Gynaecologists of, C. (2010) Recurrent urinary tract infection. J Obstet Gynaecol Can, 32, 1082-1101.

Fakhoury, G.F., Daikoku, N.H. & Parikh, A.R. (1994) Management of severe hemorrhagic cystitis in pregnancy. A report of two cases. J Reprod Med, 39, 485-488.

Fatima, N. & Ishrat, S. (2006) Frequency and risk factors of asymptomatic bacteriuria during pregnancy. J Coll Physicians Surg Pak, 16, 273-275.

Fede, T. (1983) Urinary tract infection and anemia in pregnancy. Clin Exp Obstet Gynecol, 10, 140-141.

Fihn, S.D. (2003) Clinical practice. Acute uncomplicated urinary tract infection in women. N Engl J Med, 349, 259-266.

Foxman, B. & Brown, P. (2003) Epidemiology of urinary tract infections: transmission and risk factors, incidence, and costs. Infect Dis Clin North Am, 17, 227-241.

Galajdova, L. (2010) Pulmonary dysfunction in acute antepartum pyelonephritis and other pregnancy infections. J Obstet Gynaecol, 30, 654-658.

Gilbert, G.L., Garland, S.M., Fairley, K.F. & McDowall, D.M. (1986) Bacteriuria due to ureaplasmas and other fastidious organisms during pregnancy: prevalence and significance. Pediatr Infect Dis, 5, S239-243.

Gilstrap, L.C., 3rd, Cunningham, F.G. & Whalley, P.J. (1981a) Acute pyelonephritis in pregnancy: an anterospective study. Obstet Gynecol, 57, 409-413.

Gilstrap, L.C., 3rd & Ramin, S.M. (2001) Urinary tract infections during pregnancy. Obstet Gynecol Clin North Am, 28, 581-591.

Gilstrap, L.C., Leveno, K.J., Cunningham, F.G., Whalley, P.J. & Roark, M.L. (1981b) Renal infection and pregnancy outcome. Am J Obstet Gynecol, 141, 709-716.

Golan, A., Wexler, S., Amit, A., Gordon, D. & David, M.P. (1989) Asymptomatic bacteriuria in normal and high-risk pregnancy. Eur J Obstet Gynecol Reprod Biol, 33, 101-108.

Gratacos, E., Torres, P.J., Vila, J., Alonso, P.L. & Cararach, V. (1994) Screening and treatment of asymptomatic bacteriuria in pregnancy prevent pyelonephritis. J Infect Dis, 169, 1390-1392.

Graves, C.R. (2002) Acute pulmonary complications during pregnancy. Clin Obstet Gynecol, 45, 369-376.

Gravett, M.G., Rubens, C.E. & Nunes, T.M. (2010) Global report on preterm birth and stillbirth (2 of 7): discovery science. BMC Pregnancy Childbirth, 10 Suppl 1, S2.

Guinto, V.T., De Guia, B., Festin, M.R. & Dowswell, T. (2010) Different antibiotic regimens for treating asymptomatic bacteriuria in pregnancy. Cochrane Database Syst Rev, CD007855.

Harris, R.E. & Gilstrap, L.C., 3rd (1981) Cystitis during pregnancy: a distinct clinical entity. Obstet Gynecol, 57, 578-580.

Herrera, J.A., Chaudhuri, G. & Lopez-Jaramillo, P. (2001) Is infection a major risk factor for preeclampsia? Med Hypotheses, 57, 393-397.

Hill, J.B., Sheffield, J.S., McIntire, D.D. & Wendel, G.D., Jr. (2005) Acute pyelonephritis in pregnancy. Obstet Gynecol, 105, 18-23.

Jeyabalan, A. & Lain, K.Y. (2007) Anatomic and functional changes of the upper urinary tract during pregnancy. Urol Clin North Am, 34, 1-6.

Jolley, J.A. & Wing, D.A. (2010) Pyelonephritis in pregnancy: an update on treatment options for optimal outcomes. Drugs, 70, 1643-1655.

Joseph DiPiro, R.T., Gary Yee, Gary Matzke, Barbara Wells, L. Michael Posey (2011) Pharmacotherapy: A Pathophysiologic Approach. McGraw-Hill Medical.

Kaper, J.B. (2005) Pathogenic Escherichia coli. Int J Med Microbiol, 295, 355-356.

Kass, E.H. (1962) Pyelonephritis and bacteriuria. A major problem in preventive medicine. Ann Intern Med, 56, 46-53.

Le, J., Briggs, G.G., McKeown, A. & Bustillo, G. (2004) Urinary tract infections during pregnancy. Ann Pharmacother, 38, 1692-1701.

Lee, M., Bozzo, P., Einarson, A. & Koren, G. (2008) Urinary tract infections in pregnancy. Can Fam Physician, 54, 853-854.

Lin, K. & Fajardo, K. (2008) Screening for asymptomatic bacteriuria in adults: evidence for the U.S. Preventive Services Task Force reaffirmation recommendation statement. Ann Intern Med, 149, W20-24.

Lin, K.W. & Brown, T. (2010) Screening for asymptomatic bacteriuria in adults. Am Fam Physician, 81, 508.

Lumbiganon, P., Laopaiboon, M. & Thinkhamrop, J. (2010) Screening and treating asymptomatic bacteriuria in pregnancy. Curr Opin Obstet Gynecol, 22, 95-99.

Macejko, A.M. & Schaeffer, A.J. (2007) Asymptomatic bacteriuria and symptomatic urinary tract infections during pregnancy. Urol Clin North Am, 34, 35-42.

MacLean, A.B. (2001) Urinary tract infection in pregnancy. Int J Antimicrob Agents, 17, 273-276; discussion 276-277.

Masson, P., Matheson, S., Webster, A.C. & Craig, J.C. (2009) Meta-analyses in prevention and treatment of urinary tract infections. Infect Dis Clin North Am, 23, 355-385;

McDermott, S., Callaghan, W., Szwejbka, L., Mann, H. & Daguise, V. (2000) Urinary tract infections during pregnancy and mental retardation and developmental delay. Obstet Gynecol, 96, 113-119.

McDermott, S., Daguise, V., Mann, H., Szwejbka, L. & Callaghan, W. (2001) Perinatal risk for mortality and mental retardation associated with maternal urinary-tract infections. J Fam Pract, 50, 433-437.

McIsaac, W., Carroll, J.C., Biringer, A., Bernstein, P., Lyons, E., Low, D.E. & Permaul, J.A. (2005) Screening for asymptomatic bacteriuria in pregnancy. J Obstet Gynaecol Can, 27, 20-24.

McNair, R.D., MacDonald, S.R., Dooley, S.L. & Peterson, L.R. (2000) Evaluation of the centrifuged and Gram-stained smear, urinalysis, and reagent strip testing to detect asymptomatic bacteriuria in obstetric patients. Am J Obstet Gynecol, 182, 1076-1079.

Millar, L.K. & Cox, S.M. (1997) Urinary tract infections complicating pregnancy. Infect Dis Clin North Am, 11, 13-26.

Milo, G., Katchman, E.A., Paul, M., Christiaens, T., Baerheim, A. & Leibovici, L. (2005) Duration of antibacterial treatment for uncomplicated urinary tract infection in women. Cochrane Database Syst Rev, CD004682.

Mittal, P. & Wing, D.A. (2005) Urinary tract infections in pregnancy. Clin Perinatol, 32, 749-764.

Mulvey, M.A., Schilling, J.D. & Hultgren, S.J. (2001) Establishment of a persistent Escherichia coli reservoir during the acute phase of a bladder infection. Infect Immun, 69, 4572-4579.

Naveen, R. & Mathai, E. (2005) Some virulence characteristics of uropathogenic Escherichia coli in different patient groups. Indian J Med Res, 122, 143-147.

Neal, D.E., Jr. (2008) Complicated urinary tract infections. Urol Clin North Am, 35, 13-22; v.

Nicolle, L.E. (2006) Asymptomatic bacteriuria: review and discussion of the IDSA guidelines. Int J Antimicrob Agents, 28 Suppl 1, S42-48.

Nowicki, B. (2002) Urinary Tract Infection in Pregnant Women: Old Dogmas and Current Concepts Regarding Pathogenesis. Curr Infect Dis Rep, 4, 529-535.

Nowicki, B., Sledzinska, A., Samet, A. & Nowicki, S. (2011) Pathogenesis of gestational urinary tract infection: urinary obstruction versus immune adaptation and microbial virulence. BJOG, 118, 109-112.

Oda, N., Takeuchi, K., Tanaka, A. & Maruo, T. (2008) Obstetric risk factors associated with the development of periventricular leukomalacia in preterm infants born to mothers complicated by placenta previa. Fetal Diagn Ther, 24, 345-348.

Ovalle, A. & Levancini, M. (2001) Urinary tract infections in pregnancy. Curr Opin Urol, 11, 55-59.

Ovalle, A., Silva, O., Herrera, R., Gonzalez, E. & Marin, J. (1989) [Pre-existing diseases as risk factors and prognosis of genito-urinary infection in pregnancy]. Rev Chil Obstet Ginecol, 54, 341-347.

Parsons, C.L., Shrom, S.H., Hanno, P.M. & Mulholland, S.G. (1978) Bladder surface mucin. Examination of possible mechanisms for its antibacterial effect. Invest Urol, 16, 196-200.

Pastore, L.M., Savitz, D.A. & Thorp, J.M., Jr. (1999) Predictors of urinary tract infection at the first prenatal visit. Epidemiology, 10, 282-287.

Patterson, T.F. & Andriole, V.T. (1997) Detection, significance, and therapy of bacteriuria in pregnancy. Update in the managed health care era. Infect Dis Clin North Am, 11, 593-608.

Polivka, B.J., Nickel, J.T. & Wilkins, J.R., 3rd (1997) Urinary tract infection during pregnancy: a risk factor for cerebral palsy? J Obstet Gynecol Neonatal Nurs, 26, 405-413.

Reddy, J. & Campbell, A. (1985) Bacteriuria in pregnancy. Aust N Z J Obstet Gynaecol, 25, 176-178.

Romero, R., Oyarzun, E., Mazor, M., Sirtori, M., Hobbins, J.C. & Bracken, M. (1989) Meta-analysis of the relationship between asymptomatic bacteriuria and preterm delivery/low birth weight. Obstet Gynecol, 73, 576-582.

Roos, V., Nielsen, E.M. & Klemm, P. (2006) Asymptomatic bacteriuria Escherichia coli strains: adhesins, growth and competition. FEMS Microbiol Lett, 262, 22-30.

Rosen, D.A., Hooton, T.M., Stamm, W.E., Humphrey, P.A. & Hultgren, S.J. (2007) Detection of intracellular bacterial communities in human urinary tract infection. PLoS Med, 4, e329.

Rubin, R.H., Shapiro, E.D., Andriole, V.T., Davis, R.J. & Stamm, W.E. (1992) Evaluation of new anti-infective drugs for the treatment of urinary tract infection. Infectious Diseases Society of America and the Food and Drug Administration. Clin Infect Dis, 15 Suppl 1, S216-227.

Rustveld, L.O., Kelsey, S.F. & Sharma, R. (2008) Association between maternal infections and preeclampsia: a systematic review of epidemiologic studies. Matern Child Health J, 12, 223-242.

Sahm, D.F., Thornsberry, C., Mayfield, D.C., Jones, M.E. & Karlowsky, J.A. (2001) Multidrug-resistant urinary tract isolates of Escherichia coli: prevalence and patient demographics in the United States in 2000. Antimicrob Agents Chemother, 45, 1402-1406.

Sandberg, T., Kaijser, B., Lidin-Janson, G., Lincoln, K., Orskov, F., Orskov, I., Stokland, E. & Svanborg-Eden, C. (1988) Virulence of Escherichia coli in relation to host factors in women with symptomatic urinary tract infection. J Clin Microbiol, 26, 1471-1476.

Sayres, W.G., Jr. (2010) Preterm labor. Am Fam Physician, 81, 477-484.

Santos, F., Oraichi, D., Bérard, A. (2010). Prevalence and predictors of anti-infective use during pregnancy. Pharmacoepidemiol Drug Saf, 19(4):418-427.

Santos, F., Sheehy, O., Perreault, S., Ferreira, E., Berard, A. (2010b). Exposure to anti-infective drugs during pregnancy and the risk of small-for-gestational-age newborns: a case-control study. Proceedings of the 26th International Conference on Pharmacoepidemiology and Therapeutic Risk Management, Pharmacoepidemiol Drug Saf, 19: S1–S347, Brighton, UK, Aug. 2010.

Schieve, L.A., Handler, A., Hershow, R., Persky, V. & Davis, F. (1994) Urinary tract infection during pregnancy: its association with maternal morbidity and perinatal outcome. Am J Public Health, 84, 405-410.

Schmiemann, G., Kniehl, E., Gebhardt, K., Matejczyk, M.M. & Hummers-Pradier, E. (2010) The diagnosis of urinary tract infection: a systematic review. Dtsch Arztebl Int, 107, 361-367.

Schnarr, J. & Smaill, F. (2008) Asymptomatic bacteriuria and symptomatic urinary tract infections in pregnancy. Eur J Clin Invest, 38 Suppl 2, 50-57.

Shand, D.G., Nimmon, C.C., O'Grady, F. & Cattell, W.R. (1970) Relation between residual urine volume and response to treatment of urinary infection. Lancet, 760, 1305-1306.

Sharma, P. & Thapa, L. (2007) Acute pyelonephritis in pregnancy: a retrospective study. Aust N Z J Obstet Gynaecol, 47, 313-315.

Sheffield, J.S. & Cunningham, F.G. (2005) Urinary tract infection in women. Obstet Gynecol, 106, 1085-1092.

Simmons, L.E., Rubens, C.E., Darmstadt, G.L. & Gravett, M.G. (2010) Preventing preterm birth and neonatal mortality: exploring the epidemiology, causes, and interventions. Semin Perinatol, 34, 408-415.

Smaill, F. (2000) Antibiotics for asymptomatic bacteriuria in pregnancy. Cochrane Database Syst Rev, CD000490.

Smaill, F. (2007) Asymptomatic bacteriuria in pregnancy. Best Pract Res Clin Obstet Gynaecol, 21, 439-450.

Smaill, F. & Vazquez, J.C. (2007) Antibiotics for asymptomatic bacteriuria in pregnancy. Cochrane Database Syst Rev, CD000490.

Spinillo, A., Capuzzo, E., Stronati, M., Ometto, A., De Santolo, A. & Acciano, S. (1998) Obstetric risk factors for periventricular leukomalacia among preterm infants. Br J Obstet Gynaecol, 105, 865-871.

Stamey, T.A., Fair, W.R., Timothy, M.M. & Chung, H.K. (1968) Antibacterial nature of prostatic fluid. Nature, 218, 444-447.

Tugrul, S., Oral, O., Kumru, P., Kose, D., Alkan, A. & Yildirim, G. (2005) Evaluation and importance of asymptomatic bacteriuria in pregnancy. Clin Exp Obstet Gynecol, 32, 237-240.

Turck, M., Goffe, B.S. & Petersdorf, R.G. (1962) Bacteriuria of pregnancy. Relation to socioeconomic factors. N Engl J Med, 266, 857-860.

Turiani, M. (2009) Habitos de Higiene Genital e Infeccao autorreferida no trato urinario na gravidez Escola de Enfermagem. Universidade de Sao Paulo, Sao Paulo, pp. 94.

Vazquez, J.C. & Villar, J. (2003) Treatments for symptomatic urinary tract infections during pregnancy. Cochrane Database Syst Rev, CD002256.

Verani, J.R., McGee, L. & Schrag, S.J. (2010) Prevention of perinatal group B streptococcal disease--revised guidelines from CDC, 2010. MMWR Recomm Rep, 59, 1-36.

von Dadelszen, P. & Magee, L.A. (2002) Could an infectious trigger explain the differential maternal response to the shared placental pathology of preeclampsia and normotensive intrauterine growth restriction? Acta Obstet Gynecol Scand, 81, 642-648.

Wagenlehner, F.M., Weidner, W. & Naber, K.G. (2009) An update on uncomplicated urinary tract infections in women. Curr Opin Urol, 19, 368-374.

Wax, J.R., Cartin, A. & Pinette, M.G. (2010) Biophysical and biochemical screening for the risk of preterm labor. Clin Lab Med, 30, 693-707.

Whalley, P.J., Martin, F.G. & Peters, P.C. (1965) Significance of Asymptomatic Bacteriuria Detected during Pregnancy. JAMA, 193, 879-881.

Wing, D.A. (1998) Pyelonephritis. Clin Obstet Gynecol, 41, 515-526.

Wullt, B., Bergsten, G., Samuelsson, M. & Svanborg, C. (2002) The role of P fimbriae for Escherichia coli establishment and mucosal inflammation in the human urinary tract. Int J Antimicrob Agents, 19, 522-538.

8

# Reducing the Incidence of Catheter-Associated Urinary Tract Infections in the Acute Care Setting Using Evidence-Based Guidelines

Diane Gorman
*PENN Presbyterian Medical Center*
*United States of America*

## 1. Introduction

Urinary Tract Infections (UTIs) are the most common infections acquired in the hospitalized adult patients accounting for 30-40% of all nosocomial infections and 80% of these infections are caused by indwelling catheters (Bagshaw, Laupland, 2006) (National Center of Health Statistics, CDC, 2004). The daily risk of developing a catheter-associated urinary tract infection (CA-UTI) is 3-7% in the acute care setting (Lo, Nicolle et al, 2008). Between 15-25% of hospitalized patients receive short-term indwelling catheters (CDC, 2009). Often catheters are placed for inappropriate reasons and prescribers are unaware of their presence and stay in for extended periods of time. Reported rates of UTI among patients with urinary catheters vary substantially. National data from the National Healthcare Safety Network (NHSN), designed by the Centers for Disease Control (CDC) and Prevention, previously known as the National Nosocomial Infection Surveillance System (NNISS), reported acute care hospitals in 2006 showed an average range of CA-UTI rates of 3.1-7.5 infections per 1000 catheter-days (CDC, 2009). The Centers for Medicare and Medicaid Services (CMS) identified hospital acquired urinary tract infections as one of the eight conditions for which hospitals will not receive additional reimbursement (Beaver, 2008) (CMS, 2008). The CMS regulations emphasize complications and risk with CA-UTIs which include cystitis, periurethral abscess, prostatitis, epididymitis, acute or chronic pyelonephritis, gram negative bacteremia, sepsis secondary to CA-UTI, which can be fatal in 40-60% of cases and CA-UTIs are the second most common cause of nosocomial blood stream infection (Kunin,1997,Smith, 2003,Rahn, 2008, National Center for Disease Statistics, CDC, 2004, Cravens, 2000, Warren, Damron et al 1987). The complication of a CA-UTI can increase a patient's hospital stay by 0.4 days for an asymptomatic UTI and 2 days for a symptomatic UTI (Leithauser, 2004). The CMS regulations also state the use of indwelling catheters in long-term acute care settings must be medically justified and that strategies must be in place to reduce the risk of infection for all patients and residents with catheters (CMS guidelines, 2008). An estimated 17% to 69% of CA-UTI may be preventable with recommended infection control measures, which means that up to 380,000 infections and 9000 deaths related to CA-UTI per year could be prevented CDC, 2009). This chapter will focus on methods that have demonstrated in research and recommended to help prevent CA-UTIs in the acute care setting.

Based on the 2009 Infectious Diseases Society of America Guidelines (IDSA), CA-UTI infections refer to infections occurring in persons whose urinary tract is currently catherized or has been catherized within the previous 48 hours. UTI refers to significant bacteruria in a patient with symptoms or signs attributable to the urinary tract and no alternate source. These guidelines will pertain to patients with indwelling catheters, including short term (<= 30 days) and long-term (>30 days) in the acute care setting. These guidelines in this chapter will not attend to intermittent catherization or condom catherization. Nor does it deal with patients who undergo complicated urologic catherization procedures, such as those involving ureteral stents or nephrostomy tubes. This chapter will strictly deal with the prevention of CA-UTIs in the acute care setting. The diagnosis and treatment of a CA-UTI will not be addressed.

In the acute care setting, many CA-UTIs account for many episodes of nosocomial bacteremia (Noelle, Strausbaugh, Garibaldi, 1996), (Saint, Kowalski, Kaufman, 2008). CA-bacteruria has important implications for the patients and should have high priority for infection control programs, not only for patient safety but cost issues as well. One cost analysis of UTIs estimated an additional expense ranging from $101 to $1, 727 per UTI (Tambyah, Knasinski, et al, 2002). Additional estimates have been as high as $3, 803 per infection (McConnel, 2000). In October 2008, The Centers for Medicare/Medicaid Services in the United States stopped reimbursement for healthcare acquired infections (Wald, Kramer, 2007) (Beaver, 2008) (CMS, 2008). Not surprisingly, the most effective way to reduce the incidence of CA-UTIs is removing the catheter promptly when it is no longer needed (Crouzet, Bertrand et al, 2007) (Infectious Diseases Society of America, 2009). However, despite the overwhelming link between urinary catherization and subsequent UTI, US hospitals have not widely implemented strategies to reduce hospital-acquired UTIs.

The NHSN created benchmarks for CA-UTIs based on similar hospitals. The benchmark for CA-UTI in the ICU was a rate of 4 per 1000 catheter days pooled from 300 hospitals in 2004 (Edwards, Peterson, et al, 2007). In preparation for the new CMS guidelines for healthcare acquired infections, in 2007, PENN Presbyterian Medical Center in Philadelphia, Pennsylvania, launched a campaign to decrease the incidence of CA-UTIs by adopting a set of evidence based guidelines and studied the effects of these guidelines on the rate of CA-UTIs in a pilot study done in one of the intensive care units. Before adopting these set of guidelines PENN Presbyterian Cardiac Care Unit had a CA-UTI rate of 13.1 in 2006 after 1 year, following these guidelines, the rate dropped to 6.80 by the end of 2007. Each of the University of Pennsylvania Hospitals adopted parts of these guidelines and made changes according to their specific patient populations. This chapter will outline what PENN Presbyterian did but will highlight some of the interventions utilized by all three hospitals. All three hospitals in the University of Pennsylvania Health System utilize the same order entry system therefore any changes in documentation were implemented in all three hospitals. Committees in all three hospitals met on a quarterly basis to review interventions.

The definition of practice guidelines are "systematically developed statements to assist practitioners and patients in making decisions about appropriate healthcare for specific circumstances. Attributes of high quality guidelines include validity, reliability, reproducibility, clinical applicability, clinical flexibility, clarity, multidisciplinary process, review of evidence and documentation. (IDSA, p 9. 2009). Table 1 outlines the strength of recommendation and quality of evidence as described in 1970, by the Canadian Task Force on the Periodic Health Examination. Throughout the chapter, the practice guidelines discussed will be labeled with the strength of recommendation and quality of evidence as defined by this table and recommendation from the Infectious Disease Society of America, the Centers for Disease Control and Prevention and the most current research. These guidelines will represent what was adopted by the University of Pennsylvania Health System over the past three years and also what has been studied and proven as well in these past three years since the original study that was done at PENN Presbyterian Center in 2006-2007

| **Table 1: Strength of Recommendation and Quality of Evidence** | |
|---|---|
| **Category/Grade** | **Definition** |
| **Strength of Recommendation** | |
| a. | Good Evidence to support a recommendation for or against use |
| b. | Moderate Evidence to support a recommendation for or against use |
| c. | Poor Evidence to support a recommendation for or against use |
| **Quality of Evidence** | |
| i. | Evidence from >1 properly randomized, controlled trial |
| ii. | Evidence from >1 well designed clinical trial, without randomization; from cohort or case-controlled analytic studies (preferably from >1 center); from multiple time-series; or from dramatic results from controlled experiments |
| iii. | Evidence from opinions of respected authorities, based on clinical experience, descriptive studies or reports of expert committees |

Table 1. Defines the strength of recommendation and quality of evidence adapted from the Canadian Task Force on the Periodic Health Examination 1979.

## 2. Indications for insertion and discontinuing indwelling catheters

Indwelling catheters should be placed only when they are indicated (A-III, IDSA, 2009). Institutions should develop a list of appropriate indications for inserting indwelling catheters, educate staff about indications and periodically assess adherence to the institution-specific guidelines (A-III, IDSA, 2009). Institutions should require an order in the chart before a catheter is placed (A-III, IDSA, 2009). Institutions should consider use of a portable bladder scanner to determine whether catherization is necessary for post- operative patient (B-II, IDSA, 2009).

At PENN Presbyterian, criteria for maintaining indwelling catheters were placed in a set of practice guidelines originally in 2005 and again reviewed by the policy and procedure committee in 2008 and 2009. The maintenance criteria are listed below in Table 3. These guidelines were originally adapted from *Wong and Hooton's Guidelines for the Prevention of catheter-associated urinary tract infections* from the Center for Disease Control and Prevention published in a landmark study in 1981, and modified in 2005. Most recently these guidelines were again updated and published in the 2009 International Clinical Practice Guidelines entitled *Diagnosis, Prevention and Treatment of Catheter-Associated Urinary Tract Infections in Adults* by the Infectious Diseases Society of America, led by Thomas Hooton and also by the CDC, entitled Guideline for Prevention of Cather Associated Urinary Tract Infections 2009, led by Carolyn Gould. Although the IDSA guidelines do not specifically list indications for maintaining an indwelling catheter, it stresses the need for institutions to develop their own set of criteria reducing the incidence of unnecessary catherizations making it a responsibility of the prescribers (physician, nurse practitioner, or physician's assistant) to ensure that indwelling catheters are utilized appropriately. In the CDC guidelines, listed below in table 2 there are recommendation for insertion of catheters but they are based on expert opinion and are classified as category B-I (2009).

| Examples of Appropriate Indications for Indwelling Urethral Catheter Use |
|---|
| 1. Patient has acute urinary retention or bladder outlet obstruction |
| 2. Need for accurate measurement of urinary output in critically ill patients |
| 3. Perioperative use of selective procedures: |
| - Patients undergoing urologic surgery or other surgery on contiguous structures In the genitourinary tract |
| Anticipated prolonged procedure (catheters inserted for this reason should be taken out in the recovery room) |
| Patients anticipated to receive large volume infusions or diuretics during surgery |
| Need for intraoperative monitoring of urinary output |
| 4. To assist in healing of open sacral or perineal wounds in incontinent patients |
| 5. Patients requiring prolonged immobilization (i.e. potentially unstable thoracic or lumbar spine, multiple traumatic injuries such as pelvic fractures |
| **Examples of inappropriate use of catheters** |
| 1. As a substitute for nursing care of the patient or resident with incontinence |
| 2. As a means of obtaining urine for cultures or other diagnostic test when the patient can voluntarily void |
| 3. For prolonged post-operative duration without appropriate indications (i.e. structural repair of urethra or contiguous structures, prolonged effect of epidural anesthesia etc.) |

Table 2. CDC: Guidelines for Prevention of Catheter-Associated UTIs 2009.

## 3. Prevention of catheter-associated urinary tract infections

There are many catheter factors that increase the risk for the development of CA-UTIs. Maki and Tambyah state that there are inherent risk factors that increase the risk for CA-UTIs in the acute care setting. These include being female, patients with other infections, major pre-existing chronic illnesses such as diabetes, patients suffering from malnutrition, patients with chronic renal insufficiency, insertion of a catheter outside the operating room or late in hospitalization and using a catheter to measure urine output (2001). The CDC suggests that the highest quality of evidence demonstrates that the elderly, those patients >70 years of age, patients with severe illness and finally those with prolonged catherization are at the highest risk for development of CA-UTI. This section will define factors that have and can help prevent the development of CA- UTIs in the acute care setting. Table 4 lists PENN Presbyterian's guidelines utilized to prevent catheter-associated urinary tract infections. Although most of these guidelines are based on research some guidelines in this table have been listed to help reduce the risk of CA-UTI development and may not have been proven by research but are supported by expert opinion and may need further research. These guidelines were adopted by PENN Presbyterian in 2006 and are continually reassessed

**PENN Presbyterian Medical Center Practice Guidelines for Placement and Maintaining Indwelling Catheter: Nursing Management for the Prevention of Catheter-Associated Urinary Tract Infections May 2005, Updated February 2008, updated January 2009.**

1. Patients experiencing hemodynamic instability requiring intravenous vasoactive agents or aggressive intravenous fluid resuscitation for maintenance of blood pressure and/or cerebral perfusion
2. Female patient with spinal radiographic studies that have not been cleared (thoracic or lumbar regions)
3. Patients who are incontinent with skin breakdown in the buttocks, sacral region or perineum; as this puts patients at risk for further breakdown, contamination and/or infection or with existing stage 3 or 4 sacral wounds
4. Patients who are deeply sedated (patients who are obtunded due to injury, illness or chemical induction).
5. Patients with urological requirement for indwelling catheter (for example, patients who experience surgical disruption of the urinary tract system, or patient with actual or anticipated acute urinary retention due to bladder outlet obstruction or urethral strictures for whom medical intervention is necessary to drain urine).
6. Patients who are post-operative and who will be immobile for 48 hours (indwelling catherization is only indicated for 48 hours)
7. Patients admitted with chronic indwelling catheters already in place for the diagnosis of chronic urinary retention due to spinal cord injury or disease
8. Patients who are made DNR-C with an indwelling catheter already in place (Do Not Resuscitate—Comfort Care only)
9. Patients with acute urinary retention or bladder obstruction

**The following clinical situations are NOT automatic indications for placement of an indwelling urinary catheter**

1. Presence of an epidural catheter
2. Diagnosis of acute or chronic renal failure
3. Patients who require aggressive monitoring of input and output
4. As part of the routine preparation for patients about to undergo surgical or other invasive procedures not otherwise excluded above

Table 3. PENN Presbyterian Medical Center Administration Policy Manual: The Use of Indwelling Urinary Catheters: Policy # 11.147.

yearly according to the latest evidenced- based research. This section will describe each guideline and how it was adopted into practice and describes changes made to practice since their introduction in 2006 and the strength of recommendation and quality of evidence described in the literature.

### 3.1 Insertion/maintenance of indwelling catheter in acute care setting

The CDC and IDSA make clear recommendations that indwelling catheters in the acute care setting should be placed using aseptic technique and sterile equipment (B-III, IDSA, 2009) (B-I, CDC, 2009). It is important that staff inserting catheters is properly educated and that return demonstration is conducted to ensure proper insertion to prevent CA-UTIs. It is also recommended that a closed catheter drainage system, with ports for aspiration in the distal catheter, be utilized to decrease the frequency of breakage thus reducing the risk of CA-UTIs (A-III, IDSA, 2009). Although the usage of prepackaged preconnected systems is utilized at the University of PENN Health System, there is not enough evidence to support whether such systems reduce the incidence of CA-UTIs (IDSA, 2009). Although the CDC, states that sterile, continuously closed drainage systems became the standard of care based on an uncontrolled study published in 1966 demonstrating a dramatic reduction in the risk of infection in short-term catheterized patients with the use of a closed system. Recent data also include the finding that disconnection of the drainage system is a risk factor for bacteriuria (2009). It's utilization at PENN has however decreased the incidence of breakage between the catheter and drainage system thus contributing to the lower incidence CA-UTIs.

### 3.2 Assessing the need for indwelling catheter

First and foremost is the duration of catherization that has been demonstrated to be the major independent risk factor for the development of CA-UTIs (Reilly, Sullivan, et al, 2006). Catheters left in place for >6 days have shown the most risk (Maki, Tambyah, 2001,) (A-II, IDSA, 2009). Indwelling catheters should be removed as soon as they are no longer required to reduce the risk of CA-UTIs (A-II, IDSA, 2009). Institutions should consider nurse-based or electronic physician reminder systems to reduce inappropriate urinary catherization and CA-UTIs (A-II, IDSA, 2009). This intervention has been in place since February, 2008 at all three hospitals in the University of Pennsylvania Health System. Institutions should consider automatic stop orders to reduce inappropriate urinary catherization (B-I, IDSA, 2009). An automatic stop order is placed in the University of Pennsylvania Health System order entry system after 48 hours reminding prescribers to reassess need for indwelling catheters then every 24 hours thereafter, which was introduced in February, 2010. Prescribers are stopped before any other order can be entered every 24 hours to address need for catheter and an option to place an order to discontinue the use of the catheter.

Nurses are on the frontlines of direct patient care and are the cornerstone in implementing good practice. If nurses are taught to embrace the criteria for maintenance and understand how it affects patient care and safety, assessing the need for an indwelling catheter on a routine basis becomes an easy task. At PENN Presbyterian, the focus was on nursing practice, it is simple for prescribers to enter an order to discontinue the use of an indwelling catheter but it is up to administrators, educators and infection control experts to reinforce that with concept with the nursing staff and giving timely feedback about practice good or bad. In an attempt to decrease the incidence of CA-UTIs, PENN Presbyterian's Coronary Care Unit, utilized an audit tool (table 3) to identify gaps in care. Nurses were then educated during staff meeting or individually by clinical nurse specialists and infection control specialists about noncompliance or gaps in care according to the guidelines. With this audit tool, over time, nursing began to embrace their accountability in infection prevention. They soon developed the "less is more philosophy". If nurses are convinced that they hold the key to prevention of CA-UTI typically they will embrace this concept as demonstrated in this pilot study (Gorman, 2009). Listed below is the audit tool used in Table 4. In addition, nursing was given monthly feedback about rates of infection in a monthly newsletter published by the infection control committee outlining infection rates.

### 3.3 Proper hand hygiene

It is not a new concept that proper hand hygiene before and after catheter care prevents the spread of infection. The Institution of Healthcare Improvement (IHI) 100,000 lives campaign introduced "Bundles" in December 2004. A bundle is a term developed by the IHI as a way to describe a collection of interventions to effectively care for patients undergoing particular treatments with inherent risks (IHI, 2004). Hand hygiene compliance was on the top of the list as a way to prevent infections. The Joint Commission on Accreditation of Hospital Organizations (JCAHO) recognizes hand hygiene compliance as a patient safety goal in 2004. The Center for Disease Control lists recommendations for indications for hand hygiene, hand hygiene techniques, surgical antisepsis, and selection of hand hygiene agents, skin care, health care worker (HCW) education, administrative measures and other aspects of hand hygiene. Listed below in table 5, are recommendations, including before and after handling of catheters. Because hand hygiene is the number one way to prevent the spread of any infection it was worth mentioning *all* the guidelines including those involved with an indwelling catheter. It can not be stressed enough that proper hand hygiene is the key element to infection prevention. Even if you have all other criteria in place if proper hand hygiene fails to be the number one priority, all other interventions to preventing infections are futile.

Hand hygiene compliance was and continues to be tracked monthly as well at PENN Presbyterian by anonymous observers and reported to the infection control committee with a goal of 100% compliance. Observers were and are continued to be educated to give private negative feedback so to provide a positive environment to encourage learning versus discipline. PENN Presbyterian launched an education campaign surrounding hand hygiene in 2004. To improve hand hygiene compliance, alcohol based dispensers were placed strategically around the hospital for easy access. Compliance rates started at 50-60% but presently are >90%. Clear guidelines were addressed in polices surrounding when to use alcohol based gels versus soap and water. Staff was educated explicitly on these guidelines. These guidelines are specifically outlined by the CDC.

### 3.4 Size/type of an indwelling urinary catheter

Although the IDSA does not make any recommendations on the size of an indwelling catheter it is well documented in the literature as recommended by expert opinion that size does matter when preventing a CA-UTI. The prevailing guideline for catheter size is to use the smallest diameter that will provide good drainage, typically 14-18 French unless the patient has blood clots or sediment that occlude the lumen. Larger catheters are uncomfortable and can lead to urethral erosion and impair paraurethral gland function. The paraurethral glands produce mucous that protects against ascending bacteria. Compression of these glands can result in urethritis or ascending infection (Robinson, 2001, Newman, 2007). At the University of Pennsylvania Health System, floors will only stock 14 French indwelling catheter insertion kits already attached to a drainage system. It avoids placement of any size catheter that happens to be available to staff. Specially required catheters are ordered from the store room if necessary, therefore careful thought must be taken before a larger catheter is necessary. Only if there is leakage from the catheter will a larger catheter size be considered. The IDSA suggests that in patients with short-term indwelling catheters, antimicrobial, silver alloy or antibiotic-coated catheters may be considered to reduce or delay the onset of CA-UTIs (B-II, 2009). In PENN Presbyterian, there was little difference in the rate of infection with or without the antibiotic coated catheters therefore the use was discontinued.

**PENN Presbyterian CCU Infection Control Audit (CA-UTI Section only) 2007**

**Medical Record #** ______________
**Nurse Auditing** ______________
**Nurse Audited** ______________
**Date** ________________________

**Indwelling Catheter**
How many days in place _______ Size _____
Every shift needs assessment _________
Leg Strap in place ________
Bag below Level of bladder ________
Urinalysis/culture done on admission to CCU if from outside facility________
Where was the catheter placed? ER OR OSH CCU Other ____

**Reason for Indwelling Catheter Circle all that apply**
Obstruction/Retention DNR-C (with catheter already in place), Hemodynamic instability Stage 3 or 4 sacral wound neurogenic bladder obtunded/sedated/paralyzed No reason discontinued catheter

DNR-C (Do Not Resuscitate—Comfort care only)

**Infections Present on Admission Please Circle**

UTI Pneumonia Blood Stream Infection

Table 4. PENN Presbyterian Nursing Audit Tool.

| Recommendation: | Category |
|---|---|
| **1. Indications for handwashing and hand antisepsis** | |
| d. When hands are visibly dirty or contaminated with proteinaceous material or are visibly soiled with blood or other body fluids, wash hands with either a non-antimicrobial soap and water or an antimicrobial soap and water. | IA |
| e. If hands are not visibly soiled, use an alcohol-based hand rub for routinely decontaminating hands in all other clinical situations described in 1C-J.<br>f. Alternatively, wash hands with an antimicrobial soap and water in all clinical situations described in items 1 C-J. | IA<br>**IB** |
| g. Decontaminate hands before having direct contact with patients. | IB |
| h. Decontaminate hands before donning sterile gloves when inserting a central intravascular catheter. | IB |
| i. Decontaminate hands before inserting indwelling urinary catheters, peripheral vascular catheters, or other invasive devices that do not require a surgical procedure. | IB |

| Recommendation: | Category |
|---|---|
| j. Decontaminate hands after contact with a patient's intact skin (e.g., when taking a pulse or blood pressure, and lifting a patient) | IB |
| k. Decontaminate hands after contact with body fluids or excretions, mucous membranes, nonintact skin, and wound dressings if hands are not visibly soiled. | IA |
| l. Decontaminate hands if moving from a contaminated-body site to a clean-body site during patient care. | II |
| m. Decontaminate hands after contact with inanimate objects (including medical equipment) in the immediate vicinity of the patient. | II |
| n. Decontaminate hands after removing gloves | IB |
| o. Before eating and after using a restroom, wash hands with a non-antimicrobial soap and water or a non-antimicrobial soap and water. | IB |
| p. Antimicrobial-impregnated wipes (i.e., towelettes) may be considered as an alternative to washing hands with non-antimicrobial soap and water. Because they are not as effective as alcohol-based hand rubs or washing hands with an antimicrobial soap and water for reducing the bacterial counts on the hands of HCW's, they are not a substitute for using alcohol-based hand rub or antimicrobial soap. | IB |
| q. Wash hands with non-antimicrobial soap and water or with antimicrobial soap and water it exposure to *Bacillus anthracis* is suspected or proven. The physical action of washing and rinsing hands under such circumstances is recommended because alcohols, chlorhexidine, iodophors, and other antiseptic agents have poor activity against spores. | II |
| r. No recommendation can be made regarding the routine use of nonalcohol-based hand rubs for hand hygiene in health-care settings. | Unresolved issue |
| **2. Hand-Hygiene Technique** | |
| a. When deconcontaminating hands with an alcohol-based hand rub, apply product to one hand and rub hands together, covering all surfaces of hands and fingers, until hands are dry. Follow manufacturer's recommendations regarding the volume of product to use. | IB |
| b. When washing hands with soap and water, wet hands first with water, apply an amount of product recommended by the manufacturer to hands, and rub hands together vigorously for at least 15 seconds, covering all surfaces of the hands and fingers. Rinse hands with water and dry thoroughly with a disposable towel. Use towel to turn off the faucet.<br>c. Avoid using hot water, because repeated exposure to hot water may increase the risk of dermatitis. | IB<br>IB |
| d. Liquid, bar, leaflet or powdered forms of plain soap are acceptable when washing hands with a non-antimicrobial soap and water. When bar soap is used, soap racks that facilitate the drainage and small bars of soap should be used. | II |

| Recommendation: | Category |
|---|---|
| e. Multiple-use cloth towels of the hanging or roll type are not recommended for use in health-care settings. | **II** |
| **3.** Surgical Hand Antisepsis | |
| a. Remove rings, watches, and bracelets before beginning the surgical hand scrub. | **II** |
| b. Remove debris from underneath fingernails using a nail cleaner under running water. | **II** |
| c. Surgical hand antisepsis using either an antimicrobial soap or an alcohol-based hand rub with persistent activity is recommended before donning surgical gloves when performing surgical procedures. | **IB** |
| d. When performing surgical hand antisepsis using an antimicrobial soap, scrub hands and forearms for the length of time recommended by the manufacturer, usually 2-6 minutes. Long scrub times (e.g., 10 minutes) are not necessary. | **IB** |
| e. When using an alcohol-based surgical hand scrub product with persistent activity, follow the manufacturer's instructions. Before applying the alcohol solution, prewash hands and forearms completely. After application of the alcohol-based product as recommended, allow hands and forearms to dry thoroughly before donning sterile gloves. | **IB** |
| **4. Selection of Hand Hygiene Agents** | |
| a. Provide personnel with efficacious hand-hygiene products that have low irritancy potential, particularly when these products are used multiple times per shift. This recommendation applies to products used for hand antisepsis before and after patient care in clinical areas and to products used for surgical hand antisepsis by surgical personnel. | IB |
| b. To maximize the acceptance of hand-hygiene products by HCWs, solicit input from these employees regarding the feel, fragrance, and skin tolerance of any products under consideration. The cost of hand-hygiene products should not be the primary factor for influencing product selection. | **IB** |
| c. When selecting non-antimicrobial soaps, antimicrobial soaps, or alcohol-based hand rubs, solicit information from the manufacturers regarding any know interactions between products used to clean hands, skin care products, and the types of gloves used in the institution. | **II** |
| d. Before making purchasing decisions, evaluate the dispenser systems of various product manufacturers or distributors to ensure that dispensers function adequately and deliver an appropriate volume of product. | **II** |
| e. Do not add soap to a partially empty soap dispenser. This practice of "topping off" dispensers can lead to bacterial skin contamination. | **IA** |

| Recommendation: | Category |
|---|---|
| **5. Skin Care** | |
| a. Provide HCWs with hand lotions or creams to minimize the occurrence of irritant contact dermatitis associated with hand antisepsis or hand washing. | **IA** |
| b. Solicit information from the manufacturers regarding any effects that hand lotions, creams or alcohol-based hand antiseptics may have on the persistent effects of antimicrobial soaps being used in the institution. | **IB** |
| **6. Other Aspects of Hand Hygiene** | |
| a. Do not wear artificial fingernails or extenders when having direct contact with patients at high risk (e.g., those in intensive-care units or operating rooms) | **IA** |
| b. Keep natural nail tips less than ¼ inch long.<br>c. | **II** |
| d. Wear gloves when contact with blood or other potentially infectious materials, mucous membranes, and non-intact skin should occur. | **IC** |
| e. Remove gloves after caring for the patient. Do not wear the same pair of gloves for the care of more than one patient, and do not wash gloves between uses with different patients. | IB |
| f. Change gloves during patient care if moving from a contaminated body site to a clean body site. | **II** |
| g. No recommendation can be made regarding rings in health-care settings. | Unresolved issue |
| **7. Health-care Worker Educational and Motivational Programs** | |
| a. As part of an overall program to improve hand-hygiene practices of HCWs, educate personnel regarding the types of patient-care activities that can result in hand contamination and the advantages and disadvantages of various methods used to clean their hands. | **II** |
| b. Monitor HCWs adherence with recommended hand-hygiene practices and provide personnel with information regarding their performance. | **IA** |
| c. Encourage patients and their families to remind HCWs to decontaminate their hands. | **II** |
| **8. Administrative Measures** | |
| a. Make improved hand-hygiene adherence an institutional priority and provide appropriate administrative support and financial resources. | **IB** |
| b. Implement a multidisciplinary program to improve hand-hygiene adherence of health personnel to recommended hand-hygiene practices. | **IB** |
| c. As part of a multidisciplinary program to improve hand-hygiene adherence, provide HCWs with a readily accessible alcohol-based hand rub product. | **IA** |

| Recommendation: | Category |
|---|---|
| d. To improve hand-hygiene adherence among personnel who work in areas in which high workloads and high intensity of patient care are anticipated, make alcohol-based hand rub available at the entrance to the patient's room or at the bedside, in other convenient locations, and in individual pocket-sized containers to be carried by HCWs. | **IA** |
| e. Store supplies of alcohol-based hand rubs in cabinets or areas approved for flammable materials. | **IC** |

Morbidity and Mortality Weekly Report (MMWR). Recommendations and Reports. October 25, 2002. Vol. 51, No. RR-16

Table 5. Centers for disease control and prevention.

### 3.5 Catheter securement

Although the IDSA does not make recommendations concerning the routine securement of indwelling catheters it is documented in the literature and has been apart of the practice in the University of PENN Health system. Unsecured catheters can lead to bleeding, trauma, pressure sores around the meatus and bladder spasms from pressure and traction (Hanchett, 2002). It has been recommended in the literature that the catheter be secured to the thigh for women and to the upper thigh or lower abdomen for men. The lower abdominal position in men decreases the potential for pressure necrosis and urethral erosion at the penile-scrotal junction (Cancio, Sabanegh et al, 1993). PENN Presbyterian utilizes a Velcro catheter strap around the thigh. If a patient's thigh exceeds the size limit, metapore or paper tape is used to keep the catheter in place. Both methods of securement are changed when visibly soiled, also skin assessment under each method of securement is done during each shift or whenever necessary to prevent skin breakdown or pressure sores.

### 3.6 Catheter position and drainage

Again, the IDSA does not comment on the position of the catheter but suggestions from literature have commented however that the position of the catheter is important for the prevention of CA-UTI. The University of PENN Health System has utilized this advice by expert opinion and has incorporated into their practice. Studies have demonstrated that retrograde flow of bacteria from the urine drainage bag to be a major source of bacterial contamination. A study by Maki et al, found that by allowing the tubing to drop lower than the drainage bag was associated with a significant increase risk of CA-UTI (Smith, 2007). Recently drainage bags are designed with either an anti-reflux valve or anti-reflex chamber to prevent reflux of contaminated urine from the bag back into the tubing and ultimately into the patient. Even with the new design, the University of PENN Health System believes that keeping the bag below the level of the bladder is important in the prevention of CA-UTIs (B-I, CDC, 2009). Also included into practice is not allowing the outlet tube to touch the floor or inner aspects of the drainage container to prevent contamination. Keeping the bag empty to avoid traction on the catheter from the weight of the bag is also an important part of routine practice especially when transporting patients. Finally, preventing cross contamination by positioning the drainage bag on opposite sides of any fecal management system drainage bag.

### 3.7 Meatal care

Routine care of the perineum seems obvious. Cleansing the perineum with soap and water after a bowel movement and wiping from front to back especially in female patients decreases the risk of stool contamination. PENN Presbyterian uses disposable wash cloths and non risible spray soap and educates staff to utilize multiple cloths when cleaning. Staff is educated to clean the catheter with new pair of clean gloves after a bowel movement. The motion that is advised is moving away from the meatus down the catheter towards the drainage bag. The staff is also encouraged to clean the catheter whenever visibly soiled. Enhanced meatal care with povidone-iodine solutions, silver sulfadiazine, polyantibiotic ointment or cream or green soap and water is not recommended by the IDSA to reduce CA-bacteriuria (A-I, 2009).

### 3.8 Assessing for CA-UTI

Guidelines have changed over the past couple of years as to assessing appropriately for the presence of a CA-UTI. In January, 2010, the University of PENN Health System has developed a new procedure to asses the presence of a CA-UTI as recommended by the CDC to assure that false-positive CA-UTI are minimized. If the patient has a catheter in place and develops signs and symptoms of an infection, such as leukocytosis, and fever, and there is no other obvious source for infection, a urinalysis is sent. If the urinalysis demonstrates >5-10 WBCs, and the catheter is greater than 24 hours old, the catheter is changed and a new urinalysis is obtained. The reason a catheter needs to be changed is that catheters become encrusted overtime with a biofilm which may be interpreted as an active infection and lead to the misuse of antibiotic therapy (Marklew, 2004). If the urinalysis is still positive after the change, then a urine culture is sent off of the new catheter by aspirating from the port after cleaning with an alcohol swab. If the patient is symptomatic with new symptoms such as abdominal pain, dysuria, urgency or flank pain then the catheter should be changed immediately prior to initiating antimicrobial therapy to prevent resistance and a culture is then obtained as outlined above and treated accordingly. Unfortunately, most signs and symptoms in CA-UTIs are nonspecific and place a burden on the clinician who wishes to be diligent about antimicrobial therapy. IDSA suggest a new algorithm for catheterized patients in long-term care facilities. Use of this method has resulted in no adverse events and has been shown to decrease the use of antimicrobial prescriptions (2009). Symptoms appropriate for obtaining culture and initiating antimicrobial therapy include new costovertebral tenderness, rigors or new onset of delirium (2009). If a patient develops hemodynamic instability as in a drop in blood pressure, a broad-spectrum antibiotic is also initiated then narrowed when culture data is available. The IDSA does not have a specific algorithm for hospitalized patients.

## 4. Other considerations for introduction or deletion into practice based on literature and research

The University of PENN Health System continually looks at ways to decrease the incidence of CA-UTIs. This section will describe other recommendations for future practice.

### 4.1 Catheter irrigation

Periodic irrigation is intended to prevent catheter obstruction and infection. Catheter encrustation occurs in 50% of long-term indwelling catheters and can lead to many emergency room visits and frequent catheter changes (Getliffe, 2003). Encrustation is caused by infection of the urinary tract by Proteus mirabilis or other urease-producing bacteria (Smith, 2007). The activity of the urease-producing bacteria raises the ph >7, causing precipitation of calcium and magnesium phosphates that attach to biofilm on the catheter inner and outer surfaces. Studies have demonstrated that antibiotics or antiseptic solutions are ineffective at eradicating biofilms (Stickler, Hewitt, 1991). Current recommendations or management of the encrustation and blockage include inspecting and palpating the catheter for signs of encrustation, scheduling catheter changes based on blocking history, (i.e. usual time to blockage), increasing fluid intake, keeping extra catheter kits available (Smith, 2007). At PENN Presbyterian, routine irrigation is not performed on indwelling catheters unless indicated and there are signs and symptoms of blockage (i.e. bladder distention, obvious clots). If blockage is suspected, a bladder scan is performed and irrigation is done at the site of the aspiration port. Although, utilizing a bladder scanner is not entirely proven in research it helps guide clinicians identifying bladder volumes. At PENN Presbyterian, a hemostat is placed on the tubing distal to the port the port is cleaned with alcohol and syringe filled with sterile saline is instilled into the port. If blockage is significant the entire catheter is changed, and a larger catheter is chosen. If blockage is still occurring even after the change in catheter Urology is then consulted for further evaluation and need of a closed irrigation system is specifically addressed.

### 4.2 Routine catheter change

Data is still insufficient to make recommendations as to whether routine catheter change in patients with long-term indwelling catheters reduces the risk of CA-UTIs. Catheters are often changed at routine intervals to prevent CA-UTIs but its practice is not evidenced-based (IDSA, 2009). At PENN Presbyterian, routine catheter change is not practiced nor recommended by the infection control committee.

### 4.3 Bladder scanners

The use of bladder scanners has become standard at PENN Presbyterian. Bladder scanners are present on each nursing unit to help prevent unnecessary catheter insertion. Most recently in 2009, The Michigan Health and Hospital Association Keystone Center for Patient Safety and Quality has initiated a statewide initiative to decrease the incidence of CA-UTI through the use of a "bladder bundle" (Saint, Olmsted, et al, 2009). As previously described, a bundle is a term developed by the IHI, as a way to describe a collection of interventions to effectively care for patients undergoing particular treatments with inherent risks (IHI, 2004). Their *Bladder Bundle* included 5 interventions, including bladder ultrasound to avoid unnecessary indwelling catherization. The CDC considers using a portable ultrasound device to assess urine volume in patients undergoing intermittent catheterization to assess urine volume and reduce unnecessary catheter insertions (A-II, 2009). They also suggest that further research is needed on the use of a portable ultrasound device to evaluate for obstruction in patients with indwelling catheters and low urine output. (2009). The use of bladder scanners at PENN Presbyterian has specifically been utilized in those patients that have had invasive procedures done and that have not voided in 6-8 hours post procedure to assess for acute urinary retention has been instrumental in preventing unnecessary catherization. It also has helped assess the need for reinsertion of indwelling catheters when they have been removed. What needs to be considered is the amount of urine present to prompt catherization. Currently it is up to the prescriber to determine the amount of urine which prompts the use of a catheter at PENN Presbyterian. At the Hospital of the University of Pennsylvania, staff utilizes an algorithm, which is depicted below in Table 6. It has assisted the nursing staff in the unnecessary use of indwelling catheters by utilizing the use of a portable bladder scanner. It is important that all staff is educated in the use of a bladder scanner to ensure its proper use.

### 4.4 Alternative to indwelling catheters

The CDC makes recommendations to consider the use of external catheters as an alternative to indwelling urethral catheters in cooperative male patients without urinary retention or bladder outlet obstruction (II, 2009). They also suggest intermittent catherization in spinal cord injury patient and in patients with bladder emptying dysfunction instead of the use of suprapubic catheters (II, 2009). Further research is recommended regarding the risks and benefits of suprapubic catheters as an alternative to indwelling catheters in selected patients requiring short or long term catherization, especially with respect to complications related to catheter insertion or the catheter site.

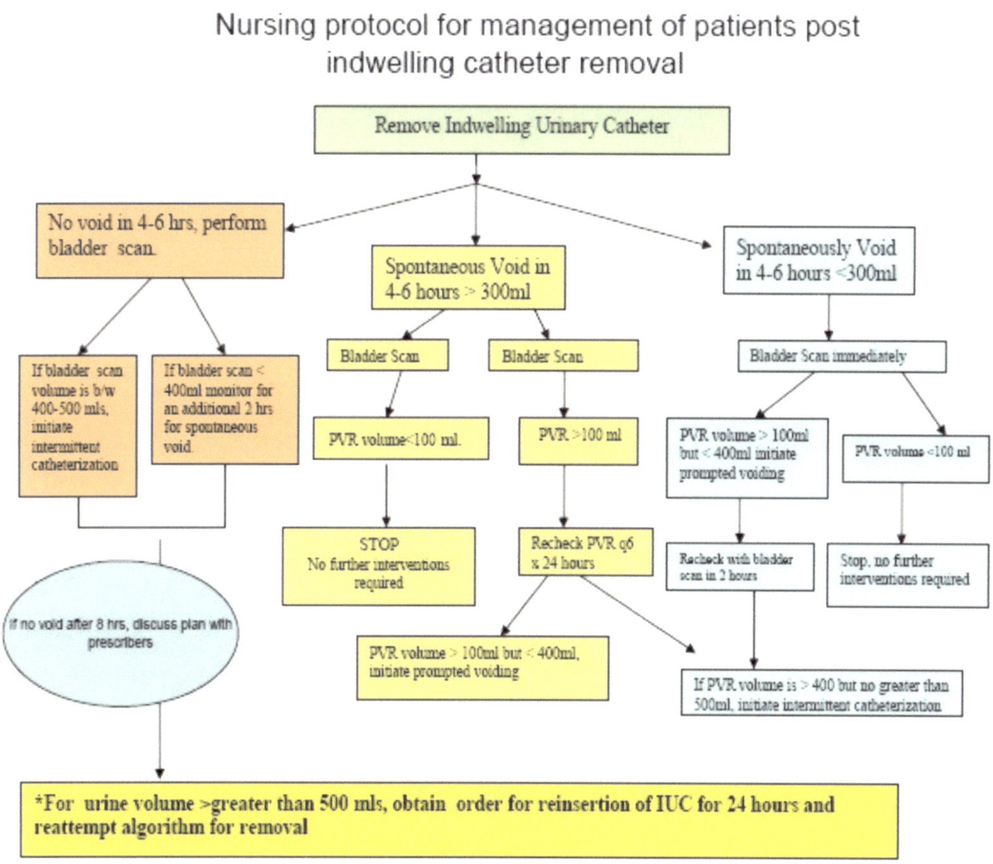


Table 6. Hospital of the University of Pennsylvania NURSING 4C-03-06 Nursing Practice Manual Clinical Practice Policy/Procedure Bladder Scanner. Patraca, K. (2005) Measure bladder volume without catheterization. Nursing 2005, 35 (4), 46-47. (PVR: post-void residual, IUC: Indwelling Urinary Catheter)

## 5. Conclusion

Although great strides in the prevention of CA-UTIs have been made, research still needs to be done to solve unanswered questions and problems surrounding CA-UTI. Specifically, around good practice and prevention, focusing on first, if a catheter is necessary, if so, then steps taken to continually assess the need for an indwelling catheter at least daily if not more often, the use of alternative approaches and adherence to good infection control practices, including proper hand hygiene. .

| Urinary Tract Infection | FY05 | FY06 | FY07 | FY08 | FY09 | FY10 | FY11 Annualized YTD | FY11 YTD | FY11Q1 | FY11Q2 | Jan-11 | Feb-11 | Mar-11 | FY11Q3 |
|---|---|---|---|---|---|---|---|---|---|---|---|---|---|---|
| **number** | | | | | | | | | | | | | | |
| HUP | 716 | 758 | 717 | 709 | 381 | 236 | **500** | **250** | 48 | 49 | 6 | 13 | 9 | 28 |
| PAH | | | 150 | 161 | 63 | 30 | **80** | **40** | 9 | 5 | 4 | 1 | 1 | 6 |
| PPMC | | | 53.00 | 35.00 | 71 | 20 | **40** | **20** | 4 | 3 | 0.00 | 3.00 | | 3 |
| UPHS | 716 | 758 | 920 | 905 | 515 | 286 | **620** | **310** | 61 | 57 | 10 | 17 | 10 | 37 |
| **denominator** | | | | | | | | | | | | | | |
| HUP | 48,424 | 51,495 | 51,441 | 52,712 | 45,405 | 45,733 | **131,252** | **65,626** | 10909 | 11095 | 3,713 | 3,337 | 3,759 | 10809 |
| PAH | | | 24,160 | 23,848 | 22,249 | 21,339 | **60,908** | **30,454** | 5081 | 5022 | 1,871 | 1,566 | 1,687 | 5124 |
| PPMC | | | 5,396 | 5,262 | 10,548 | 11,803 | **29,028** | **14,514** | 2806 | 2644 | 870 | 937 | | 1807 |
| UPHS | 48,424 | 51,495 | 80,997 | 81,822 | 78,202 | 78,875 | **221,188** | **110,594** | 18796 | 18761 | 6,454 | 5,840 | 5,446 | 17740 |
| **Urinary Tract Infection Rate** | **FY05** | **FY06** | **FY07** | **FY08** | **FY09** | **FY10** | **FY11 Annualized YTD** | **FY11 YTD** | **FY11Q1** | **FY11Q2** | **Jan-11** | **Feb-11** | **Mar-11** | **FY11Q3** |
| HUP | 14.79 | 14.72 | 13.94 | 13.45 | 8.39 | 5.16 | **3.81** | **3.81** | 4.40 | 4.42 | 1.62 | 3.90 | 2.39 | 2.59 |
| PAH | | | 6.21 | 6.75 | 2.83 | 1.41 | **1.31** | **1.31** | 1.77 | 1.00 | 2.14 | 0.64 | 0.59 | 1.17 |
| PPMC | | | 9.82 | 6.65 | 6.73 | 1.69 | **1.38** | **1.38** | 1.43 | 1.13 | 0.00 | 3.20 | | 1.66 |
| UPHS | 14.79 | 14.72 | 11.36 | 11.06 | 6.59 | 3.63 | **2.80** | **2.80** | 3.25 | 3.04 | 1.55 | 2.91 | 1.84 | 2.09 |

Table 7. UPHS CAUTI rates from Fiscal Year 2005-2011.

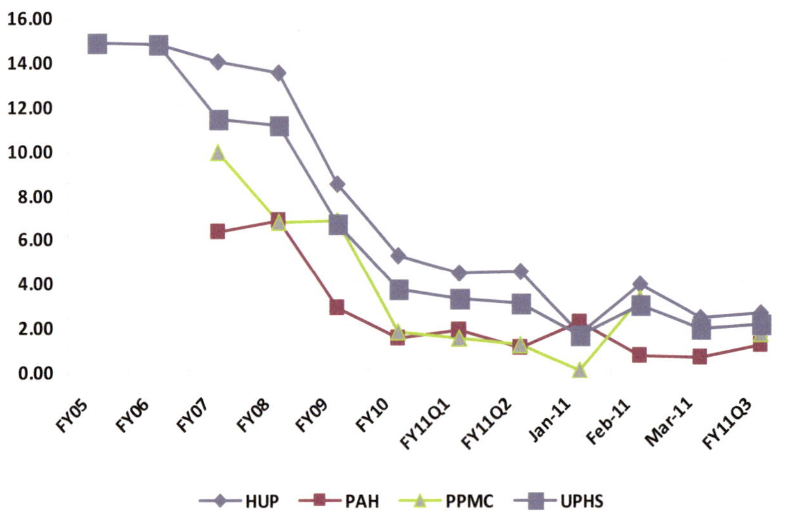


Table 7-7a. Reproduced with permission from the (UPHS) University of Pennsylvania Health System Infection Control Department 2011 (HUP): Hospital of the University of Pennsylvania, (PAH): Pennsylvania Hospital, (PPMC): Penn Presbyterian Medical Center. Rate per 1000 catheter days, (FY) Fiscal Year, (Q) Quarter

The focus also needs to be on continually reassessing gaps in care and re-educating staff as the need arises. Table 7 and 7a depicts the rates of CA-UTI since 2005 in all three University of Pennsylvania Health System hospitals. The rates of CA-UTIs started at about 6-15 infections in 1000 catheter days in 2005 and have been progressively going down over the past seven years to a rate of 0-2 infections in 1000 catheter days. Which demonstrates with hard work and perseverance rates can come down

## 6. Acknowledgment

I would like to thank Dr. Jack Ende and the PENN Presbyterian Department of Medicine for funding this text book chapter, my first. I would also like to thank Drs. Judy O'Donnell, Neil Fishman (Heads of Infectious Diseases at PENN Presbyterian and University of Pennsylvania respectively and Kevin Fosnocht at the time Chief Patient Safety Officer now Chief Medical Officer, for supporting my research and standing behind the CA-UTI policy when it was being developed and enforced. The infection control department especially, Georganne Ryan, for always having infection control data at hand and finally the CCU nursing staff , Julie Galen, nurse manager, for being participants in the research project from 2006-2007 when I asked them to be advocates even when they received push back from various services . Finally, my family, my husband Brian, my children Danny, Madeline, Gwen and Jacquelyn for standing behind me on all my projects. I am very proud of the work that was accomplished at PENN Presbyterian Medical Center and the University of Pennsylvania Health System.

## 7. References

Bagshaw, S., Laupland, K. (2006) Epidemiology of Intensive Care Unit-Acquired Urinary Tract infections. *Current Opinion Infectious Disease*, November, volume 19: 67-71. Retrieved from PENN Presbyterian Health Sciences Library, February 21, 2011.

Beaver M., CMC reimbursement changes put on spotlight on prevention of catheter-related infections (2008) *Infection Control Magazine* retrieved from www.infectioncontroltoday.com/articles/402/cmc-regulations-catheter-infections.html accessed on October 12, 2008.

Cancio, L., Sabanegh, E., Thompson, I., Managing the Foley catheter (1993) *American Family Physician* volume 48 (5) 829-836. Retrieved from http://www.ncbi.nlm.nih.gov/pubmed/8213413 on February 27, 2011

Centers for Disease Control and Prevention. Healthcare Infection Control Practices Advisory Committee (HICPAC) Guidelines for Prevention of Catheter-Associated Urinary Tract Infections (2009) Webpage: http://www.cdc.gov/hipac/index/html. February 10, 2011.

Centers for Medicare and Medicaid Services (CMS) Hospital Acquired Conditions (2008) Retrieved from www.cmc.hhs.gov/hospitalacqcond/01overview.asp#topofpage on February 21, 2011.

Cravens, D. Zweig, S. Urinary Catheter management (2000) *American Family Physician* 61: 369-376.
http://www.wocn.org/pdfs/WOCN_Library/Fact_Sheets/cauti_fact_sheet.pdf

Crouzet, J., Bertrand, X., Venier, A., Badoz, M., Husson, C., Talon, D. Control of the Duration of urinary catherization: impact on catheter-associated urinary tract infection (2007). *Journal of Hospital Infection* August 67, 253-257. Retrieved from http://www.ncbi.nlm.nih.gov/pubmed/17949851 on February 22, 2011

Edwards, J., Peterson, K., Andrus, M., Tolson, J., Goulding J., Dubeck M., NHSN report Summary for 2006. Issued June 2007. *American Journal of Infection Control* 35 (5) 290-301. Retrieved from http://www.ncbi.nlm.nih.gov/pubmed/17577475

Getliffe, K., Managing recurrent urinary catheter blockage: problems, promises, and practicalities (2003) *Wound Ostomy Continence* volume 30 (3) 146-151. Retrieved from http://www.ncbi.nlm.nih.gov/pubmed/12761486 on February 27, 2011

Gorman, D. Reducing the Incidence of Catheter-Associated Urinary Tract Infections Through the adoption of an evidenced-based protocol in the Cardiac Care Unit (2009) *Infectious Disease in Clinical Practice* volume 17: 157-160. Original Article

Hooton, T., Bradley, S., Cardenas, D., Colgan, R., Geerlins, S. Rice, J., Saint, S., Schaeffer, J., Tambayh, P., Tenke, P., Nicolle, L., IDSA Guidelines: Diagnosis, Prevention, and Treatment of Catheter-Associated Tract Infections in Adults (2009). International Clinical Practice Guidelines from the Infectious Disease Society of America. *Clinical Infectious Diseases* February 2010, 50: 625-663. http://www.ncbi.nlm.nih.gov/pub/20175247 Institution of Healthcare Improvement 2004 Prevention of HAI through Bundle Care retrieved from http://www.ihi.org/IHI/Programs/Campaign/mentor_registry_cauti.htm http://www.ihi.org/imap/tool/#Process=f0e22d9b-e08d-4d96-9f5b-181fe63743d8

Kunin, C. Nosocomial Urinary Tract Infections and the Indwelling Catheter: What is New? What is True? (2001) *Chest (120) 10-15.* http://chestjournal.chestpubs.org/content/120/1/10.full.pdf+html

Leithhauser, D., Urinary Tract Infections (2004) *Associate Professionals Infection Control Epidemiology 25: 1-15.* Retrieved from PENN Presbyterian Health Sciences Library on January 15, 2011.

Lo, E., Nicolle L., Classen, D. et al. Strategies to Prevent Catheter-Associated Urinary Tract Infections in Acute Care Hospitals. (2008). *Infection Control Hospital Epidemiology.* 29 Supplement 1: 41-50. Retrieved from http://www.guideline.gov/content.aspx?id=13394 on April 2, 2011. February 21, 2011.

Maki, D., Knasinski, V., Halvorson, K., Tambyah, P., Risk factors for catheter-associated Urinary tract infection: a prospective study showing the minimal effect of catheter care Violations on the risk of CAUTI. (2000) *Infection Control Hospital Epidemiology 21: 165.* Retrieved from http://www.ncbi.nlm.nih.gov/pubmed/10069349 on February 2, 2011.

Maki, D. Tambyah, P., Knasinski, V. The direct costs of nosocomial catheter-associated Urinary tract infection in the era of managed-care. (2002) *Infection Control Hospital Epidemiology* August (23) 27-31. Retrieved from http://www.ncbi.nlm.nih.gov/pubmed/11868889

Maki, D., Tambyah P., Engineering out the risk for infection with urinary Catheters.(2001) *Emerging Infectious Diseases.* April volume 20 (4): 260-262. Retrieved http://wwww.cdc.gov/ncidod/eid/vol7no2/maki.htm on February 12, 2011.

McConnell, J. New Catheters decrease nosocomial infections. (2000) Nursing Management June volume 31: 52-55. Retrieved from PubMed http://www.ncbi.nlm.nih.gov/pubmed/15127533 February 23, 2011.

Marklew, A., Urinary Catheter Care in the Intensive Care Unit (2004) Nursing Critical Care September volume 1: 21-27. Retrieved from http://www.ncbi.nlm.nih.gov/pubmed?term=Marklew%2C%20A.%2C%20Urinary%20Catheter%20Care%20in%20the%20Intensive%20Care%20Unit%20(2004)%20Nursing%20Critical%20Care%20 on February 27, 2011

National Nosocomial Infection Surveillance System Report, data summary from January 1992 through June 2004, (2004). *American Journal of Infection Control* 8:32 470-485. Retrieved from http://www.cdc.gov/ncidod/dhqp/pdf/nnis/NNIS_2004.pdf on September 2007.

Newman, D., The Indwelling Catheter: Principles for Best Practice (2007) *Journal of Wound Ostomy Continence Nursing* November/December volume 34 (6) 655-661. Retrieved from http://www.ncbi.nlm.nih.gov/pubmed/18030105 on February 27, 2011.

Noelle, L., Strausbaugh, L., Garibaldi, R. Infections and Antibiotic Resistance in Nursing Homes (1996). *American Society of Microbiology* January volume 9: 1-17. Retrieved from http://cmr.asm.org/cgi/reprint/9/1/1

Patraca, K. Measure Bladder Volume without catherization (2005). *Nursing* April 35 (4) 46-47. Retrieved from http://www.ncbi.nlm.nih.gov/pubmed/15818254

Rahn, D., Urinary tract Infections: contemporary management (2008) *Urological Nursing* 28:334. Retrieved from http://www.nursingcenter.com/ library/ static.asp? pageid=930205

Reilly L., Sullivan P., Ninni S., Fochesto, D., Williams, K, Fetherman, B., Reducing Foley Catheter days in the Intensive care unit; using the evidence to change practice (2006). *AACN Advance Critical Care.* Volume 17: 272-283. Retrieved from http://www.ncbi.nlm.nih.gov/pubmed?term=Reilly%20L.%2C%20Sullivan%20P.%2C%20Ninni%20S.%2C%20%20et%20al%20Reducing%20Foley%20catheter%20device%20days%20in%20the%20 on February 22, 2011.

Robinson, J. Urethral Catheter Selection (2001) *Nursing Standard* volume 15 (25): 39-42. Retrieved from http://www.ncbi.nlm.nih.gov/pubmed/12211824 on February 23, 2011

Saint S., Kowalski C, Kaufman S., Hofer, T., Kauffman, C., Olmsted, R., Forman, J., Basaszak-Holl, J., Damschroder, L., Krein, S., Preventing hospital-acquired urinary Tract infections in the United States: A National Study (2008) *Clinical Infectious Disease* January, Volume 46: 243-250. Retrieved from
http://www.cid.oxfordjournals.org at University of Pennsylvania Health Sciences Library.

Saint, S., Olmsted, R., Fakih, M., Kowalski, C., Watson, S., Sales, A., Krein, S., Translating Health care-associated urinary tract infection prevention into practice via the bladder Bundle (2009). *Journal of quality patient safety* September volume 35 (9) 449-55 Retrieved From PubMed: http://www.ncbinlm.nih.gov/pubmed/19769204 on March 28, 2011.

Smith, J. Indwelling Catheter Management: from Habit-based to Evidenced-base Practice (2003). *Ostomy/wound management* December volume 49: 39-45. Retrieved from http://www.om-com/article/2272 on November 21, 2007.

Smith, P., Bennett, G., Bradley, S SHEA/APIC guidelines: infection prevention and control in the long-term care facility (2008) *Infection Control Hospital Epidemiology* July 29

785-14. Retrieved from http://www.ncbi.nlm.nih.gov/pubmed/18767983 on January 11, 2011

Stickler, D., Hewitt P. Activity of antiseptics against biofilms of mixed bacterial species Growing on silicone surfaces (1991) *Europe Journal of Clinical Microbiology Infectious Diseases.* June 10: 416-421. Retrieved from http://www.ncbi.nlm.nih.gov/pubmed/1905626 on March 22, 2011.

Wald, H., Krammer, A., Nonpayment for harms resulting from medical care: Catheter-associated urinary tract infections. (2007). *JAMA* 298 volume 23: 2782-2784. Retrieved from http://www.ncbi.nlm.nih.gov/pubmed on February 22, 2011.

Warren J., Damron D., Tenny, J. Fever, Bacteremia and Death as complications of Bacteriuria in women with long-term urethral catheters (1987) *Journal of Infectious Diseases* volume 155: 1151-1158. PENN Presbyterian health Sciences Library January 15, 2011.

9

# The Formation of Poly-Microbial Biofilms on Urinary Catheters

Veronika Hola and Filip Ruzicka
*Faculty of Medicine, Masaryk University, Brno*
*Czech Republic*

## 1. Introduction

The number of catheter associated urinary tract infections (CAUTIs) increases every year. The increasing number of CAUTIs bears on fact that urinary catheters became second most often used foreign body inserted into human body. Over 40% of nosocomial infections are infections of urinary tract, especially infections of catheterised patients (Gorman & Jones, 1991). Despite good aseptic management, circa 50% of patients have bacteriuria in first 10–14 days of catheterisation (Morris & Stickler, 1998). The risk of urinary tract infections is significantly higher in long-term inserted catheters (28 days); the percentage of infected catheters in these patients gets near to 100% (Morris & Stickler 1998).

The high number of CAUTIs is associated with biofilm mode of growth of microbes. The biofilm mode of growth is advantageous from several reasons. The artificial surface of the implants facilitates adhesion of bacteria, which can therefore form biofilm. The bacteria in biofilm are protected against drying, mechanical damage and other influences of the outer environment. In the human body the bacteria in biofilm are protected against the immunity system and antibiotic treatment (Stewart & Costerton, 2001). The higher resistance of biofilm bacteria to antimicrobials is a serious problem and the reason of common therapy failure. The extracellular polysaccharide matrix plays the key role in the resistance of biofilm to the antibiotics. It prevents the diffusion of the antibiotics to the bacterial cells, it is the reason of the higher concentration of antibiotic-reducing enzymes in the bacterial surroundings and it partakes on the change of microenvironment in the deeper layers of biofilm. These features play an important role in antibiotics resistance because the low pH reduces effect of some antibiotics (such as aminoglycosides) and the nutrition and oxygen deficiency leads to the growth stasis of bacteria (e.g. the beta-lactam antibiotics become ineffective).

The biofilms grow easily also on the surface of other implants, such as venous, prosthetic of heart valves, orthopaedic devices etc. (Stewart et al., 2001). It's estimated, that biofilms are associated with about 65 % of nosocomial infections (Licking 1999).

With the inserted catheter, the bacteria can more easily attack urinary tract and urinary bladder (Tunney et al., 1999). There are also other complications that are linked with bacterial colonisation of urinary tract and catheters, e.g. blockage of catheters with crystallic deposits of bacterial origin, generation of gravels and pyelonephritis (Gorman & Tunney, 1997). The obstruction of the urine flow in catheters with crystallic deposits meets circa 50% of long-term catheterised patients; and there is no method of prevention of these deposits nowadays. Except of crystallic deposits that are result of metabolic dysfunction, there are also crystallic deposits of bacterial origin, caused mainly by urease-positive species of bacteria. The bacteria account to 15-20% of all gravels and these gravels are often connected with biofilm colonisation of long-term inserted urinary catheter or stent.

### 1.1 Colonisation of urinary catheters with biofilm-positive microbes

Adhesion of bacteria to the catheter depends on many factors, e.g. surface charge, hydrophobicity or hydrophility of the catheter and bacterial cell, on specific genes for adhesion etc. (Liedl, 2001). The risk of infection depends on the length of catheterisation and catheter management.

#### 1.1.1 Intermittent catheterisation and risk of urinary infections

In patients with single or intermittent catheterisation is the risk of UTI significantly lower in comparison with indwelling catheters (Gorman & Jones, 1991). Many studies showed that intermittent catheterisation decreases risk of UTI up to 50% in comparison with indwelling catheterisation and is the preferred method of bladder drainage (Perkas & Giroux, 1993; de Ruz et al., 2000; Larsen et al., 1997; and others). However, intermittent catheterisation can be cause of urethral trauma or stricture, hematuria, epididymitis in men, and other complications. As far as sterile intermittent catheterisation (SIC) and clean intermittent catheterisation (CIC) are concerned, the US National Institute on Disability and Rehabilitation Research published that the CIC does not pose a greater risk of infection than SIC and is much more economic (NIDRR, 1993). Many studies reported CIC to be as safe as SIC (Lemke et al., 2005; King et al., 1992; and others) and the CIC is widely accepted to be appropriate method of catheterisation. However, the SIC is essential in the hospital setting because of the presence of wide spectrum highly antibiotic-resistant pathogens.

The bacteria that are present in the bladder during intermittent catheterisation reach only low numbers and the stream of the urine does not allow them to adhere. It is assumed, that most of the bacteria are flushed away with the urine and the rest is killed by immune system.

#### 1.1.2 Long-therm catheterisation and risk of urinary infections

The presence of catheter in urinary tract facilitates the bacterial adhesion and colonisation of this niche. The permanent presence of artificial surface help bacteria to colonise the urinary system in the short- and long-term indwelling catheters.

In long-term catheterised patients (weeks or longer), e.g. in patients with chronic urinary incontinence, chronic obstruction of urinary tract or neurogenic urinary bladder, the bacteriuria is common; the number of bacteria in one millilitre of the urine is commonly higher that $10^5$ (Mobley & Warren, 1987). Nevertheless, the CAUTI are rarely associated with significant clinical symptoms and more than 90% of these infections are asymptomatic (Tambyah & Maki, 2000). It is widely accepted that such colonisation of the catheter (without signs of pyelonephritis or septicaemia) is not necessary to treat (Warren, 1994). The colonisation of the catheter often cannot be proved by common cultivation of catheterised urine, but it can be proved by the cultivation of extracted catheter. The results of the study of Farsi et al. (1995) show the difference between bacteriuria (present only in 30% of patients) and real colonisation of the catheter (present in 68% of the same set of patients).

There are three main ways, how the bacteria can reach the urinary bladder of long-term catheterised patients - bringing the bacterial contamination during insertion of the catheter; extraluminar migration of the bacteria present in urethra; and migration of bacteria in the lumen of the catheter from contaminated drainage system. The intraluminar invasion to the urinary tract is faster (32-48 hrs) in comparison with extraluminar (72-168 hrs). The intraluminar upstream movement of *Pseudomonas aeruginosa* was 1-2 cm per hour (Nickel et al., 1985).

The longer has the patient catheter, the higher diversity shows the biofilm microflora. Catheter infections of urinary tract are caused most commonly by faecal microflora - gram-negative rods (*Escherichia coli, Klebsiella pneumoniae, Enterobacter* sp., *Pseudomonas aeruginosa, Proteus mirabilis* etc.) and enterococci (esp. *Enterococcus faecalis*) (Tenke et al., 2006). Less often the urinary infections cause other species of bacteria, e.g. *Staphylococcus epidermidis, Streptococcus agalactiae,* and yeasts (*Candida albicans*). Higher pathogenicity of these microbes is caused by the presence of many virulence factors, esp. the ability to form biofilm, the ability to co-aggregate or ability to withstand effect of antibiotics. Some of uropathogenic bacteria, those with hydrophobic surface, adhere better to hydrophobic materials of catheters (e.g. *Enteroccus faecalis*), some other, which are rather hydrophilic, adhere better to hydrophilic surfaces of catheters (e.g. *Escherichia coli*).

The diversity of the microbial biofilm can be shown by the use of sonication techniques, as discussed further. The sonication of catheters followed by isolation, determination and biofilm assessment of particular microbial strains can discriminate particular causative agents of infections of urinary tract and their importance as biofilm-formers in the microbial community of the urinary catheter. The examination of other virulence factors, e.g. different types of motility, urease production etc., also helps with interpretation of importance of particular strains.

### 1.2 Bacterial encrustation and mineralization of biofilm on catheters

Clinical complication of the CAUTIs is obstruction of the urinary flow in the catheters by crystallic deposits. The problem of crystallic deposits meet c. 50% of long-term catheterised patients (Getliffe & Mulhall, 1991); and there is no method of prevention of these deposits nowadays (Stickler et al., 2002). The manipulation with the catheter with crystallic deposits, thus even its removal, traumatizes the mucosa of the urinary bladder and urethra which helps to further bacterial colonisation of the mucosa of urinary tract.

Crystallic deposits can evolve by several mechanisms in the urinary tract, and be of different composition. In practice there are five types of crystallic deposits. There are deposits on the basis of uric acid, calcium oxalate, calcium phosphate, cystine, and magnesium ammonium phosphate ($MgNH_4PO_4{*}6H_2O$). Calcium phosphate encrustation may present as brushite ($CaHPO_4$), hydroxyapatite [$Ca_{10}(PO_4)_6(OH)_2$], or carbonate-apatite [$Ca_{10}(PO_4)_6CO_3$] complexes. The first four types listed are often referred to as metabolic encrustation, as they normally result from metabolic dysfunction, whereas magnesium ammonium phosphate encrustation (struvite) has an infectious origin (Tunney et al. 1999, as cited in Gorman & Jones 2003). Urinary stones of microbial origin are often associated with long-term inserted catheters and form approx. 15 - 20% of all urinary stones.

Morris & Stickler (1998) described origin of microbial crystallic deposits by several phases:

- Infection of urinary tract by urease-positive bacteria
- Bacterial adhesion to the catheter surface and biofilm formation
- Increase of the pH of the urine by reason of present bacteria
- Chemical interactions of negatively charged matrix of the biofilm with positively charged ions of magnesium and calcium
- Crystallization of calcium and magnesium phosphates

One of the factors, leading to the urinary stone formation, is colonisation of the catheter by urease-positive bacteria (Cox et al., 1989; Morris et al., 1999). Urease, main reason of incrustations on the catheters, is produced by approx. 200 bacterial species. From the point of view of the CAUTIs, the most clinically significant are *Proteus vulgaris* (urease produce >90% of strains), *Morganella morganii* (>90%), *Providencia stuarti* (>90%), *Klebsiella pneumoniae* (>60%), *Pseudomonas aeruginosa* (>30%) and *Serratia marcescens* (~29%).
The present urease hydrolyses urea and increases pH of urine. Urine analysis of patients with heavy mineral deposits showed its increased pH. The magnesium ammonium phosphate and hydroxyapatite were present in higher amounts (Keane et al., 1994). Chemically, the change of urine pH and formation of crystallic deposits has several steps (Griffith 1978, as cited in Gorman & Jones, 2003). The urease hydrolyses urea and catalyses formation of ammonium and carbon dioxide (1). The ammonium becomes ammonium ion in neutral or slightly acidic pH (pH of normal urine); which induces alcalization of the urine (2). Carbon dioxide reacts with water and forms carbonic acid (3). Depending on the pH of the urine, the carbonic acid may dissociate (4).

$$NH_2CONH_2 + H_2O \rightarrow 2NH_3 + CO_2 \quad (1)$$

$$NH_3 + H_2O \rightarrow NH_4^+ + OH^- \quad (2)$$

$$CO_2 + H_2O \rightarrow H_2CO_3 \quad (3)$$

$$H_2CO_3 \leftrightarrow HCO_3^- + H^+ \leftrightarrow CO_3^{2-} + H^+ \quad (4)$$

Production of ammonium leads to increase of pH and precipitation of poorly soluble magnesium and calcium salts in form of magnesium ammonium phosphate, hydroxyapatite, and carbonite apatite, which leads to crystalline formation (Gorman & Tunney, 1997; McLean et al., 1991). The mineral deposits, formed on the basis of microbial infection, are mineralised biofilms, so the process of biofilm formation is also process of crystalline deposits formation. Urethral stents, which enable urinary drainage in patients with obstructive uropathy, meet same problems with crystallic deposits and biofilm formation as urinary catheters, especially in patients with long-term stent drainage. According to Keane et al. (1994), nearly 75% of stents gets obstructed within 24 weeks from insertion. The formation of crystallic deposits and stones on the surface of these devices is the main problem of their management (Choong et al., 2001). These deposits may lead to obstruction of the lumen of catheter or stent, to the retention of urine, bacteriuria, and rarely to other complications, such as pyelonephritis and septicaemia. Moreover, the hardness of the crystals of these deposits (c. 5 according to Mohr's scale) may lead to permanent damage of urethral epithelium.
Important role in the mineral deposit formation have the bacterial capsule and other extra-cellular polysaccharides. The chemical interactions and polarization between negatively charged biofilm matrix and positively charged calcium and magnesium ions lead to over-saturation of the environment by these ions in the close proximity of the biofilm layer and their subsequent precipitation. These capsular exopolysaccharides may also bind magnesium in the struvite crystals (ammonium magnesium phosphate), which leads to full or partial immersion of struvite crystals in the biofilm matrix (Dumanski et al., 1994; Gorman & Tunney, 1997).

## 2. Sonication and biofilm protocol

For the better understanding of poly-microbial infections, the cultivation and identification of microbial species is of particular interest. The best way for isolation of wide spectrum of pathogens from urinary catheter biofilm, the sonication seems to be most appropriate method (Hola et al., 2010). The catheter must be aseptically withdrawn into empty sterile test tube and sent immediately for microbial examination. Due to number of microbial species and their different growing speed, the immediate examination is of particular interest. Otherwise the results can be distorted by overgrowing of some fast-growing species (Hola et al., 2010).

### 2.1 Sonication protocol

The sonication protocol is based on procedure as previously described by Sherertz et al. (1990) for blood stream catheters, with several modifications. The sonication protocol, as it is described here, is used in our laboratory for four years with good results. The sonication of the catheter itself comprises of several subsequent steps, which include sonication, vortexing and diluting. The cut part of the catheter (2 cm; ~7,5 $cm^2$) is sonicated in 5 mL of Brain-Heart Infusion (BHI) for 5 minutes, than vortexed for 2 minutes and sonicated for another 5 minutes. The repeated sonication together with vortexing leads to more accurate results of the procedure. According to our findings, the sonication alone shows worse results (lower number of microbes and lower number of microbial species) in comparison with sonication-vortex-sonication protocol. The suspension is subsequently diluted 10- and 100-times and inoculated to solid media. This step is necessary for accurate quantification and isolation of individual strains (Hola et al., 2010). The set of solid media used in our laboratory comprises of Blood Agar, UriSelect 4 (BioRad), Endo Agar, Blood Agar with 10% of NaCl, Blood Agar with Amikacine (32mg/1L) and Sabouraud Agar with Vankomycine (5mg/1L) and Amikacine (20mg/1L). The quantification is performed on Blood Agar, the UriSelect helps with quantification of mixed cultures and also with species isolation and preliminary identification, the other four media are used for species isolation and preliminary identification; Endo Agar for selective cultivation of most of Gram negative rods, BA with NaCl for selective cultivation of staphylococci, BA with Amikacine for selective cultivation of streptococci and Sabouraud Agar for selective cultivation of yeasts. All isolated strains are identified by the conventional biochemical tests to the species/genus level (Micro-LA-tests, Lachema, CZ and/or API Biomerieux, FR).

### 2.2 Biofilm protocol

Prior to biofilm production assay, the strains are cultured on Blood Agar and incubated overnight aerobically at 37°C. After verifying purity of the tested strain, several colonies with identical morphology are suspended in sterile physiological saline. The turbidity of the bacterial suspension is adjusted to 0,5 of the McFarland standard (~1,5 x $10^8$ CFU/ml) using a photometric device. The obtained suspension is vortexed for 1 min and subsequently diluted 1:100 with fresh medium. The inoculum size should be carefully determined, because the size of the inoculum considerably influences the amount of biofilm produced, i.e. biofilm density increases with increaseing initial inoculum (Stepanovic et al. 2003).

All strains are cultivated in triplicate in flat-bottomed microtiter tissue culture plates (Fig. 1) in the temperature 37°C for 24 hours in the Brain-Heart Infusion with 4% of glucose (200 μL per well). The choice of the medium depends on planned experiments. For the biofilm formation, the Brain Heart Infusion with 4% of glucose seems to be good choice for most of the microbial species. The negative control wells contain pure culture medium. After cultivation, the wells of microtiter plates are washed three times with sterile phosphate-buffered saline (PBS; pH 7,2). With every washing step, the wells should be emptied by flicking the plates. The biofilm layer is fixed by air-drying (Stepanovic et al. 2007).

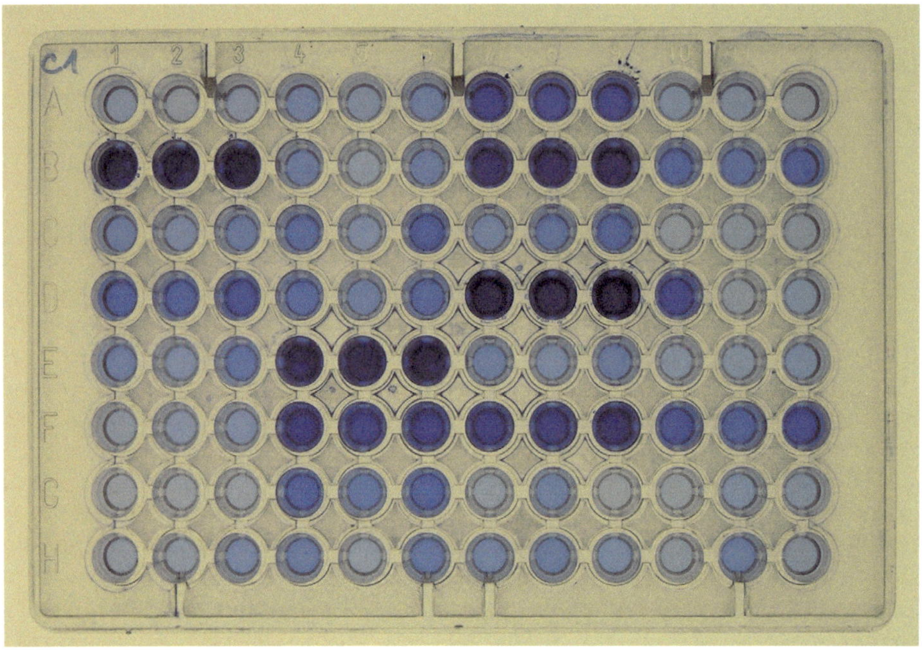

Fig. 1. Biofilm formation assay.

The fixed biofilm layer is stained with crystal violet for 15 min at room temperature. After staining, the stain is aspirated with a pipette and excess stain is rinsed off by placing the microtiter plate under running tap water. The washing continues until the water from the plate remains clean. After the microplate is air dried at room temperature, the dye bound to the cells is resolubilized with 150 µL of 95% ethanol per well. Ethanol should be added gently. Thereafter the microtiter plate covered with the lid (to minimize evaporation) is left at room temperature for approx. 30 min (Stepanovic et al. 2007) and the biofilm-positivity is assessed quantitatively by means of optical density (OD) assessment (595 nm).
For all tested strains and negative controls, the average OD values are calculated (from the inoculated triplets). The cut-off value ($OD_c$) should be established; the $OD_c$ is defined as three standard deviations (SD) above the mean OD of the negative control (5). The OD value of the tested strain is expressed as average OD value of the strain reduced by $OD_c$ value (6). $OD_c$ value should be calculated for each microtiter plate separately.

$$OD_c = \varnothing\, OD_{negative\ control} + 3 \times SD_{negative\ control} \tag{5}$$

$$OD = \varnothing\, OD_{tested\ strain} - OD_c \tag{6}$$

For easier interpretation of the results, strains may be divided into the following categories (Stepanovic et al. 2000): strain no producing biofilm (7), strain weakly producing biofilm (8), strain moderately producing biofilm (9) and strain strongly producing biofilm (10). This categorization should be based of the previously calculated OD values (for this type of data interpretation the OD value of the strain should not be reduced by $OD_c$ value).

$$OD \leq OD_c \tag{7}$$

$$OD_c < OD \leq 2x\ OD_c \tag{8}$$

$$2x\ OD_c < OD \leq 4x\ OD_c \tag{9}$$

$$4x\ OD_c < OD \tag{10}$$

As the control, biofilm-positive strains deposited in several culture collections may be used, e.g. *Staphylococcus epidermidis* strains No. ATCC 35981, ATCC 35982, ATCC 35983 and ATCC 35984 or *S. epidermidis* CCM 7221, deposited in the Czech Collection of Microorganisms in Brno (Christensen et al. 1985; Ruzicka et al. 2004).

## 3. Antibiotic susceptibility testing

Biofilm, as an important factor of virulence, enables microbes to colonise surfaces and increases their resistance to the antimicrobial agents. For the study of resistance of biofilm isolates to antimicrobials, three assays should be performed, the minimum inhibitory concentration assay (MIC), the minimum biofilm inhibitory concentration assay (MBIC) and minimum biofilm eradication concentration assay (MBEC). The results of these three assays can show the actual susceptibility/resistance of particular strains to antimicrobials.

The methods of the minimum biofilm inhibition concentration (MBIC) and minimum biofilm eradication concentration (MBEC) assessment, together with minimum inhibitory concentration assessment, are applicable for the evaluation of the differences in the antibiotic resistance in planktonic and biofilm forms of growth and for the evaluation of differences in the biofilm-positive and biofilm-negative strains (Hola et al., 2004 a).

In our studies we examined coagulase-negative staphylococci and the set of anti-staphylococcal and wide-spectrum antibiotics: penicillin, oxacillin, ampicillin-sulbactam, chloramphenicol, tetracycline, co-trimoxazole, erythromycin, clindamycin, ciprofloxacin, gentamicin, teicoplanin and vancomycine. To the commercially available microtiter plates with serial dilutions of antibiotics covering break-point concentration, we prepared second microtiter plate with serial dilutions of the same antibiotics, which linked up with increasing concentrations of tested antibiotics to cover the MBIC and MBEC values. For the concentrations of diluted antibiotics see Table 1.

### 3.1 Minimum inhibitory concentration assay

Minimum inhibitory concentration assay (MIC) was proved by the microdilution method according to the European Standards as they are implemented in the Czech Microbiological Standards (Urbášková, 1998). Briefly, fresh 24-hrs culture of the strain cultured on Blood Agar is suspended in physiological saline to the optical density equal to 0,5 according to McFarland Standard. This suspension is inoculated in the wells of microtiter plate with serial (logarithmic) dilutions of tested antibiotics in Mueller-Hinton Broth (commercially available from Trios Ltd., Prague, CZ). The final concentration of cells of the tested strain is equal to 500 000 CFU/ml. After 18 hrs of cultivation the minimum inhibitory concentration is assessed.

| Standard antibiotic concentrations (mg/L) | | | | | | | | | | | |
|---|---|---|---|---|---|---|---|---|---|---|---|
| PEN | OXA | AMS | CMP | TET | COT | ERY | CLI | CIP | GEN | TEI | VAN |
| 0,015 | 0,125 | 2 | 0,125 | 0,125 | 0,5 | 0,063 | 0,063 | 0,063 | 0,063 | 0,25 | 0,25 |
| 0,031 | 0,25 | 4 | 0,25 | 0,25 | 1 | 0,125 | 0,125 | 0,125 | 0,125 | 0,5 | 0,5 |
| 0,063 | 0,5 | 8 | 0,5 | 0,5 | 2 | 0,25 | 0,25 | 0,25 | 0,25 | 1 | 1 |
| 0,125 | 1 | 16 | 1 | 1 | 4 | 0,5 | 0,5 | 0,5 | 0,5 | 2 | 2 |
| 0,25 | 2 | 32 | 2 | 2 | 8 | 1 | 1 | 1 | 1 | 4 | 4 |
| 0,5 | 4 | 64 | 4 | 4 | 16 | 2 | 2 | 2 | 2 | 8 | 8 |
| 1 | 8 | 128 | 8 | 8 | 32 | 4 | 4 | 4 | 4 | 16 | 16 |
| 2 | 16 | 256 | 16 | 16 | 64 | 8 | 8 | 8 | 8 | 32 | GC |
| Increased antibiotic concentrations (mg/L) | | | | | | | | | | | |
| PEN | OXA | AMS | CMP | TET | COT | ERY | CLI | CIP | GEN | TEI | VAN |
| 4 | 32 | 512 | 32 | 32 | 128 | 16 | 16 | 16 | 16 | 64 | 32 |
| 8 | 64 | 1024 | 64 | 64 | 256 | 32 | 32 | 32 | 32 | 128 | 64 |
| 16 | 128 | 2048 | 128 | 128 | 512 | 64 | 64 | 64 | 64 | 256 | 128 |
| 32 | 256 | 4096 | 256 | 256 | 1024 | 128 | 128 | 128 | 128 | 512 | 256 |
| 64 | 512 | 8192 | 512 | 512 | 2048 | 256 | 256 | 256 | 256 | 1024 | 512 |
| 128 | 1024 | 16384 | 1024 | 1024 | 4096 | 512 | 512 | 512 | 512 | 2048 | 1024 |
| 256 | 2048 | 32768 | 2048 | 2048 | 8192 | 1024 | 1024 | 1024 | 1024 | 4096 | 2048 |
| 512 | 4096 | GC | 4096 | 4096 | 16384 | 2048 | 2048 | 2048 | 2048 | 8192 | 4096 |

PEN – penicillin; OXA – oxacillin; AMS – ampicillin-sulbactam; CMP – chloramphenicol; TET – tetracycline; COT – co-trimoxazole; ERY – erythromycin; CLI – clindamycin; CIP – ciprofloxacin; GEN – gentamicin; TEI – teicoplanin; VAN – vancomycine, GC – growth control

Table 1. Used concentrations of antibiotics.

### 3.2 Minimum biofilm inhibitory concentration and minimum biofilm eradication concentration assays

The resistance/susceptibility was assessed on the hardened-polystyrene pegged plates that fit into standard microtiter plates. These pegged plates enable the biofilm cultivation on all 96 pegs simultaneously, so they prompt and simplify the manipulation with the biofilms (see Fig. 2). For better cell-adhesivity, the surface of the pegged plate was modified by poly-L-lysine (Hola et al. 2004 c). The wells of the microtiter plate were filled with *S. epidermidis* culture (precultured in BHI supplemented with 4% of glucose) and the pegs were submerged in it. The primary adhesion was performed for 90 minutes. Then the pegged plates were removed into fresh sterile Brain Heart Infusion (BHI) and cultivated at 37 °C for 24 hours.

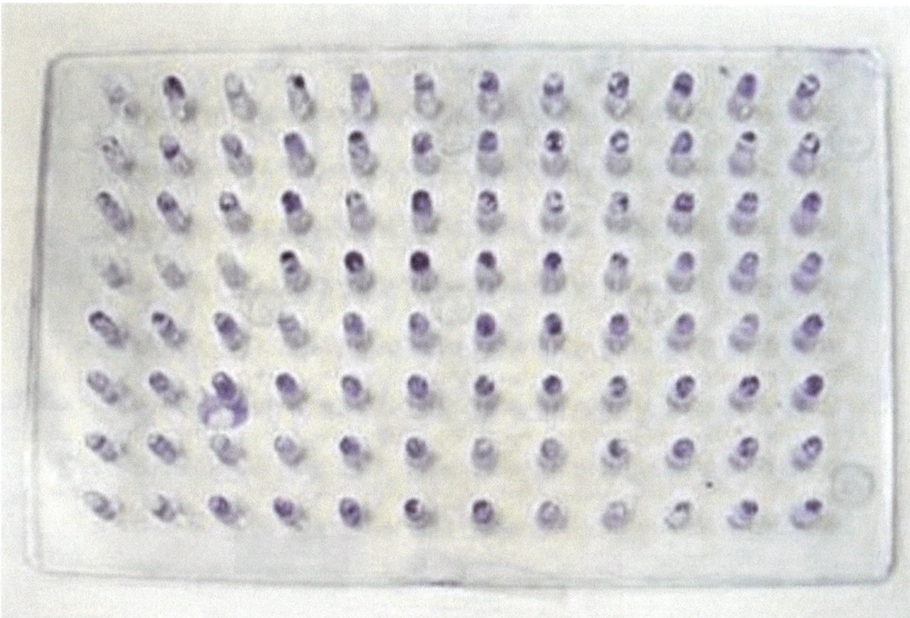

Fig. 2 - Pegged plate with grown biofilm; the biofilm layer was fixed by drying and stained with crystal violet.

In the MBIC assessment, the biofilm grown on the pegs of the pegged plate was exposed to the action of antibiotics by submerging into the medium with antibiotics compounds (concentrations listed in Table 1). The MBIC value was assessed after 18 hours of cultivation on the basis of presence of turbidity in the wells. After the exposure of the pegs with grown biofilm to the antibiotics (18 hours of cultivation) the pegs were three times washed by the sterile phosphate buffered saline (pH 7,4) and moved into the colorimetric medium, which changes the colour in the presence of living cells. After next 18 hours of cultivation the MBEC was assessed on the basis of colour change of the medium, the presence or absence of turbidity in the well being of no importance (Hola et al., 2004 a).

### 3.3 Minimum Inhibitory Concentration in biofilm-positive and biofilm-negative strains

Figure 3 shows average values of MIC of biofilm-negative and biofilm-positive strains of tested antibiotics. The biofilm-positive strains have higher average values of MICs. The median values of MICs of both groups of strains are shown in Table 2. The differences between biofilm-positive and biofilm-negative strains were statistically significant in oxacillin, tetracycline, co-trimoxazole, ciprofloxacin, gentamicin and clindamycin ($P \leq 0,05$, $n = 88$). All strains were susceptible to teicoplanin and vancomycine in both tested groups. Despite the fact, that the MIC value is defined for planktonic form of growth, there is significant difference between biofilm-positive and biofilm-negative strains of microbes (Hola et al., 2004 b).

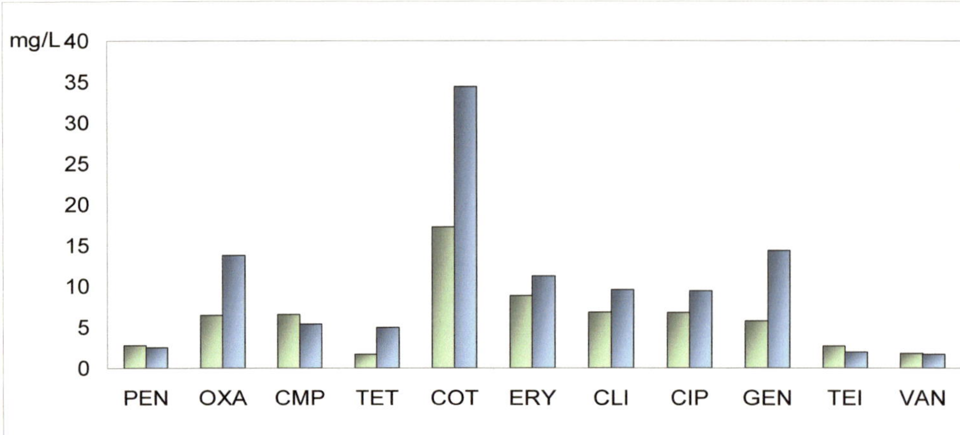


PEN - penicillin; OXA - oxacillin; AMS - ampicillin-sulbactam; CMP - chloramphenicol; TET - tetracycline; COT - co-trimoxazole; ERY - erythromycin; CLI - clindamycin; CIP - ciprofloxacin; GEN - gentamicin; TEI - teicoplanin; VAN - vancomycine, blue - biofilm-positive, green - biofilm-negative

Fig. 3. Mean values of MICs in biofilm-positive and biofilm-negative strains.

One of the factors, increasing the resistance of biofilm-positive strains to antibiotics, is the extracellular polysaccharide, in staphylococci presented as polysaccharide intercellular adhesine (PIA). The PIA is inherent compound of the biofilm layer and covers staphylococcal cells as slimy layer. The PIA facilitates bacterial adhesion to solid surfaces and co-aggregation of the bacterial cells. The mechanisms of resistance of cells covered by PIA to antibiotics are not yet fully understood, but it is widely accepted, that they differ from mechanisms of resistance of individual cells (enzyme production, change of bonding place etc.) (Costerton et al., 1995).

| | Biofilm-positive strains | | | Biofilm-negative strains | | |
|---|---|---|---|---|---|---|
| | Mean | SE | Median | Mean | SE | Median |
| PEN | 2,516 | 0,243 | 2 | 2,788 | 0,234 | 4 |
| OXA | 13,777 | 2,321 | 8 | 6,439 | 1,432 | 2 |
| CMP | 5,360 | 1,258 | 2 | 6,535 | 1,596 | 2 |
| TET | 4,942 | 1,446 | 1 | 1,695 | 0,316 | 0,5 |
| COT | 34,419 | 4,513 | 32 | 17,267 | 3,428 | 4 |
| ERY | 11,225 | 1,211 | 16 | 8,826 | 1,171 | 16 |
| CLI | 9,540 | 1,596 | 8 | 6,785 | 1,695 | 0,125 |
| CIP | 9,426 | 1,136 | 16 | 6,753 | 0,960 | 8 |
| GEN | 14,387 | 1,956 | 16 | 5,735 | 1,824 | 0,125 |
| TEI | 1,953 | 0,205 | 2 | 2,680 | 0,275 | 2 |
| VAN | 1,686 | 0,074 | 2 | 1,802 | 0,087 | 2 |

SE - standard error; PEN - penicillin; OXA - oxacillin; AMS - ampicillin-sulbactam; CMP - chloramphenicol; TET - tetracycline; COT - co-trimoxazole; ERY - erythromycin; CLI - clindamycin; CIP - ciprofloxacin; GEN - gentamicin; TEI - teicoplanin; VAN - vancomycine

Table 2. Mean and median of MICs in biofilm-positive and biofilm-negative strains.

The bonding of the molecules of antibiotic to the negatively charged chemical compounds present in biofilm layer may be the reason of the increased gentamicin resistance. The change of physico-chemical conditions may affect tetracycline and the production of enzymes degrading antibiotics may affect action of oxacilline.
The higher resistance to antibiotics of biofilm-positive strains even in their planktonic form can be explained by influence of weak biofilm layer covering the cells and formation of micro-colonies surrounded by PIA. However, the layer of the polysaccharides is still relatively weak. This, together with the absence of resistance factors that act in the layer of matured biofilm (decreased growth rate inside biofilm layer, strong changes in the inner environment including acidification, lack of oxygen etc.), leads to the observed differences between MIC values of biofilm-positive and values of biofilm-negative strains.

### 3.4 MIC, MBIC and MBEC in biofilm-positive strains

Figure 4 shows average values of MICs, MBICs and MBECs of biofilm-positive strains to tested antibiotics. The minimum concentrations of antibiotics, which are able to penetrate biofilm, in most cases exceed the minimum inhibitory concentrations (MIC) measured for planktonic form of the bacteria by several orders. Comparing the minimum inhibitory concentrations with concentrations affecting the cells in the biofilm (MBIC, MBEC), the all the differences were statistically significant ($P \leq 0,01$). For summary results see Table 3.

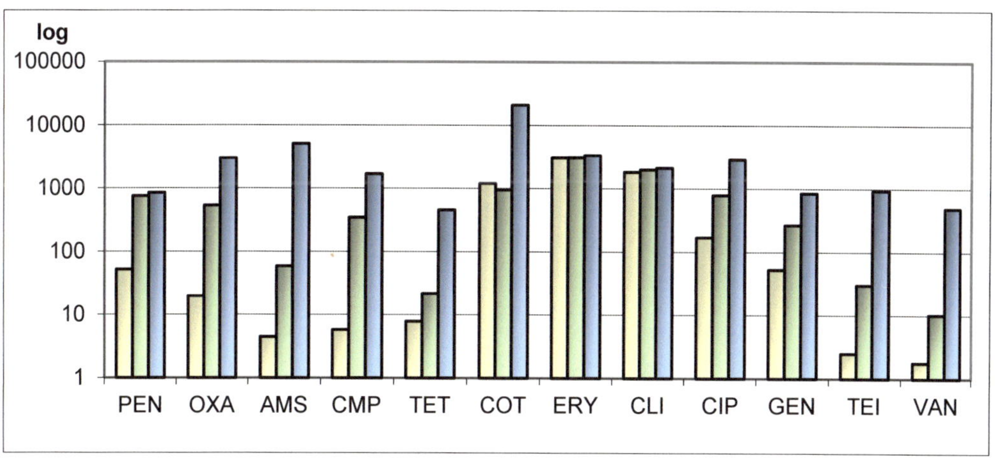


PEN - penicillin; OXA - oxacillin; AMS - ampicillin-sulbactam; CMP - chloramphenicol; TET - tetracycline; COT - co-trimoxazole; ERY - erythromycin; CLI - clindamycin; CIP - ciprofloxacin; GEN - gentamicin; TEI - teicoplanin; VAN - vancomycine; MIC - yellow; MBIC - green; MBEC - blue

Fig. 4. Comparison of MIC, MBIC and MBEC values (log).

The results show, that the MIC values did not correspond with the values that are able eradicate the biofilm. The biofilm layer act as a barrier for antibiotic diffusion to the cells, e.g. glycopeptides, with their large molecules have very low effect on staphylococci in the biofilm layer, because their large molecules cannot penetrate the biofilm layer (König et al., 2001). Another mechanism of resistance is chemical bonding of the positively charged antibiotics to the negatively charged compounds of the biofilm layer (aminoglycosides) (Lewis, 2001). The diffusion barrier formed by the biofilm layer acts also in the opposite direction - the enzymes such as beta-lactamases cannot diffuse from the close proximity of the bacterial cells, so the concentration of these enzymes in the bacterial surrounding is relatively high (Stewart, 1996). The accumulation of waste products and defection of nutrients may lead to the change of physico-chemical conditions in micro-colonies. Such environment decreases efficiency of aminoglycosides. These entire factors act in combination, which enhances their effect (Lewis, 2001) and similar mechanisms can be found also for other antimicrobial compounds.

| | MIC | | MBIC | | MBEC | |
|---|---|---|---|---|---|---|
| | Mean | Median | Mean | Median | Mean | Median |
| PEN | 2,21 | 2 | 931 | 1024 | 936 | 1024 |
| OXA | 11,1 | 4 | 219 | 256 | 2420 | 2048 |
| AMS | 5,6 | 2 | 34,2 | 32 | 1979 | 2048 |
| CMP | 8,27 | 2 | 37,8 | 4 | 698 | 512 |
| TET | 6,68 | 0,5 | 25,3 | 1 | 1002 | 128 |
| COT | 16,9 | 4 | 289 | 16 | 15639 | 2048 |
| ERY | 14,9 | 16 | 4096 | 4096 | 4096 | 4096 |
| CLI | 9,17 | 16 | 2283 | 4096 | 2340 | 4096 |
| CIP | 9,96 | 16 | 922 | 256 | 3377 | 4096 |
| GEN | 10,4 | 0,25 | 80,8 | 64 | 182 | 128 |
| TEI | 2,02 | 2 | 10,4 | 8 | 558 | 512 |
| VAN | 1,64 | 2 | 7,09 | 4 | 209 | 256 |

PEN - penicillin; OXA - oxacillin; AMS - ampicillin-sulbactam; CMP - chloramphenicol; TET - tetracycline; COT - co-trimoxazole; ERY - erythromycin; CLI - clindamycin; CIP - ciprofloxacin; GEN - gentamicin; TEI - teicoplanin; VAN - vancomycine

Table 3. Average MIC, MBIC and MBEC values.

The results of our studies confirm the importance of biofilm-positive bacteria as causative agents of biofilm infections of catheters and implants and indicate increased risk of failure of conventional antimicrobial therapy caused by increased resistance of such strains.

## 4. Poly-microbial biofilms and their composition

In our studies we presented the difference in results of microbial assessment based on use of pre-cultivation and sonication techniques (Hola et al., 2010). Our results showed that the sonication technique is more reliable for examination of biofilm infections of catheters, because it detects wider number of microbial species. Another advantage of sonication technique is quantification of isolated microbes, which can be very helpful for the treatment of the infection and for more detailed knowledge about mixed-species biofilm community. The sonication technique also solves problem of over-growing of some fast-growing microbes, such as *Pseudomonas aeruginosa*. The over-growing is often present in "classic" pre-cultivation technique and can suppress growth of other species and thus lead to the lower sensitivity of these techniques. From all above-mentioned reasons, the infection can be misinterpreted as single- or dual-species infection only (Hola et al., 2010).

The CAUTI are rarely single-species. More often these infections are poly-microbial. The number of isolated strains from one catheter/stent ranges between one and seven, where the mono-species infection is present only in 16,2% of catheters. Most of the CAUTI are three-species biofilms - c. 30%, less often two- and four-species biofilms (see Fig. 5).

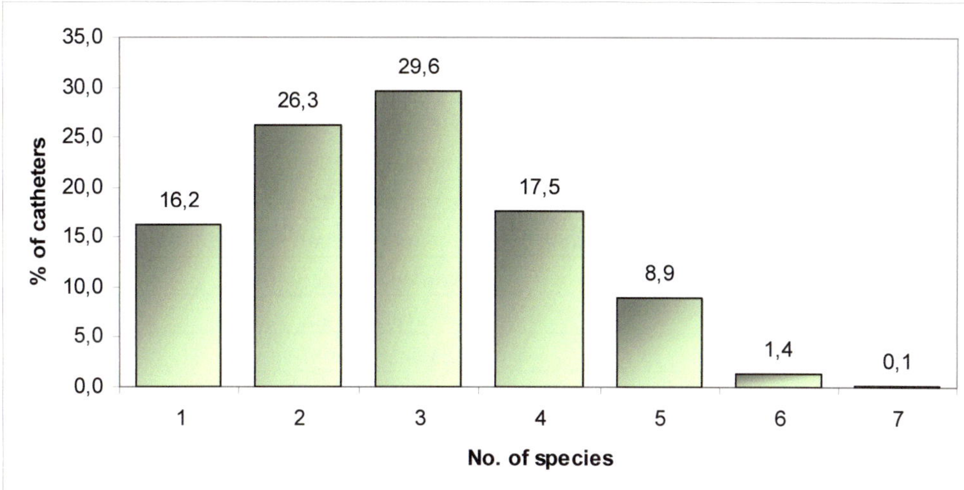


Fig. 5. Number of strains isolated from one catheter.

In these mixed-species biofilm communities, several microbial species are very often present, although the species composition of catheter is variable. Such species are *Escherichia coli* (present in 76,5% of poly-microbial catheter infections), *Enterococcus* sp. (at least one species present in 76,5% of poly-microbial catheter infections), *Candida* sp. (at least one species present in 64,7% of poly-microbial catheter infections) and *Klebsiella* sp. (at least one species present in 41,1% of poly-microbial catheter infections). The composition of other microbial species in the biofilm community is variable (Hola et al., 2008). Up to now we isolated 47 different microbial taxa from urinary tract catheters. Most often we isolated *Enterococcus faecalis, Escherichia coli, Pseudomonas aeruginosa, Klebsiella pneumoniae, Staphylococcus epidermidis* and *Candida albicans*. These microbial species presented over 65% of total microbial isolates. For the full list of microbial taxa present in poly-microbial CAUTIs see Table 4.

The ability to form biofilm is present in most of our isolates. Very often, circa in 70% of the isolates, we can prove strong biofilm production.

Only very low number of strains isolated from IUC is not able to form biofilm (less than 5%). The biofilm formation also differs among particular microbial species. Some species show high ratio of biofilm-positive strains whereas other show lower. The differences in the biofilm formation among microbial species were statistically significant (ANOVA, $p = 0,0031$). The highest ratios of strong biofilm-positive strains have species *Enterococcus faecalis* (95%), *Proteus mirabilis* (94%), *Candida tropicalis* (91%) and *Staphylococcus aureus* (100%). Low ratio of strong biofilm-positive strains had e.g. *Escherichia coli* (35%).

| Microbial taxa present in poly-microbial CAUTIs | |
|---|---|
| *Acinetobacter baumannii* | *Klebsiella sp.* (other) |
| *Burkholderia cepacia* | *Kluyvera cryocrescens* |
| *Candida albicans* | *Morganella morganii* |
| *Candida glabrata* | *Ochrobactrum anthropi* |
| *Candida krusei* | *Pantoea agglomerans* |
| *Candida parapsilosis* | *Pantoea* sp. |
| *Candida tropicalis* | *Proteus mirabilis* |
| *Citrobacter koseri* | *Proteus vulgaris* |
| *Citrobacter freundii* | *Providencia rettgeri* |
| *Citrobacter* sp. (non-*freundii*, non-*koseri)* | *Providencia stuartii* |
| *Corynebacterium* sp. | *Pseudomonas aeruginosa* |
| *Enterococcus faecium* | *Pseudomonas* sp. |
| *Enterococcus faecalis* | *Ralstonia picketii* |
| *Enterobacter aerogenes* | *Raoultella terrigena* |
| *Enterobacter cloacae* | *Serratia marcescens* |
| *Enterobacter dissolvens* | *Serratia odolifera* |
| *Enterobacter kobei* | *Streptococcus agalactiae* |
| *Enterobacter* sp. (other) | *Streptococcus* sp. (alpha-haemolytic) |
| *Escherichia coli* | *Streptococcus pyogenes* |
| *Hafnia alvei* | *Staphylococcus aureus* |
| *Klebsiella ornithinolytica* | *Staphylococcus epidermidis* |
| *Klebsiella oxytoca* | *Staphylococcus haemolyticus* |
| *Klebsiella ozanae* | *Staphylococcus hominis* |
| *Klebsiella pneumoniae* | |

Table 4. List of microbial taxa isolated from poly-microbial CAUTIs in St. Anne's University Hospital during years 2007-2010.

The strong biofilm forming strains seem to be responsible for biofilm production in mixed-species biofilms. These species seem to be primary colonisers and co-aggregate with other species or just provide refuge to other species that are only weak biofilm-producers building up the mixed-species biofilm community.

The other virulence factors, which can be present in bacteria, play important role in the mixed-species biofilms. These virulence factors affect the microenvironment in the biofilm niche, e.g. urease production increases pH of the biofilm layer; the production of beta-lactamases protect whole mixed-species community etc.

Also presence of microbes in different stages and forms plays important role in the mixed-species biofilm formation, for example the *Candida* species form pseudohyphae in their biofilm mode of growth; the strains of the genus *Proteus* may profit from close contact with each other, because in the formation of parallel cells they are capable of faster movement on the catheter surface and they produce higher amount of extra-cellular polysaccharides (Stickler & Hughes, 1999), which protects the microenvironment in the biofilm layer.

## 5. Prevention of biofilm infections of urinary tract

Progress in the area of prevention of urinary catheter–associated infections is very limited and the preventive procedures used nowadays rather only prolong the "abacterial window" then really prevent the infection. There are only few effective preventive strategies available for prevention of CAUTIs. These include avoiding unnecessary catheterisation, selecting alternative catheterisation procedures, maintaining the closed drainage system, and eliminating bacterial colonisation of the patient (Jacobsen et al., 2008).

Every from above-mentioned preventive strategies are bound onto well-informed personnel, which plays the key role in the prevention of biofilm infections of urinary tract.

The prolongation of the catheterisation or even unnecessary flat catheterisation are the first steps which can be changed in the course of prevention of the CAUTIs. More attention to the selective and limited catheter use can lead to reduction of the number of CAUTIs. Once it is determined that a patient requires urinary catheterisation, the risk of developing CAUTI is affected by the duration of the catheterisation (Jacobsen et al., 2008). To reduce the risk of infection; the urinary catheter should be changed approx. every 8 days (Rudra & Rudra, 2002) and drainage bags should be emptied minimally every 4 hours to prevent bacteria reaching the lumen of catheter (Newman, 1998). To the minimization of inappropriate prolongation of the catheterisation may help various reminder systems (Blodgett, 2009; Jacobsen et al., 2008).

The use of a closed drainage system rather than open collection container, reduces the incidence of bacteriuria to approximately 50% at 11 days of continuous catheterisation in comparison with 95% presence of significant bacteriuria in patients with open catheter drainage for 96 hours (Trautner & Darouiche, 2004). The drainage system should be dependent at all times. The presence of the drainage tube and/or collection bag above the level of the urinary bladder is associated with an increased risk of CAUTIs, as well as the presence of the drainage tube below the level of the collection bag (Maki & Tambyah, 2001). The differences in bacterial colonisation of the urinary tract with intermittent catheterisation and with indwelling catheters are discussed in chapter 1.1.1 and 1.1.2.

There are many ways of surface treatment of catheters, which have been examined during last decade. These techniques of catheter surface treatment should prevent bacterial adhesion to the artificial surface ant thus prevent formation of biofilm infection. These procedures include e.g. incorporation of the antimicrobial compound into the catheter material (without chemical bond), increase of surface concentration of antimicrobial compounds by means of catheter soaking, chemical bonding of antimicrobial compounds to the surface of the catheter, chemical bonding of antimicrobial compounds in polymer structure of the material or use of new anti-adherent coatings. These procedures lead to significantly higher concentrations of antibiotic, which can act directly in the place of origin of the biofilm focus (Jansen & Peters, 1991).

These methods, such as antimicrobial-impregnated urinary catheters rather only prolong the "abacterial window" then really prevent the infection and the colonising microflora one day anyway appears. Study performed in patients with acute spinal cord injury, who received long-term urinary catheters, showed that the silver-coated catheters delayed but did not prevent the onset of bacteriuria (Schaeffer et al., 1988). The in vitro laboratory study of colonisation of different types of catheters showed no differences among silicone and silver-coated catheters (Hola et al., 2009) The same problem is in antibiotic impregnation of urinary catheters - the onset of bacterial colonisation is later, but is always present (Darouiche at al., 1999; Guay, 2001; Johnson et al., 1999). In general, the antimicrobial-coated urinary catheters may be beneficial in hospitalized patients that undergo short-term bladder colonisation (Trautner & Darouiche, 2004). Additionally, all antibiotic-impregnated urinary catheters have same problem - the subinhibitory levels of the antimicrobial agent that is eluted into the urine may induce resistance in the resident organisms, especially in patients with prolonged catheter use (Stickler, 2002).

The consensus of antimicrobial treatment of CAUTIs is, that systemic antibiotics are not recommended in general for patients with asymptomatic bacteriuria (Warren, 1994). The systemic dosage of antibiotic should be used only in cases with clear indication of antimicrobial therapy (signs of septicaemia, pyelonephritis etc.).

## 6. Treatment of biofilm infections of urinary tract

The antibiotic treatment cannot efficiently affect bacteria embedded in the biofilm layer. *In vivo* the antibiotics can suppress symptoms of the infection by the eradication of planktonic cells, but they fail in the eradication of the cells embedded in the biofilm. After antibiotic treatment the biofilm can act as the focus of the infection and cause recurrence of the infection. It is well known, that biofilm-associated infections commonly persist, until the colonised surface is removed from the patient's body (Stewart & Costerton, 2001).

Comparison of the antibiotic resistance of planktonic and biofilm form of microbes causing CAUTIs showed, that bacterial biofilms may survive several orders higher concentrations of antibiotic (Hola et al. 2004 c; Souli & Giamarellou, 1998; Mah & O'Toole, 2001). It is obvious, that the presence of biofilm on the urinary catheter leads to therapy failure. There are many mechanisms of biofilm resistance against antibiotics, which supply and overlap.

Some mechanisms of biofilm resistance were discussed above. The most important type of the biofilm resistance is the diffusion barrier formed by biofilm matrix (Ishida et al., 1998). The penetration potential differs among different antibiotics and depends also on the infectious agents present in the biofilm layer (Vrany et al., 1997).

The chemical bonding of antibiotics and increased concentration of antibiotic-degrading enzymes in the close proximity of bacterial cells are other two mechanisms, which can suppress action of beta-lactam antibiotics (Lewis, 2001; Stewart, 1996).

Another mechanism is based on changes in the biofilm layer, the absence of nutrients and decreased levels of oxygen. These conditions may lead to the starvation of cells in the biofilm layer. The starving cells grow more slowly or don't grow at all. Such slowly growing cells show increased resistance to beta-lactams (Spoering & Lewis, 2001; Schierholz & Beuth, 2001). The accumulation of waste products, which changes physico-chemical properties inside the biofilm layer, decreases efficiency of aminoglycosides and tetracyclines (Lewis, 2001).

Spatial heterogeneity of the cells in the biofilm layer is another important form of biofilm resistance. The spatial heterogeneity is important survival strategy, because minimally part of the cells, which represent wide scale of different metabolic states, have always chance to survive every metabolically targeted attack (Costerton et al., 1999). Because of these unique and changing properties of the biofilm-positive microbes, it is extremely difficult to find simple antimicrobial compound, which would be capable of getting over most of strategies

of biofilm resistance. Despite the antibiotic treatment, the infections of the implants often persist until the device is removed (Schierholz & Beuth, 2001).
To the particular recommendations for the treatment of biofilm infection of uropoetic system belong replacement of colonised catheter (and by this way removal of the biofilm nidus) and, if necessary for successful treatment, increased dosage of antibiotics. On the other side, if the patient has no signs of septicaemia or pyelonephritis, the colonisation of the catheter is not necessary to be treated (Warren, 1994).

## 7. Acknowledgment

The research was funded by grants IGA MZ 9678, MSMT 1M0528 and MSMT INGO LA10037.

## 8. References

Blodgett TJ. Reminder systems to reduce the duration of indwelling urinary catheters: a narrative review. Urol Nurs. 2009; 29 (5): 369-378.

Choong, S, Wood, S, Fry, & C, Whitfield, H: Catheter associated urinary tract infection and encrustation. Int. J. Antimicrob. Agents. 2001, 17, 305-310.

Christensen GD, Simpson WA, Younger JJ, Baddour LM, Barrett FF, Melton DM, et al. Adherence of coagulase-negative staphylococci to plastic tissue culture plates: a quantitative model for the adherence of staphylococci tomedical devices. J ClinMicrobiol 1985;22:996–1006.

Costerton, J. W., Stewart, P. S., Greenberg, E. P.: Bacterial biofilms: a common cause of persistent infections. Science, 284, 1999, 1318-1322.

Costerton, J. W., Lewandowski, Z., Caldwell, D. E., Korber, D. R., & Lappin-Scott, H. M.: Microbial biofilms. Annu. Rev. Microbiol., 49, 1995, 711-745.

Cox, A.J., Hukins, D.W., Sutton, T.M.: Infection of catheterised patients: bacterial colonisation of encrusted Foley catheters shown by scanning electron microscopy. Urol. Res. 17, 1989, 349-352.

Darouiche R, Smith J, Hanna H, et al. Efficacy of antimicrobial-impregnated bladder catheters in reducing catheter-associated bacteriuria: a prospective, randomized, multicenter clinical trial. Urology 1999; 54: 976–981.

de Ruz AE, Leoni EG, Cabrera RH. Epidemiology and risk factors for urinary tract infection in patients with spinal cord injury. J Urol. 2000; 164: 1285–1289.

Dumanski, A. J., Hedelin, H., Edin-Liljegren, A., Beauchemin, D., & McLean, R. J.: Unique ability of the *Proteus mirabilis* capsule to enhance mineral growth in infectious urinary calculi; Infect.Immun. 62, 1994, 7, 2998-3003.

Farsi, H. M., Mosli, H. A., Al Zemaity, M. F., Bahnassy, A. A., & Alvarez, M.: Bacteriuria and colonization of double-pigtail ureteral stents: long-term experience with 237 patients, J. Endourol. 1995, 9; 6: p. 469-472.

Getliffe, K. A., Mulhall, A. B.: The encrustation of indwelling catheters; Br.J.Urol. 1991, 67, 4, 337-341.

Gorman, S.P., Jones, D.S.: Biofilm complications of urinary tract devices. In: Wilson M, Devine D (eds.): Medical Implications of Biofilms. Cambridge University Press, Cambridge 1991, 136-170.

Gorman, S.P., Tunney, M.M.: Assessment of encrustation behaviour on urinary tract biomaterials. J. Biomater. Appl. 1997, 12, 136-166.

Gorman SP, Jones DS: Biofilm complications of urinary tract devices. In: Wilson M, Devine D (eds.): Medical Implications of Biofilms. Cambridge University Press, Cambridge, 2003. p. 136-170.

Guay D. An update on the role of nitrofurans in the management of urinary tract infections. Drugs 2001; 61: 353–364.

Holá V., Růžička F., Tejkalová R., & Votava M.: [Determination of sensitivity of biofilm-positive forms of microorganisms to antibiotics]; Klinická mikrobiologie a infekční lékařství; 2004 a, vol. 10; 5; p. 218–222.

Holá V., Růžička F., Votava M.: [Differences in antibiotic sensitivity in biofilm-positive and biofilm-negative strains of *Staphylococcus epidermidis* isolated from blood cultures]; Epidemiologie, mikrobiologie a imunologie; 2004 b; 53; č. 2; p. 66 - 69.

Holá V., Růžička F., Votava M.: Impact of surface coating on the adherence of slime producing and nonproducing *Staphylococcus epidermidis*; Microbiologica; 2004 c; vol. 27; 3, p. 305-308.

Holá V, Růzicka F.: [Urinary catheter biofilm infections]. Epidemiol Mikrobiol Imunol. 2008; 57 (2): 47-52.

Hola V, Ruzicka F, Horka M.: Microbial diversity in biofilm infections of the urinary tract with the use of sonication techniques. FEMS Immunol Med Microbiol. 2010, 59(3):525-8.

Holá V., Růžička F., Tejkalova R., Kadlec R. The surface charge of the urinary catheters and biofilm adhesion. ASM Conference Biofilms. 2009; Cancún, Mexico; Abstract book, p. 151.

Ishida, H., Ishida, Y., Kurosaka, Y., Otani, T., Sato, K., & Kobayashi, H.: In vitro and in vivo activities of levofloxacin against biofilm-producing *Pseudomonas aeruginosa*, Antimicrobial Agents and Chemotherapy 1998, 42, 7, 1641-1645.

Jacobsen SM, Stickler DJ, Mobley HL, Shirtliff ME. Complicated catheter-associated urinary tract infections due to *Escherichia coli* and *Proteus mirabilis*. Clin Microbiol Rev. 2008; 21 (1): 26-59.

Jansen, B., Peters, G.: Modern strategies in the prevention of polymer-associated infections; J. Hosp. Infect. 1991, 19, 2, 83-88.

Johnson J, Delavari P, Azar M. Activities of a nitrofurazone-containing urinary catheter and a silver hydrogel catheter against multidrug-resistant bacteria characteristic of catheter-associated urinary tract infection. Antimicrob Agents Chemother 1999; 43: 2990–2995.

Keane, P.F., Bonner, M.C., Johnston, S.R., Zafar, A., & Gorman, S.P.: Characterization of biofilm and encrustation on ureteric stents in vivo, Br. J. Urol. 1994, 73, 687-691.

King RB, Carlson CE, Mervine J, Wu Y and Yarkony GM. Clean and sterile intermittent catheterisation methods in hospitalized patients with spinal cord injury. Arch Phys Med Rehabil. 1992, 73: 798-802.

König, C., Schwank, S., Blaser, J.: Factors compromising antibiotic activity against biofilms of *Staphylococcus epidermidis*. Eur. J. Clin. Microbiol. Infect. Dis., 20, 2001, s. 20-26.

Larsen LD, Chamberlin DA, Khonsari F, Ahlering TE. Retrospective analysis of urologic complications in male patients with spinal cord injury managed with and without indwelling urinary catheters. Urology. 1997; 50: 418–422.

Lemke, J.R., Kasprowicz, K., & Worral, S. Intermittent catheterisation for patients with a neurogenic bladder: Sterile versus clean: Using evidence-based practice at the staff nurse level. Journal Nursing Care Quality. 2005, 20, 302-306.

Lewis, K.: Riddle of biofilm resistance. Antimicrob. Agents Chemother., 45, 2001, s. 999-1007.

Licking E. Getting a grip on bacterial slime. Bussiness Week 1999;13:98 - 100.

Liedl B.: Catheter-associated urinary tract infections. Curr. Opin. Urol. 2001, 11, 75-79.

Mah, T. F., O'Toole, G. A.: Mechanisms of biofilm resistance to antimicrobial agents ; Trends Microbiol. 2001, 9, 1, 34-39.

Maki D., Tambyah P. Engineering out the risk of infection with urinary catheters. Emerg. Infect. Dis. 2001; 7: 1–13.

McLean, R.J., Lawrence, J.R., Korber, D.R., & Caldwell, D.E.: *Proteus mirabilis* biofilm protection against struvite crystal dissolution and its implications in struvite urolithiasis. J. Urol. 1991, 146, 1138-1142.

Mobley, H. L., Warren, J. W.: Urease-positive bacteriuria and obstruction of long-term urinary catheters; J.Clin.Microbiol. 1987, 25, 11, 2216-2217.

Morris, N.S., Stickler, D.J.: Encrustation of indwelling urethral catheters by *Proteus mirabilis* biofilms growing in human urine. J. Hosp. Infect. 1998, 39, 227-234.

Morris, N.S., Stickler, D.J., McLean, R.J.: The development of bacterial biofilms on indwelling urethral catheters. World J. Urol. 1999, 17, 345-350.

National Institute on Disability and Rehabilitation Research: The prevention and management of urinary tract infections among people with spinal cord injuries. National Institute on Disability and Rehabilitation Research consensus statement. January 27-29, 1992. SCI Nurs. 1993, 10: 49-61.

Newman, D. K. 1998. Managing indwelling urethral catheters. Ostomy. Wound Manage. 44: 26–28, 30, 32.

Nickel, J.C., Grant, S.K., Costerton, J.W.: Catheter-associated bacteriuria. An experimental study. Urology, 1985, 26, 369-375.

Perkash I, Giroux J. Clean intermittent catheterisation in spinal cord injury patients: a followup study. J Urol. 1993; 149: 1068–1071.

Rudra, A., and P. Rudra. 2002. Nosocomial infections in intensive care unit. Ind. J. Crit. Care Med. 6: 127–138.

Růžička, F., Holá, V., Votava, M., Tejkalová, R., Horváth, R., Heroldová, M., & Woznicová, V. 2004. Biofilm detection and the clinical significance of *Staphylococcus epidermidis*. Folia Microbiologica. 49 : 596-600.

Schaeffer AJ, Story KO, Johnson SM. Effect of silver oxide/trichloroisocyanuric acid antimicrobial urinary drainage system on catheter-associated bacteriuria. J Urol 1988; 139: 69–73.

Schierholz, J. M., Beuth, J.: Implant infections: a haven for opportunistic bacteria; Journal of Hospital Infection 2001, 49, 2, 87-93.

Sherertz RJ, Raad II, Belani A, Koo LC, Rand KH, Pickett DL, Straub SA, & Fauerbach LL: Three-year experience with sonicated vascular catheter cultures in a clinical microbiology laboratory. J Clin Microbiol 1990, 28: 76-82.

Souli, M., Giamarellou, H.: Effects of slime produced by clinical isolates of coagulase-negative staphylococci on activities of various antimicrobial agents; Antimicrob.Agents Chemother. 1998, 42, 4, 939-941.

Spoering, A. L., Lewis, K.: Biofilms and planktonic cells of *Pseudomonas aeruginosa* have similar resistance to killing by antimicrobials; Journal of Bacteriology, 2001, 183, 23, 6746-6751.

Stepanovic S, Djukic N, Opavski N, & Djukic S. Significance of inoculum size in biofilm formation by staphylococci. NewMicrobiol 2003; 26:129–32.

Stepanović S, Vuković D, Hola V, Di Bonaventura G, Djukić S, Cirković I, Ruzicka F. Quantification of biofilm in microtiter plates: overview of testing conditions and practical recommendations for assessment of biofilm production by staphylococci. APMIS 2007 ; 115: 891-9.

Stewart, P. S.: Theoretical aspects of antibiotic diffusion into microbial biofilms. Antimicrob. Agents Chemother., 40, 1996, s. 2517-2522.

Stewart, P. S., Costerton, J. W.: Antibiotic resistance of bacteria in biofilms. Lancet, 358, 2001, s. 135-138.

Stickler D. Susceptibility of antibiotic-resistant Gram-negative bacteria to biocides: a perspective from the study of catheter biofilms. J Appl Microbiol 2002; 92: 163S–170S.

Stickler, D.J., Evans, A., Morris, N., & Hughes, G.: Strategies for the control of catheter encrustation. Int. J. Antimicrob. Agents 2002, 19, 499-506.

Stickler, D., Hughes, G.: Ability of *Proteus mirabilis* to swarm over urethral catheters; Eur.J.Clin.Microbiol.Infect.Dis. 1999, 18, 3, 206-208.

Tambyah, P. A., Maki, D. G.: Catheter-associated urinary tract infection is rarely symptomatic: a prospective study of 1,497 catheterized patients; Arch.Intern.Med. 2000, 160, 5, 678 -682.

Tenke, P., Kovacs, B., Jackel, M., & Nagy, E.: The role of biofilm infection in urology. World J. Urol. 2006, 24, 13-20.

Trautner BW, Darouiche RO. Catheter-associated infections: pathogenesis affects prevention. Arch Intern Med. 2004; 164 (8): 842-50.

Tunney, M.M., Jones, D.S., Gorman, S.P.: Biofilm and biofilm-related encrustation of urinary tract devices. Methods Enzymol. 1999, 310, 558-66.

Urbášková P. Resistance of bacteria to antibiotics. Selected methods. Praha, Trios, 1998:100.

Vrany, J. D., Stewart, P. S., Suci, P. A.: Comparison of recalcitrance to ciprofloxacin and levofloxacin exhibited by *Pseudomonas aeruginosa* biofilms displaying rapid-transport characteristics; Antimicrobial Agents and Chemotherapy 1997, 41, 6, 1352-1358.

Warren, J. W.: Catheter-associated bacteriuria in long-term care facilities; Infect. Control Hosp. Epidemiol. 1994, 15, 8, 557-562.

10

# Urinary Tract Infections in Psychiatric Patients

Teresita Sáinz Espuñes, Maria Elisa Drago Serrano and Jaime Amadeo Bustos Martínez
*Universidad Autónoma Metropolitana-Unidad Xochimilco*
*México*

## 1. Introduction

Urinary tract infections (UTIs) are widely extended among ambulatory and hospitalized patients under psychiatric treatment in all around the world in developed and developing countries. There are few reports about UTIs in this special type of patients, most of them are hospital inpatients and stay for very long periods of time, while others are hospitalized and discharged several times during years of treatment as their illness evolves. Several factors associated to UTIs including age, gender, type of psychiatric disease, use of invasive devices such as catheter, and recently genetic background has been considered. Despite innate mechanical safeguards against microbial infection of the intact human urinary tract, specific organisms are capable of colonizing and persisting in this environmental niche. Most infections in the urinary tract are caused by Gram negative including uropathogenic *Escherichia coli* (UPEC) and *Proteus mirabilis*, and Gram positive bacteria such as *Staphyloccous aureus* carrying a wide array of virulence factors. A main concern of the frequent antibiotic treatment prescribed for the therapy to combat UTIs is the growing generation of bacterial resistance. Application of antimicrobial agents for treatment of UTIs produces clinically relevant adverse reaction because of their interactions with psychotropic drugs prescribed to psychiatric patients. The pharmaceutical surveillance for tracking adverse reactions represents the main goal in the prevention and control of UTIs in psychiatric patients.

In spite of pathogenic protozoa like *Thrichomonas vaginalis* and yeasts such as *Candida albicans* are usually associated to UTIs this chapter is focused on the bacterial pathogens. Therefore this work reviews the UTIs associated to bacteria in psychiatric patients, a group scarcely analyzed in spite of their clinical relevance. The scope of this study is to contribute on the understanding of the treatment for UTIs to prevent their spreading among patients and the medical care workers, due to their special conditions.

## 2. Distribution of UTIs in psychiatric patients

Surveillance of infections in psychiatric hospitals has faced operational difficulties owing to require of strategies based on available standard criteria to the unique needs of these patient population (Loving et al., 1992). Some epidemiologic studies of infections in hospitals reported that the urinary tract infections (UTIs) are the most frequent infections in psychiatric inpatients (Haenen et al., 1997; Hoving et al., 1981; Reilly et al., 2008; Muller et. al., 1997). The results from a survey to estimate the prevalence of health care associated infections (HAI) indicated that UTIs were the most common type of HAI in acute and non-acute hospital inpatients; moreover, in non-acute hospital, 5% of psychiatric inpatients was affected by a HAI (Reilly et al., 2008). According to a prevalence survey done in Norway of infections among hospitalized patients, the psychiatry ward presented the lowest rate of hospital infections and the UTIs were the most common infections among inpatients (Hoving et al., 1981). In a cross sectional study performed to assess the prevalence of infections in psychiatric institutes in Belgium, reported that the UITs were the most common infections moreover, a statistically significant association with infection prevalence were found with the psychiatric diagnosis and duration of hospitalization (Haenen et al., 1997).

In spite of epidemiologic assessment of UTIs has been difficult because are not reportable diseases (Foxman, 2002), reports of their incidence have been recorded in subpopulations that are at increased risk. At present, a special attention has been devoted to the study of nosocomial infections in long term care facilities (Nicolle, 2000) which include chronic diseases hospitals, rehabilitation centers, psychiatric hospitals, institutions for the mentally retarded and nursing homes.

Nursing homes are a type of geriatric clinic that provide varying levels care (including psychiatric) for aged people, who for personal, social, health or other reasons, can not longer live alone or with their families (Chen et al., 2008) regrettably in some places, these clinics are not equipped with facilities and qualified personal as found in health institutions (Alameida & Pedroso, 1999). In fact, most of research on UTIs among the elderly has done on patients who are institutionalized in nursing homes (Chen et al., 2008; Nicolle, 2002) and hospitals (Foxmann, 2002). In elderly persons, the UTIs are usually asymptomatic i.e. the isolation of bacteria from urine in significant quantities is consistent with the infection, but without the local or systemic genitourinary signs or symptoms. Unlike the symptomatic patients with UTIs, in asymptomatic patients a positive urine culture does not confirm a diagnosis of UTI among this population. Further in geriatric patients, UTIs can be either uncomplicated infections that can occur in a normal genitourinary tract (Nicolle, 2000) or complicated infections characterized by structural or functional abnormalities by instrumentation such as indwelling urinary catheters (Hazeleltt et al., 2006).

The prevalence surveys in nursing homes of different countries report that the frequency of asymptomatic bacteruria is 15-30% of men and 25-50% of women and symptomatic episodes contributed to morbidity in this population (Nicolle, 2000). The high frequency is favored by chronic comorbid conditions including mental deterioration, incontinence of bladder and bowel. The latter can associated to degenerative mental disorders such as Parkinson´s and Alzheimer diseases which impaired bladder empty and uretric reflux which favored to the high frequency of bacteriuria (Nicolle, 2000).

Urinary tract infections are commonly present in several psychiatric disorders in elderly people such as depression, psychosis (Woo et al., 2003), Huntington´s disease (Dubinsky, 2005), Parkinson´s disease (Woodford & Walker, 2005) and dementia (Hewer & Stark, 2010; Manepalli et al., 1990). Urinary tract infections have been the most frequent unrecognized medical disorder in geriatric patients with depression and psychosis (Woo et al., 2003) and also they have been commonly associated to hospital admission of patients with Huntington´s disease (Dubinsky, 2005) and idiopathic Parkinson´s disease (Woodford & Walker, 2005). They are associated to falls in geriatric women with mental disturbances

(Ericksson et al., 2009) and medical interventions in geriatric inpatients with dementia (Hewer & Stark, 2010).

In a study in hospitalized geriatric patients, UTIs were found as a risk factor associated to delirium (Khurana et al., 2002). A retrospective analysis involving 407 patients discharged over a 2 year period from a psycho-geriatric unit found that 83 (20.4%) had UTIs and 54 (13.3%) had delirium diagnoses at admission. Of the 54 with delirium, 14 (25.9%) had UTIs from which only 14 (42.8%) showed symptoms of UTIs. In this study was concluded that UTIs can precipitate delirium especially in geriatric patients with pre-existing cognitive impairment (Manepalli et al., 1990).

The efficacy of routine admission urine analysis in psychiatric hospitals has been questioned by its little impact on the care of psychiatric patients (Berber & McFeely, 1991) therefore, in the clinical practice the diagnosis of UTIs in geriatric patients in most cases depends on the judgment of signs and symptoms of infection (Nicolle, 2002; Anderson, 1981). A contributing medical practice which affects the reported cases of UTIs is that in some cases the UTIs are not recognized in patients with psychiatric illness because doctors may be more likely to ascribe symptoms to psychiatric cause (Mulder & de Reus, 2001). So this problem deserves attention for doctors to take in account somatic diseases which usually affect psychiatric patients such UTIs by analyzing clinical presentation, urinalysis and bacteriological culture of urine to get an accurate diagnosis (Foxman, 2002).

The infants represent a population at high risk of susceptibility of UTIs whose incidence is approximately 3% and 1% of pre-puberal girls and boys, respectively. The risk of UTIs increases with the age in girls but decreases with the age in boys. In pediatric girls, UTIs are associated with high morbidity and long-term consequences including impaired renal function, hypertension, and complications of pregnancy in adulthood. Pediatric girls are highly vulnerable to recurrent UTIs which may increase their progression to pyelonephritis and subsequent risk of renal scarring (Shortliffe & McCue, 2002). The risk of UTIs is also high in psychiatric children with behavior dysfunctions. The incidence of UTIs in patients of pediatric population has been documented in psychiatric conditions related with diurnal and night miction (Berg et al., 1977), urinary incontinence (Lettgen et al., 2002; von Gontard et al., 2004), urinary retention (Lettgen et al., 2002; Wan et al., 2010) and encopresis (von Gontard et al., 2004). A clinical study found that either boys or girls who wet both during the day and at night are more in risk of suffering psychiatric disturbances. No urinary infections were found in boys and girls who wet at bedtime. Only one case of urinary infection was reported in boys with day and night wetting in contrast, bacteriuria occurred in a 50% of girls who wet at day and night. The occurrence of UTIs in girls was associated to the persistent wet of perineum which favored bacterial proliferation (Berg et al., 1977). A study focused to analyze the behavioral and somatic symptoms in children suffering of eneuresis (bedwetting), urinary incontinence (daytime wetting with or without bedwetting) and encopresis (habitual inability to defecate in the appropriate place) found that the more common behavioral disturbances were hyperkinetic syndromes, emotional and conduct disorders but the rates of previous UTIs were higher although not significant (von Gontard et al., 2004). Other reports indicated that children with urge incontinence are in higher risk of suffering UTIs than children with void postponement however, the latter present a wide variety of behavioral symptoms such as aggresivity, delinquent, withdrawn and attention problems (Lettgen et al., 2002). Urinary tract infection was also associated with psychogenic urinary retention as it was indicated in a case report on a 6 year old girl (Wan et al., 2010).

According to the above described, in children with behavior disturbances, the accurate psychiatric evaluation and supportive psychoteraphy along with studies of imaging, ultrasound, uroflowmetry and a reliable bacteriologic diagnosis of UTIs are required for their fully rehabilitation.

Urinary tract infections are very common in female population in fact, approximately, 50% of women have suffered a symptomatic UTI during their lifetime and many have recurrent episodes. About 33% of women with acute uncomplicated UTI have recurrent episodes; during pregnancy asymptomatic or symptomatic UTIs often progress to pielonephritis and increase the risk of premature delivery, fetal mortalility or pregnancy induced hypertension (Stamm, 2002). In the particular case of psychiatric morbidity in pregnant women, UTIs have been associated to abortion, preterm delivery and perinatal mortality moreover; psychiatric pathologies contribute as risk factors (Ovalle et al., 1989). On other hand, UITs have been commonly found in disorders like disuria (painful or difficult of urination) and nocturia (frequent urination during the night) in women (18-55 age) under high levels of distress (Sumners et al., 1992). Although, psychological factors may be involved in clinic symptoms of UTIs, studies in female patients (21-84 age) with recurrent UTIs found that, the associated symptoms such as urinary urgency and frequency and chronic urethral and or pelvic pain decreased with doxycycline treatment and psychiatric or psychological treatment was skipped (Burkhard et al., 2004). Urinary tract infections are the most common bacterial infections in women of all ages but the incidence increases with older age (Foxman, 2002; Shortliffe & McCue, 2002). In very old women UTIs have been associated with delirium (Eriksson et al., 2011) and they seem to be independently associated with low morale (Eriksson et al., 2010b) and multi-infarct dementia (Eriksson et al., 2010a) which might indicate that they are not harmless diseases. Prevention, diagnosis and treatment of UTIs may help for wellbeing in the old women population.

## 3. Risk factors associated to UTIs in psychiatric patients

Specific subpopulations at increased risk of UTI include infants, pregnant women, the elderly, patients with spinal cord injuries and/or catheters, patients with diabetes or multiple sclerosis, patients with acquired immunodeficiency disease syndrome/human immunodeficiency virus, and patients with underlying urologic abnormalities. However, there has been found some factors related with the mental status of the patients (Juthani-Mehta et al., 2009; Rees & Farhoumand, 1977; Sumners et al., 1992; Wood et al., 2009)

A wide range of risk factors have been identified that can increase susceptibility to UTI, which can be grouped into genetic, biological, and modifiable behavioral factors.

### 3.1 Genetic factors

Within the genetic factors that have been studied are those related with the interactions among the microorganisms and their host, in these cases the influence of blood group on the availability of receptors for attachment of uropathogenic bacteria, where depending on the tape of the blood group there is an enhanced attachment of bacteria to the cells (Lomberg, 1986).

Recently the search of genes among risk populations that could be related to UTIs development was performed. Some relevant founding in particular the heat shock protein (HSPA1B), IL-8 receptor genes (CXCR1 and 2), toll-like receptors (TLRs), and transforming growth factor-beta 1 (TGF-β1) genes seem to be associated with an alteration of the host response to UTIs at various levels.

#### 3.1.1 Interleukin-8 (IL-8) and IL-8 receptor genes (CXCR1 and CXCR2)
Several clinical studies have demonstrated IL-8 chemokine in the urine of individuals with acute, symptomatic UTI (Hawn et al., 2009). The CXCR1 and CXCR2 genes encode human chemokines receptors genes for IL-8. CXCR1 is the most important gene that seems to be involved in susceptibility to recurrent UTI. A reduced CXCR1 expression was observed in both children and adults with recurrent UTI (Foxman, 2002). CXCR1 polymorphisms were associated with asymptomatic bacteriuria (ASB) and a CXCR1 variant was associated with urine IL-8 levels (Hawn et al., 2009). This is important for schizophrenic patients were higher levels of constitutively IL-8 were found (Reale et al., 2011), raising the risk among these patients to develop UTIs.

#### 3.1.2 Heat shock protein (HSPA1B) gene
HSPA1B gene encodes a 70 kDa heat shock protein (HSP) that is a member of the HSP70 family. Patients with recurrent UTIs showed a high prevalence of the HSPA1B 1267G allele (Foxman, 2002). These is important for psychiatric patients because polymorphism in HSP70 protein gene might be implicated in the development of schizophrenia (Kim et al., 2008; Pae et al., 2009).

#### 3.1.3 Toll-like receptors (TLRs) pathway genes
TLRs are a family of germline-encoded receptors that orchestrate the innate immune response and recognize Pathogen-Associated Molecular Patterns (PAMPs) such as bacterial flagellin (TLR5), lipopolysaccharide (LPS) (TLR4), and bacterial lipopeptides (TLR1/2/6). Polymorphisms in TLRs 1, 4, and 5 are associated with altered risks of UTI in adult women (Hawn et al., 2009). The 896/AG genotype and the 896G allele of the TLR4 gene showed a higher prevalence among UTI patients and TLR4 expression was reduced in children with recurrent UTIs (Foxman, 2002). Polymorphism TLR2-G2258A, a variant associated with decreased lipopeptide-induced signaling, was associated with increased ASB risk (Hawn et al., 2009). Differences in the expression of TLR genes have been associated with autism and schizophrenia (Chang et al., 2010; Enstrom et al., 2010).

#### 3.1.4 Transforming growth factor-beta 1 (TGF-β1) gene
TGF-β1 gene appears to be a key cytokine involved in the regulation of cell proliferation, differentiation, extracellular matrix formation and immune response. TGF-β1 genes seem to be associated at various levels with an alteration of the host response to the UTI. TGF-β1-509T allele showed a protective role in predisposition to recurrent UTIs because they were less frequent in children with recurrent UTIs (Foxman, 2002). It has been observed that changes in the TGF-β1 gene expression could be related to a major depressive disorder (Kim, 2007).
The main genes involved in UTIs are also related to psychiatric disorders, so it is expected that the risk of UTIs among these patients will be enhanced.

### 3.2 Biological factors
#### 3.2.1 Gender
Women are significantly more likely to experience UTI than men (Foxman, 2002; Laupland et al., 2005; Zaffanello et al., 2010). UTIs are extremely common infections in women, affecting an estimated 1 in 3 women before the age of 24 years. Approximately 50% of

women have at least 1 symptomatic UTI during their lifetime, and many have recurrent episodes. Infections in men are uncommon until the age of 50 years, when increasing prostatic hypertrophy may obstruct urinary flow (Stamm, 2002).

#### 3.2.2 Age

Patients at increased risk of urinary tract infection are pediatric and elderly patients (Nicolle, 2009). UTIs are one of the most common infections in pediatric patients, 3% in prepubertal girls and 1% prepubertal boys (Shortliffe & McCue, 2002). In noninstitutionalized elderly populations, UTIs are the second most common form of infection (after respiratory tract infection), accounting for nearly 25% of all infections (Foxman, 2002; Shortliffe & McCue, 2002).

#### 3.2.3 Diabetes

Diabetes increases the risk of UTI and bacteriuria among female but not male patients. Patients with diabetes generally have a 2-fold to 4-fold increased incidence of bacteriuria over patients without diabetes. However diabetes does not appear to increase the risk of ASB among men (Foxman, 2002). Furthermore, diabetic patients with a UTI more often develop severe and rare complications, such as emphysematous cystitis and papillary necrosis (Schneeberger et al., 2008).

HIV/AIDS: The incidence of UTI among both women and men who are seropositive for HIV is greater than among women and men who are HIV seronegative (Foxman, 2002).

#### 3.2.4 Urologic abnormalities

Functional and anatomic predispositions associated with UTI are commonly observed in elderly patients. Changes in prostatic function in men, as well as an increased risk of obstructive uropathy in both men and women, may increase susceptibility to UTI. Anatomic changes related to childbearing and/or reproductive surgery, as well as mucosal and smooth muscle changes related to postmenopausal estrogen deficiency with resultant changes in the vaginal flora, can predispose the postmenopausal woman to UTI. Similarly, postmenopausal women with urinary incontinence, cystocele, postvoiding residual urine, or a history of premenopausal UTI are at increased risk of recurrent UTI (Shortliffe & McCue, 2002).

#### 3.2.5 Pregnant patients

UTIs are the most common bacterial infections during pregnancy, and pyelonephritis is the most common severe bacterial infection complicating pregnancy (Foxman, 2002).

#### 3.2.6 Multiple sclerosis

The risk of UTI and bacteriuria is significantly increased (90% and 74%, respectively) among patients with multiple sclerosis. UTI frequently precedes multiple sclerosis relapse, and recurrent UTI is associated with acute exacerbation and neurologic progression of the disease (Foxman, 2002).

#### 3.2.7 Spinal cord injuries

Patients with spinal cord injuries (SCIs) are predominantly young males. UTIs are very common among patients with SCIs and are always complicated in nature (Foxman, 2002). SCIs could cause psychiatric damages increasing UTIs risk in these patients.

### 3.3 Modifiable behavioral factors

Frequency of sexual intercourse and use of diaphragms, condoms and/or spermicides for contraception, and use of antimicrobials among premenopausal women, increases subsequent susceptibility to UTI (Foxman, 2002; Stamm, 2002).

Catheters: A special mention for the catheters, because catheter-associated UTI is the most common nosocomial infection (Foxman, 2002; Trautner & Darouiche, 2004). The risk of UTI increases with increasing duration of catheterization (Foxman, 2002), the majority of cases of nosocomial UTI are associated with an indwelling urinary catheter (Trautner, 2010). The elderly with indwelling urinary catheters are at especially high risk of acquiring UTIs. It has been suggested that UTIs are caused by organisms in the patient's urethra that contaminate the drainage tube and bag (Kane et al., 1985).

Biofilm forms on the surfaces of indwelling catheters, is central to understanding the pathogenesis of infection of these devices. The first step in formation of catheter-associated biofilm is deposition of a conditioning film on the surface of the device. Urine deposits organic molecules such as Tamm-Horsfall glycoprotein, a slimy protein of renal origin. The host proteins deposited from urine may facilitate attachment to the catheter by uropathogens. Lately catheter became colonized. Attached, or *sessile*, organisms divide to form microcolonies and then begin to secrete the extracellular polysaccharide matrix that forms the architectural structure of the biofilm. Sessile organisms can detach and become free-floating, or *planktonic*. The presence of planktonic organisms in the urine can lead in turn to symptomatic host infection (Trautner & Darouiche, 2004).

### 3.4 Psychiatric status

Clinical assessment of UTIs in nursing home residents usually are associated to mental conditions like changes in level of consciousness, periods of altered perception, disorganized speech, or lethargy (Juthani-Mehta et al., 2009).

Studies of women in urology clinics indicated that the urethral syndrome is not associated with increased psychiatric morbidity. Patients with the urethral syndrome are no more neurotic than those with significant bacteriuria and that both groups require tolerance for the distress generated by their condition (Sumners et al., 1992).

Women particularly suffering anxiety with recurrent cystitis have significantly more psychiatric symptoms than the population as a whole (Rees & Farhoumand, 1977).

Psychological stress can impact on visceral function with pathological consequences, one study found that social stress produces marked changes in bladder structure and function induced bladder disorders (Wood et al., 2009).

It has also been noticed that neurologic and other chronic diseases that cause incontinence and weakness increase the risk of UTI. For example, Alzheimer disease is associated with incontinence, often a form of neurologic dysmotility syndrome that could predispose to UTI and asymptomatic bacteriuria (ASB). Similarly, such drugs as antibiotics, anticholinergics, and psychotropics may have a negative effect on bladder function (Shortliffe & McCue, 2002).

## 4. Common microorganisms causing UTIs in psychiatric patients

Psychiatric patients commonly suffer from a variety of infections and may be, more frequently than other populations, and the prevalence may vary substantially among different countries. It has been reported among acute psychiatric patients the prevalence of viral infections caused by human immunodeficiency, hepatitis B and hepatitis C viruses, monitored by serological tests (Rosenberg et al., 2001; Fernández-Egea et al., 2002). Borna disease virus infections were also found in psychiatric patients (Fukuda et al., 2001). Intestinal parasitosis was also studied among psychiatric patients in several countries (Haghighi et al., 2002; Cheng et al., 2005; Meza et al., 2005; Alvarado et al., 2008).

Urinary tract infections (UTIs) are widely extended among ambulatory and hospitalized patients under psychiatric treatment in all around the world. After respiratory tract infections UTIs were the most common reported infections (Haenen et al., 1997; Sáinz et al., 2008). UTIs among psychiatric patients may be complicated by comorbidities as well as the baseline presence of asymptomatic bacteriuria and benign urinary symptoms that can complicate diagnosis (Shortliffe & McCue 2002). In addition, the great diversity in psychiatric patients ranging from non dependent ones to the long-term care institutionalized patients, affects the etiology, diagnosis and management of UTIs within these special kinds of patients.

The most frequently isolated bacteria strains in psychiatric patients with UTIs were *Escherichia coli, Proteus mirabilis, Klebsiella* spp. *Pseudomonas aeruginosa* and *Staphylococcus aureus, Morganella morganii, Protteus vulgaris* and *Citrobacter freundii* were also found (Gabastou et al., 1995; Sáinz et al., 2008). In a recent study among inpatients of a Psychiatric Hospital in Mexico (Sáinz et al., 2008) in order to investigate *E. coli* serotypes associate to UTIs, it was found that the most frequent serogroups were O75, O1 and O2, being O75:H44 the most common serotype, followed by O1:HNM. All these serotypes belong to the UPEC pathotype as reported by JR Johnson (Johnson, 1991). *Klebsiella pneumoniae* and *Morganella morganii* strains were also isolated.

Among the main virulence factors associated with *E. coli* strains that cause UTIs are: adherence to solid substrates of host structures, in order to avoid being swept along by the normal flow of body fluids like urine (Johnson, 1991), and P fimbriae. In the late 1970s it was recognized for the first time that strains of *E. coli* causing UTIs typically agglutinate human erythrocytes, despite the presence of mannose therefore these strains are known as mannose resistant hemagglutination, (MRHA). The close association observed in individual strains between epithelial-cell adherence and MRHA was explained by the discovery that among most urinary isolates, both properties are mediated by fimbriae. Type 1 and P fimbriae are commonly investigated in *E. coli* UTIs strains (Johnson, 1991).

PCR techniques have been utilized in order to investigate several virulence genes like *papA* and also important autotransporter (SPATE's) toxin genes like *sat* and *pic* present in many *E. coli* UTIs strains (Sáinz et al., 2008). In the study carried out in Mexico in all the UPEC (Uropathogenic *E. coli*) strains the three genes were present and also they were identified in serotypes O134:HNM, O139:H10 (Sáinz et al., 2008). *Proteus mirabilis* was also isolated from urine samples of the psychiatric patients studied in Mexico and a DNA probe designed from a conserved sequence of some SPATEs proteins, identified some genes in these strains.

### 4.1 Antibacterial therapy and bacterial resistance

First-line treatment of acute uncomplicated UTI has traditionally involved a regimen of trimethoprim-sulfametoxazole (TMP-SMX) or TMP alone for patients with sulfa allergies (Karpman & Kurzrock, 2004; Nicolle, 2002). Increasing resistance among *Escherichia coli* to TMP-SMX worldwide has led to the reassessment of the most appropriate empiric therapy for these infections. Alternative first-line agents include the fluoroquinolones, nitrofurantoin, cephalothin and fosfomycin (Nicolle, 2002; Gupta, 2002). *Enterobacteriaceae* are progressively becoming resistant to aminopenicillines, but remain sensitive to third generation cephalosporines. A study of antibiotic susceptibility of strains isolated from five hospitals in Paris reported that at least 30% of the *P. aeruginosa* strains are resistant to ciprofloxacine (Gabastou et al., 1995). In the Mexican study *E. coli* isolated strains showed resistance to TMP-SMX, amoxicillin, piperaciline, ciprofloxacine and norfloxacine (Sáinz et al., 2008). Resistant phenotypes to antibiotics of the strains isolated in patients from psychiatric hospitals are located between those observed in outpatients and in patients from non psychiatric hospitals. However, we noticed a worrying evolution of resistance to those encountered in psychiatric hospitals. Therefore, a multiresistant strains emergence monitoring must be carried out regularly.

## 5. Interaction of antibiotics with drugs used for psychiatric treatment

Surveillance of adverse effects of psychotropic drugs is a major concern of health systems (Aagaard et al., 2010; Lin et al., 2010; Wysowski et al., 2005; Moore et al., 2007) in fact, psychiatric patients mainly elderly represent a high risk population of being affected by drug interactions (Janchawee et al., 2005; Hosia-Randell et al., 2008). Interactions of psychotropic drugs and antibiotics are potentially dangerous because sometimes cause adverse events which result in life threatening to patients. In contrast with patients with acute illness who require short-term therapy with one medication, psychiatric patients suffering chronic illness (for instance, depression) which require prolonged treatment with psychotropic drug and medications for other comorbid symptoms. Therefore, they are more exposed to the consequences of drug interactions (Ereshefsky et al., 2009). In psychiatric patients, treatment of UTIs requires the choice of an accurately selection of antibiotics in order to maximize their effectiveness and minimize collateral interactions with the psychotropic drugs prescribed for them. Therapy for uncomplicated or complicated symptomatic UTIs is based in the application of antibiotics including quinolones, cephalosporines, betalactamics, nitrofurantoin, fosfomycin, trimethoprim (TMP) alone or in combination with sulfamethoxazol (TMP-SMX). Nevertheless antibiotics are invaluable for the control of pathogens causing UTIs (Nicolle, 2002) an intrinsic toxicity is associated to their administration. Toxic effect of antibiotics applied for UTIs therapy including for example, hepatoxicity (sulphonamides), nephrotoxicity (cephalosporines, sulphonamides, quinolones), hepatoxicity (fluoroquinolones, sulphonamides), neurotoxicity and cardiotoxicity (fluoroquinolones) (Wawruch et al., 2002). The growing rate of resistance to antibiotics like TMP-SMX, has lead to the use of quinolones mainly those from fluoroquinolone group. In clinical practice, fluoroquinolones most widely use are ciprofloxacin, gatifloxacin and levofloxacin and those of limited use include norfloxacin and ofloxacin (Schaeffer, 2002). At present, fluoroquinolones are used as the first choice for the treatment of complicated UTIs in patients from all ages who cannot tolerate sulphonamides or TMP, those who has risk factors for TMP-SMX resistance or who lives in geographical areas of high spreading of bacterial resistance to TMP/SMX (Schaeffer, 2002). However, adverse effects are commonly reported with fluoroquinolones (Louro et al., 2007; Owens, 2005). Drug interactions with psychotropic drugs focused antibiotics commonly prescribed for UTIs are described next.

Ciprofloxacin is a fluoroquinolone widely prescribed in patients with uncomplicated UTIs, complicated UTIs or acute uncomplicated pyelonephritis (Blondeau, 2004) but some adverse effects have been reported. In psychiatric patients under electroconvulsive therapy (ECT) ciprofloxacin prolonged the electroconvulsive therapy seizures which are serious adverse effects of ECT as it was reported in cases reports of schizophrenia (Saito et al., 2008) and depression postpartum in a woman with UTIs (Kisa et al., 2005). Moreover ciprofloxacin displays intrinsic toxic such as thrombocytopenia as it was reported in a patient diagnosed with UTIs (Starr et al., 2005). Additionally, use of fluoroquinolones leads to the risks of adverse effects of interactions with psychotropic drugs (Fish, 2001). Ciprofloxacin apparently does not alter the elimination of some tranquilizers drugs like diazepam (Wijnands et al., 1990) however, causes clinically interaction with clozapine (Markowitz et al., 1997) , an anti-psychotropic drug usually prescribed for treatment of schizophrenia, bipolar disorder, psychotic refractory depression and Parkinson´s disease in psychotic patients (Solanki et al., 2007). As reported in a randomized double blind cross over study in schizophrenic inpatients, ciprofloxacin strongly inhibited clozapine metabolism associated to the increase in serum levels of clozapine and a metabolic derivative, N-desmethylclozapine, (Raaska et al., 2000). In a case report of one patient with urosepsis under clozapin therapy, treatment with ciprofloxacin followed by rhabdomyolisis i.e. destruction of skeletal muscle and subsequent leaking of muscle protein into the urine, was caused by a toxic accumulation of clozapin associated to the inhibition of cytochrome P450 (CYP) enzymes1A2 and 3A4 (Brouwers et al., 2009). The high serum levels of clozapin caused by ciprofloxacin in patients with symptomatic UTI under clozapin therapy produce some toxic effects including dizziness, somnolence (Sandson et al., 2007) myocarditis (Brownlowe, 2008). On other hand, serotonin syndrome caused by excessive serotoninergic activity of neurones is a potential life threatening disorder caused by the interaction of ciprofloxacin with serotonin re-uptake inhibitors drugs used as antidepressant (Montané et al., 2009) such as venlafaxine (Lee, 2009). Levofloxacin is a fluoroquinolone with epileptogenic properties causing of seizures (Bellon et al., 2009) and displays toxic effects in combination with lithium (Takahashi et al., 2000), used to treat the episodes of manic depression. Other fluoroquinolone antibiotic, i.e. gatifloxacin causes exacerbation of psychotic symptoms in patients with schizoaffective disorder when is concurrently administered with quetiapine, an antipsychotic drug, and with setraline, a selective serotonin-reuptake inhibitor commonly prescribed as an anti-depressant and with risperdal used in the treatment of paranoid schizophrenia (Reeves, 2007).

Betalactamic antibiotics used as second choice agents for UTIs antimicrobial treatment (Shortliffe & McCue, 2002) and specially prescribed for pielonephritis (Nicolle, 2002), have been associated to adverse effects. In psychiatric patients under ECT, piperacillin (synthetic penicillin derivative) and cefotiam (a cephalosporine) displayed epileptogenic effects causing of tardive seizure (Saito et al., 2008). Convulsive neurotoxic effect resulting from the interaction of penicillin derivatives in combination with flunitrazapam, a sedative benzodiazepine, has been associated to the affinity of penicillin derivatives with benzodiazepine receptor (Antoniadis et al., 1980). Additionally, a case of serotonin syndrome after single doses of *co-amoxiclav* a trade mark to denote the combination of amoxicillin and clavulanic acid (betalactamic derivatives) was reported in a patient taking venlafaxine as maintenance treatment for depression (Connor, 2003). In a study with patients chronically treated with anticonvulsants or chlorpromazine an antipsychotic drug and hetacillin a betalactamic antibiotic no interaction on the metabolism of these psychotropic drugs was observed (Galanopoulou et al., 1990).

Other antibiotics like trimethoprim, sulfamethoxazol prescribed for uncomplicated UTIs, pyelonephritis (Nicolle, 2002) and acute UTIs (Shorthliffe & McCue, 2002), have been associate to the increase of toxic levels of clozapine in a patient with maniac and paranoid syndrome with urosepsis (Jecel et al., 2005). It has also been reported that nitrofurantoin, trimetroprim and sulfamethoxazol could cause adverse reactions including gastrointestinal disturbances, cutaneous reactions, pulmonary toxicity, hepatic and haematological toxicity (Karpman & Kurzrock, 2004).

## 6. Conclusions

UTIs are a common bacterial complication that is associated with morbidity but not mortality in psychiatric patients mainly the elderly. There is a relative paucity of research about the prevalence of UTIs in psychiatric population because UTIs are not always reportable diseases.

The etiology of UTIs is also affected by underlying host factors that complicate UTI, such as age, diabetes, catheterization and psychiatric conditions like lethargy, anxiety and Alzheimer disease. Currently genetic factors that may be involved in UTIs are also present in patients with mental problems, where the same gene is altered enhancing the risk of a UTIs, that is the case for schizophrenic patients with IL-8 or HSPA1B polymorphic genes that are also implicated in the development of these infections.

The microbial etiology of urinary infections has been regarded as well established and reasonably consistent. *Enterobacteriaceae* family members like *Escherichia coli* remain the predominant uropathogen isolated in acute uncomplicated infections. Moreover other genders like *Klebsiella, Enterobacter* and *Proteus* species frequently cause complicated UTIs. Other common uropathogens include *Pseudomonas* and *Staphylococcus* spp. The pathogens traditionally associated with UTI are changing many of their features, particularly because of antimicrobial resistance.

The advances in molecular biology may facilitate the identification of new etiologic agents for UTI. A renewed interest in the etiology and management of UTI has surfaced over the past few years. The need for accurate and updated population surveillance data is apparent, particularly in light of concerns regarding antimicrobial resistance.

Antimicrobial treatment of symptomatic UTIs should be carefully prescribed and supported with laboratory diagnostic, in order to ensure the effectiveness of the antibiotic, and to avoid bacterial resistances. Drug surveillance should reduce the possibility of side effects or interactions with the psychotropic drugs that are prescribe in clinical illness that affects the psychiatric patients.

More studies are needed to better define the epidemiology and management of these infections in this special type of patients.

## 7. References

Aagaard, L. & Hansen, E. (2010). Adverse Drug Reactions from Psychotropic Medicines in the Pediatric Population: Analysis of Reports to the Danish Medicines Agency over a decade. *BMC Research Notes*, Vol. 3, (June 23, 2010), pp. 176-182, ISSN 1756-0500

Almeida, R.C. & Pedroso, E.R.P. (1999). Nosocomial Infection in Long Term Care Facilities. A survey in a Brazilian Psychiatric Hospital. *Revista do Instituto de Medicina Tropical de São Paulo*, Vol. 41, No. 6, (November-December 1999), pp. 365-370, ISSN 0036-4665

Alvarado, C.; Arreola, M.A.; Rodríguez, A.; Alanis, O.; Estrada, S.; Luevanos, C.; Martínez, L.; Martínez, S.; Ramírez, E.; Ibarra, I. & González, C. (2008). Seroprevalence of Selected Viral, Bacterial and Parasitic Infections Among Inpatients of a Public Psychiatric Hospital of Mexico. *Journal of the São Paulo Institute of Tropical Medicine,* Vol.50, No.3, (May 2008), pp. 161-164, ISSN 0036-4665

Anderson, J, E. (1981). Initial Treatment Decisions in Urinary Tract Infection. *Canadian Family Physician,* Vol. 27, No.12 (December 1981), pp. 1909-1912, ISSN 0008-350X

Antoniadis, A.; Muller, W.E. & Wollert, U. (1980). Benzodiazepine Receptor Interactions May Be Involved in the Neurotoxicity of Various Penicillin Derivatives. *Annals of Neurology,* Vol. 8, No. 1, (July 1980), pp. 71-73, ISSN 0364-5134

Bellon, A.; Perez-Garcia, G.; Coverdale, J.H. & Chacko, R.C. (2009). Seizures Associated with Levofloxacin: Case Presentation and Literature Review. *European Journal of Clinical Pharmacology,* Vol. 65, No. 10 (October 2009), pp. 959-962, ISSN 0031-6970

Berber, M.J. & McFeely, N. (1991). Efficacy of Routine Admission Urinalyses in Psychiatric Hospitals. *Canadian Journal of Psychiatry,* Vol.36, No. 3, (April 1991), pp.190-193, ISSN 0706-7437

Berg, I.; Fielding, D. & Meadow, R. (1977). Psychiatric Disturbance, Urgency, and Bacteriuria in Children with Day and Night Wetting. *Archives of Diseases in Childhood,* Vol. 52, No. 8, (August 1977), pp. 651-657, ISSN 1743-0585

Blondeau, J.M. (2004). Current Issues in the Management of Urinary Tract Infections: Extended-release Ciprofloxacin as a Novel Treatment Option. *Drugs,* Vol. 64, No. 6, (March 2004), pp. 611-628. ISSN 0012-6667

Brouwers, E.E.; Söhne, M.; Kuipers, S.; van Gorp, E.C.; Schellens, J.H.; Koks, C.H.; Beijnen, J.H. & Huitema, A.D. (2009). Ciprofloxacin Strongly Inhibits Clozapine Metabolism: Two Case Reports. *Clinical Drug Investigation,* Vol. 29, No. 1, (January, 2009), pp 59-63, ISSN 1173-2563

Brownlowe, K. (2008). Clozapine Toxicity in Smoking Cessarion and with Ciprofloxacine. *Psychosomatics,* Vol. 49, No. 2, (March-April 2008), pp. 176, ISSN 0033-3182

Burkhard, F.C.; Blick, N.; Hochreiter, W.W. & Studer, U.E. (2004). Urinary Urgency and Frequency, and Chronic Urethral and/or Pelvic Pain in Females. Can do Doxycycline Help? *The Journal of Urology,* Vol. 172, No. 1, (July 2004), pp. 232-235, ISSN 0022-5347

Chang, S.H.; Chiang, S.Y.; Chiu, C.C.; Tsai, C.C.; Tsai, H.H.; Huang, C.Y.; Hsu, T.C. & Tzang, B.S. (2010). Expression of Anti-cardiolipin Antibodies and Inflammatory Associated Factors in Patients with Schizophrenia. *Psychiatry Research,* (May 2010), doi:10.1016/ j.psychres. 2010.04.049. ISSN 0165-1781

Chen, H.; Chiu, A.; Lam, PSS.; Poon, W.K.; Chow, S.M.; Ng, W.P. & Yung R.W.H. (2008). Prevalence of Infections in Residential Care Homes for Elderly in Honk Kong. *Hong Kong Medical Journal,* Vol. 14, No. 6, (December 2008), pp. 444-450, ISSN 1024-2708

Cheng, H.S. & Wang, L.C. (2005). Intestinal Parasites May Not Cause Nosocomial Infections in Psychiatric Hospital. *Parasitology Research,* Vol.95, No.5, (March 2005), pp. 358-362, ISSN 0932-0113

Connor, H. (2003). Serotonine Syndrome After Single Doses of Co-amoxiclav During Treatment with Venflaxine. *Journal of the Royal Society of Medicine,* Vol. 96, No. 5, (May 2003), pp. 233-234, ISSN 0141-0768

Dubinsky, R.M. (2005). No Going Home for Hospitalized Huntington´s disease patients. *Movement Disorders,* Vol. 20, No. 10, (October 2005), pp. 1316-1322, ISSN 0885-3185

Enstrom, A.M.; Onore, C.E.; Van de Water, J.A. & Ashwood, P. (2010). Differential Monocyte Responses to TLR Ligands in Children with Autism Spectrum Disorders. *Brain,Behavior, and Immunity,* Vol. 24. No. 1, (January 2010), pp. 64-71. ISSN 0889-1591

Ereshefsky, L. & Sloan, D.M. (2009). Drug-Drug Interactions with the Use of Psychotropic Medications. *Question and Answer Forum,* Vol. 14, No. 8, (August 2009), pp. 1-8. Available from http://www.cnsspectrums.com/userdocs/0809cns_q_a_ereshefsky.pdf

Ericksson, I.; Gustafson, Y.; Fagerström, L. & Olofsson, B. (2010a). Prevalence and Factors Associated with Urinary Tract Infections (UTIs) in Very Old Women. *Archives of Gerontology Geriatrics,* Vol. 50, No. 2, (March-April 2010), pp. 132-135, ISSN 0167-4943

Ericksson, I.; Gustafson, Y.; Fagerström, L. & Olofsson, B. (2010b). Do Urinary Tract Infections Affect Morale Among Very Old Women? *Health and Quality of Life Outcomes,* Vol. 8, (July 22, 2010), pp. 73, ISSN 1477-7525

Ericksson, I.; Gustafson, Y.; Fagerström, L. & Olofsson, B. (2011). Urinary Tract Infection in Very Old Women is Associated with Delirium. *International Psychogeriatrics,* Vol. 23, No. 3, (April 2011), pp. 496-502, ISSN 1041-6102

Ericksson, S.; Strandberg, S.; Gustafson, Y. & Lundin-Olsson, L. (2009). Circumstances Surrounding Falls in Patients with Dementia in a Psychogeriatric Ward. *Archives of Gerontology Geriatrics,* Vol. 49, No. 1, (July-August 2009) pp. 80-87, ISSN 0167-4943

Fernández-Egea, E.; Gómez, G. E.; Corbella, S. B.; Salamero, B. M.; Blanch, A.J.; & Valdés, M. M. (2002). Serological Testing and Prevalence of Human Immunodeficiency, Hepatitis B and C Viruses Infections Amongst Acute Psychiatric Inpatients. *Medicina Clínica,* Vol.119, No.18, (November 2002), pp. 690-692, ISSN 0025-7753

Fish, D.N. (2001). Fluoroquinolone Adverse Effects and Drug Interactions. *Pharmacotherapy,* Vol. 21, No. 10 Pt 2, (October 2001), pp. 253S-272S, ISSN 0277-0008

Foxman, B. (2002). Epidemiology of Urinary Tract Infections: Incidence, Morbidity, and Economic Costs. *The American Journal of Medicine,* Vol. 113, Suppl. 1A, (July 2002), pp. 5S–13S. ISSN 0002-9343

Fukuda, K.; Takahashi, K.; Iwata, Y.; Mori, N.; Gonda, K.; Ogawa, T.; Osonoe, K.; Ogata, S.; Horimoto, T.; Sawasa, T.; Tashiro, M.; Yamaguchi, K.; Niwa, S.; & Shigeta, S. (2001). Immunological and PCR Analyses for Borna Disease Virus in Psychiatric Patients and Blood Donors in Japan. *Journal of Clinical Microbiology,* Vol.39, No.2, (February 2001), pp. 419-429, ISSN 0095-1137

Gabastou, J.M.; Chouaki, T. ; Mangeot, J. ; Zemir, A.; Lepitre, M.; Gravisse, J.; Cornel, E.; Denis-Jacquot, N.; & Mahuzier, G. (1995). Phenotypes of Resistance to Antibiotics of the Most Frequently Isolated Strains in Five Specialized Hospital Centers. Multicenter Study. *Pathologie et Biologie,* Vol.43, No.4, (April 1995), pp. 320-323, ISSN 0369-8114

Galanopoulou, P.; Karageorgiuo, C. & Dimakopoulou, K. (1990). Effect of Enzyme Induction on Bioavailability of Hetacillin in Patients Treated with Anticonvulsants and Chlorpromazine. *European Journal of Drug Metabolism and Pharmacokinetics,* Vol. 15, No. 1, (January-March 1990), pp. 15-18, ISSN 0378-7966

Gupta, K. (2002). Addressing Antibiotic Resistance. *The American Journal of Medicine,* Vol.113, No.1A, (July 2002), pp. 29S-34S, ISSN 0002-9343

Haenen, R.; Moens, G. & Jacques P. (1997). The Prevalence of Infections in Psychiatric Institutes in Belgium. *The Journal of Hospital Infection,* Vol. 37, No. 4, (December 1997), ISSN 0195-6701

Haghighi, A.; Kobayashi, S.; Takeuchi, T.; Gohta, M.; & Nozaki, T. (2002). Remarkable Genetic Polymorphism among *Entamoeba histolytica* Isolates from a Limited Geographic Area. *Journal of Clinical Microbiology,* Vol.40, No.11, (November 2001), pp. 419-429, ISSN 0095-1137

Hawn, T.R.; Scholes, D.; Wang, H.; Li, SS.; Stapleton, A.E.; Janer, M.; Aderem, A.; Stamm, W.E.; Zhao, L.P. & Hooton, T.M. (2009). Genetic Variation of the Human Urinary Tract Innate Immune Response and Asymptomatic Bacteriuria in Women. *Public Library of Science One,* Vol. 4, No. 12, e8300, (December 2009), doi:10.1371/journal.pone.0005990. ISSN 1932-6203

Hazelett, S.E.; Tsai, M.; Gareri, M. & Allen, K. (2006).The Association Between Indwelling Urinary Catheter Use in the Elderly and Urinary Tract Infections in Acute Care. *BMC Geriatrics,* Vol. 6, (October 12, 2006) pp.15-22, ISSN 1471-2318

Hewer, W. & Stark, H.W. (2010). General Medical Interventions in Patients with Dementia Treated in a Psychogeriatric Unit. *Zeitschrift für Gerontologie und Geriatrie,* Vol. 43, No. 3, (June 2010), pp. 180-182, ISSN 0948-6704

Hosia-Randell, H.M.; Muurinen, S.M. & Pitkälä, K.H. (2008). Exposure to Potentially Inappropriate Drugs and Drug-Drug Interactions in Elderly Nursing Home Residents in Helsinki, Finland: a Cross Sectional Study. *Drug Aging,* Vol. 25, No. 8, (August, 2008), pp. 683-692, ISSN 1170-229X

Hoving, B.; Lystad, A. & Opsjøn, H. (1981). A Prevalence Survey of Infections Among Hospitalized Patients in Norway. *National Institute of Public Health Annals,* Vol. 4 No. 2, (December 1981), pp. 49-60, ISSN 0332-5652

Janchawee, B.; Wongpoowarack, W.; Owatranporn, T. & Chongsuvivatwong, V. (2005). Pharmacoepidemiologic Study of Potential Drug Interactions in Outpatients of a University Hospital in Thailand. *Journal of Clinical Pharmacy and Therapeutics,* Vol. 30, No. 1, (February 2005), pp. 13-20, ISSN 0269-4727

Jecel, J.; Michel, T.M.; Gutknecht, L.; Schmidt, D.; Pfuhlmann, B. & Jabs, B.E. (2005). Toxic Clozapine Serum Levels During Acute Urinary Tract Infection: a Case Report. *European Journal of Clinical Pharmacology,* Vol. 60, No. 12, (February, 2005), pp. 909-910, ISSN 0031-6970

Johnson, J. R. (1991). Virulence Factors in *Escherichia coli* Urinary Tract Infection. *Clinical Microbiology Reviews,* Vol.4, No.1, (January 1991), pp. 80-128, ISSN 0893-8512

Juthani-Mehta, M.; Quagliarello, V.; Perrelli, E.; Towle, V.; Phil, M.; Van Ness, P.H. & Tinetti, M. (2009). Clinical Features to Identify UTI in Nursing Home Residents: A Cohort Study. *Journal of the American Geriatrics Society,* Vol. 57, No.6, (June 2009), pp. 963–970. ISSN 0002-8614

Kane, R.L.; Kane, R.A. & Arnold, S.B. (1985). Prevention and the Elderly: Risk Factors. *Health Services Research,* Vol. 19, No. 6 Pt2, (February 1985), pp. 945-1006. ISSN 0017-9124

Karpman, E. & Kurzrock, E.A. (2004).Adverse Reactions of Nitrofurantoin, Trimethoprim and Sulfamethoxazole in children. *The Journal of Urology,* Vol. 172, No. 2 (August 2004), pp. 448-453, ISSN 0022-5347

Khurana, P.S.; Sharma, P.S.V.N. & Avasthi A. (2002). Risk Factors in Delirious Geriatric General Medical Inpatients. *Indian Journal of Psychiatry*, Vol. 44, No. 3 (July 2002), pp. 266-272, ISSN 0019-5545

Kim, J.J.; Mandelli, L.; Lim, S.; Lim, H.K.; Kwon, O.J.; Pae, C.U.; Serretti, A.; Nimgaonkar, V.L,.; Paik, I.H. & Jun, T.Y. (2008). Association Analysis of Heat Shock Protein 70 Gene Polymorphisms in Schizophrenia. *European Archives of Psychiatry and Clinical Neuroscience*, Vol. 258, No. 4, (June 2008), pp. 239-244. ISSN 0940-1334

Kim, Y.K.; Na, K.S.; Shin, K.H.; Jung, H.Y.; Choi, S.H. & Kim, J.B. (2007). Cytokine Imbalance in the Pathophysiology of Major Depressive Disorder. *Progress in Neuro-psychopharmacology & Biological Psychiatry*, Vol. 31, No. 5, (June 2007), pp. 1044-1053. ISSN 0278-5846

Kisa, C.; Yildirim, S.G.; Aydemir, C.; Cebeci, S. & Goka, E.(2005). Prolonged Electroconvulsive Therapy Seizure in a Patient Taking Ciprofloxacin. *Journal of ECT*, Vol. 21, No. 1 (March 2005), pp. 43-44, ISSN 1095-0680

Laupland, K.B.; Bagshaw, S.M.; Gregson, D.B.; Kirkpatrick, A.W.; Ross, T. & Church, D.L. (2005). Intensive Care Unit-Acquired Urinary Tract Infections in a Regional Critical Care System. *Critical Care*, Vol. 9, No. 2, (April 2005), pp. R60-R65. ISSN 1364-8535

Lee, J. (2009). Serotonin Syndrome in a Chronic-Pain Patient Receiving Concurrent Methadone, Ciprofloxacin, and Venlafaxine. *Psychosomatics*, Vol. 50, No. 6 (November-December 2009), pp. 638-639, ISSN 0033-3182

Lettgen, B.; vonGontard, A.; Olbing, H.; Heiken-Löwenau, C.; Gaebel, E. & Schmitz, I. (2002). Urge Incontinence and Voiding Postponement in Children: Somatic and Psychosocial Factors. *Acta Paediatrica*, Vol. 91, No. 9, (September, 2002), pp. 978-984, ISSN 0803-5253

Lin, R.Y.; Heacock, L. C. & Fogel, J.F. (2010). Drug Induced, Dementia-Associated and Non-Dementia, Non-Drug Delirium Hospitalizations in the United States, 1998-2005: an Analysis of the National Inpatient Sample. *Drugs Aging*, Vol. 27, No. 1 (January 2010), pp. 51-61, ISSN 1170-229X

Lomberg, H.; Cedergren, B.; Leffler, H.; Nilsson, B.; Carlstrom, A.S. & Svanborg-Eden, C. (1986). Influence of Blood Group on the Availability of Receptors for Attachment of Uropathogenic Escherichia coli. *Infection and Immunity*, Vol. 51, No. 3, (March 1986), pp. 919-926. ISSN 0019-9567

Louro, E.; Romano-Lieber, N, S. & Ribiero, E. (2007). Adverse Events to Antibiotics in Inpatients of a University Hospital. *Revista de Saúde Pública*, Vol 41, No. 6 (December, 2007), pp. 1-6, ISSN 0034-8910

Loving, P.; Porter, S.; Stuifbergen, A.; Houfek, J. & Collins, P. (1992). Surveillance of Nosocomial Infection in Private Psychiatric Hospitals: an Exploratory Study. *American Journal of Infection Control*, Vol. 20, No. 3, (June 1992), pp. 149-155, ISSN 0196-6553

Manepalli, J.; Grossberg, G.T. & Mueller, C. (1990). Prevalence of Delirium and Urinary Tract Infections in a Psychogeriatric Unit. *Journal of Geriatric Psychiatry and Neurology*, Vol. 3, No. 4 (October-December 1990), pp. 198-202, ISSN 0891-9887

Markowitz, J.S.; Gill, H.S.; Devane, C.L.& Mintzer, J.E. (1997). Fluoroquinolone Inhibition of Clozapine Metabolism, T*he American Journal of Psychiatry*, Vol. 154, No. 6, (June 1997), pp. 881, ISSN 0002-953X

Meza, N.W.; Rossi, N.E.; Galeazzi, T.N.; Sánchez, N.M.; Comenares, S. J.; Medina, O.D.; Uzcategui, N.L..; Alfonzo, N.; Arango, C. & Urdaneta, H. (2005). Cysticercosis in Chronic Psychiatric Inpatients from a Venezuelan Community. *American Journal of Tropical Medicine and Hygiene*, Vol.73, No.3, (September 2005), pp. 504-509, ISSN 0002-9637

Montané, E.; Barrriocanal, A.; Isern, I.; Parajon, T. & Costa, J. (2009). Multiple Drug Interactions-Induced Serotonine Sindrome: a Case Report. *Journal of Clinical Pharmacy and Therapeutics,* Vol. 34, No. 4, (August 2009), pp. 485-487, ISSN 0269-4727

Moore, T.J.; Cohen, M, R. & Furberg, C, D. (2007). Serious Adverse Drug Events Reported to the Food and Drug Administration, 1998-2005. *Archives of Internal Medicine,* Vol. 167, No. 16, (September 2007), pp. 1752-1759, ISSN 0003-9926

Mulder, T. & de Reus, R. (2001). Psychiatric Illness does not Protect Against a Somatic Disease. *Nederlands tijdschrift voor geneeskunde,* Vol. 145, No. 28, (July 2001), pp. 1333-1336, ISSN 0028-2162

Muller, J.P.; Alix, L. & Castel, O. (1997). Nosocomial Infections in Psychiatry:Myth of Reality? *Encephale,* Vol. 23, No. 5, (September-October 1997), pp. 375-379, ISSN 0013-7006

Nicolle, L.E. (2000). Urinary Tract Infections in Long Term Care Facility Residents. *Clinical Infectious Diseases*, Vol. 31, No.3, (September 2000) pp. 757-761, ISSN 1058-4838

Nicolle, L.E. (2002). Urinary Tract Infection: Traditional Pharmacologic Therapies. *The American Journal of Medicine,* Vol.113, No.1A, (July 2002), pp. 35S-44S, ISSN 0002-9343

Nicolle, L.E. (2009). Urinary Tract Infections in the Elderly. *Clinics in Geriatric Medicine*, Vol. 25, No. 3, (August 2009), pp. 423-436, ISSN 0749-0690

Ovalle, A.; Silva, O.; Herrera, R.; González, E. & Marín, J. (1989). Pre-existing Diseases as Risk Factors and Prognosis of Genito-urinary Infection in Preganancy. *Revista Chilena de Obstetricia y Ginecología*. Vol. 54, No. 6, pp. 341-347. ISSN 0048-766X

Owens, R.C. & Ambrose, P.G. 2005. Antimicrobial Safety: Focus on Fluoroquinolones. *Clinical Infectious Diseases*, Vol. 41, Suppl 2, (July 2005), pp. S144-S157, ISSN 1058-4838

Pae, C.U.; Drago, A.; Kim, J.J.; Mandelli, L.; De Ronchi, D. & Serretti, A. (2009). The Impact of Heat Shock Protein 70 Gene Variations on Clinical Presentation and Outcome in Schizophrenic Inpatients. *Neuropsychobiology*, Vol. 59, No. 3, (May 2009), pp. 135-41. ISSN 0302-282X.

Raaska, K. & Neuvonen, P.J. (2000). Ciprofloxacine Increases Serum Clozapine and N-desmethylclozapine: a Study in Patients with Schizophrenia. *European Journal of Clinical Pharmacology*, Vol. 56, No. 8, (November 2000), pp. 585-589, ISSN 0031-6970

Reale, M.; Patruno, A.; De Lutiis, M.A.; Pesce, M.; Felaco, M.; Di Giannantonio, M.; Di Nicola, M. & Grilli, A. (2011). Dysregulation of Chemo-cytokine Production in Schizophrenic Patients Versus Healthy Controls. *BMC Neuroscience*, Vol. 12, (January 2011), pp. 13-22. ISSN 1471-2202

Rees, D.L. & Farhoumand, N. (1977). Psychiatric Aspects of Recurrent Cystitis in Women. *British Journal of Urology*, Vol. 49, No. 7, pp. 651-658. ISSN 0007-1331

Reeves, R.R. (2007). Exacerbation of Psychotic Symptoms Associated with Gatifloxacin. *Psychosomatics*, Vol. 48, No. 1, (January-February 2007), pp. 87, ISSN 0033-3182

Reilly, J.; Stewart, S.; Allardice, G.A.; Noone, A.; Robertson, C.; Walker, A, & Coubrough, S. (2008). Results from the Scottish National HAI Prevalence Survey. *The Journal of Hospital Infection*, Vol. 69, No. 1, (May 2008), pp. 62-68, ISSN 0195-6701

Rosenberg, S.D.; Goodman, L.A.; Osher, F.C.; Swartz, M. S.; Essock, S. M.; Butterfield, M. I.; Constantine, N. T.; Wolford, G. L.; & Salyers M.P. (2001). Prevalence of HIV, Hepatitis B, and Hepatitis C in People With Severe Mental Illness. *American Journal of Public Health*, Vol.91, No.1, (January 2001), pp. 31-37, ISSN 0090-0036

Sáinz, E.T.R; Reyes, M.V.; Vicente, P.J.; Serapio, A.R.; Zárate, M.P.; Navarro, A.; & Eslava C.C. (2008). Antimicrobial Resistance of *E. coli* Strains of Different Serotypes Isolated From Patients of a Psychiatric Hospital. *Revista Mexicana de Ciencias Farmacéuticas*, Vol.39, No.4, (October-December 2008), pp. 18-25, ISSN 1870-0195

Saito, T.; Nakamura, M.; Watari, M. & Isse, K. (2008). Tardive Seizure and Antibiotics: Case Reports and Review of Literature. *Journal of electroconvulsive therapy*, Vol. 24 No. 4, (December 2008), pp. 275-276, ISSN 1095-0680

Sandson, N.B.; Cozza, K.L.; Armstrong, S.C.; Eckermann, G.; Fisher, B.A. & Phillips, B. (2007). Clozapine Case Series. *Psychosomatics*, Vol. 48, No. 2, (March-April 2007) pp. 170-175, ISSN 0033-3182

Schaeffer, A.J. (2002). The Expanding Role of Fluroquinolones. *The American Journal of Medicine*, Vol. 113, Suppl. 1A, (July 2002), pp. 45S-54S, ISSN 0002-9343

Schneeberger, C.; Stolk, R.P.; Devries, J.H.; Schneeberger, P.M.; Herings, R.M. & Geerlings, S.E. (2008). Differences in the Pattern of Antibiotic Prescription Profile and Recurrence Rate for Possible Urinary Tract Infections in Women With and Without Diabetes. *Diabetes Care*, Vol. 31, No. 7 (July 2008), pp. 1380–1385. ISSN 0149-5992

Shortliffe, L.M. & McCue, J.D. (2002). Urinary Tract Infection at the Age Extremes: Pediatrics and Geriatrics. *The American Journal of Medicine*, Vol.113, No.1A, (July 2002), pp. 55S-66S, ISSN 0002-9343

Solanki, R.K.; Singh, P. & Swami, M.K. (2007). Clozapine: Current Perspective. *Indian Journal of Psychiatry*, Vol. 49, No. 4 (October-December 2007), pp. 271-278, ISSN 0019-5545

Stamm, W.E. (2002). Scientific and Clinical Challenges in the Management of Urinary Tract Infections. *The American Journal of Medicine*, Vol.113, No.1A, (July 2002), pp. 1S-4S, ISSN 0002-9343

Starr, J.A. & Ragucci, K.R. (2005). Thrombocytopenia Associated with Intravenous Ciprofloxacin. *Pharmacotherapy*, Vol. 25, No. 7 (July 2005), pp. 1030-1034, ISSN 0277-0008

Sumners, D.; Kelsey, M. & Chait, I. (1992). Psychological Aspects of Lower Urinary Tract Infections in Women. *British Medical Journal*, Vol. 304, No. 6818, (January 1992), pp. 17-19. ISSN 0959-8138.

Takahashi, H.; Higuchi, H. & Shimizu, T. (2000). Severe Lithium Toxicity Induced by Combined Levofloxacin Administration. *The Journal of Clinical Psychiatry*, Vol. 61, No. 12, (December 2000), pp. 949-950. ISSN 0160-6689

Trautner, B.W. & Darouiche, R.O. (2004). Catheter-Associated Infections: Pathogenesis Affects Prevention. *Archives of Internal Medicine*, Vol. 164, No. 8, (April 2004), pp. 842–850, ISSN 0730-188X

Trautner, B.W. (2010). Management of Catheter-Associated Urinary Tract Infection (CAUTI). *Current Opinion Infectious Diseases*, Vol. 23, No. 1, (February 2010), pp. 76–82, ISSN 0951-7375

Von Gontard, A. & Hollmann, E. (2004). Comorbility of Functional Urinary Tract Incontinence and Encopresis: Somatic and Behavioral associations. *The Journal of Urology*, Vol. 171, No. 6 Pt 2, (June 2004), pp. 2644-2647, ISSN 0022-5347

Wan, K,S.; Liu, N.H. & Hwang, I.Z. (2010). Psychogenic Urinary Retention in Children: a Case Report. *Pediatrics and neonatology*, Vol. 51, No. 5, (October 2010), pp. 300-302, ISSN 1875-9572

Wawruch, M.; Bozekova, L.; Kremery, S. & Kriska, M. (2002), Risks of Antibiotic Treatment, *Bratislavské lekárske listy*, Vol. 103, No. 7-8, pp. 270-275, ISSN 0006-9248

Wijnands, W.J.; Trooster, J.F.; Teunissen, P.C.; Cats, H.A. & Vree, T.B. (1990). Ciprofloxacin Does not Impair the Elimination of Diazepam in Humans. *Drug Metabolism and Disposition*, Vol. 18, No. 6, (November-December 1990), pp. 954-957, ISSN 0090-9556

Woo, B.K.; Daly, J.M.; Allen, E.C.; Jeste, D.V. & Sewell, D.D. (2003). Unrecognized Medical Disorders in Older Psychiatric Inpatients in a Senior Behavioral Health Unit in a University Hospital. *Journal of Geriatric Psychiatry and Neurology*, Vol. 16, No. 2, (June 2003), pp. 121-125, ISSN 0891-9887

Wood, S.K.; Baez, M.A.; Bhatnagar. S. & Valentino, R.J. (2009). Social Stress-Induced Bladder Dysfunction: Potential Role of Corticotropin-Releasing Factor. *American Journal of Physiology. Regulatory, Integrative and Comparative Physiology*, Vol. 296, No. 5, (May 2009), pp. R1671-1678, ISSN 0363-6119.

Woodford, H. & Walker, R. (2005) Emergency Hospital Admissions in Idiopathic Parkinson´s Disease. *Movement Disorders*, Vol. 20, No. 9, (September 2005), pp. 1104-1108, ISSN 0885-3185

Wysowski, D.K. & Swartz L. (2005). Adverse Drug Event Surveillance and Drug Withdrawals in United States, 1969-2002. *Archives of Internal Medicine*, Vol.165, No. 12, (June 2005), pp. 1363-1369, ISSN 0003-9926

Zaffanello, M.; Malerba, G.; Cataldi, L.; Antoniazzi, F.; Franchini, M.; Monti, E. & Fanos, V. (2010). Genetic Risk for Recurrent Urinary Tract Infections in Humans: A Systematic Review. *Journal of Biomedicine & Biotechnology*, Vol. 2010, Article ID 321082, (March 2010), 9 pages. doi:10.1155/2010/321082, ISSN 1110-7251

# Part 2

# Antibiotics and Other Strategies of Prevention/Treatment

# 11

# Antibiotic Resistance in Urinary Tract Infections: Current Issues and Future Solutions

David W. Hilbert
*Femeris Women's Health Research Center, Medical Diagnostic Laboratories, A Division of Genesis Biotechnology Group, Hamilton NJ United States of America*

## 1. Introduction

### 1.1 Incidence and costs

UTIs are a major source of morbidity and associated healthcare costs in the United States (US). Community-acquired UTIs largely affect women of reproductive age, with 11% of women experiencing infections each year, one-third of women having an infection by the age of 26, and 60% experiencing at least one infection during their lifetime (Foxman *et al.*, 2000). In 1997, the last year for which epidemiological data is available, these infections resulted in 7 million physician office visits and 1 million emergency room visits (Foxman, 2002). Treatment of these infections cost $1.6 billion in 1995 (Foxman et al., 2000), which is the equivalent of $2.2 billion in inflation-adjusted 2009 dollars. UTIs are also a major health problem for hospitalized patients, especially those undergoing long-term catheterization. Catheter-associated UTIs account for >40% of nosocomial infections, with over 1 million cases per year at a cost of $451 million (Jacobsen *et al.*, 2008).

### 1.2 Diagnosis

UTIs are defined clinically by the presence of a significant level of bacteria in the urine (i.e. bacteriuria). Guidelines vary, but typically a pure culture of between $10^4$-$10^6$ colony forming units (CFUs)/milliliter (mL) of urine is indicative of a UTI. Patient symptoms are painful, urgent and frequent urination, along with malodorous and/or cloudy urine. Signs of infection include the presence of blood (hematuria) or white blood cells (pyuria) in urine. UTIs comprise a spectrum of diseases of varying severity, with different outcomes and treatment guidelines. Asymptomatic infections are referred to as asymptomatic bacteriuria (ABU), whereas symptomatic infections are classified as either cystitis if they are confined to the bladder or pyelonephritis if the infection has spread to the kidneys. Due the absence of symptoms, ABU is often only discovered through a positive urine culture, and does not require treatment unless risk factors for complication are present (e.g. pregnancy, kidney transplantation). Most catheter-associated nosocomial UTIs can be categorized as ABU, since the presence of a urinary catheter obscures patient symptoms. Cystitis is normally treated on an out-patient basis with oral antimicrobial therapy, although recurrence is a major problem, with 27% of patients experiencing another episode within 6 months and 44%

experiencing another episode within 1 year (Foxman, 1990, Ikaheimo *et al.*, 1996). In addition to the symptoms of cystitis, pyelonephritis is characterized by fever, flank pain and vomiting. Pyelonephritis is a serious and potentially life-threatening condition that frequently results in hospitalization—nearly 200,000 such cases in were reported in the US in 1997 (Foxman *et al.*, 2003). Pyelonephritis patients are at very high risk of developing sepsis (i.e. urosepsis), and 25% of all sepsis cases originate from a UTI (Wagenlehner *et al.*, 2008).

### 1.3 Etiology

The source of UTI pathogens is generally considered to be the patient's own flora. UTIs are preceded by colonization of the vagina and periurethral area by uropathogens from the GI tract (Hilbert, 2011). Women are much more susceptible than men to community-acquired UTIs, in part, due to the female anatomy in that a much shorter urethra allows pathogens easier access to the bladder. Uropathogenic *Escherichia coli* (UPEC) is responsible for >80% of community-acquired UTIs, with most other infections caused by *Staphylococcus saprophyticus, Klebsiella pneumoniae, Proteus mirabilis* and *Enterococcus faecalis* (Ronald, 2003). UPEC is the cause of between one-third and one-half of all nosocomial UTIs, which in addition to the previously mentioned uropathogens, are also caused by *Enterobacter* spp., *Pseudomonas aeruginosa,* Group B streptococci and fungal pathogens (e.g. *Candida* spp.) (Mathai *et al.*, 2001, Gordon & Jones, 2003, Hidron *et al.*, 2008). Eighty percent of nosocomial UTIs are catheter-associated, as insertion of the catheter introduces fecal microbes and genital flora into the urinary tract (Jacobsen et al., 2008).

## 2. Treatment

### 2.1 Community-acquired UTIs

Community-acquired symptomatic UTIs are treated with empirical antimicrobial therapy upon diagnosis based on patient symptoms. Urine cultures are recommended for complicated and recurrent cases, and may be performed for uncomplicated cases, although physician guidelines vary. Since treatment will precede identification of the pathogen, local trends for antibiotic resistance must be accounted for. The recommended first-line antibiotic therapy for cystitis is either 100 milligrams (mg) of nitrofurantoin per day for 5 days or 160 mg-800 mg of trimethoprim-sulfamethoxazole (SXT) per day for 3 days. Nitrofurantoin should be avoided if pyelonephritis is suspected, as this drug only reaches an effective concentration in the bladder. SXT should be avoided if resistance in the area is >20% or if the patient has been treated with this antibiotic in the last three months. Another option for treatment is Pivmecillinam (400 mg daily for 3-7 days), but this drug is not approved for use in North America and some European countries. Fosfomycin (3 gram single dose) can also be used, but some studies suggest it is less effective than nitrofurantoin or SXT. Although amoxicillin and ampicillin should be avoided due to endemic resistance, 3-7 day courses of the β-lactam-β-lactamase inhibitor combination amoxicillin-clavulanic acid, as well as cephalosporins such as cefaclor, cefdinir and cefpodoxime proxetil, may be used. However, they exhibit less effectiveness and are associated with more adverse effects than the recommended front-line therapies (nitrofurantoin and SXT). Fluoroquinolones (e.g. ciprofloxacin, ofloxacin and levofloxacin) are highly effective in 3-day courses, resistance is minimal and they are well-tolerated, but are only recommended as second-line therapies as they are highly useful for more serious infections and their judicious use will delay the rise of resistance. Pyelonephritis is a much more serious conditions, often requiring hospitalization and paranteral administration of antibiotics—either ceftriaxone (400 mg) or a consolidated twenty-four hour dose (i.e. 7 mg drug/kg body weight) of an aminoglycoside (gentaminicin or tobramycin), in addition to oral ciprofloxacin (Gupta *et al.*, 2011).

### 2.2 Pregnant patients

Although pregnant women are not at an increased risk for UTIs in general, they are more likely to develop pyelonephritis than non-pregnant women. Approximately 4-6% of both pregnant and non-pregnant women exhibit ABU. For otherwise healthy non-pregnant women, there is no need for treatment. However, if ABU is left untreated during pregnancy, 20-40% of these women will develop pyelonephritis, often during the third trimester (Macejko & Schaeffer, 2007). As a consequence, The American College of Obstetricians and Gynecologists recommends screening for ABU in all pregnant women at sixteen weeks of gestation (Millar & Cox, 1997), and patients with positive cultures should be treated. The most important consideration in treatment is that it must be safe for both mother and fetus. Therefore, fluoroquinolones and trimethoprim should not be used, as they are assigned to the US Food and Drug Administration (FDA) pregnancy risk "C" category (gestational risk in animal studies and no adequate human studies performed). As with non-pregnant patients, nitrofurantoin can be used as a front-line therapy. As noted previously, nitrofurantoin is not recommended for treatment of pyelonephritis due to poor tissue penetration. Patients should have a follow-up urine culture one week later to determine if treatment was successful, as 20-30% of patients will require additional treatment. In addition, up to one-third of pregnant women will suffer a recurrent infection during pregnancy. Therefore, after the initial episode, either administration of prophylactic antimicrobial therapy (50-100 mg of nitrofurantoin nightly) or frequent urine cultures should be performed throughout the pregnancy (Macejko & Schaeffer, 2007). Any pregnant patient who develops pyelonephritis should be admitted and treated with paranteral antimicrobial therapy (see above). Complications of pyelonephritis during pregnancy include low fetal birth weight and neonatal death, as well as maternal anemia, hypertension, renal failure and sepsis.

### 2.3 Catheter-associated UTIs

Nosocomial UTIs are usually associated with catheterization, and asymptomatic infections are not normally treated unless additional complications are present. For symptomatic patients, the recommended procedure is replacement of the catheter combined with a 7-14 days of treatment with an agent to which the pathogen is susceptible (e.g. SXT). Specifically, it has been found that a 5-day course of levofloxacin (oral or paranteral) is an appropriate treatment for patients who are not severely ill. Unlike community-acquired UTIs, culturing of a urine sample to identify the uropathogen and determination of antimicrobial sensitivities is recommended prior to treatment, due to the diversity of nosocomial uropathogens and high rates of resistance (Hooton *et al.*, 2010).

## 3. Antimicrobial resistance

### 3.1 Uropathogenic *E. coli* (UPEC)

#### 3.1.1 β-lactam antibiotics

β-lactams antibiotics are the oldest and most broadly used class of antibiotics. They exert a bactericidal effect by inhibiting bacterial cell wall synthesis and are administered both orally and parenterally to treat a wide variety of bacterial infections. These antibiotics fall into three major structural categories—penicillins, cephalosporins and carbapenems. Penicillins, such as ampicillin and amoxicillin, were used previously as front-line therapies for UTIs. Resistance to these agents is mediated by β-lactamases which degrade them, and these enzymes play an important role in antibiotic-refractory UTIs. The TEM, SHV and OXA classes of β-lactamases hydrolyze penicillin β-lactam antibiotics (e.g. amoxicillin) and are widely distributed among UPEC (Simpson *et al.*, 1980), resulting in 38-48% of these isolates being ampicillin-resistant (Schito et al., 2009, Zhanel et al., 2006). The genes encoding these β-lactamases are usually found on plasmids that are horizontally transferred between bacteria. Penicillin β-lactam resistance can be overcome by combining the penicillin β-lactam with a β-lactamase inhibitor, such as ampicillin-sulbactam, amoxicillin-clavulanic acid or piperacillin-tazobactam. However, inhibitor-resistant TEM β-lactamases have evolved, leading to emerging UPEC resistance—the Antimicrobial Resistance Epidemiological Survey (ARESC) of nine European countries and Brazil collected 2,315 UPEC isolates and found that 3.8% were resistant to amoxicillin-clavulanic acid (Schito et al., 2009). Similarly, the SENTRY antimicrobial resistance surveillance program analyzed 1,316 nosocomial UPEC isolates in North America, Latin America and Europe and found 5% resistance to this combination (Gordon & Jones, 2003). Mutant TEM and SHV β-lactamases have emerged that hydrolyze not only penicillins but also third-generation extended-spectrum cephalosporin β-lactam antibiotics (e.g. ceftriaxone). These enzymes are referred to as extended-spectrum β-lactamases (ESBLs). UPEC resistant to cerufoxime, and therefore expressing ESBLs, are responsible for 2.4% of community-acquired infections and 4% of nosocomial infections (Schito et al., 2009, Gordon & Jones, 2003). In addition, the US National Healthcare Safety Network analyzed 2,009 UPEC isolates from catheter-associated UTIs and found that 5.5% of isolates expressed ESBLs (defined by resistance to ceftriaxone or ceftazidime) (Hidron et al., 2008). Another class of β-lactamases is CTX-M, which originated by horizontal transfer of a chromosomal β-lactamase gene from the non-pathogenic genus *Kluyvera*. The epidemic UPEC clone O25:H4-ST131 encodes CTX-M-15, rendering it cephalosporin-resistant (Nicolas-Chanoine *et al.*, 2008). The most recent evolution in β-lactam resistance is the emergence of carbapenemases, enzymes that hydrolyze carbapenem of β-lactam antibiotics, which are resistant to degradation by other ESBLs. Carbapenemases are already a problem among catheter-associated UTIs, with 4% of isolates resistant to imipenem, meropenem or ertapenem (Hidron et al., 2008). In addition, the New Delhi metallo--β-lactamase-1 (NDM-1) carbapenemase, has been identified in a O25:H4-ST131 UPEC isolate (Peirano *et al.*, 2011). Although β-lactam-β-lactamase inhibitor combinations, cephalosporins and carbapenems remain effective for UTI treatment, epidemiological trends suggest that emerging resistance will be problematic. For example, a study analyzing 11,407 UPEC isolates from community-acquired infections determined that the prevalence of ESBLs increased from 0.21% in 2003 to 3% in 2008 (Qi et al., 2010).

### 3.1.2 Trimethoprim-sulfamethoxazole (SXT)

Trimethoprim and sulfamethoxazole are both inhibitors of bacterial folate synthesis, which is required for *de novo* synthesis of thymidine, and therefore DNA synthesis. They are administered orally in combination as a 1:5 ratio (SXT). Traditionally a front-line therapy for UTIs, their utility has decreased in certain areas due to increasing resistance. In general, guidelines state that SXT should be avoided once resistance reaches 15-20%(Gupta et al.,

2011). The North American Urinary Tract Infection Collaborative Alliance (NAUTICA) study analyzed resistance among 1,142 UPEC isolates from outpatients at 40 medical centers and found that 21% were resistant to SXT (Zhanel et al., 2006). Similarly, the ARESC study found that 29% of UPEC isolates were resistant (Schito et al., 2009). Trimethoprim and sulfamethoxazole inhibit dihydrate folate reductase, and dihydropteroate synthetase, respectively, and resistance to SXT can be mediated by horizontal transfer of genes encoding resistant versions of these enzymes. A study of 305 SXT-resistant UPEC isolates found that 66% of them encoded a *dfr* allele encoding a trimethoprim-resistant dihydrate folate reductase, and 96% of them had a *sul* gene encoding a sulfamethoxazole-resistant dihydropteroate synthetase. The presence of these genes on integrons and plasmids facilitates their spread among bacterial populations (Blahna *et al.*, 2006).

### 3.1.3 Fluoroquinolones

Fluoroquinolones, such as ciprofloxacin and levofloxacin, target bacterial DNA gyrase and topoisomerases, enzymes responsible for DNA unwinding during DNA replication. They are currently recommended for use as second-line agents for uncomplicated UTIs, and front-line therapy for nosocomial UTIs and pyelonephritis (Gupta et al., 2011, Hooton et al., 2010). Resistance to these agents is largely due to mutations in the *gyrA* gene encoding the gyrase enzyme. (Weigel *et al.*, 2002). The NAUTICA, ARESC and SENTRY studies reported UPEC resistance rates of 5-6%, 8% and 11%, respectively (Gordon & Jones, 2003, Schito et al., 2009, Zhanel et al., 2006). Alarmingly, 25% of UPEC from catheter-associated UTIs are fluoroquinolone-resistant (Hidron et al., 2008). The rate of UPEC fluoroquinolone resistance appears to be increasing rapidly. Between 1998 and 2005, a four-fold increase in levofloxacin prescriptions for UTIs at one medical center was correlated with an increase in resistance from 1% to 9% (Johnson *et al.*, 2008). Similarly, a comparison of 2073 nosocomial UPEC isolates from 1990-1994 to 3112 isolates from 2000-2004 found that resistance to ciprofloxacin increased from 0.9% to 9.8% (Klevens *et al.*, 2008).

### 3.1.4 Nitrofurantoin

Nitrofurantoin is currently recommended as a front-line agent for the treatment of community-acquired cystitis (Gupta et al., 2011). The NAUTICA and ARESC studies of community-acquired UTIs found only 1.1% and 1.6% of UPEC isolates were nitrofurantoin resistant, respectively (Schito et al., 2009, Zhanel et al., 2006). Nitrofurantoin is a pro-drug, and when reduced it becomes highly reactive, damaging bacterial DNA. A laboratory study identified mutations in the nitroreductase-encoding genes *nsfA* and *nsfB* that led to resistance. However, the presence of these mutations was associated with poor bacterial growth, thus explaining why they are not commonly identified in resistant clinical isolates (Sandegren *et al.*, 2008). Nitrofurantoin is often recommended for treatment of pregnant patients, as there are concerns about the safety of fluoroquinolones and trimethoprim for this population (Macejko & Schaeffer, 2007). However, it is important to note that nitrofurantoin is not useful for the treatment of pyelonephritis, and also that many uropathogens other than *E. coli*, such as *K. pneumoniae*, *P. mirabilis* and *P. aeruginosa*, are non-susceptible.

### 3.1.5 Fosfomycin

Fosfomycin is a broad-spectrum *Streptomyces*-produced antibiotic that inhibits bacterial cell wall synthesis, and is currently recommended as a front-line therapy for community-acquired UTIs (Gupta et al., 2011). *In vitro* studies found high rates of spontaneous resistance, but these mutants grew poorly, suggesting that clinical resistance should be rare (Nilsson *et al.*, 2003). Indeed, the ARESC study found that only 0.6% of UPEC isolates were resistant (Schito et al., 2009). In addition, a recent meta-study analyzing 1657 ESBL-producing *E. coli* isolates, most of which were UPEC, found that 97% of them were susceptible to fosfomycin (Falagas *et al.*, 2010). Therefore, fosfomycin may have significant utility in combating emerging UPEC antibiotic resistance.

### 3.1.6 Multi-drug resistant UPEC clones

In addition to general trends of increasing antibiotic resistance, specific multidrug-resistant UPEC clones have emerged. A year-long outbreak of O15:K52:H1 *E. coli* occurred in London in 1986-7, causing up to 13% of UTIs in this area during this time period. Most of these isolates were resistant to SXT, ampicillin, chloramphenicol, streptomycin and tetracycline (Phillips *et al.*, 1988, O'Neill *et al.*, 1990). Analysis of 100 different O15:K2:H1 clones, isolated over a span of 30 years, revealed that SXT resistance first emerged in this lineage in 1986 and fluoroquinolone resistance in 1995 (Olesen *et al.*, 2009). A separate group of isolates (also related to O:15:K2:H1), termed clonal Group A (CGA), accounted for 50% of SXT-resistant, and 11% of total, cystitis isolates from three geographically distinct sites in the US. These isolates typically had similar O (lipopolysaccharide) antigens, encoded similar virulence factors and were frequently multidrug resistant (Manges *et al.*, 2001). CGA isolates also comprise 34% of SXT-resistant, and 7% of total, SXT-resistant pyelonephritis isolates (Johnson *et al.*, 2002). The third major antibiotic-resistant UPEC clone is O25:H4-ST131, which expresses the CTX-M-15 ESBL rendering it resistant to third-generation cephalosporins (Nicolas-Chanoine *et al.*, 2008). These three clonal groups accounted for 37% of total UPEC isolates, 44% of SXT-resistant isolates and 64% of fluoroquinolone-resistant isolates in Canada from 2002-4 (Johnson *et al.*, 2009). One-third of ciprofloxacin-resistant UPEC clones in a European study belonged to the O15:K2:H1 or O25:H4-ST131 groups (Cagnacci *et al.*, 2008). There are also reports that the O25:H4-ST131 lineage has acquired the NDM-1 carbapenemase (Peirano et al., 2011) in North America and fosfomycin resistance in Spain (Oteo *et al.*, 2009), indicating that this lineage will continue to evolve multi-drug resistance and be a major public health issue.

## 3.2 Resistance of other uropathogens

### 3.2.1 *Staphylococcus saprophyticus*

*S. saprophyticus* is a responsible for 2-6% of uncomplicated UTIs (Kahlmeter, 2003, Schito et al., 2009). The ARESC study found resistance rates of 36% for ampicillin and 10% for SXT (Schito et al., 2009). An earlier study analyzing isolates from sixteen European countries and Canada obtained different results, with only 2% of isolates resistant to ampicillin and none resistant to SXT (Kahlmeter, 2003). However, both studies found that >99% of isolates were sensitive to amoxicillin-clavulanic acid.

### 3.2.2 *Klebsiella pneumoniae*

*K. pneumoniae* is responsible for 1-6% of uncomplicated UTIs (Kahlmeter, 2003, Schito et al., 2009). In addition to being intrinsically resistant to ampicillin and nitrofurantoin, resistance to other antibiotics is very common among these isolates. One study found non-susceptibility rates to be 23% for SXT, 21% for cefuroxime (a second-generation cephalosporin), 12% for fosfomycin and 6% for ciprofloxacin (Schito et al., 2009). An earlier study found a similar resistance pattern, although overall prevalence was lower (Kahlmeter, 2003). In both studies, 94-99% of isolates were susceptible to ciprofloxacin and 91-96% were susceptible to amoxicillin-clavulanic acid. In addition, *K. pneumoniae* is the cause of 8-11% of nosocomial catheter-associated UTIs, and 17-21% of these isolates are resistant to extended-spectrum cephalosporins and 10% are resistant to carbapenems (Hidron et al., 2008, Gordon & Jones, 2003).

### 3.2.3 *Proteus mirabilis*

*P. mirabilis* is the cause of 3-5% of uncomplicated UTIs. *P. mirabilis* is intrinsically non-susceptible to nitrofurantoin, and also has high levels of non-susceptibility to other common UTI therapies—15-38% for SXT, 16-33% for ampicillin and up to 14% for fosfomycin and 10% for ciprofloxacin. The lowest levels of non-susceptibility were observed for amoxicillin-clavulanic acid (1-6%) and first (cefadroxil) or second generation (cefuroxime) cephalosporins (4-7%) (Schito et al., 2009, Kahlmeter, 2003). *P. mirabilis* is also the cause of 5% of nosocomial UTIs and 10%of catheter-associated UTIs (Gordon & Jones, 2003, Hidron et al., 2008); however, no extensive studies of antimicrobial resistance for these isolates has been performed

### 3.2.4 *Enterococcus* spp.

*Enterococcus* spp. are responsible for 13% of nosocomial UTIs. Resistance rates were found to be 5% for vancomycin, 12% for ampicillin and ampicillin-clavulanic acid, 37% for SXT and 50% for ciprofloxacin. Only 1% of isolates were resistant to nitrofurantoin (Gordon & Jones, 2003). A study of catheter-associated UTIs in the US found that 15% of them were due to *Enterococcus* spp., and these isolates exhibited a much higher rate of vancomycin resistance (29%) than nosocomial isolates in general (5%). Most of the resistance was due to *E. faecium*, which was only responsible for 24% of infections but accounted for 72% of vancomycin-resistant isolates. In addition, 89% of catheter-associated UTI *E. faecium* isolates were ampicillin-resistant. In contrast only 6% of *E. faecalis* isolates were vancomycin-resistant and only 3% were ampicillin resistant (Hidron et al., 2008).

### 3.2.5 *Pseudomonas aeruginosa*

*P. aeruginosa* accounts for 8% of nosocomial UTIs, and is intrinsically resistant to ampicillin,, ampicillin-clavulanic acid, SXT, nitrofurantoin and cefuroxime. In addition, 59% of isolates were ciprofloxacin-resistant (Gordon & Jones, 2003). Ten percent of catheter-associated UTIs are caused by *P. aeruginosa*, and resistance rates were found to be 34% for fluoroquinolones, 25% for carbapenems (imipenem and meropenem), 11-13% for cephalosporins (cefepime and ceftazidime), and 17% for piperacillin (extended-spectrum β-lactam), alone or in combination with tazobactam (a β-lactamase-inhibitor) (Hidron et al., 2008).

## 3.3 Newer UTI therapies

### 3.3.1 Recently approved therapies

Doripenem is a broad-spectrum injectable carbapenem β-lactam, approved by the FDA in 2007 for treatment of complicated UTIs, including pyelonephritis. Analysis of 1,772 clinical

*E. coli* isolates (many from complicated UTIs) found that 99.8% of them were susceptible to doripenem, including all 30 ESBL-producers (Pillar *et al.*, 2008). Analysis of 6 Phase III clinical trials demonstrated that doripenem was as effective as levofloxacin, imipenem, meropenem and piperacillin-tazobactam in treatment of patients with complicated UTIs due to ciprofloxacin-resistant and ESBL-producing *Enterobacteriaceae* (largely UPEC) (Kaniga *et al.*, 2010). Prulifloxacin is a fluoroquinolone approved for treatment of UTIs in Italy and Japan, but not yet approved in the US. A study of 257 patients with complicated UTIs showed it was as effective as ciprofloxacin (Carmignani *et al.*, 2005).

### 3.3.2 Clinical therapeutic candidates

ACHN-490 is a next-generation therapeutic belonging to the aminoglycoside family of antibiotics that inhibit bacterial protein synthesis. It has demonstrated efficacy *in vitro* against carbapenemase-expressing *E. coli* and *K. pneumoniae* (with the exception of NDM-1-expressing isolates) (Livermore *et al.*, 2011). It is currently being evaluated in a Phase II clinical trial for treatment of complicated UTIs. NXL104 is a novel inhibitor of CTX-M β-lactamases (Livermore *et al.*, 2008), and patients are being recruited for a Phase II trial to test its efficacy as a combination therapy with ceftaroline (fifth-generation cephalosporin) for the treatment of complicated UTIs. There is anecdotal evidence that tigecycline, a glyclcycline bacterial protein synthesis inhibitor, may be useful in treating complicated UTIs due to multi-drug resistant UPEC (Geerlings *et al.*, 2010). Although tigecycline is not approved for treatment of complicated UTIs, it has been suggested that it should be evaluated for this indication (Bhattacharya *et al.*, 2009)

### 3.3.3 Experimental therapies

A number of other compounds are still being developed experimentally, and although far from the clinic, they provide promise as potential future therapies. One new approach to treating UPEC infections is rather than attempting to prevent growth or kill the pathogen, is instead to inhibit its virulence properties so that an infection cannot persist (i.e. antivirulence therapies). This approach has focused on type 1 fimbriae that are required by UPEC to adhere to the bladder epithelium during infection (Hilbert, 2011). The FimH adhesin of type 1 fimbriae normally binds mannose, and related compounds, such as butyl α-D-mannoside, bind with much higher affinity, and therefore may be useful as decoys to saturate FimH and impair UPEC adherence to the bladder epithelium (Bouckaert *et al.*, 2005). Type 1 fimbriae are assembled through the chaperone-usher pathway, and ring-fused 2-pyridone peptidomimics (i.e. pilicides) impair this pathway, thereby preventing fimbrial expression, bacterial adherence and virulence in a mouse model of infection (Pinkner *et al.*, 2006, Klein *et al.*, 2010). Future studies are necessary to determine if antivirulence therapies will be useful in the clinic.

## 4. Prevention

### 4.1 Cranberry juice

In addition to improving therapy, another major area of research is the prevention of UTIs. As is the case for treatment, both traditional and novel strategies are being evaluated. Consumption of cranberry juice is a traditional folk method of UTI prevention and treatment. Roughly a dozen studies have been performed examining the ability of cranberry products to prevent UTIs (Raz *et al.*, 2004), but only two were randomized placebo-controlled studies with significant patient populations (150 women with a history of UTI). One study found that daily consumption of cranberry juice concentrate reduced the risk of UTI to 16% over a six month period, compared to 36% in the placebo group. A one-year study found that <20% of women who consumed cranberry juice or tablets experienced UTIs, compared to 32% in the placebo group (Kontiokari *et al.*, 2001, Stothers, 2002). As for the mechanism of action, studies have found that cranberry juice extracts inhibited the ability UPEC to adhere to vaginal and bladder epithelial cells (Hilbert, 2011). Identification of the inhibitory cranberry constituent could facilitate the development of a novel antivirulence therapy for UTIs.

### 4.2 Vaginal probiotics

As vaginal and periurethral colonization with UPEC is strongly associated with UTIs (Hilbert, 2011), another prevention strategy is to use vaginal probiotics to prevent colonization. Small pilot studies have found that vaginal colonization with *Lactobacillus* spp. helps to prevent recurrent UTIs (Bruce & Reid, 1988, Uehara *et al.*, 2006, Reid *et al.*, 1992). A Phase I trial on the use of vaginal *Lactobacillus* suppositories to prevent recurrent UTIs has been completed with minimal patient side effects (Czaja *et al.*, 2007), paving the way for future trials and the possible use of probiotics clinically to prevent UTIs.

### 4.3 Antimicrobial catheters

Different strategies are used to prevent catheter-associated nosocomial UTIs. One approach is the development of catheters coated with silver alloy or nitrofurazone (similar to nitrofurantoin) to prevent attachment by uropathogens. A meta-analysis of eight clinical trials since 1995 found that the use of these catheters reduced the risk of bacteriuria by up to 12% when compared to uncoated catheters (Johnson *et al.*, 2006). Another strategy for long-term catheterization (e.g. patients with neurogenic bladder) is bacterial interference, where the bladder is deliberately colonized with an ABU *E. coli* isolate (ABU 83972) to prevent symptomatic infection. A randomized, double-blind placebo-control study found that over a period of one year, patients successfully colonized with ABU 83972 had an average 1.6 UTIs, whereas the placebo group experienced an average of 3.5 infections (Darouiche *et al.*, 2005).

### 4.4 Immuno-stimulation

Polyvalent mixtures of killed uropathogens have been tested for their ability to prevent UTIs. UroVaxom (OM-89) is a lyophilized extract of 18 UPEC strains that is taken orally in Europe to prevent recurrent UTIs. It provides immunity to mice in experimental studies (Sedelmeier & Bessler, 1995). A meta-analysis of five placebo-controlled double-blind studies found that oral consumption of UroVaxom reduced the risk of UTI by 36% over 6 months (Naber *et al.*, 2009). These findings were replicated in a large multicenter study (453 patients) that found a 34% reduction in UTIs over 1 year (Bauer *et al.*, 2005). A related product is SolcoUrovac, a vaginal suppository containing lyophilized extract from six UPEC strains and one strain each of *P. mirabilis*, *Morganella morganii*, *K. pneumoniae* and *E. faecalis*. A Phase II randomized, double-blind placebo-control trial of 75 women with recurrent UTIs over 160 days observed a recurrence rate of 70% for the placebo arm and 27.5% for the vaccination plus booster arm of the study (Hopkins *et al.*, 2007). Although these products appear useful to prevent recurrent UTIs, they are not vaccines *per se* as they require frequent administration. The clinical trial for UroVaxom had patients take one pill daily for 3 months, no treatment for the next 3 months, then one pill daily for the first 10 days of each of the next 3 months followed by another 3 month cessation (Bauer et al., 2005). Similarly, the SolcoUrovac trial gave patients one suppository each week for the first three weeks, followed by an additional suppository each month for 3 months (Hopkins et al., 2007). Therefore, these treatments fall under the category of immuno-stimulation, rather than vaccination.

### 4.5 Vaccine development

Development of a UTI vaccine has also been a major research area. Vaccination of cynomolgus monkeys with type 1 fimbrial components protected them from UTIs (Langermann *et al.*, 2000), as did vaginal immunization with formalin-killed UPEC (Uehling *et al.*, 1987). Vaccination of baboons and cynomolgus monkeys with another UPEC adhesin, purified P fimbriae, or components thereof, protected them from pyelonephritis (Roberts *et al.*, 1989, Roberts *et al.*, 2004). Immuno-correlates for successful vaccination appear to be antigen-specific serum IgG, as well as vaginal and urinary antibodies (Hilbert, 2011). Although these experimental studies of UPEC vaccination are promising, none of these candidates has progressed to clinical testing in humans.

## 5. Conclusion

In summary, rising antibiotic resistance among uropathogens, and especially the emergence of multi-drug resistant clonal groups, has provided urgency to the development of novel preventative and therapeutic strategies. Some older drugs, such as fosfomycin, may prove to be very useful in treating antimicrobial-refractory UTIs, especially those due to ESBL-producers. Newer drugs, such as the recently approved doripenem, have proven highly effective in the clinic to treat complicated UTIs. Research into novel anti-virulence therapies, such as inhibiting the production of, or adherence by, UPEC fimbriae is still an early stage but holds promise for future development. The use of probiotics to prevent vaginal UPEC colonization and the use of an immuno-stimulatory uropathogen extract (SolcoUrovac), are currently in clinical trials to determine efficacy in preventing recurrent UTIs. Another preventative strategy is vaccination, and experimental vaccines have been developed that are effective in preventing UTIs in primates. In summary, a combination of traditional and innovative prevention and treatment strategies is being deployed to combat the threat of emerging antibiotic resistance among uropathogens.

## 6. References

Bauer, H. W., S. Alloussi, G. Egger, H. M. Blumlein, G. Cozma & C. C. Schulman, (2005) A long-term, multicenter, double-blind study of an *Escherichia coli* extract (OM-89) in female patients with recurrent urinary tract infections. *Eur Urol* 47: 542-548; discussion 548.

Bhattacharya, M., A. Parakh & M. Narang, (2009) Tigecycline. *J Postgrad Med* 55: 65-68.

Blahna, M. T., C. A. Zalewski, J. Reuer, G. Kahlmeter, B. Foxman & C. F. Marrs, (2006) The role of horizontal gene transfer in the spread of trimethoprim-sulfamethoxazole resistance among uropathogenic *Escherichia coli* in Europe and Canada. *J Antimicrob Chemother* 57: 666-672.

Bouckaert, J., J. Berglund, M. Schembri, E. De Genst, L. Cools, M. Wuhrer, C. S. Hung, J. Pinkner, R. Slattegard, A. Zavialov, D. Choudhury, S. Langermann, S. J. Hultgren, L. Wyns, P. Klemm, S. Oscarson, S. D. Knight & H. De Greve, (2005) Receptor binding studies disclose a novel class of high-affinity inhibitors of the *Escherichia coli* FimH adhesin. *Mol Microbiol* 55: 441-455.

Bruce, A. W. & G. Reid, (1988) Intravaginal instillation of lactobacilli for prevention of recurrent urinary tract infections. *Can J Microbiol* 34: 339-343.

Cagnacci, S., L. Gualco, E. Debbia, G. C. Schito & A. Marchese, (2008) European emergence of ciprofloxacin-resistant *Escherichia coli* clonal groups O25:H4-ST 131 and O15:K52:H1 causing community-acquired uncomplicated cystitis. *J Clin Microbiol* 46: 2605-2612.

Carmignani, G., A. F. De Rose, L. Olivieri, E. Salvatori, M. T. Rosignoli & P. Dionisio, (2005) Prulifloxacin versus ciprofloxacin in the treatment of adults with complicated urinary tract infections. *Urol Int* 74: 326-331.

Czaja, C. A., A. E. Stapleton, Y. Yarova-Yarovaya & W. E. Stamm, (2007) Phase I trial of a Lactobacillus crispatus vaginal suppository for prevention of recurrent urinary tract infection in women. *Infect Dis Obstet Gynecol* 2007: 35387.

Darouiche, R. O., J. I. Thornby, C. Cerra-Stewart, W. H. Donovan & R. A. Hull, (2005) Bacterial interference for prevention of urinary tract infection: a prospective, randomized, placebo-controlled, double-blind pilot trial. *Clin Infect Dis* 41: 1531-1534.

Falagas, M. E., A. C. Kastoris, A. M. Kapaskelis & D. E. Karageorgopoulos, (2010) Fosfomycin for the treatment of multidrug-resistant, including extended-spectrum beta-lactamase producing, *Enterobacteriaceae* infections: a systematic review. *Lancet Infect Dis* 10: 43-50.

Foxman, B., (1990) Recurring urinary tract infection: incidence and risk factors. *Am J Public Health* 80: 331-333.

Foxman, B., (2002) Epidemiology of urinary tract infections: incidence, morbidity, and economic costs. *Am J Med* 113 Suppl 1A: 5S-13S.

Foxman, B., R. Barlow, H. D'Arcy, B. Gillespie & J. D. Sobel, (2000) Urinary tract infection: self-reported incidence and associated costs. *Ann Epidemiol* 10: 509-515.

Foxman, B., K. L. Klemstine & P. D. Brown, (2003) Acute pyelonephritis in US hospitals in 1997: hospitalization and in-hospital mortality. *Ann Epidemiol* 13: 144-150.

Geerlings, S. E., K. A. van Donselaar-van der Pant & I. Keur, (2010) Successful treatment with tigecycline of two patients with complicated urinary tract infections caused by extended-spectrum beta-lactamase-producing *Escherichia coli. J Antimicrob Chemother* 65: 2048-2049.

Gordon, K. A. & R. N. Jones, (2003) Susceptibility patterns of orally administered antimicrobials among urinary tract infection pathogens from hospitalized patients in North America: comparison report to Europe and Latin America. Results from the SENTRY Antimicrobial Surveillance Program (2000). *Diagn Microbiol Infect Dis* 45: 295-301.

Gupta, K., T. M. Hooton, K. G. Naber, B. Wullt, R. Colgan, L. G. Miller, G. J. Moran, L. E. Nicolle, R. Raz, A. J. Schaeffer & D. E. Soper, (2011) International clinical practice guidelines for the treatment of acute uncomplicated cystitis and pyelonephritis in women: A 2010 update by the Infectious Diseases Society of America and the European Society for Microbiology and Infectious Diseases. *Clin Infect Dis* 52: e103-120.

Hidron, A. I., J. R. Edwards, J. Patel, T. C. Horan, D. M. Sievert, D. A. Pollock & S. K. Fridkin, (2008) NHSN annual update: antimicrobial-resistant pathogens associated with healthcare-associated infections: annual summary of data reported to the National Healthcare Safety Network at the Centers for Disease Control and Prevention, 2006-2007. *Infect Control Hosp Epidemiol* 29: 996-1011.

Hilbert, D. W., (2011) Uropathogenic *Escherichia coli*: The Pre-Eminent Urinary Tract Infection Pathogen. *In MM Rogers and ND Peterson (Ed.) E. coli Infections: Causes, Treatment and Prevention. Nova Science Publishers, Hauppauge, NY (pp. 1-67)*

Hooton, T. M., S. F. Bradley, D. D. Cardenas, R. Colgan, S. E. Geerlings, J. C. Rice, S. Saint, A. J. Schaeffer, P. A. Tambayh, P. Tenke & L. E. Nicolle, (2010) Diagnosis, prevention, and treatment of catheter-associated urinary tract infection in adults: 2009 International Clinical Practice Guidelines from the Infectious Diseases Society of America. *Clin Infect Dis* 50: 625-663.

Hopkins, W. J., J. Elkahwaji, L. M. Beierle, G. E. Leverson & D. T. Uehling, (2007) Vaginal mucosal vaccine for recurrent urinary tract infections in women: results of a phase 2 clinical trial. *J Urol* 177: 1349-1353; quiz 1591.

Ikaheimo, R., A. Siitonen, T. Heiskanen, U. Karkkainen, P. Kuosmanen, P. Lipponen & P. H. Makela, (1996) Recurrence of urinary tract infection in a primary care setting: analysis of a 1-year follow-up of 179 women. *Clin Infect Dis* 22: 91-99.

Jacobsen, S. M., D. J. Stickler, H. L. Mobley & M. E. Shirtliff, (2008) Complicated catheter-associated urinary tract infections due to *Escherichia coli* and Proteus mirabilis. *Clin Microbiol Rev* 21: 26-59.

Johnson, J. R., M. A. Kuskowski & T. J. Wilt, (2006) Systematic review: antimicrobial urinary catheters to prevent catheter-associated urinary tract infection in hospitalized patients. *Ann Intern Med* 144: 116-126.

Johnson, J. R., A. R. Manges, T. T. O'Bryan & L. W. Riley, (2002) A disseminated multidrug-resistant clonal group of uropathogenic *Escherichia coli* in pyelonephritis. *Lancet* 359: 2249-2251.

Johnson, J. R., M. Menard, B. Johnston, M. A. Kuskowski, K. Nichol & G. G. Zhanel, (2009) Epidemic clonal groups of *Escherichia coli* as a cause of antimicrobial-resistant urinary tract infections in Canada, 2002 to 2004. *Antimicrob Agents Chemother* 53: 2733-2739.

Johnson, L., A. Sabel, W. J. Burman, R. M. Everhart, M. Rome, T. D. MacKenzie, J. Rozwadowski, P. S. Mehler & C. S. Price, (2008) Emergence of fluoroquinolone resistance in outpatient urinary *Escherichia coli* isolates. *Am J Med* 121: 876-884.

Kahlmeter, G., (2003) An international survey of the antimicrobial susceptibility of pathogens from uncomplicated urinary tract infections: the ECO.SENS Project. *J Antimicrob Chemother* 51: 69-76.

Kaniga, K., R. Flamm, S. Y. Tong, M. Lee, I. Friedland & R. Redman, (2010) Worldwide experience with the use of doripenem against extended-spectrum-beta-lactamase-producing and ciprofloxacin-resistant *Enterobacteriaceae*: analysis of six phase 3 clinical studies. *Antimicrob Agents Chemother* 54: 2119-2124.

Klein, T., D. Abgottspon, M. Wittwer, S. Rabbani, J. Herold, X. Jiang, S. Kleeb, C. Luthi, M. Scharenberg, J. Bezencon, E. Gubler, L. Pang, M. Smiesko, B. Cutting, O. Schwardt & B. Ernst, (2010) FimH antagonists for the oral treatment of urinary tract infections: from design and synthesis to in vitro and in vivo evaluation. *J Med Chem* 53: 8627-8641.

Klevens, R. M., J. R. Edwards & R. P. Gaynes, (2008) The impact of antimicrobial-resistant, health care-associated infections on mortality in the United States. *Clin Infect Dis* 47: 927-930.

Kontiokari, T., K. Sundqvist, M. Nuutinen, T. Pokka, M. Koskela & M. Uhari, (2001) Randomised trial of cranberry-lingonberry juice and Lactobacillus GG drink for the prevention of urinary tract infections in women. *BMJ* 322: 1571.

Langermann, S., R. Mollby, J. E. Burlein, S. R. Palaszynski, C. G. Auguste, A. DeFusco, R. Strouse, M. A. Schenerman, S. J. Hultgren, J. S. Pinkner, J. Winberg, L. Guldevall,

M. Soderhall, K. Ishikawa, S. Normark & S. Koenig, (2000) Vaccination with FimH adhesin protects cynomolgus monkeys from colonization and infection by uropathogenic *Escherichia coli*. *J Infect Dis* 181: 774-778.

Livermore, D. M., S. Mushtaq, M. Warner, C. Miossec & N. Woodford, (2008) NXL104 combinations versus *Enterobacteriaceae* with CTX-M extended-spectrum beta-lactamases and carbapenemases. *J Antimicrob Chemother* 62: 1053-1056.

Livermore, D. M., S. Mushtaq, M. Warner, J. C. Zhang, S. Maharjan, M. Doumith & N. Woodford, (2011) Activity of aminoglycosides, including ACHN-490, against carbapenem-resistant *Enterobacteriaceae* isolates. *J Antimicrob Chemother* 66: 48-53.

Macejko, A. M. & A. J. Schaeffer, (2007) Asymptomatic bacteriuria and symptomatic urinary tract infections during pregnancy. *Urol Clin North Am* 34: 35-42.

Manges, A. R., J. R. Johnson, B. Foxman, T. T. O'Bryan, K. E. Fullerton & L. W. Riley, (2001) Widespread distribution of urinary tract infections caused by a multidrug-resistant *Escherichia coli* clonal group. *N Engl J Med* 345: 1007-1013.

Mathai, D., R. N. Jones & M. A. Pfaller, (2001) Epidemiology and frequency of resistance among pathogens causing urinary tract infections in 1,510 hospitalized patients: a report from the SENTRY Antimicrobial Surveillance Program (North America). *Diagn Microbiol Infect Dis* 40: 129-136.

Millar, L. K. & S. M. Cox, (1997) Urinary tract infections complicating pregnancy. *Infect Dis Clin North Am* 11: 13-26.

Naber, K. G., Y. H. Cho, T. Matsumoto & A. J. Schaeffer, (2009) Immunoactive prophylaxis of recurrent urinary tract infections: a meta-analysis. *Int J Antimicrob Agents* 33: 111-119.

Nicolas-Chanoine, M. H., J. Blanco, V. Leflon-Guibout, R. Demarty, M. P. Alonso, M. M. Canica, Y. J. Park, J. P. Lavigne, J. Pitout & J. R. Johnson, (2008) Intercontinental emergence of *Escherichia coli* clone O25:H4-ST131 producing CTX-M-15. *J Antimicrob Chemother* 61: 273-281.

Nilsson, A. I., O. G. Berg, O. Aspevall, G. Kahlmeter & D. I. Andersson, (2003) Biological costs and mechanisms of fosfomycin resistance in *Escherichia coli*. *Antimicrob Agents Chemother* 47: 2850-2858.

O'Neill, P. M., C. A. Talboys, A. P. Roberts & B. S. Azadian, (1990) The rise and fall of *Escherichia coli* O15 in a London teaching hospital. *J Med Microbiol* 33: 23-27.

Olesen, B., F. Scheutz, M. Menard, M. N. Skov, H. J. Kolmos, M. A. Kuskowski & J. R. Johnson, (2009) Three-decade epidemiological analysis of *Escherichia coli* O15:K52:H1. *J Clin Microbiol* 47: 1857-1862.

Oteo, J., B. Orden, V. Bautista, O. Cuevas, M. Arroyo, R. Martinez-Ruiz, M. Perez-Vazquez, M. Alcaraz, S. Garcia-Cobos & J. Campos, (2009) CTX-M-15-producing urinary *Escherichia coli* O25b-ST131-phylogroup B2 has acquired resistance to fosfomycin. *J Antimicrob Chemother* 64: 712-717.

Peirano, G., P. C. Schreckenberger & J. D. Pitout, (2011) The characteristics of NDM-1-producing *Escherichia coli* that belong to the successful and virulent clone ST131. *Antimicrob Agents Chemother.*

Phillips, I., S. Eykyn, A. King, W. R. Gransden, B. Rowe, J. A. Frost & R. J. Gross, (1988) Epidemic multiresistant *Escherichia coli* infection in West Lambeth Health District. *Lancet* 1: 1038-1041.

Pillar, C. M., M. K. Torres, N. P. Brown, D. Shah & D. F. Sahm, (2008) In vitro activity of doripenem, a carbapenem for the treatment of challenging infections caused by gram-negative bacteria, against recent clinical isolates from the United States. *Antimicrob Agents Chemother* 52: 4388-4399.

Pinkner, J. S., H. Remaut, F. Buelens, E. Miller, V. Aberg, N. Pemberton, M. Hedenstrom, A. Larsson, P. Seed, G. Waksman, S. J. Hultgren & F. Almqvist, (2006) Rationally designed small compounds inhibit pilus biogenesis in uropathogenic bacteria. *Proc Natl Acad Sci U S A* 103: 17897-17902.

Qi, C., V. Pilla, J. H. Yu & K. Reed, (2010) Changing prevalence of *Escherichia coli* with CTX-M-type extended-spectrum beta-lactamases in outpatient urinary E. coli between 2003 and 2008. *Diagn Microbiol Infect Dis* 67: 87-91.

Raz, R., B. Chazan & M. Dan, (2004) Cranberry juice and urinary tract infection. *Clin Infect Dis* 38: 1413-1419.

Reid, G., A. W. Bruce & M. Taylor, (1992) Influence of three-day antimicrobial therapy and lactobacillus vaginal suppositories on recurrence of urinary tract infections. Clin Ther 14: 11-16.

Roberts, J. A., M. B. Kaack, G. Baskin, M. R. Chapman, D. A. Hunstad, J. S. Pinkner & S. J. Hultgren, (2004) Antibody responses and protection from pyelonephritis following vaccination with purified *Escherichia coli* PapDG protein. *J Urol* 171: 1682-1685.

Roberts, J. A., M. B. Kaack, G. Baskin, T. K. Korhonen, S. B. Svenson & J. Winberg, (1989) P-fimbriae vaccines. II. Cross reactive protection against pyelonephritis. *Pediatr Nephrol* 3: 391-396.

Ronald, A., (2003) The etiology of urinary tract infection: traditional and emerging pathogens. *Dis Mon* 49: 71-82.

Sandegren, L., A. Lindqvist, G. Kahlmeter & D. I. Andersson, (2008) Nitrofurantoin resistance mechanism and fitness cost in *Escherichia coli*. *J Antimicrob Chemother* 62: 495-503.

Schito, G. C., K. G. Naber, H. Botto, J. Palou, T. Mazzei, L. Gualco & A. Marchese, (2009) The ARESC study: an international survey on the antimicrobial resistance of pathogens involved in uncomplicated urinary tract infections. *Int J Antimicrob Agents* 34: 407-413.

Sedelmeier, E. A. & W. G. Bessler, (1995) Biological activity of bacterial cell-wall components: immunogenicity of the bacterial extract OM-89. *Immunopharmacology* 29: 29-36.

Simpson, I. N., P. B. Harper & C. H. O'Callaghan, (1980) Principal beta-lactamases responsible for resistance to beta-lactam antibiotics in urinary tract infections. *Antimicrob Agents Chemother* 17: 929-936.

Stothers, L., (2002) A randomized trial to evaluate effectiveness and cost effectiveness of naturopathic cranberry products as prophylaxis against urinary tract infection in women. *Can J Urol* 9: 1558-1562.

Uehara, S., K. Monden, K. Nomoto, Y. Seno, R. Kariyama & H. Kumon, (2006) A pilot study evaluating the safety and effectiveness of Lactobacillus vaginal suppositories in patients with recurrent urinary tract infection. *Int J Antimicrob Agents* 28 Suppl 1: S30-34.

Uehling, D. T., W. J. Hopkins, J. Jensen & E. Balish, (1987) Vaginal immunization against induced cystitis in monkeys. *J Urol* 137: 327-329.

Wagenlehner, F. M., A. Pilatz, K. G. Naber & W. Weidner, (2008) Therapeutic challenges of urosepsis. *Eur J Clin Invest* 38 Suppl 2: 45-49.

Weigel, L. M., G. J. Anderson & F. C. Tenover, (2002) DNA gyrase and topoisomerase IV mutations associated with fluoroquinolone resistance in Proteus mirabilis. *Antimicrob Agents Chemother* 46: 2582-2587.

Zhanel, G. G., T. L. Hisanaga, N. M. Laing, M. R. DeCorby, K. A. Nichol, B. Weshnoweski, J. Johnson, A. Noreddin, D. E. Low, J. A. Karlowsky & D. J. Hoban, (2006) Antibiotic resistance in *Escherichia coli* outpatient urinary isolates: final results from the North American Urinary Tract Infection Collaborative Alliance (NAUTICA). *Int J Antimicrob Agents* 27: 468-475.

12

# Identification and Antibiotic Sensitivity of UTI Pathogens Using Raman Spectroscopy

Evdokia Kastanos[1], Alexandros Kyriakides[2],
Katerina Hadjigeorgiou[2] and Costas Pitris[2]
[1]*University of Nicosia,*
[2]*University of Cyprus*
*Cyprus*

## 1. Introduction

Conventional methods of Urinary Tract Infection (UTI) diagnosis require determining the concentration and identity of the involved bacteria, as well as their susceptibility to various antibiotics, the so-called antibiogram. Such assays require repeated culturing of a sample and need at least 48 hours in order for bacterial colonies to be grown, counted, and exposed to antibiotics. However, the patient cannot remain untreated during this rather prolonged period before definitive diagnosis of the suspected infection becomes available. As a result, physicians prescribe broad spectrum antibiotics prior to antibiogram availability. This practice has many undesirable consequences, both short term and long term: (i) unsuccessful treatments leading to chronic infections, (ii) increased health care costs, and, most importantly, (iii) increased antibiotic resistance by a growing number of bacterial strains (Gruneberg, 1994; Casadevall, 1996; Cosgrove, S. & Carmeli, 2003; Alanis, 2005). Given these concerns, it is obvious that rapid and accurate identification of UTI pathogens as well as determination of their susceptibility to antibiotics would offer significant clinical benefits. Such methodologies are currently being developed and include the promising application of Raman spectroscopy for the diagnosis of UTIs.

Recently, rapid diagnosis methods based on polymerase chain reaction (PCR) have been developed in order to bypass the need for culturing (Mothershed & Whitney, 2006) as well as to identify genes that confer antibiotic resistance (Rolain et al., 2004). Although such PCR assays are fast and very sensitive, they typically require species and strain specific probes that may or may not be available for a particular organism. In addition, amplification methods, like PCR, suffer from contamination problems, complex interpretation of results, as well as high costs. Mass Spectrometry is another method that has been proposed as an alternative approach for bacterial diagnostics without culturing (Chen et al., 2008). However, like the PCR approach, Mass Spectrometry also depends on prior knowledge of the pathogen under study and suffers from increased complexity and cost.

Vibrational spectroscopies, like Raman spectroscopy, have been used, for the last few years, to detect bacteria with minimal sample manipulation (Maquelin et al., 2000; Schuster, 2000a, 2000b). Classification of bacterial species, as well as of subspecies, has been achieved with great accuracy and speed, especially with Surface Enhanced Raman Spectroscopy (SERS) (Kneipp et al., 2006) which allows enhancement of the inherently weak Raman signal. More recently, it was shown that bacterial susceptibility to antibiotics can also be determined using Raman spectroscopy and SERS (Liu et al., 2009; Kastanos et al., 2010; Kastanos et al., 2011).

### 1.1 Raman spectroscopy

Whole organism fingerprinting is a relatively recent approach for the identification of pathogens based on their unique chemical characteristics with minimal sample preparation (Magee, 1993). Some of the techniques that are being evaluated for such fingerprinting include vibrational spectroscopic methods such as Fourier-Transform Infrared spectroscopy (FTIR), Raman Spectroscopy, and UV resonance Raman spectroscopy (UVRR). Vibrational spectroscopic features arise from the loss or gain of energy by photons which are inelastically scattered from a vibrating sample. This energy change results in an alteration of the photons' wavelength which, in the case of organic molecules, is directly related to the vibrational states of its chemical bonds. Therefore, quantitative biochemical information can be extracted from the spectra.

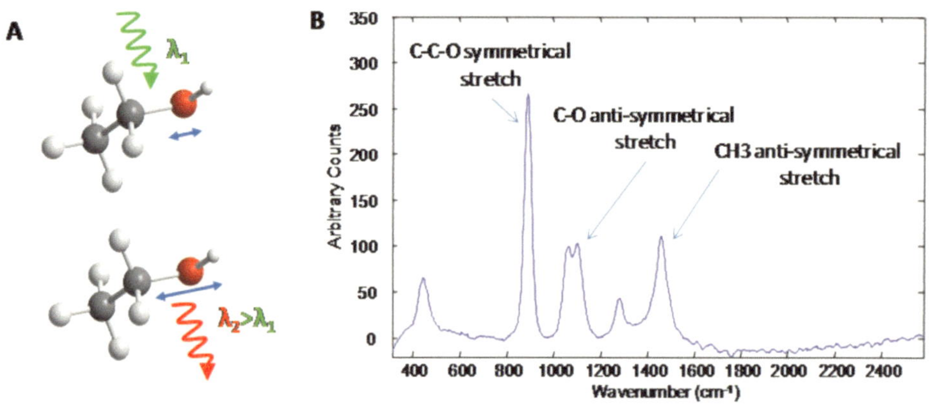


Fig. 1. A. Schematic showing the inelastic scattering of photons from an ethanol molecule. Energy from the incident light (green wave) is transferred to the molecule (top) causing a larger vibration (blue arrows) resulting in scattered light (bottom) with less energy and a longer wavelength (red wave). B. Raman spectrum of ethanol, indicating some of the major peaks and their relationship to the molecular bonds of that molecule.

The Raman effect is observed when a very small number of photons incident on a molecule (about 1 in $10^7$) are inelastically scattered, i.e. scattered at different frequencies than the frequency of the incident photons (Mahadevan-Jansen, 2002). A Raman spectrum is a plot of the intensity of scattered light versus the energy difference between the incident photons and the Raman scattered photons, and contains information about the chemical composition and the molecular structure of a substance (Fig. 1). A major limitation of Raman spectroscopy is the weakness of the Raman effect which results in very low signals, often below the limit of detection for dilute biological samples. In addition, Raman spectroscopy is not very selective with respect to the various molecules present in complex biological samples, resulting in highly congested spectra. Finally, Raman spectroscopy suffers from a strong fluorescence background which significantly decreases the dynamic range of the measurement. Even though FTIR is much more sensitive than Raman, its use in biological systems is very limited due to the strong absorbance of water at those wavelengths. However, several publications have come out in the last few years that show discrimination of bacteria using FTIR and also quite complex classification analysis methods (Preisner et al., 2008; Forrester et al., 2009). UVRR is also more sensitive than normal Raman and suffers from almost no fluorescence background. It has already been exploited for the discrimination of UTI bacteria (Jarvis & Goodacre, 2004b). The highly energetic nature of UV photons, however, can cause photochemical or burning effects on a sample and limits its use as a routine method for bacterial analysis. Additionally, excitation in the UV is not very useful for the discrimination of different species of bacteria as it mostly identifies nucleic acid bases which are not expected to vary significantly between different bacterial species. The widespread adoption of UVRR is also limited by the high cost and complexity of the equipment required.

Raman spectroscopy has also been successfully applied to bacterial identification in the configuration of a Raman microscope which allows collection of spectra from single cells and enhances sensitivity. The group of Hutsebaut et al. have used Raman microscopy to identify samples belonging to 3 different *Bacillus* species (Hutsebaut et al., 2004). Xie et al., successfully classified 6 different bacterial species (Xie et al., 2005). Studies by Harz et al. (Harz et al., 2005) have shown that discrimination of different Staphylococcus species can be achieved with 95-97% accuracy not only at species but also at strain level. The same group have successfully discriminated 29 strains of bacteria derived from a variety of species (Schmid et al., 2009). Despite increased sensitivity, studies using Micro-Raman spectroscopy have to face a few unique challenges. First, the fact that imaging individual bacteria is a time consuming process that leads to inadequate evaluation of large samples. Second, the increased variability between spectra of individual cells, mostly due to variations in the growth stage of each cell, usually necessitates the use of classification methods of increased complexity.

### 1.2 Surface enhanced Raman spectroscopy

Surface Enhanced Raman Spectroscopy (SERS) is a variation of Raman spectroscopy which offers significant enhancement of the signal (up to theoretical $10^{14}$ times) thus making detection faster, simpler, and more accurate. The enhancement is a direct effect of plasmon resonance, i.e. the unison oscillation of electrons on the surface of a metallic nanostructure as a result of incident light of the right, resonant, frequency. These oscillations produce an enhanced electromagnetic field in the proximity of the surface (Fig. 2.). If a sample is within a few nanometers (nm) from the nanostructure, it will experience this enhanced field and exhibit a stronger Raman signal (Kneipp et al., 1997; Nie & Emory, 1997; Moskovits, 1985; Vo-Dinh et al., 2005).

SERS spectra also exhibit reduced data congestion compared to normal Raman spectra since the enhancement is significant only for molecules found on, or very close to, the SERS substrate. This method also significantly improves the dynamic range of the measurement due to the ability of SERS-active substrates to quench fluorescence. Finally SERS can be performed using simple, mobile and relatively inexpensive equipment providing a significantly improved signal at high speed and low cost.

One of the first groups to work on the identification of bacteria by SERS is the team of Efrima et al. (Efrima & Bronk, 1998; Zeiri et al., 2002; Zeiriet al., 2004; Efrima & Zeiri, 2009). The SERS-active substrates they employed were mostly silver but also gold colloids. What is unique about their methodology is that they usually produced the colloid in the presence of

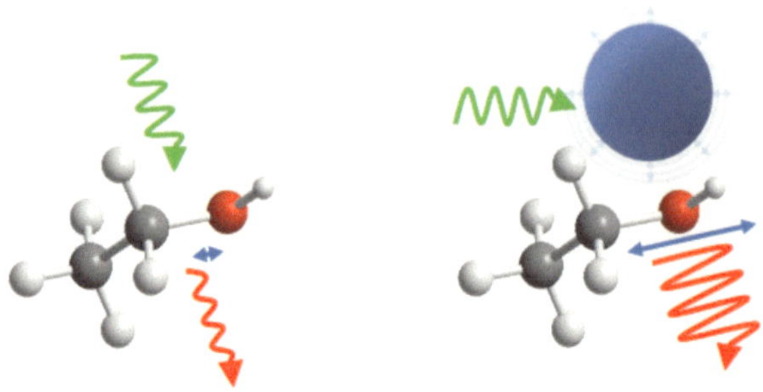

Fig. 2. Surface Enhanced Raman Spectroscopy (SERS). The proximity to a metallic surface or nanostructure exhibiting plasmon resonance (right) results in a much stronger Raman signal than the molecule alone (left.)

the bacteria and not mixing pre-formed colloid with the sample. In addition, they demonstrated growth of colloids in the interior or the exterior of bacterial cells obtaining different spectra in each case. As far as the collection of SERS spectra is concerned, they have done it under a large variety of conditions, including various preparations of their substrates, using different fractions of bacterial cells, and different excitations, ranging from the UV to the NIR (250-800 nm). Jarvis et al. is another group with significant contributions to the area of SERS and identification of bacteria. Specifically, they investigated UTI involved bacteria, using silver colloids in combination with different types of Raman microscopes (Jarvis & Goodacre, 2004a; Jarvis et al., 2004; Jarvis et al., 2006; Jarvis et al., 2008; Jarvis & Goodacre, 2008). They were also one of the first groups to successfully apply various advanced classification techniques to the SERS spectra. The group of Premasiri et al. have used gold-cluster-covered silicon substrates and a Raman microscope to discriminate SERS spectra of bacteria (Premasiri et al., 2005) as well as to classify the bacteria down to the subspecies level (Patel et al., 2008). A very recent study by Walter et al. uses silver colloids and a microfluidic device and greatly minimizes sample volume and exposure time for obtaining SERS spectra of *E. coli* which are classified with high accuracy (Walter et al., 2011). A major limitation of SERS in the identification of bacteria are the spectral variations present, even between spectra from the same sample, since the technique is very sensitive to substrate, sample preparation, as well as local field conditions. Despite these limitations SERS is definitely much more sensitive for identifying and classifying bacteria than normal Raman and is now the preferred route for developing rapid methods of UTI diagnosis.

### 1.3 Raman instrumentation

A Raman spectrometer setup is conceptually simple. It consists of a light source, light focusing optics, a spectrograph, and a detector (Fig. 3.) Modern Raman spectrometers may be classified roughly into multichannel Raman spectrometer systems, with variable laser sources and a charge-coupled device (CCD) detector, and small compact Raman systems, with fixed excitation wavelength and a CCD detector. In most cases, a laser is used as the excitation source. Light can be delivered to and collected from the sample either directly or via fiber-optic probes. The Raman scattered signal is directed to a spectrograph where it is analyzed to its constituent wavelengths and projected onto the CCD, allowing the latter to acquire a Raman spectrum. The data is collected in raw digital form for further processing on a computer. Raman systems are commercially available in a variety of sizes and configurations. Depending on the accuracy and sensitivity requirements of the application, the complexity of a Raman system can vary from a simple handheld device to a custom experimental setup. The Raman apparatus can also be seamlessly integrated with an optical microscope to perform Raman microscopy.

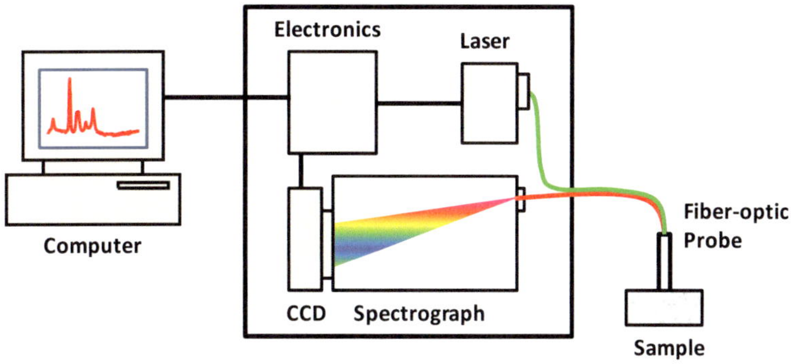


Fig. 3. Basic Raman instrumentation with a single laser source, fiber-optic delivery probe, spectrograph, CCD, and necessary electronics for power supply and computer interfacing.

## 2. Data processing, classification, and evaluation

Raman spectra from simple and concentrated solutions, of single or few chemical constituents, are easy to measure and interpret. However, as the concentration decreases or the samples become more complex, e.g. tissue or bacteria, the extraction of useful information from the weak and noisy Raman spectra becomes more challenging. The two major factors which make Raman signals difficult to classify are the fact that they are usually obscured by a large amount of noise and that the signals have a great deal of variance even between spectra which originate from the same sample. Both these problems (noise and high variance) must be rigorously addressed when attempting to classify the Raman spectra of UTI involved pathogens.

Classification is the exercise of assigning a class to an object. In the case of analyzing Raman spectra for UTI, the objects are the Raman spectra themselves, and the class of each spectrum is the species or subspecies of the bacteria that yielded the specific measurement. The procedure for performing classification can be broken down into four main steps. The first step is pre-processing which attempts to remove noise and to normalize the Raman spectra. The second step is feature creation which uses the de-noised and normalized spectra in order to create features which will be fed to the classification algorithm. In statistical terms, the features can be considered to be the "independent variables." The "dependent variable" is the class. The third step in the classification process is the use of the features by the classification algorithm to yield the estimated class of the sample. The final step is the evaluation of the classification to determine its accuracy.

Although these four steps describe the overall picture of the classification process well, it is not always the case that all steps are necessary or even separable. For example, in some procedures the de-noising, normalization and feature creation can be conceptualized as one step. Furthermore, in one of the most successful techniques presented for the classification of Raman spectra (Kyriakides et al., 2010), no explicit normalization is performed in the pre-processing step, but instead, the normalization is accomplished by the distance metric used to compare the feature vectors.

## 2.1 Pre-processing

### 2.1.1 Noise removal

The weak nature of the Raman effect results in spectra with very low signal-to-noise ratio (SNR). Noise in Raman spectra takes one of three forms: (i) High frequency noise, (ii) Low frequency noise, and (iii) Cosmic spikes (Fig. 4).

High frequency noise comes from the acquisition electronics and other sources of system variation. Median filtering can be used to remove this type of noise (Harz et al., 2005). Another technique commonly used is wavelet-based denoising (Ehrentreich & Sümmchen, 2001). Both these techniques work well and using at least one of them is recommended. Low frequency noise arises from ambient light entering the spectrograph and fluorescence emission from the sample which, in the case of biological samples, can significantly reduce the dynamic range of the measurement. This is seen as a background baseline which is present in the spectra. Iterative curve-fitting or low pass filtering can be used to estimate and remove the background baseline (Mahadevan-Jansen, 2002). Removing the low frequency noise can help improve the accuracy of the classification, but it is not always necessary. Using the first and second derivatives of the spectrum as features for the classification by itself removes the baseline since the derivatives indicate changes and curvature and not background (see section "Feature Creation" below). Cosmic spikes are spurious, very narrow, spikes appearing in the Raman spectra. They are an artefact of the detection electronics. The techniques used to filter out high frequency noise can also be used to remove cosmic spikes. For example, it has been shown that median filtering is an effective way to remove this type of noise too (Kastanos et al., 2010). Cosmic spikes can produce outliers which can be detrimental to the accuracy of several classification methods. It is therefore highly recommended that cosmic spikes are always removed before initiating any classification process.

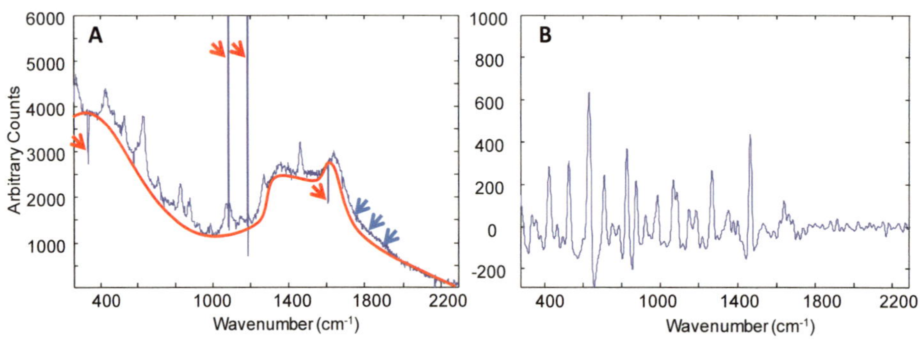


Fig. 4. A. Raman spectrum of fructose exhibiting cosmic spikes (red arrows), background fluorescence (red curve), and high frequency noise (blue arrows). B. The same spectrum after pre-processing.

### 2.1.2 Normalization

Raman spectra acquired sequentially or intermittently from exactly the same sample can exhibit a large amount of variance. This is usually in the form of an additive or multiplicative shift. These variations, in certain cases, can adversely affect the classification and should be eliminated by normalizing the spectra. Two of the most common techniques used are normalization using the highest peak (Liu et al., 2009), and vector normalization

(Dörfer et al., 2010). In the first case, all the spectra are modified so that they have the same minimum and maximum values. In the case of vector normalization the samples are considered to be multi-dimensional vectors and are modified so that their magnitudes are equal.

### 2.1.3 Considerations and caveats

It is important to note that the pre-processing step greatly affects the accuracy of the classification results. A sufficient amount of pre-processing must be performed in order to increase the classification accuracy. At the same time, however, it is imperative to understand that too much pre-processing can introduce user bias and over-fitting effects, which will decrease the accuracy of the results when truly unknown samples are subsequently classified. A classification algorithm which is self-normalizing (Kyriakides et al., 2010) avoids the pitfalls of too much pre-processing and therefore improves the classification accuracy of the technique.

### 2.2 Feature creation

Once the noise removal and normalization have been completed, features must be created to be subsequently used by the classification algorithm. The most common technique of feature creation is Principal Component Analysis (Jollife, 2002) which uses a linear transformation to represent the original data into a new coordinate space. The dimensions of this new space are in the directions of maximum variance of the features. The first principal component captures the dimension of maximum variance, the second principal component captures the dimension of the second greatest variance, and, similarly, the subsequent principal components capture the dimensions of successively decreasing variances. It is common to choose only a subset of these principal components as features. Usually the first few principal components are used, although this is not always the best approach (Jollife, 1982). An important benefit of selecting only a subset of the principal components is that the dimensionality of the data is reduced. This can be advantageous for the classification process for several reasons. The reduced number of features might capture the differences between classes more effectively, thus increasing the classification accuracy. In addition, the reduced number of variables might decrease the complexity of the classification, lower the computational cost, and improve the speed of the classification procedure. In methods such as Discriminant Analysis (DA, discussed below), dimensionality reduction is sometimes required in order to remove features which are highly correlated. In the DA algorithm, such features produce a singular matrix with no inverse, and thus DA cannot be performed.

Using the first and second derivatives is also a commonly used technique (Ferraro et al., 2003; Loethen et al., 2004; Navas et al., 2010) for feature creation. This method has the advantage of capturing the successive intensity differences of the Raman spectrum (first derivative), or the successive rates of change of the differences in the spectrum (second derivative). These measures have proven very successful in the analysis of Raman data and have been widely adopted. An additional advantage of taking the derivatives of the spectrum is that the baseline is removed without introducing bias or human error which would occur if the baseline was removed manually.

Another technique, which was shown to be successful in feature creation, is the use of spectral band ratios (Kyriakides et al., 2010). Each spectrum is broken down into segments, each consisting of a small band of wavenumbers. The mean intensity of each segment is found, and the ratio of the mean intensity of each segment to every other segment in the

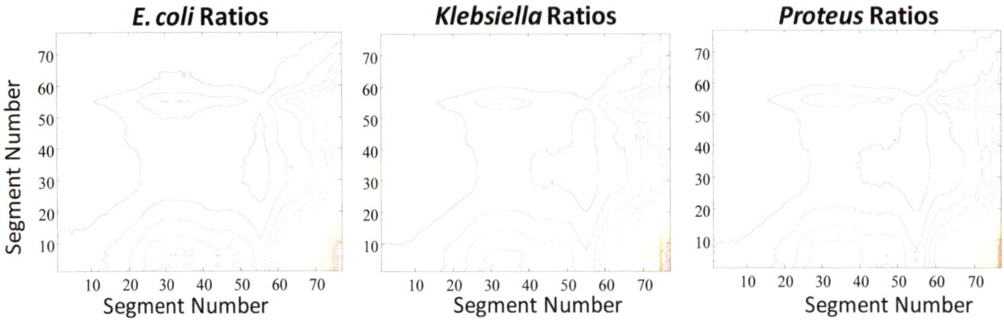


Fig. 5. Contour plots of the ratios between different segments of the average Raman spectra from several samples of *E. coli*, *Klebsiella*, and *Proteus*. Differences between the species are evident.

spectrum is then calculated. These ratios are then used as features for the classification of the data. This technique has two significant advantages. First, normalization is inherently achieved since the intensity of one part of the spectrum is compared to the intensity of other parts of the same spectrum. In this way, even if the intensity of the whole spectrum uniformly varies, the ratios of intensities remain the same. Second, the number of features is much less than the original number of data points thus achieving a reduction in the dimensionality of the data. The success of this method implies that classification can still achieve good accuracy even when using a low resolution spectrum, an important deduction supporting the use of clinically viable, commercial, low cost, low resolution systems.

### 2.3 Classification

Accurate classification of Raman spectra is crucial if the technique is ever to have a clinical application and, more importantly, affect disease diagnosis and prognosis. The range of classification techniques in the literature is extensive. However, certain methods appear to perform well when applied to Raman spectra and those will be covered in this section. Classification can be either supervised or unsupervised. Unsupervised classification methods group the data points into clusters without using any information about the class (label) of each data point. Supervised classification methods on the other hand require a set of data points which are labeled, i.e. their class is known *a priory*. These labeled data points are used to train the algorithm, using the known information about the class (label) of each point, to create a model of the data. Once the supervised model has been trained, it can be used to classify data points which were not in the training set, by assigning them to one of the classes described in the training set.

#### 2.3.1 Unsupervised classification (Clustering)

In Raman spectroscopy, Hierarchical Cluster Analysis (HCA) is the most commonly used unsupervised classification method (Baker & Hubert, 1975). Being an unsupervised method, it does not require *a priori* labeling of the data points. During the training phase clusters are formed and, subsequently, HCA can be used to classify a new data point by determining into which cluster this new data point falls. The results of HCA are easy to interpret and can be easily visualized as a dendrogram (Fig. 6). This ease of interpretation has made HCA very popular. However, this method does not provide good classification performance on data points which are "out-of-sample," i.e. not in the training set. HCA is relatively unstable because clusters formed in the lower levels of the hierarchy can constrain the clusters formed at higher levels of the hierarchy. This constraint can make the analysis unreliable.

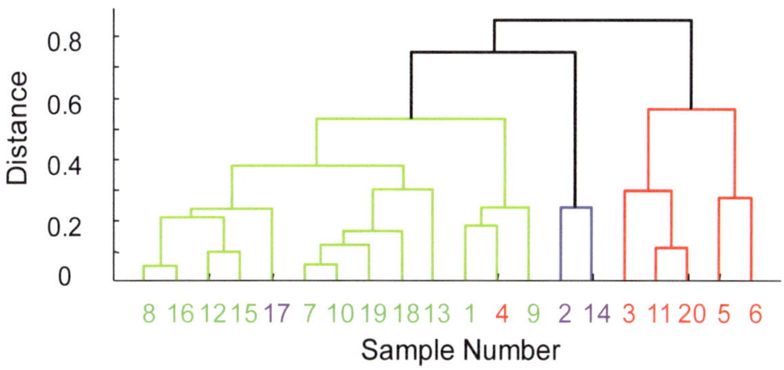


Fig. 6. Example dendrogram clustering 20 samples according to their "color" property. Below is the sample number indicating the true "color" of each sample. Notice that samples 17 and 4 have been misclassified.

The most important consideration when performing cluster analysis is the similarity metric (distance metric) which is used to compare data points. The most commonly used distance metric is the Euclidean distance, but this might not be the most appropriate in the case of Raman spectra. A general disadvantage of cluster analysis is the assumption that clusters do actually exist. This assumption is not always true. Furthermore, it is not always clear how many clusters should be formed. The number of clusters is a prominent concern when performing this type of analysis.

### 2.3.2 Supervised classification

In supervised classification, the goal is to assign data points, which were not seen before, into classes learned from a training set assuming that each data point belongs to one of the known classes. For example, Raman spectra obtained from bacteria can be labeled and classified based on the species of the bacterium from which they originated. Each spectrum is a data point, and it belongs to one class. Supervised learning requires that the class of some data points is known (labeled data points). Those points are used as a training set to create a model which can then be used to predict the label of unlabeled data points ("out-of-sample" data points) whose class is not known. Semi-supervised methods, which do not require all data points to be labeled, do exist. However, in this section, we will only deal with supervised methods in which all the data points are labeled. Some of the most commonly used supervised learning methods, applicable to the classification of Raman spectra, are listed below including a brief discussion of their advantages and disadvantages.

**Nearest Neighbor**: The nearest neighbour approach is very simple and does not explicitly require any training. The data points in the training set are used to predict future unlabeled data points by finding the distance between unlabeled data points and the labeled data points in the training set. The unlabeled data point is predicted to belong to the class of the data point in the training set to which it is closest. In the simplest case, the class is determined by the one data point which is closest, the so-called 1-nearest neighbor (1NN). It is possible to perform the classification using more nearest neighbors. For example, if the three data points in the training set closest to the unlabeled data point are used, then the approach is called 3-nearest neighbor (3NN). In the general case, when K nearest neighbors are used, the approach is called K-nearest neighbor (KNN). A disadvantage of this method is that the prediction could be slow because unlabeled data points must be compared to all data points in the training set. Therefore, the prediction speed depends on the size of the training set. KNN models have been shown to work well in certain applications although the 3NN approach is usually preferred. It is a very simple technique to implement. The most serious disadvantage of this method is that it is very sensitive to outliers. It is also very sensitive to irrelevant features which might be present in the data points.

**Discriminant Analysis**: Linear discriminant analysis (LDA) is one of the most commonly-used classification methods, mainly due to its simplicity and low computational cost (Krzanowski, 2000). It is a parametric technique which assumes that the independent variables (features) follow a multivariate normal distribution. The training data is used to find the parameters of the normal distribution which describes each class. These distributions are then used to create a discriminant model. In LDA, the assumption is that the different classes are described by identical covariance matrices. If this assumption is removed, then the different classes are allowed to have different covariances. In this way, the separating functions become quadratic, and this is called Quadratic Discriminant Analysis (QDA). It is important to choose either LDA or QDA depending on the characteristics of the data. DA is highly sensitive to outliers since they can greatly affect the shape of the calculated distributions. If it is obvious that a data point is an outlier it is best to remove it before carrying out DA. DA can be advantageous since (Tufféry, 2011):

- It is very fast because it requires very little computation.
- It is optimal when the assumptions of normality hold true.
- The models produced are concise and are easily implemented.
- It is a good technique for detecting global phenomena.
- It is widely implemented so it is easy to find and use.

However, DA may be suboptimal in some cases since:

- If using LDA, only linear phenomena can be detected.
- It is sensitive to outliers.
- It makes assumptions of normality on the features (independent variables). If this assumption does not hold, then the accuracy of the results will be greatly reduced. This is the main and most serious disadvantage of DA.

DA is a simple technique that only performs well on data points which are well-separated and on features which follow a normal distribution. If one of the independent variables (features) is highly correlated with another, or is a function of another set of features, then the calculations for finding the discriminant function will fail. This case is very common when the number of features (independent variables) is much greater than the number of observations (data points). For this reason it is better to first transform the features before applying DA. The two most commonly used methods for transforming the Raman data are Principal Component Analysis (PCA), and Partial Least squares (PLS). This leads to the two classification methods known as PC-DFA (Principal Component Discriminant Function Analysis) and PLS-DA (Partial Least Squares Discriminant Analysis).

Principle Components Discriminant Function Analysis (PC-DFA) uses Principal Component Analysis to first transform the data into a new space in order to maximize the variance in each dimension before performing DA. Each dimension is called a principal component.

This method can often lead to good results. However, in cases where the variance of the features is not a good criterion for class separability, it is best to use another method, such as PLS-DA.

Partial Least Squares Discriminant Analysis (PLS-DA) is a method which attempts to increase the separation of groups (classes) by representing the data points in a new space (Barker & Rayens, 2003). The key difference between PLS and PCA is that PCA aims to find directions of maximum variance, whereas PLS aims to find directions which maximize group separability. In some cases the two coincide, that is when group separability is well described by the variance of the features. In other cases it is best to use PLS instead of PCA. An advantage of PLS-DA is that it can describe complex relationships between features (Weston & Watkins, 1999). However, it has been shown that PLS-DA has issues with over-fitting (Westerhuis et al., 2008). For this reason, it might produce good results when performing cross validation, but its accuracy on "out-of-sample" data can be low when over-fitting on the training data occurs. This is a good example of how cross-validation accuracy fails to capture the expected classification accuracy on future "out-of-sample" data.

**Support Vector Machines (SVMs)**: A Support Vector Machine is a binary classifier which aims to distinguish between two classes of instances by finding the maximum separating hyperplane between them (Vapnik, 1998). For this reason it tends to generalize better than the much simpler DA-based approaches. By design, SVM's can only discriminate between two classes. In order to allow for the classification of more than two classes, one can employ more than one SVM's. SVM's, in their simple form, are linear classifiers. It is possible however to create non-linear SVM's by increasing the dimensionality of the feature space by using the so-called "kernel trick" (Schölkopf et al., 1998; Cristianini & Shawe-Taylor, 2004), which employs a kernel function to transform the data. It is thus possible to find a separating hyperplane in higher dimensions where such a hyperplane would not exist in lower dimensions. There are many choices for the type of kernel function to use (Cristianini & Shawe-Taylor, 2004). The standard choices are the linear kernel (dot-product kernel), the polynomial kernel, and the Gaussian Kernel. The best results can be obtained by using an appropriate kernel. It has been shown that for the classification of Raman Spectra, the correlation kernel (Kyriakides et al., 2010) can give high accuracy on "out-of-sample data."

SVM's have several advantages (Tufféry, 2011):

- By using a kernel the power of the SVM can be greatly increased so that it can model non-linear phenomena.
- SVM's are non parametric. They do not make any assumptions about the distribution of the data.
- They can generalize well. This results in good predictive performance on "out-of-sample" data.
- With the choice of the appropriate kernel, one can put more stress on the desired characteristics of the data which are used for discrimination.
- The uniqueness of the solution is guaranteed.
- Only the most important data points (support vectors) of the training set are used in making predictions, making the classifier more robust to noise and outliers.

Disadvantages of SVM's include:

- The SVM model is not transparent. Due to its non-parametric nature the results cannot be presented in a way which can be easily interpreted for further analysis to gain further insight.
- SVM's are sensitive to the choice of kernel parameters.

- They require a lot of computation to find the best parameters during training.

### 2.4 Evaluation of the classification results

In order to evaluate the performance of a classifier, the most commonly used techniques are cross-validation and performance on a "hold-out set." Cross-validation uses only the training set which is broken down into smaller parts, or "folds". It is often preferred to use 10 folds to perform so-called 10-fold cross-validation. All the folds, except one, are used for training. Testing consists of predicting the class of each data point in the fold which was left out. The cross-validation procedure performs training and testing as many times as there are folds. Each time, a different fold is left out for testing. In this way, a prediction is made on the class of all the data points in the training set. In the extreme case, each fold can consist of only one data point. This is called Leave-One-Out Cross Validation, and is most often used when the training set is small. Cross-validation generally results in a good estimate, but this is not always the case. Classification algorithms which do not generalize well can sometimes perform well in cross-validation and not so well on "out-of-sample data" (Kyriakides et al., 2010). For this reason it is best to test the classification on a "hold-out set" consisting of data points which were not used for training but whose class label is known. The performance of the classifier on such a test set is a good indication of the performance on future unseen ("out-of-sample") data.

## 3. Raman spectroscopy for UTI diagnosis

For Raman spectroscopy to become a viable clinical tool the following key diagnostic objectives must be addressed and successfully accomplished:

1. Classification of urine samples as positive or negative for UTI based on the bacterial load.
2. Identification of the pathogen involved in the positive samples.
3. Determination of the antibiogram, i.e. antibiotic sensitivity, of the bacteria involved.

Recent research results indicate that it may indeed be possible to achieve all three of the above objectives with Raman or SERS enabling rapid and accurate UTI diagnosis using low cost, turn-key equipment.

### 3.1 Classification of bacterial samples as positive or negative

Most of the work published on Raman spectroscopy of bacteria has focused on identification of bacterial species or subspecies with but a few studies are available on quantification of samples using these techniques. Escoriza et al. used Raman spectroscopy to quantify filtered waterborne bacteria but ran into problems because of the high fluorescence background from the alumina or silver membrane filters they used (Escoriza, 2006). There are also some studies on quantification of viruses using SERS (Fan, 2010; Wang, 2010)

Raman spectroscopy and, in particular, SERS are sensitive enough to detect bacteria at concentrations considered normal and pathologic for UTIs. This can be verified by performing quantification studies of known bacterial concentrations. For example, *E. coli* bacteria were cultured and their concentration in solution was determined using their optical density. Samples were diluted serially with sterile deionized water to obtain the following concentrations: $10^3$, $10^4$, $10^5$, $10^6$, $10^7$ and $10^8$ bacteria/ml. 10 µl of each sample were mixed with an equal volume of concentrated gold nanoparticles, spotted on glass slides and allowed to dry. SERS spectra were collected form 22 samples using a portable commercial Raman spectrometer at 785 nm excitation wavelength and 4.5 $cm^{-1}$ resolution. Spectra were preprocessed by filtering to remove the background and high frequency noise. Figure 7 shows the spectra after pre-processing. The feature vector for each sample contained the pre-processed Raman spectrum as well as its first and second derivatives. Each sample was assigned a class of 0 for no infection (concentrations of $\leq 10^4$ bacteria/ml) or 1 for infection (concentration $\geq 10^5$ bacteria/ml.) The outcome showed that ~ 82% of the samples were correctly classified as negative (class 0) or positive (class 1) for UTI (Kastanos et al., 2011).

These results are, of course, very preliminary and much more work is required to develop the technique. They do indicate, however, that it is possible to examine a urine sample and determine whether it is negative or positive for UTI based on its Raman spectral properties.

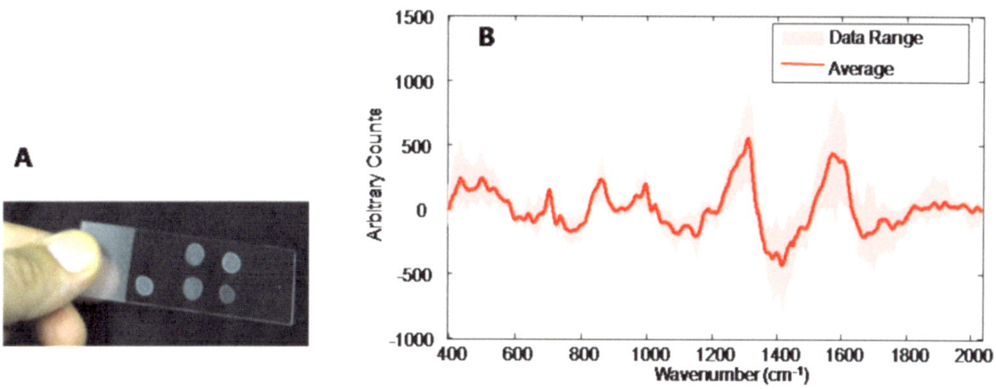


Fig. 7. A. Bacteria (*E. coli*) and gold nanoparticles spotted on a glass slide for SERS measurement. B. SERS spectra for different *E.coli* samples after pre-processing, indicating the average spectrum and the range of values, i.e. inter-sample variability.

### 3.2 Identification of the pathogen in a positive sample

As mentioned in the chapter's introduction, several investigators are evaluating the use of Raman spectroscopy as a tool for bacterial classification. Recent studies have shown that employing novel feature creation techniques, such as the ratios of different Raman bands (Fig. 5) yields high-quality results even when using a low cost, low resolution Raman system (Kastanos et al., 2010). The power of Raman spectroscopy for UTI diagnosis can be verified experimentally. For example, clinical bacterial isolates from patients with UTI (n =75), previously identified by conventional tests as positive, were collected from clinical laboratories. Specifically, spectra from 25 samples of *E. coli*, 25 of *K. pneumoniae* and 25 of *Proteus spp.* were acquired using a portable commercial Raman spectrometer at 785 nm excitation wavelength and 4.5 $cm^{-1}$ resolution. No filtering of the spectra was performed. Each spectrum was broken up into 25 $cm^{-1}$ segments and the mean intensity for each segment was determined. Ratios of each segment's mean intensity to every other segment's mean intensity were calculated. The classification method used was Linear Discriminant Analysis with a Principal Components transformation to reduce the dimensionality of the data. A leave-one-out cross-validation procedure was performed to verify the performance of the classifier. The overall accuracy of the technique was 95%. Very high sensitivity (88-

100%) and specificity (94-100%) values for classification of the three species of bacteria were obtained.

The use of SERS can further enhance the sensitivity and specificity of bacterial classification providing accurate results for more than three species at a time. To verify this, clinical bacterial isolates from patients with UTI (n = 46) were obtained from clinical laboratories after being identified as positive using conventional tests. Specifically, 10 samples of *E. coli*, 9 of *K. pneumoniae*, 9 of *Proteus spp.*, 9 of *Enterococcus spp.* and 9 of *Citrobacter spp.* were obtained for SERS using the same spectrometer as before. Ratio features, PCA, DA, and a leave-one-out cross-validation procedure were performed as before. Classification was originally done for 3 species (*E.coli, K. pneumonia, Proteus spp.*) and then for all 5 species of bacteria. Table 1 illustrates the results of the classification analysis of the SERS spectra. These results suggest that classification of bacteria belonging to 3 classes using SERS is as accurate (93%) as classification using normal Raman spectra (95%). However, much more accurate classification of bacteria belonging to 5 classes is achieved using SERS (91%) compared to using normal Raman spectra (73%). A wavenumber band of 25 $cm^{-1}$ was proved to be a better choice for providing more accurate classification of the 5 classes of bacteria using the ratios method.

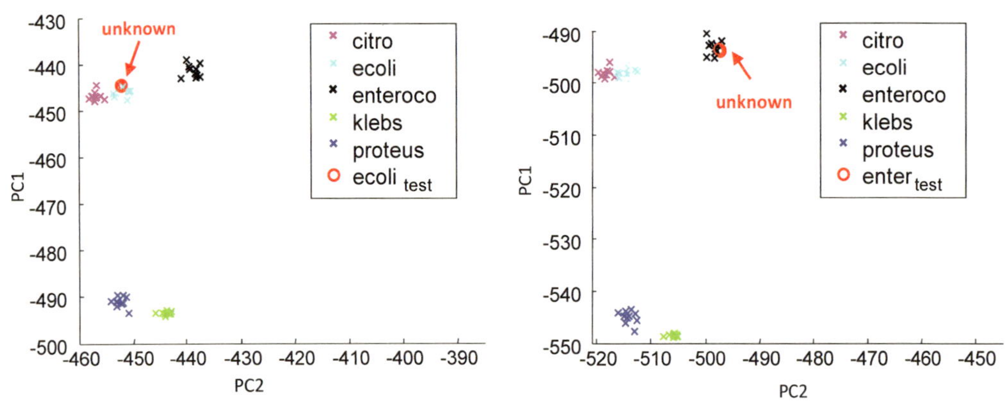


Fig. 8. SERS classification of two unknowns, *E. coli*, (A) and *Enterococcus spp*, (B). The first two principal components (PC1 & PC2), that contained the most information, were plotted against each other for visualization purposes. Each of the unknowns clearly falls in the correct species cluster. Note that the plots differ since the training sets differ by one member.

| Classes | Band Size (cm-1) | Correct Classification |
|---|---|---|
| 3 | 50 | 28/30 (93%) |
| 3 | 25 | 28/30 (93%) |
| 5 | 50 | 40/46 (87%) |
| 5 | 25 | 42/46 (91%) |

Table 1. Results of classification analysis of SERS spectra from 3 or 5 classes of bacteria.

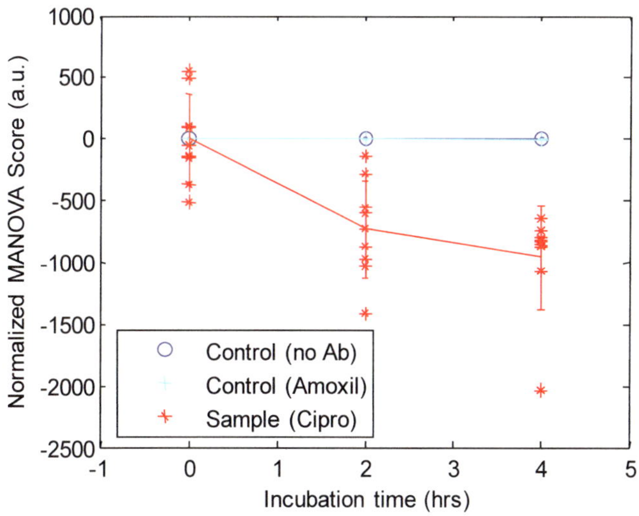


Fig. 9. Normalized MANOVA score of SERS spectra of *E. coli*, *K. pneumonia*, and *Proteus spp.* strains after their incubation in the presence of 0.128 µg/ml Ciprofloxacin (*), in the presence of 64 µg/ml Amoxicillin (+), or in the absence of any antibiotic (○).

### 3.3 Antibiotic sensitivity of bacterial samples

In order for the diagnosis of a UTI to be complete, the antibiotic sensitivity of the involved pathogen must be determined. Most of the studies, in the past, involved the use of Raman for distinguishing live bacteria from bacteria that were killed by heating (Baek et al., 1988; Grow et al., 2003), desiccation (Robertson et al., 1992; Deng & Cliver, 1999), or UV irradiation (Lorenzo-Lorenzo et al. , 1993; Belosevic et al., 2001). More recent work by Liu et al (Liu et al., 2009) shows very clear differences between the spectra of bacteria that are sensitive and the spectra of bacteria that are resistant to an antibiotic. However, no classification of samples as sensitive or resistant to an antibiotic was done by this group. The current hypothesis is that exposure of bacteria to an antibiotic to which they are sensitive will cause either external or internal molecular changes, depending on the mechanism of action of the antibiotic. It is expected that the short life cycle of bacteria will allow the visualization of these changes in their Raman spectra within a few hours of exposure to an antibiotic.

In a recent study (Kastanos et al., 2010), Raman spectra were collected from 27 strains of bacteria, belonging to the species *E. coli, K. pneumonia*, and *Proteus spp.*, shown to be sensitive to Ciprofloxacin and resistant to Amoxicillin by conventional antibiograms. The spectra were collected after treatment in the presence or absence of each of the two antibiotics for 0, 2 and 4 hours. Spectra were collected using a portable, commercial, Raman spectrometer at 785 nm excitation wavelength and 4.5 $cm^{-1}$ resolution. The spectra were filtered and the fluorescence background was subtracted. The Raman spectrum, as well as the first and second derivatives, were included in the feature vector. A principal components (PCs) transformation was used and only PCs describing the highest variance were retained. The data was, then, analyzed using the MANOVA algorithm which calculated a score for each sample which would provide maximum separation between a group of bacteria which were sensitive to an antibiotic with the groups of bacteria which were resistant or were not treated with antibiotic. Figure 9 shows that the MANOVA score of bacteria incubated with

Ciprofloxacin is significantly lower than that of untreated bacteria or bacteria treated with Amoxicillin even as early as 2 hours after incubation with the antibiotics. These results suggest that Raman spectroscopy could be used to determine the antibiotic susceptibility of bacteria even after a very short treatment with the antibiotic. The study was repeated using SERS with similar results indicating that the advantages of SERS, such as increased sensitivity and improved speed, can be exploited in antibiotic testing as well. These studies are currently being expanded to include more bacteria and more antibiotics.

## 4. Conclusion

In this chapter, a review of the current state of the application of Raman spectroscopy in bacterial identification and, more specifically, UTI diagnosis is presented. Raman spectroscopy and SERS, in particular, offer the possibility to develop highly versatile and powerful diagnostic tools. They can provide complex biochemical information which, in conjunction with advanced analysis and classification techniques, can lead to rapid and accurate diagnosis of UTIs. Recent advances in the instrumentation, experimental techniques, analysis, and classification, have enabled the fast and accurate quantification and identification of bacterial populations as well as the determination of their sensitivity to antibiotics. These results are still preliminary and must be significantly expanded. However, there is great interest in the area and the research community actively strives to improve the yield and accuracy of Raman-based diagnostics. In the future, a simple, point-of-care, device is envisioned which will provide a complete UTI diagnosis, from a single urine sample, within a few hours. Such a technology could have significant short and long term benefits for public health by reducing the cost of diagnosis, improving prognosis, and reducing the unnecessary use of antibiotics and, therefore, bacterial resistance.

## 5. Acknowledgment

Some of the research presented in this chapter was partially supported by the KIOS Research Center for Intelligent Systems and Networks of the University of Cyprus and the Research Promotion Foundation of Cyprus. The authors also wish to thank all their collaborators at P. Hadjikoumis Microbiology Laboratory and the Limassol General Hospital for their support.

## 6. References

Alanis, A. (2005). Resistance to Antibiotics: Are we in the Post-Antibiotic Era? *Archives of Medical Research*, Vol. 36, pp. 697-705.

Baek, M., Nelson, W., Britt, D. & Sperry, J. (1988). UV-Excited Resonance Raman Spectra of Heat Denatured Lysozyme and Staphylococcus epidermidis. *Applied Spectroscopy*, Vol. 42, pp. 1312-1314.

Baker, F.B., & Hubert, L.J. (1975). Measuring the Power of Hierarchical Cluster Analysis. Journal of the American Statistical Association, Vol. 70, No. 349, (March 1975), pp. 31-38.

Barker, M., & Rayens, W. (2003). Partial least squares for discrimination. *Journal of Chemometrics*, Vol. 17, No. 3, (2003), pp. 166-173, ISSN: 1099-128X.

Belosevic, M., Craik, S. A., Stafford, J. L., Neumann, N. F., Kruithof, J. & Smith, D. W. (2001), Studies on the resistance/reactivation of Giardia muris cysts and Cryptosporidium parvum oocysts exposed to medium-pressure ultraviolet radiation. *FEMS Microbiology Letters*, Vol. 204, pp. 197–203.

Casadevall, A. (1996). Crisis in Infectious Diseases: Time for a New Paradigm?. *Clinical and Infectious Disease*, Vol. 23, p. 790.

Chen, W., Tsai, P. & Chen, Y. (2008). Functional Nanoparticle-Based Proteomic Strategies for Characterization of Pathogenic Bacteria. *Analytical Chemistry*, Vol. 80, pp. 9612-9621.

Cheng, H., Huan, S., Wu, H., Shen, G. & Yu, R. (2009). Surface-Enhanced Raman Spectroscopic Detection of a Bacteria Biomarker Using Gold Nanoparticle Immobilized Substrates. *Analytical Chemistry*, Vol. 81, pp. 9902-9912.

Cristianini, N., & Shawe-Taylor, J. (2004). *An introduction to support Vector Machines: and other kernel-based learning methods*, Cambridge University Press, ISBN: 0521780195, UK.

Cosgrove, S. & Carmeli, Y. (2003). The impact of antimicrobial resistance on health and economic outcomes. *Clinical and Infectious Disease*, Vol. 36, pp. 1433-1437.

Demirel, M., Kao, P., Malvadkar, N., Wang, H., Gong, X., Poss, M. and Allara, D. (2009). Bio-organism sensing via surface enhanced Raman spectroscopy on controlled metal/polymer nanostructured substrates. *Biointerphases*, Vol. 4, No. 2, (June 2009), pp. 35-41.

Deng, M. & Cliver, D. (1999). Cryptosporidium parvum studies with dairy products. *International Journal of Food Microbiology*, Vol. 46, pp. 113-121.

Dörfer, T., Schumacher, W., Tarcea, N., Schmitt, M., & Popp, J. (2010). Quantitative mineral analysis using Raman spectroscopy and chemometric techniques. *Journal of Raman Spectroscopy*, Vol. 41, No. 6, (2010), pp. 684-689, ISSN: 1097-4555.

Efrima, S. & Bronk, B. (1998). Silver Colloids Impregnating or Coating Bacteria. *Journal of Physical Chemistry B*, Vol. 102, pp. 5947-5950.

Efrima, S. & Zeiri, L. (2009). Understanding SERS of bacteria. *Journal of Raman Spectroscopy*, Vol. 40, pp. 277-288.

Ehrentreich, F., & Sümmchen L. (2001). Spike removal and denoising of Raman spectra by wavelet transform methods. *Analytical Chemistry*, Vol. 73, No. 17, (2001), pp. 4364-4373, ISSN: 0003-2700.

Escoriza, M., VanBriesen, J., Stewart, S., Maier, J. & Treado, P. (2006). Raman spectroscopy and chemical imaging for quantification of filtered waterborne bacteria. *Journal of Microbiological Methods*, Vol. 66, pp. 63-72.

Fan, C., Hu, Z., Riley, L., Purdy, G., Mustapha, A. & Lin, M. (2010). Detecting Food- and Waterborne Viruses by Surface-Enhanced Raman Spectroscopy. *Journal of Food Science*, Vol. 75, pp. M302-M307.

Ferraro, J.R., Nakamoto, K., & Brown, C.W. (2003). *Introductory Raman Spectroscopy (Second Edition)*, Elsevier Science, ISBN: 978-0-12-254105-6 , USA.

Forrester, J., Valentine, N., Su, Y. & Johnson, T. (2009). Chemometric analysis of multiple species of Bacillus bacterial endospores using infrared spectroscopy: Discrimination to the strain level. *Analytical Chimica Acta*, Vol. 651, pp. 24-30.

Gruneberg, R. (1994). Changes in urinary pathogens and their antibiotic sensitivities, 1971-1992. *Journal of Antimicrobial Chemotherapy*, Vol. 33 (Suppl. A), p. 1.

Grow, A., Wood, L., Claycomb, J. & Thompson, P. (2003). New biochip technology for label-free detection of pathogens and their toxins. *Journal of Microbiological Methods*, Vol. 53, pp. 221-233.

Guzelian, A., Sylvia, J., Janni, J., Clauson, S. &, Spencer, K. (2002). SERS of whole-cell bacteria and trace levels of biological molecules. *Proceedings of SPIE*, Vol. 4577, p. 182.

Harz, M., Rösch, P., Peschke, K., Ronneberger, O., Burkhardt, H. & Popp, J. (2005). Micro-Raman spectroscopic identification of bacterial cells of the genus Staphylococcus and dependence on their cultivation conditions. *Analyst*, Vol. 130, No. 11, (2005), pp. 1543-1550.

Hennigan, S., Driskell, J., Dluhy, R., Zhao, Y., Tripp, R., Waites, K. & Krausee, D. (2010). Detection of Mycoplasma pneumonia in Simulated and True Clinical Throat Swab Specimens by Nanorod Array-Surface-Enhanced Raman Spectroscopy. *PLOS ONE*, Vol. 5, No. 10, e13633.

Hutsebaut, D., Maquelin, K., De Vos, P. Vandenabeele, P., Moens, L. & Puppels, G. (2004). Effect of Culture Conditions on the Achievable Taxonomic Resolution of Raman Spectroscopy Disclosed by Three *Bacillus* Species. *Analytical Chemistry*, Vol. 76, pp. 6274-6281.

Jarvis, R. & Goodacre, R. (2004). Discrimination of bacteria using surface-enhanced Raman spectroscopy. *Analytical Chemistry*, Vol. 76, pp. 40-47.

Jarvis, R. & Goodacre, R. (2004). Ultra-violet resonance Raman spectroscopy for the rapid discrimination of urinary tract infection bacteria. *FEMS Microbiology Letters*, Vol. 232, pp. 127-132.

Jarvis, R. & Goodacre, R. (2008). Characterization and identification of bacteria using SERS. *Chemical Society Reviews*, Vol. 37, pp. 931-936.

Jarvis, R., Brooker, A. & Goodacre, R. (2004). Surface-enhanced Raman spectroscopy for bacterial discrimination utilizing a scanning electron microscope with a Raman spectroscopy interface. *Analytical Chemistry*, Vol. 76, pp. 5198-5202.

Jarvis, R., Brooker, A. & Goodacre, R. (2006). Surface-enhanced Raman scattering for the rapid discrimination of bacteria. *Faraday Discussions*, Vol. 132, pp. 281-292.

Jarvis, R., Law, N., Shadi, I., O' Brien, P,. Lloyd, J. & Goodacre, R. (2008). Surface-Enhanced Raman Scattering from Intracellular and Extracellular Bacterial Locations. *Analytical Chemistry*, Vol. 80, pp. 6741-6746.

Jolliffe, I.T. (1982). A Note on the Use of Principal Components in Regression. *Journal of the Royal Statistical Society. Series C (Applied Statistics)*, Vol. 31, No. 3, (1982), pp. 300-303, ISSN: 0035-9254.

Jollife, I.T. (2002). *Principal component analysis (Second edition)*, Springer, ISBN: 0-387-95442-2, New York.

Kastanos E., Kyriakides A., Hadjigeorgiou K. & Pitris C. (2010). A Novel Method for Urinary Tract Infection Diagnosis and Antibiogram Using Raman Spectroscopy. *J. of Raman Spectroscopy*, DOI 10.1002/jrs.2540.

Kastanos E., Hadjigeorgiou K., Kyriakides A. & Pitris C. (2011) Classification of bacterial samples as negative or positive for a UTI and antibiogram using surface enhanced raman spectroscopy. *Proc. SPIE 7911*, 791107.

Knauer, M., Ivleva, N., Liu, H., Niessner, R. & Haisch, C. (2010). Surface-Enhanced Raman Scattering-Based Label-Free Microarray Readout for the Detection of Microorganisms. *Analytical Chemistry*, Vol. 82, pp. 2766-2772.

Kneipp, K., Wang, Y., Kneipp, H., Perlman, L. &, Itzkan, I. (1997). Single Molecule Detection Using Surface-Enhanced Raman Scattering (SERS). Physics Reviews Letters, Vol. 78, p. 1667.

Kneipp, K., Moskovits, M, Kneip, H. (2006). Surface-Enhanced Raman Scattering: *Physics and Applications Topics in Applied Physics*. Vol. 103, pp. 1-464.

Krzanowski, W.J. (2000). *Principles of multivariate analysis: a user's perspective (Revised edition)*, Oxford University Press, ISBN: 0198507089, USA.

Kyriakides, A., Kastanos, E., Hadjigeorgiou, K., & Pitris, C. (2010). Classification of Raman spectra using the correlation kernel. *Journal of Raman Spectroscopy, DOI 10.1002/jrs.2809*.

Liu, T.T., Lin, Y.H., Hung, C.S., Liu, T.J., Chen, Y., Huang, Y.C., Tsai, T.H., Wang, H.H., Wang, D.W., Wang, J.K., Wang, Y.L., & Lin, C.H. (2009). A high speed detection platform based on surface-enhanced Raman scattering for monitoring antibiotic-induced chemical changes in bacteria cell wall. *PLoS ONE*, Vol. 4, No. 5, (May 2009), pp. E5470, ISSN: 1932-6203.

Loethen, Y.L., Zhang, D., Favors, R.N., Basiaga, S.B.G., & Ben-Amotz, D. (2004). Second-derivative variance minimization method for automated spectral subtraction. *Applied spectroscopy*, Vol. 58, No. 3, (2004), pp. 272-278.

Lorenzo-Lorenzo, M., Ares-Mazas, M., Villacorta-Martinez de Maturana, I. & Duran-Oreiro, D. (1993). Effect of Ultraviolet Disinfection of Drinking Water on the Viability of Cryptosporidium parvum Oocysts. *Journal of Parasitology*, Vol. 79, pp. 67-70.

Magee J. (1993) Whole-organism fingerprinting. In: *Handbook of New Bacterial Systematics*, Goodfellow, M. & O'Donnell, A. (Eds.), pp. 383- 427, Academic Press, London.

Mahadevan-Jansen, A. (2002). Raman Spectroscopy from Benchtop to Bedside, In: *Biomedical Photonics Handbook*, Vo-Dinh, T. (Ed.), pp., CRC Press, ISBN, London.

Maquelin, K., Choo-Smith, L., Vreeswijk, T., Endtz, H., Smith, B, Bennett, R., Bruining, H.,Puppels, G. (2000). Raman spectroscopic method for identification of clinically relevant microorganisms growing on solid culture medium. *Analytical Chemistry*, Vol. 72, p. 12.

Moskovits, M. (1985). Surface-enhanced Spectroscopy. *Reviews in Modern Physics*, Vol. 57, pp. 783-826.

Mothershed, E. & Whitney, A. (2006). Nucleic acid-based methods for the detection of bacterial pathogens: present and future considerations for the clinical laboratory. *Clinical and Chimica Acta*, Vol.363, No., (Month 2006), pp. 206-220, ISSN

Navas, N., Romero-Pastor, J., Manzano, E., & Cardell, C. (2010). Raman spectroscopic discrimination of pigments and tempera paint model samples by principal component analysis on first-derivative spectra. *Journal of Raman Spectroscopy*, Vol. 41, No. 11, (2010), pp. 1196-1203, ISSN: 1196-1203.

Nie, S. & Emory, S. (1997). Probing Single Molecules and Single Nanoparticles by Surface-Enhanced Raman Scattering. *Science*, Vol. 275, p. 1102.

Pal, A., Isola, N., Alarie, J., Stokes, D. & Vo-Dinh, T. (2006). Synthesis and characterization of SERS gene probe for BRCA-1 (breast cancer). *Faraday Discussions*, Vol. 132, pp. 293-301.

Patel, I., Premasiri, W., Moir, D. & Ziegler, L. (2008). Barcoding bacterial cells: a SERS-based methodology for pathogen identification. *Journal of Raman Spectroscopy*, Vol. 39, pp. 1660-1672.

Preisner, O., Lopes, J. & Menezes, J. (2008). Uncertainty assessment in FT-IR spectroscopy based bacteria classification models. *Chemometrics and Intelligent Laboratory Systems*, Vol. 94, pp. 33-42.

Premasiri, W., Moir, D., Klempner, M., Krieger, N., Jones, G. II & Ziegler, L. (2005). Characterization of the surface enhanced raman scattering (SERS) of bacteria. *Journal of Physical Chemistry B*, Vol. 109, pp. 312-320.

Robertson, L., Campbell, A. & Smith, H. (1992). Survival of Cryptosporidium parvum oocysts under various environmental pressures. Applied Environmental Microbiology, Vol. 58, pp. 3494-3500.

Rolain, J., Mallet, M., Fournier, P., Raoult, D. (2004). Real-time PCR for universal antibiotic susceptibility testing. *Journal of Antimicrobial Chemotherapy*, Vol. 54, No., (Month 2004), pp. 538-541, ISSN

Schmid, U., Rosch, P., Krause, M., Harz, Popp, J. & Baumann, K. (2009). Gausssian mixture discriminant analysis for the single-cell differentiation of bacteria using micro-Raman spectroscopy. *Chemometrics and Intelligent Laboratory Systems*, Vol. 96, pp. 159-171.

Schuster, K.C., Reese, I., Urlaub, E., Gapes, J.R. & Lendl, . (2000). Multidimensional Information on the Chemical Composition of Single Bacterial Cells by Confocal Raman Microspectroscopy. *Analytical Chemistry,* Vol. 72, pp. 5529-5534
Schuster, K.C., Urlaub, E. & Gapes, J.R. (2000). Single-cell analysis of bacteria by Raman microscopy: spectral information on the chemical composition of cells and on the heterogeneity in a culture. *Journal of Microbiological Methods,* Vol. 42, pp. 29-38
Schölkopf, B., Burges, C.J.C, & Smola, A.J. (Ed(s).). (1998). *Advances in kernel methods - support vector learning,* MIT Press, ISBN: 978-0-262-19416-7, USA.
Sengupta, A., Laucks, M., Dildine, N., Drapala, E. & Davis, J. (2005). Bioaerosol characterization by surface-enhanced Raman spectroscopy (SERS). *Journal of Aerosol Science,* Vol. 36, pp. 651-664.
Sengupta, A., Mujacic, M. & Davis, E. (2006). Detection of bacteria by surface-enhanced Raman spectroscopy. *Analytical and Bioanalytical Chemistry,* Vol. 386, pp. 1379-1386
Shanmukh, S., Jones, L., Zhao, Y., Driskell, J., Tripp, R. & Dluhy, R. (2008). Identification and classification of respiratory syncytial virus (RSV) strains by surface-enhanced Raman spectroscopy and multivariate statistical techniques. *Analytical and Bioanalytical Chemistry,* Vol. 390, pp. 1551-1555.
Tufféry, S. (2011). *Data Mining and Statistics for Decision Making.* John Wiley & Sons Ltd, ISBN: 978-0-470-68829-8, UK.
Vapnik, V.N. (1998). *Statistical learning theory,* Wiley-Interscience, New York.
Vo-Dinh, T., Yan, F., & Stokes, D. (2005). Plasmonics-based nanostructures for surface-enhanced Raman scattering bioanalysis. *Methods in Molecular Biology,* Vol. 300, pp. 225-283.
Walter, A., Marz, A., Schumacher, W., Rosch, P. & Popp, J. (2011). Towards a fast, high specific and reliable discrimination of bacteria on strain level by means of SERS in a microfluidic device. *Lab Chip,* Vol. 11, pp. 1013-1021.
Wang, X., Li, Y., Wang, H., Fu, Q., Peng, J., Wang, Y., Du, J., Zhou, Y. & Zhan, L. (2010). Gold nanorod-based localized surface plasmon resonance biosensor for sensitive detection of hepatitis B virus in buffer, blood serum and plasma. *Biosensors and Bioelectronics,* Vol. 26, pp. 404-410.
Westerhuis, J.A., Hoefsloot, H.C.J., Smit, S., Vis, D.J., Smilde, A.K., van Velzen, E.J.J., van Duijnhoven, J.P.M., & van Dorsten, F.A. (2008). Assessment of PLSDA cross validation. *Metabolomics,* Vol. 4, No. 1, (January 2008), pp. 81-89, ISSN: 1573-3882.
Weston, J., & Watkins (1999). Support vector machines for multi-class pattern recognition. *Proceedings of the seventh European symposium on artificial neural networks,* Belgium, April 1999.
Xie, C., Mace, J., Dinno, M., Li, Y., Tang, W., Newton, R. & Gemperline, P. (2005). Identification of Single Bacterial Cells in Aqueous Solution Using Confocal Laser Tweezers Raman Spectroscopy. *Analytical Chemistry,* Vol. 77, pp. 4390-4397.
Yonzon, C., Haynes, C., Zhang, X., Walsh, J. Jr. & Van Duyne, R. (2004). A glucose biosensor based on surface-enhanced Raman scattering: improved partition layer, temporal stability, reversibility, and resistance to serum protein interference. *Analytical Chemistry,* Vol. 76, pp. 78-85.
Zeiri, L., Bronk, B., Shabtai, Y., Czege, J. & Efrima, S. (2002). Silver metal induced surface enhanced Raman of bacteria. *Colloids Surface A.,* Vol. 208, pp. 357-362.
Zeiri, L., Bronk, B., Shabtai, Y., Eichler, J. & Efrima, S. (2004). Surface-enhanced Raman spectroscopy as a tool for probing specific biochemical components in bacteria. *Applied Spectroscopy,* Vol. 58, pp. 33-40.

13

# Natural Approaches for Controlling Urinary Tract Infections

Mary Anne Roshni Amalaradjou[1] and Kumar Venkitanarayanan[2]
[1]*Department of Food Science, Purdue University, West Lafayette, IN,*
[2]*Department of Animal Science, University of Connecticut, Storrs, CT,*
*USA*

## 1. Introduction

Urinary Tract Infections (UTIs) account for nearly 8 million physician visits and 1.5 million visits to emergency rooms annually in the United States (Foxman, 2003; Litwin et al., 2005; Stamm and Hooton, 1993). It is the second most common infection of any organ and is one of the most common infections in humans (Tabiban et al., 2008). UTIs account for a total annual cost of more than $ 3.5 billion in the United States (Litwin et al., 2005). UTI refers to the presence of clinical signs and symptoms arising from the genitourinary tract associated with the presence of one or more microorganisms (Guay, 2009). UTIs are usually localized to the bladder, kidneys or prostate. The term UTI in this chapter refers to infections of the lower urinary tract that involve the bladder and urethra. *Escherichia coli* is the predominant uropathogen responsible for roughly 80% of all UTI cases, followed by *Staphylococcus, Klebsiella, Enterobacter, Proteus* and *Enterococci* species (Ronald, 2003).
There are several approaches to the treatment and management of UTIs. Accurate classification of cases is the foremost and critical step in the clinical management of UTIs. UTIs may be primarily distinguished between the two anatomic locations of the infection, namely upper and lower tract infections. In majority of cases, the infection is associated with the lower part of the tract (Najar et al., 2009). Additionally, the infection may also be classified as complicated and uncomplicated based on the level of tissue involvement. Uncomplicated infections engross an episode of cysto-urethritis associated with bacterial colonization of the ureteral and bladder mucosa. Complicated infections involve pyelonephritis or prostitis and often occur as a result of obstruction or instrumentation in the tract (Huland and Busch, 1984; Najar et al., 2009). UTIs may also be classified as recurrent infection, reinfection or relapse (Najar et al., 2009). Reinfection is recurring infection due to a different microorganism that is usually drug susceptible, whereas relapse is a return of infection due to the same microorganism which is drug resistant. A relapse implies that there has been a failure to eradicate the infection (Cattell, 1973).
Traditionally, the treatment of UTIs consists of antimicrobial therapy administered in a regimen appropriate to the clinical situation, freqently administered temporally either as a prophylactic to reduce the risk of UTI or as a therapeutic approach. Several antibiotics such as penicillins, sulfanilamide, nitrofurantoin and cephalexin have been used in therapy (Nicolle, 2002). The customary UTI treatment involves a short course of antimicrobials such as a 3-day regimen of trimethorpim-sulfamethoxazole combination (Nickel, 2005a). This

initial therapy is based on knowledge of the predominant pathogens and their antimicrobial susceptibility (Perez-Lopez et al., 2009). Besides the therapeutic approach, preventive treatment with antibiotics are also administered to susceptible populations, including the elderly, children and women with recurrent UTIs. However, one major drawback to the use of antibiotics is the potential for development of antibiotic resistance among uropathogens (Head et al., 2008). The increasing prevalence of antibiotic resistant bacteria, escalating costs of antibiotic therapy and unsatisfactory therapeutic alternatives in recurrent UTIs have stimulated an interest in novel, non-antibiotic based methods for preventing and controlling UTIs (Vaughan, 2007; Smith et al., 2006).

## 2. Alternative treatment options

UTIs have been a common illness in humans long before bacteria were recognized as the causative agents. Initial therapy for UTIs was primarily the use of herbal treatments to ameliorate urinary symptoms, as recorded in the Ebers papyrus from ancient Egypt (Nickel, 2005b). The early 19$^{th}$ century provided detailed descriptions of UTIs with treatment that included hospitalization, bed rest, attention to diet, plastics, narcotics, herbal enemas, douches and surgery for stones, abscess and retention (Nickel, 2005b). However, with the advent of modern medicine, the use of select antibacterial agents and antibiotics for the treatment of UTIs was put into practice. Although the effectiveness of antibiotics was validated in clinical practice, the continued use of select agents in the prophylaxis and therapy of UTIs led to the emergence of antibiotic resistant uropathogens (Nickel, 2005c). This triggered an interest in the application of alternative, non-antibiotic approaches for preventing and controlling UTIs. This chapter discusses the various alternative approaches that are currently available and are being evaluated to control UTIs. These include the use of plant derived antimicrobials, probiotics, and vaccines targeting specific proteins in uropathogens.

### 2.1 Plant derived antimicrobials

Historically, plants have served as a basis for development of novel drugs, thereby contributing to human health and well-being. A variety of plant-derived polyphenols serve as dietary constituents as well as active components in a number of herbal and traditional medicines (Wollenweber, 1988). In excess of 5000 plant polyphenols have been identified, and several of them exhibit a wide spectrum of biological effects, including anti-inflammatory, antimicrobial, and anti-carcinogenic properties (Beretz et al., 1978). Several of them have been also used in the treatment and control of UTIs. These include cranberry, blueberry, berberine, bearberry, cinnamon and other herbs. Since several plant antimicrobials contain different functional groups in their structure, their antimicrobial activity is attributed to multiple mechanisms (Burt, 2004). Therefore, unlike antibiotics, the potential for bacteria to develop resistance to plant antimicrobials is relatively smaller (Ohno et al., 2003).

#### 2.1.1 *Vaccinium macrocarpon* (Cranberry)

A significant body of literature exists on the positive effects of dietary intake of berry fruits on human health, performance and disease (Seeram, 2008). The ripe fruit of the cranberry is the part of the plant that is most commonly used for medicinal purposes. Cranberries are composed of 80-88% water and approximately 10% carbohydrates. Flavanoids, anthocyanins, catechin, triterpenoids, organic acids and ascorbic acid are the other constituents that make up the rest of the 10% (Siciliano, 1996; Raz et al., 2004). Cranberry products such as the juice and tablets have been used as an alternative medicine to prevent UTIs in humans for decades.

Clinical and epidemiological studies support the use of cranberry in maintaining a healthy urinary tract (Perez-Lopez et al., 2009). The first controlled clinical trial demonstrating the use of cranberry juice in reducing the presence of bacteria in urine was conducted by Avorn and others (1994). This study included 192 participants, where baseline urine samples, followed by monthly samples were collected over a six month period, during which participants regularly consumed 300 ml of cranberry juice daily. The results of this study revealed that bacteriuria and pyuria occurred in 28% of the placebo group in comparison to only 14% in the cranberry juice group. Following this initial study, there have been several other investigations that demonstrated the antimicrobial property of cranberries against uropathogens. Although several studies have tested the antimicrobial effect of cranberries against multiple uropathogens, it was found to be most effective against uropathogenic *E. coli* (UPEC).

Di Martino et al (2005) investigated the effect of cranberry juice on UPEC biofilm population in a small group of human subjects. Similarly, Bailey et al (2007) conducted a study in women with recurrent UTI to evaluate the effects of a daily dose of concentrated cranberry extracts for a period of 12 weeks. In another study conducted by Bohbot (2007), a comparison was made between the use of proanthocyanidins (PAC) and cranberry total components. The results of the study demonstrated that components other than PAC also contribute to the UTI preventive effect of cranberries.

No definitive mechanism of action has been identified to explain the antimicrobial effect of cranberries against uropathogens. The initial hypothesis suggested that cranberry acidity produces the antibacterial effect in the body, but it was later disproved (Blatherwick and Long, 1923). Cranberries exert anti-adhesive effects on certain uropathogens (Ohnishi et al., 2006) and this effect is specific to certain components of cranberry (Ofek et al., 1991). Cranberries contain three different flavonoids (flavonols, anthocyanins and PAC), catechins, hydroxycinnamic and other phenolic acids and triterpenoids. The anthocyanins are absorbed in the human circulatory system and transported without any chemical change to the urine (Perez-Lopez et al., 2009). Cranberry products do not inhibit bacterial growth, but inhibit bacterial adherence to uroepithelial cells, thereby reducing the development of UTI. The anti-adhesive effects of p-fimbriated UPEC to uroepithelial cells are related to A-linked PAC as compared with lack of anti-adhesion activities of B-linked PAC from grape, apple juice, green tea and chocolate (Howell et al., 2005). The A-type PAC in cranberries enhance the anti-adhesive effects *in vitro* and in urine. PAC binds to lipopolysaccharide in gram negative bacteria. When *E. coli* was grown in the presence of cranberry components, the bacterial morphology changed to a more spherical cell-like form. These changes cause them to be repelled by the human cells (Liu et al., 2006).

Lavigne et al (2008) investigated the effect of cranberry capsules on bacterial adherence to urinary tract. Participants who consumed cranberry capsules showed a significant dose-dependent reduction in bacterial adherence to urinary epithelial cells compared to placebo. Another potential mechanism of action of cranberry against UPEC is the non-enzymatic generation of nitric oxide under mildly acidic conditions (MacMiking et al., 1997). Nitric oxide possesses potent antimicrobial activities that are both time and dose-dependent.

Although, cranberry has demonstrated potential against UTIs, dose administration recommendations of cranberry products have been poorly defined (Perez-Lopez et al., 2009). Available products include sweetened cranberry juice (OceanSpray®), which is 25% pure juice. Recommended doses vary from 4 to 32 oz/day. Recommended doses of the dried concentrated juice range from 600 to greater than 1200 mg/day (Ross, 2006; Lynch, 2004).

Cranberry has undergone extensive evaluation in the management of UTIs. Currently, there is no evidence that cranberry can be used to treat UTIs. Hence, the focus has been on its use as a prophylactic agent in the prevention of UTIs (Guay, 2009). The consumption of cranberry juice can help to prevent the adhesion of UPEC to the uroepithelium and thereby help reduce the incidence of UTIs. With rising concerns of antibiotic resistance among UPEC, cranberry could serve as an effective alternative in controlling UTIs.

#### 2.1.2 *Vaccinium myrtillus* (Bilberry; Blueberry)

Blueberry extracts possess constituents similar to that found in cranberry extracts. Although extensive studies have not been performed on the antimicrobial effects of blueberry extracts, evidence indicates that blueberry extracts possess similar anti-adhesive effects against uropathogenic bacteria (Head, 2008). When compared to other fruit extracts such as guava, mango, orange, grapefruit or pineapple, blueberry constituents were reported to bind to the same uroepithelial cells where bacteria attach (Ofek et al., 1991; 1996). These studies demonstrated that the constituents in blueberry extracts like those in cranberry inhibited UPEC from adhering to the uroepithelial cells using the mannose-resistant adhesins. Similarly, Weiss et al (2002), compared the effect of cranberry, mango, melon, peach, plum and raspberry extracts on the ability of oral bacteria to aggregate and colonize the oral mucosa. It was found that only members of the *Vaccinium* genus were able to inhibit the bacterial aggregation. Cranberry extract was found to be most effective followed by blueberry, thus suggesting that blueberry may also serve as an alternative to the use of antibiotics in preventing UTIs.

#### 2.1.3 Berberine

Berberine is an alkaloid present in many plants, including *Hydrastis canadensis* (goldenseal), *Coptis chinensis* (Coptis or goldenthread), *Berberis aquifolium* (Oregon grape), *Berberis vulgaris* (barberry) and *Berberis aristata* (tree turmeric). Berberine is present in the root, rhizome, and stem bark of the plants. Berberine extracts have been shown to be effective against a variety of organisms, including bacteria, viruses, fungi, protozoans, helminthes and Chlamydia (Head, 2008). Research using berberine demonstrated its inhibitory effect on the growth of several bacterial pathogens such as *Staphylococcus aureus, Pseudomonas aeruginosa, , E. coli, and Bacillus subtilis* (Cernakova and Kostalova, 2002). Supporting this finding, another study revealed that alkaloids from *Hydrastis* sp. possessed antibacterial activity against *E. coli*, *S. aureus* and *P. aeruginosa* (Scazzocchio et al., 2001). The antimicrobial effect of the ingredient alkaloids in the order of potency was berberine > coptisine > palmatine (Yan et al., 2008). Although the mechanisms behind antimicrobial property of berbine is not completely understood, it was reported to target the FtsZ protein involved in the first stage of bacterial cell division (Domadia et al., 2008).

In controlling UTIs, the antibacterial effect of berberine was attributed to its ability to inhibit bacterial adhesion to uroepithelial cells. Sun et al (1988a) demonstrated that growth of clinical isolates of *E. coli* in the presence of berberine sulfate completely inhibited fimbrial synthesis. Likewise, berberine sulfate was found to inhibit the capacity of *Streptococcus pyogenes* to adhere to host cells (Sun et al., 1988b). Since *E. coli* infection in the urinary tract has been attributed to the migration of the pathogen from the gut, a reduction of *E. coli* load in the gut can indirectly reduce UTIs (Rabbani et al., 1987). In this context, berberine has been demonstrated to reduce *E. coli* induced diarrhea in human and animal subjects through its anti-secretory effects, thereby reducing the likelihood of bacterial migration into the urinary tract (Sach and Froehlich, 1982).

### 2.1.4 *Arctostaphylos uva ursi* (Bearberry)

This is another fruit commonly used for its antimicrobial property in controlling UTIs (Head, 2008). The active antimicrobial ingredient in bearberry is an aglycone hydroquinone which is released in alkaline urine (Uva ursi, 2004). A study conducted by Schindler et al (2002) involving human subjects who consumed a dried leaf extract of uva ursi showed that 64.8% of arbutin consumed in tablet form and 66.7% of arbutin ingested in aqueous solution were released in the urine. This significant level of the fruit extract in urine was attributed to its antimicrobial effect. Frohne (1970) and Kedzia et al (1975) conducted clinical studies with human subjects in which urine from patients given extracts of uva ursi or isolated arbutin was evaluated. The urine from the treatment group demonstrated significant antimicrobial activity against *E. coli, P. mirabilis, P. aeruginosa, S. aureus* and 70 other urinary bacteria. Frohne (1970) also demonstrated that the crude extract of uva ursi was more effective against bacteria than arbutin by itself. The one and only clinical study to investigate the effect of uva ursi in controlling UTIs was conducted by Larsson et al (1993). This study involved 57 women with chronic UTIs who were assigned to uva ursi extract or placebo for a period of one month and subsequently followed for a year. A statistically significant reduction in the incidence of UTIs was noted in the treatment group when compared to that in the placebo group, thereby demonstrating its efficacy as an antimicrobial against UTIs. The antimicrobial activity of uva ursi was attributed to its ability to change microbial cell surface characteristics. Supporting this, a study by Turi et al (1997) demonstrated that growth of clinical isolates of *E. coli* in the presence of uva ursi extracts increased the microbial cell surface hydrophobicity, thereby decreasing their ability to adhere to host cells. Additionally, uva ursi has diuretic and anti-inflammatory effects that indirectly aid in its use as an antimicrobial to control UTIs (Beaux et al., 1999; Kubo et al., 1990).

### 2.1.5 Trans-cinnamaldehyde

Trans-cinnamaldehyde (TC) is a major component of the bark extract of cinnamon (Adams et al., 2004). It is a generally recognized as safe (GRAS) molecule approved for use in foods by the Food and Drug Administration (FDA). The U. S. Flavoring Extract Manufacturers' Association reported that TC has a wide margin of safety between conservative estimates of intake and no observed adverse effect levels, from sub-chronic and chronic studies (Adams *et al.*, 2004). The report also indicated no genotoxic or mutagenic effects due to TC. The antibacterial activity of TC against *Clostridium botulinum* (Bowles and Miller, 1993), *S. aureus* (Bowles *et al.*, 1995), *E. coli* O157:H7 and *Salmonella* Typhimurium (Helander *et al.*, 1998) has been previously reported. Although, cinnamon or cinnamon oil has been used for ages in the treatment of UTIs, no scientific study was undertaken to investigate its antimicrobial efficacy against uropathogens. Amalaradjou et al (2010) were the first to demonstrate the ability of trans-cinnamaldehyde to inactivate and inhibit UPEC biofilm formation on urinary

catheters. A follow up study conducted by the same group (Amalaradjou et al., 2011) indicated that trans-cinnamaldehyde inhibited the adhesion and invasion of uroepithelial cells by UPEC by downregulating major virulence genes in the pathogen. These results indicate the potential use of trans-cinnamaldehyde as an antimicrobial for controlling UTIs.
The antimicrobial effect of TC could be attributed to multiple mechanisms. A critical property of essential oils or their components, including TC is their hydrophobicity, which helps them to target the lipid-containing bacterial cell membrane and mitochondria (Sikkema et al., 1994). This makes these membranes more permeable, leading to leakage of ions and other cell contents. In addition to the effect on cell membranes, TC is also believed to kill bacteria by inhibiting energy generation and glucose uptake (Gill and Holey, 2006). Yet another mechanism by which cinnamon oil and its components kill microorganisms is by their inhibitory effect on enzymes such as amino acid decarboxylases (Wendakoon and Sakaguchi, 1995). It is also known that plant essential oils and their components, including that from cinnamon are capable of inhibiting the production of virulence factors, and modulating bacterial pathogenesis (Smith-Palmer et al., 2002). For example, Smith-Palmer and coworkers (2004) reported that sub-inhibitory concentrations of oils of cinnamon, bay, clove and thyme significantly decreased the production of enterotoxin A and α-toxin, two virulence factors in *S aureus*. The authors concluded that since the essentials oils did not directly inactivate or prevent export of α-toxin from the cells, their inhibitory activity could be at the transcriptional or translational level. Similarly, low concentrations of cinnamaldehyde were reported to inhibit quorum sensing (QS) or cell-density dependent regulation of gene expression in *E. coli* and biofilm synthesis in *Vibrio* spp. without inhibiting bacterial growth (Brackman et al., 2008). Amalaradjou et al (2011) demonstrated that trans-cinnamaldehyde reduced the expression of several virulence genes essential for UPEC motility, host cell attachment and invasion. Thus, the ability of trans-cinnamaldehyde to inhibit bacteria through multipronged mechanisms makes it a potential candidate for use as an antimicrobial agent for controlling UTIs.

### 2.1.6 Other herbs

Essential oil extracted from *Salvia officinalis* (Garden sage; common sage) has been shown to be inhibitory against several uropathogens obtained from the urine samples of individuals with UTIs. Sage oil completely inhibited several pathogens, including *Klebsiella, Enterobacter* species, *E. coli* , *Proteus mirabilis* and *Morganella morganii* (Pereira et al., 2004). *Barosma betulina* (bachu) is another herb which has been used in the treatment of urinary tract infection, catarrhal cystitis and urethritis for a long time (Barnes et al., 2007). *In vitro* studies have demonstrated its antimicrobial effect against uropathogens (Mills and Bone, 2000). In addition to its antimicrobial effect, bachu also has diuretic properties (Simpson, 1998). Several other herbs that are used for the treatment of UTIs but lack scientific basis include *Agrimonia eupatoria* (agrimony), *Althea officinalis* (marshmallow), *Apium graveolens* (celery seed), *Arctium lappa* (burdock), *Elymus repens* (couchgrass), *Hydrangea aborescens* (hydrangea), *Juniperus communis* (juniper), *Mentha piperita* (peppermint), *Taraxacum officinalis* leaf (dandelion), *Ulmus fulva* (slippery elm) and *Zea mays* (corn silk).

## 2.2 Dietary interventions

Besides the use of antimicrobials, several nutrients have been used in the management, prevention and treatment of UTIs. These include vitamins, salts, and sugars.

### 2.2.1 Vitamins

Ochoa et al (2007) investigated the efficacy of vitamin C for its effect on UTIs in pregnant women. The study consisted of 110 pregnant women who were divided into two groups. One group received a dose of 100 mg vitamin C daily while the other group was used as a control for a period of three months. Urine sample was collected from the subjects and evaluated for presence of uropathogens. The results of this study revealed that the vitamin C group had a significantly lower incidence of UTIs than the control group. Similarly, the use of vitamin A in the management of UTIs in children was evaluated by Yilmaz et al (2007). This study tested 24 children, 12 in the vitamin A group who received 200,000 IU of vitamin A, in addition to antimicrobial therapy for 10 days and 12 in the control group who just received the antimicrobial. The subjects were followed for one year and continued on antibiotic prophylaxis. It was observed that the children in the vitamin A group had a significantly lower incidence of UTIs than the control group.

### 2.2.2 Citrate salts

The purpose behind the use of citrate salts in the management of UTIs is to alkalinize the urine, since alkaline urine can provide significant benefit for UTI symptoms such as dysuria. In a study conducted by Spooner (1984), it was shown that intake of sodium citrate in women with UTI for a period of 48 hours significantly improved symptoms in 80 percent of the subjects with bacteriuria. In addition to improving symptoms like dysuria, alkalinity in the urine aids to provide an effective environment for certain antimicrobials such as uva ursi and berberine to function (Head, 2008). Potassium and sodium citrate have also been found to be effective against urinary candidiasis, a mold infection associated with the presence of indwelling catheters. Strassner and Friesen (1995), in a clinical study with hospitalized patients, demonstrated that oral intake of potassium-sodium-hydrogen-citrate for a period of two days to one month resulted in a significant increase in urinary pH and simultaneous disappearance of Candida in the urine.

### 2.2.3 D- mannose

Simple sugars like D-mannose prevent adherence of bacteria to uroepithelial cells. Ofek and Beachey (1978) identified a mannose-specific lectin on the surface of adherent strains of *E. coli*. Mannose functions as the primary bladder cell receptor site for UPEC to bind. Likewise, Hung et al (2002) reported that the first step in the adhesion of UPEC to the uroepithelial cells is the binding of FimH adhesin to the bladder epithelium via interaction with mannose moieties on the host cell surface. Thus the use of mannose or mannose analogs can help to block adhesion of *E. coli* to the bladder epithelium.

Several studies have also investigated the efficacy of alpha-glycosides of mannose and D-mannose in controlling UTIs (Firon et al., 1987; Schaeffer et al., 1984). An *in vivo* study conducted in mouse demonstrated that D-mannose not only blocked adhesion of *E. coli* to the urinary tract epithelium, but also prevented bacterial invasion and subsequent biofilm formation (Wellens et al., 2008). Growth of *E. coli* strains isolated from women with recurrent UTIs in the presence of D-mannose inhibited the adherence of *E. coli* by 42% (Schaffer et al., 1984). Similarly in a study of urinary tract epithelial cells collected from voided urine of healthy women, use of a 2.5% solution of D-mannose, D- mannitol or alpha-methyl-D-mannoside completely inhibited *E. coli* adherence to the uroepithelium. However, when a similar concentration of D-lyxose, D-arabinose, D-fructose and D-glyceraldehyde

were used, only a partial inhibition of bacterial adhesion was noticed. Additionally, the use of lower concentrations (0.1-1.0%) of mannose, mannitol and mannoside also resulted in a partial inhibition of bacterial adhesion to urinary tract epithelial cells (Schaffer et al., 1980).
In addition to the use of naturally existing mannose residues and its derivatives in the control of UTIs, Klein et al (2010) synthesized and evaluated the efficacy of several mannosides in blocking bacterial-host interaction. Among the different mannosides developed and evaluated using a mouse UTI model, para substituted biphenyl derivative of D-mannose was found to be the most effective in controlling UTIs. Following oral administration of this mannoside, bacterial numbers were reduced by 2 orders and 4 orders of magnitude in the urine and bladder, respectively. This FimH antagonist thus provides an alternative approach with a new class of orally available antimicrobials for effective treatment of UTIs.

### 2.3 Probiotics

Probiotics are live organisms which when administered in adequate amounts confer a health benefit on the host (FAO/WHO, 2001). The rationale for the use of probiotics is based on the gastrointestinal and genitourinary regulatory role played by the commensal microflora, and the need for restoration of this microbial ecosystem after an imbalance or infection (Barrons and Tassone, 2008). For use as a probiotic in controlling UTIs, the candidate culture must exhibit adequate antibacterial properties. For example, an important attribute of an ideal probiotic culture such as lactobacilli is the ability to maintain a low pH $\leq 4.5$, where the acidic environment provides lactobacilli a favorable environment to multiply and produce additional antibacterial molecules, including bacteriocin and hydrogen peroxide (Aroutcheva et al., 2001). In a study investigating the defense factors against infection in 22 lactobacilli strains isolated from healthy human vaginal ecosystems, moderate to high production of hydrogen peroxide and bacteriocin was observed in 82% and 68% of the strains (Aroutcheva et al., 2001).
Besides their ability to produce acid, hydrogen peroxide and bacteriocins, lactobacilli may also offer protection against UTIs through the production of biosurfactants. Biosurfactants inhibit growth of uropathogens by inhibiting the adhesion of these pathogens to the uroepithelium (Velraeds et al., 1996). A study conducted using 15 strains of lactobacilli showed that the strains produced varying amounts of biosurfactants providing up to 82% inhibition of *Enterococcus fecalis* adhesion to a glass surface (Velraeds et al., 1996). Moreover, lactobacilli co-aggregate with uropathogens to block their adhesion and/or displace previously adherent uropathogens from the urinary tract. This co-aggregation can create a microenvironment in which the inhibitory substances produced by the lactobacilli can concentrate on the pathogens and inhibit them (Mastromarino et al., 2002).
Osset et al (2001) conducted an *in vitro* study in which the antimicrobial ability of 15 *Lactobacillus* species against pathogens was investigated. *Lactobacillus crispatus* was found to be the species that demonstrated the strongest ability to block pathogen adhesion. Another *in vitro* study examined the antagonistic effect of five probiotic species against six pathogenic bacteria. The results revealed that a pyelonephritic *E. coli* strain was sensitive to *Lactobacillus rhamnosus* GG, *Bifidobacterium lactis* Bb 12 and *Bifidobacterium longus* 46 (Hutt et al., 2006).
Several clinical studies have investigated the effect of probiotic suppositories for the prevention of UTIs. Reid et al (1992) investigated the effect of probiotic lactobacill in controlling infection in women with acute UTIs (Reid et al., 1995). These patients were

treated with antibiotics for three days and recurrence occurred in 41% of the patients. These individuals were randomly assigned to Lactobacillus suppositories or placebo suppositories twice weekly for two weeks, then once a month for the next two months. Recurrence was 21 percent in the Lactobacillus group compared to 47% in the placebo group. The same group of researchers conducted a follow-up study comparing the effects of suppositories containing the Lactobacillus species with suppositories containing Lactobacillus growth factor. The subjects were administered with either one of the suppositories once weekly for 12 months. At the end of the 12 months, both the groups exhibited a 73% reduction in the incidence of UTIs (Reid et al., 1995).

Studies were also conducted to evaluate the efficacy of oral probiotics in controlling UTIs. In order for an oral probiotic to be effective, it must be able to colonize the intestinal and/or urogenital region. *L. rhamonosus* GR-1 and *L. fermentum* RC-14 were administered twice daily for 14 days and the bacterial recovery from the vaginal tissue was monitored (Reid et al., 2001). It was observed that the vaginal epithelium was colonized with lactobacilli within one week of the oral administration (Reid et al., 2001). Similarly studies in pediatric populations revealed that administration of *L. rhamnosus* GG orally for 50 days resulted in a reduction in UTI incidence rate compared to the placebo group (Dani et al., 2002). Taken together, results from these aforementioned studies suggest the potential benefit of probiotics in controlling UTIs.

## 2.4 Hormone therapy

In postmenopausal women, hormone waning results in thinning of the vaginal and urethral mucosa, disruption of the normal vaginal flora and an increased risk for UTIs (Head, 2008). Therefore administration of estrogen in such patients has been reported to reduce UTIs. A randomized study including postmenopausal women evaluated the effect of intravaginally administered estriol in reducing UTIs. The results of this study showed a significant reduction in the incidence of UTIs compared to the placebo group. It was also observed that Lactobacilli that were absent in the vaginal cultures of subjects at the beginning of the trial reappeared in 61 percent of the estriol group (Raz and Stamm, 1993).

## 2.5 Vaccines

As with other infectious diseases, UTIs can also be controlled using vaccines. Wieser et al.(2010) reported that an ideal vaccine target against uropathogens should be (i) exposed on the bacterial surface and (ii) widely distributed among clinical isolates but not among commensal strains of the gut flora, (iii) possess epitopes that are conserved across diverse strains, and (iv) elicit a protective immune response. Additional desirable characteristics of an effective vaccine target include increased expression at the site of infection and a role in the pathogenesis of disease (Wieser et al., 2010).

Several studies have investigated the use of potential antigens as targets for vaccine development against UPEC. Initial studies for vaccine candidates consisted of single target protein or whole cells. Langermann et al (1997) evaluated the use of an adhesion based vaccine targeting the FimH protein on the surface of UPEC. Immunization with FimH reduced *in vivo* bacterial colonization of the bladder mucosa by more than 99 percent in a murine cystitis model, and immunoglobulin G to FimH was detected in the urinary samples from protected mice. Additionally, passive systemic administration of immune sera to FimH also resulted in reduced bladder colonization by UPEC. A similar study by Li et al (2004) developed an intranasal vaccine against *Proteus mirabilis* infections in the urinary tract. The mice were vaccinated with formalin-killed bacteria or purified mannose-resistant Proteus-like fimbriae (MR/P), a surface antigen expressed by *P. mirabilis* during UTI. Four different routes of administration, including subcutaneous, intradermal, intranasal and trans urethral were evaluated in this study, where intranasal administration of MR/P elicited the most protective immune response against *P. mirabilis* UTI.

Alteri et al (2009) investigated the use of six novel vaccine candidates against UPEC. These candidates were indentified using bioinformatics, functional genomics, transcriptomic and proteomic analyses. All the six proteins belonged to the class of outer membrane iron receptors that are upregulated in an iron restricted environment. Intranasal administration of these antigens in mice elicited both systemic and mucosal immune responses that included the production of antigen-specific IgM, IgG and IgA antibodies, cytokine responses and protection against UTI in the mouse model (Alteri et al., 2009). A similar study was also conducted by Wieser et al (2010), where they evaluated the use of a subunit vaccine against extra intestinal *E. coli*. Using a novel approach of computer-aided design, two completely artificial genes were created, both encoding eight peptide domains derived from these extra intestinal *E. coli* proteins. In mice, the vaccine was highly immunogenic, eliciting both strong humoral and cellular immune responses. Nasal application of the vaccine resulted in high secretory immunoglobulin A (sIgA) production, which was detectable on the mucosal surface of the urogenital tract. Finally, it bestowed protection, as shown by a significant reduction of bacterial load in a mouse model of extra intestinal *E. coli* peritonitis.

Besides the use of immunogenic antigens as vaccines, immunotherapy for UTIs can also be accomplished using immunomodulants. A study carried by Krcmery et al (2010) investigated the efficacy of two immunomodulatory agents (Urovaxom and luivac) for the management of recurrent UTIs in women over a 12 month period. The results indicated that a combined treatment using immunotherapy and chemoprophylaxis significantly reduced the occurrences of UTI relapses in these women.

## 3. Conclusion

Infections of the genitourinary tract are common occurrences in individuals especially in young women, during pregnancy and in post menopausal women. The conventional use of antibiotics in the prevention and treatment of acute and chronic recurring infections contribute to gut and vaginal dysbiosis and bacterial antibiotic resistance. In an attempt to control the increasing trends in infections with antibiotic resistant uropathogens, there is a renewed interest in the use of non-antibiotic based intervention strategies against UTIs. Several studies have investigated the use of natural substances in the prevention and treatment of UTIs. Nutrients and botanicals such as cranberry, berberine, cinnamaldehyde, probiotics and vaccines have demonstrated the greatest effectiveness. While most clinical research has evaluated the antimicrobial potential of these natural substances, their mechanism of action and the clinical experience of health care practitioners are critical for evaluating their effectiveness (Head, 2008). Use of these alternatives in the control of UTIs would help to circumvent dysbiosis and microbial drug resistance induced by the repeated use of antibiotics.

## 4. References

Adams, T. B., Cohen, S. M., Doull, J., Feron, V. J., Goodman, J. I., Marnett, L. J., Munro, I, C., Portoghese, P. S. Smith, R. L., Waddell, W. J. & Wagner, B. M. (2004). The FEMA GRAS assessment of cinnamyl derivatives used as flavor ingredients. *Food Chemistry and Toxicology*, Vol. 42, No. 2,(February 2004), pp.157-185 ISSN 0278-6915

Alteri, C. J., Hagan, E. C., Sivick, K. E., Smith, S. N. & Mobley, H. L. (2009). Mucosal immunization with iron receptor antigens protects against urinary tract infection. *PLoS Pathog*, Vol. 5, No. 9, (September 2009), pp.e1000586 ISSN 1553-7374

Amalaradjou, M. A., Narayanan, A. & Venkitanarayanan, K. 2011. Trans-cinnamaldehyde decreases attachment and invasion of uropathogenic *Escherichia coli* in urinary tract epithelial cells by modulating virulence gene expression. J Urol, Vol. 185, No. 4, (April 2011), pp.1526-1531 ISSN 0022-5347

Amalaradjou, M. A., Narayanan, A., Baskaran, S. A. & Venkitanarayanan, K. 2010. Antibiofilm effect of trans-cinnamaldehyde on uropathogenic *Escherichia coli*. *J Urol*, Vol. 184, No. 1, (July 2010), pp.358-363 ISSN 0022-5347

Aroutcheva, A., Gariti, D., Simon, M., Shott, S., Faro, J., Simoes, J. A., Gurguis, A. & Faro, S. (2001). Defense factors of vaginal Lactobacilli. *Am J Obstet Gynecol*, Vol. 185, No. 2, (August 2001), pp.375-379 ISSN 0002-9378

Avorn, J., Monane, M., Gurwitz, J. H., Glynn, R. J., Choodnovskiy, I. & Lipsitz, L. A. (1994). Reduction of bacteriuria and pyuria after ingestion of cranberry juice. *JAMA*, Vol. 271, No. 10, (March 1994), pp. 751-754 ISSN *0098-7484*

Bailey, D. T., Dalton, C., Joseph Daugherty, F. & Tempesta, M. S. (2007). Can a concentrated cranberry extract prevent recurrent urinary tract infections in women? A pilot study. *Phytomedicine*, Vol. 14, No. 4, (April 2007), pp. 237-241 ISSN 0944-7113

Barnes, J., Anderson, L. A. & Phillipson, J. D. (2007). *Herbal Medicines*. 3rd ed. Grayslake, IL: Pharmaceutical Press ISBN 0853696233

Barrons, R. & Tassone, D. (2008). Us eof Lactobacillus probiotics for bacterial genitourinary infections in women: A review. *Clinical Therapeutics*, Vol. 30, No. 3, (November 2008), pp.453-468 ISSN 0149-2918

Beaux, D., Fleurentin, J. & Mortier, F. (1999). Effect of extracts of *Orthosiphon stamineus Benth, Hieracium pilosella L., Sambucus nigra L.* and *Arctostaphylos uva-ursi* (L.) Spreng. in rats. *Phytother Res*, Vol. 13, No. 3, (May 1999), pp.222-225 ISSN 0951-418X

Beretz, A., Anton, R. & Stoclet, J. C. (1978). Flavonoid compounds are potent inhibitors of cyclic AMP phosphodiesterase. *Experientia*, Vol. 34, No. 8, (August 1978) pp. 1054-1055 ISSN 0014-4754

Blatherwick, N. R. & Long, M. L. (1923). Studies of urinary acidity. II. The increased acidity produced by eating prunes and cranberries. *J Biol Chem*, Vol. 57, No. 3, (October 1923), pp. 815-818 ISSN 0021-9258

Bohbot, J. M. (2007). Resultas d'une etude randomisee en double aveugle sur la prevention des cystitis recidivants par GynDelta. *La Revue Pract Gynecol Obstetr*,No. 3, pp. 3-6 ISSN 0035-290X

Borchert, D., Sheridan, L., Papatsoris, A., Faruquz, Z., Barua, J. M., Junaid, I., Pati, Y., Chinegwundoh, F. & Buchholz, N. (2008). Prevention and treatment of urinary tract infection with probiotics: Review and research perspective. *Indian J Urol*, Vol. 24, No. 2, (April 2008), pp. 139-144 ISSN 0970-1591

Bowles, B. L. & Miller, A. J. (1993). Antibotulinal properties of selected aromatic and aliphatic aldehydes. *J Food Prot*, Vol. 5, pp.788-794 ISSN 0362-028X

Bowles, B. L., Sackitey, S. K. & Williams, A. C. 1995. Inhibitory effects of flavor compounds on *Staphylococcus aureus* WRRC B124. Journal of Food Safety, Vol. 15, pp.337-347 ISSN 1745-4565

Brackman, G., Defoirdt, T., Miyamoto, C., Bossier, P., Van Calenbergh, S., Nelis, H. & Coenye. T. (2008). Cinnamaldehyde and cinnamaldehyde derivatives reduce virulence in *Vibrio* spp. by decreasing the DNA-binding activity of the quorum sensing response regulator LuxR. *BMC Microbiol*, Vol. 8, pp.149, ISSN 1471-2180

Burt, S. (2004). Essential oils: their antibacterial properties and potential applications in foods - a review. *Intl J Food Microbiol,* Vol. 94, No. 3, (August 2004), pp. 223-253 ISSN 0168-1605

Catell, W. R. (1973). The localization of urinary tract infection and its relationship to relapse, reinfection and treatment. IN. Brumfitt, W. & Asscher, A. W. *Urinary Tract Infection.* ISBN 0387901477, London: Oxford University Press; 1973. Pp. 206-214.

Cernáková, M. & Kostálová, D. (2002). Antimicrobial activity of berberine - a constituent of *Mahonia aquifolium*. *Folia Microbiol*, Vol. 47, No. 4, (August, 2002), pp. 375-378 ISSN 0015-5632

Dani, C., Biadaioli, R., Bertini, G., Martelli, E. & Rubaltelli, F. F. (2002). Probiotics feeding in prevention of urinary tract infection, bacterial sepsis and necrotizing enterocolitis in preterm infants. A prospective double-blind study. *Biol Neonate*, Vol. 82, No. 2, (August 2002), pp.103-108 ISSN 0006-3126

Di Martino, P., Agniel, R., Gaillard, J. L. & Denys, P. (2005). Effects of cranberry juice on uropathogenic *Escherichia coli in vitro* biofilm formation. *J Chemother*, Vol. 17, No. 5, (October 2005), pp. 563-565 ISSN 1120-009X

Domadia PN, Bhunia A, Sivaraman J, Swarup S, Dasgupta D. (2008). Berberine targets assembly of *Escherichia coli* cell division protein FtsZ. *Biochemistry*, Vol. 47, No. 10, (March 2008), pp.3225-3234 ISSN *0006-2960*

FAO/WHO. (2001). Report of a joint FAO/WHO expert consultation on health and nutritional properties of probiotics in food including powder milk with live lactic acid bacteria. American Cordoba Park Hotel, Cordoba, Argentina, 1-4 October 2001 http://www.who.int/foodsafety/publications/fs_management/en/probiotics.pdf . Accessed April 02, 2010

Firon, N., Ashkenazi, S., Mirelman, D., Ofek, I. & Sharon, N. (1987). Aromatic alpha-glycosides of mannose are powerful inhibitors of the adherence of type 1 fimbriated *Escherichia coli* to yeast and intestinal epithelial cells. *Infect Immun*, Vol. 55, No. 2, (February 1987), pp.472-476 ISSN 0019-9567

Foxman, B. (2003). Epidemiology of urinary tract infections: incidence, morbidity, and economic costs. *Dis. Mon.*, Vol. 49, No. 2, (February 2003), pp. 53-70 ISSN 0011-5029

Frohne, D. (1970). The urinary disinfectant effect of extract from leaves uva ursi. *Planta Med*, Vol. 18, No. 1, (January 1970), pp. 1-25 ISSN 0032-0943

Gill, A. O. & Holley, R. A., 2006. Disruption of *Escherichia coli, Listeria monocytogenes* and *Lactobacillus sakei* cellular membranes by plant oil aromatics. *Int J Food Microbiol,* Vol. 108, pp.1-9 ISSN 0168-1605

Guay, D. R. P. (2009). Cranberry and urinary tract infections. *Drugs,* Vol. 69, No. 7, (May 2009), pp. 775-807 ISSN 0012-6667

Head, K. A. (2008). Natural approaches to prevention and treatment of the lower urinary tract. *Alternative Medicine Review,* Vol. 13, No. 3, (September 2008), pp. 227-244 ISSN 1089-5159

Helander, I. M., Alakomi, H. L., Latva-Kala, K., Mattila-Sandholm, Y., Pol, L., Smid, E. J., Gorris, L. G. M. & von Wright, A., 1998. Characterization of the action of selected essential oil components on gram-negative bacteria. *J Agric Food chem,* Vol. 46, pp.3590-3595 ISSN

Howell, A. B., Reed, J. D., Krueger, C. G., Winterbottom, R., Cunningham, D. G. & Leahy, M. (2005). A-type cranberry proanthocyanidins and uropathogenic bacterial anti-adhesion activity. *Phytochemistry,* Vol. 66, No. 18, (September 2005), pp. 2281-2291 ISSN 0031-9422

Huland, H. & Busch, R. (1984). Pyelonephritic scarring in 213 patients with upper and lower urinary tract infections: long-term follow-up. *J Urol,* Vol. 139, No. 5, (November 1984), pp. 936-939 ISSN 0022-5347

Hung, C. S., Bouckaert, J., Hung, D., Pinkner, J., Widberg, C., DeFusco, A., Auguste, C. G., Strouse, R., Langermann, S., Waksman, G. & Hultgren, S. J. 2002. Structural basis of tropism of *Escherichia coli* to the bladder during urinary tract infection. *Mol Microbiol,* Vol. 44, No. 4, (May 2002), pp.903-915 ISSN 0950-382X

Hütt, P., Shchepetova, J., Lõivukene, K., Kullisaar, T. & Mikelsaar, M. (2006). Antagonistic activity of probiotic Lactobacilli and Bifidobacteria against entero- and uropathogens. *J Appl Microbiol,* Vol. 100, No. 6, (June 2006), pp.1324-1332 ISSN 1365-2672

Kedzia, B., Wrociński, T., Mrugasiewicz, K., Gorecki, P. & Grzewińska, H. (1975). Antibacterial action of urine containing products of arbutin metabolism. *Med Dosw Mikrobiol,* Vol. 27, No. 3, pp.305-314 ISSN 0025-8601

Klein, T., Abgottspon, D., Wittwer, M., Rabbani, .S, Herold, J., Jiang, X., Kleeb, S., Lüthi, C., Scharenberg, M., Bezençon, J., Gubler, E., Pang, L., Smiesko, M., Cutting, B., Schwardt, O. & Ernst, B. (2010). FimH antagonists for the oral treatment of urinary tract infections: from design and synthesis to in vitro and in vivo evaluation. *J Med Chem,* Vol. 53, No. 24, (December 2010), pp.8627-8641 ISSN *1520-4804*

Krcméry, S., Hromec, J., Gábrisová, Z. & Tahotný, R. (2010). Immunotherapy and long-term chemoprophylaxis in prevention of recurrent urinary infections in women. *Vnitr Lek,* Vol. 56, No. 9, (September 2010), pp.955-960 ISSN 0042-773X

Kubo, M., Ito, M., Nakata, H. & Matsuda, H. (1990). Pharmacological studies on leaf of *Arctostaphylos uva-ursi* (L.) Spreng. I. Combined effect of 50% methanolic extract from Arctostaphylos uva-ursi (L.) Spreng. (bearberry leaf) and prednisolone on immuno-inflammation. *Yakugaku Zasshi,* Vol. 110, No. 1, (January 1990), pp.59-67 ISSN 1347-5231

Langermann, S., Palaszynski, S., Barnhart, M., Auguste, G., Pinkner, J. S., Burlein, J., Barren, P., Koenig, S., Leath, S., Jones, C. H. & Hultgren, S. J. (1997). Prevention of mucosal *Escherichia coli* infection by FimH-adhesin-based systemic vaccination. *Science*, Vol. 276, No. 5312, (April 1997), pp.607-611 ISSN 0036-8075

Larsson, B., Jonasson, A. & Fianu, S. (1993). Prophylactic effect of UVA-E in women with recurrent cystitis: a preliminary report. *Curr Ther Res*, Vol. 53, No. 4, (July 1993), pp. 441-443 ISSN 0011-393X

Lavigne, J. P., Bourg, G., Combescure, C., Botto, H. & Sotto, A. (2008). In-vitro and in-vivo evidence of dose-dependent decrease of uropathogenic *Escherichia coli* virulence after consumption of commercial Vaccinium macrocarpon (cranberry) capsules. *Clin Microbiol Infect*, Vol. 14, No. 4, (April 2008), pp.350-355 ISSN 1198-743X

Li, X., Erbe, J. L., Lockatell, C. V., Johnson, D. E., Jobling, M. G., Holmes, R. K. & Mobley, H. L. (2004). Use of translational fusion of the MrpH fimbrial adhesin-binding domain with the cholera toxin A2 domain, coexpressed with the cholera toxin B subunit, as an intranasal vaccine to prevent experimental urinary tract infection by *Proteus mirabilis*. *Infect Immun*, Vol. 72, No. 12, (December 2004), pp.7306-7310 ISSN 0019-9567

Litwin, M. S., Saigal, C. S., Yano, E. M., Avila, C., Geschwind, S. A. & Hanley, J. M. (2005). Urologic diseases in America project: analytical methods and principal findings. *J. Urol.*, Vol. 173, No. 3, (March 2005), pp. 933-937 ISSN 0022-5347

Liu, Y., Black, M. A., Caron, L. & Camesano, T. A.(2006). Role of cranberry juice on molecular-scale surface characteristics and adhesion behavior of *Escherichia coli*. *Biotechnol Bioeng*, Vol. 93, No. 2, (February 2006), pp. 297-305 ISSN *0006-3592*

Lynch, D. M. (2004). Cranberry for prevention of urinary tract infections. *Am Fam Physician*. Vol. 70, No. 11, (December 2004), pp.2175-2177 ISSN *0002-838X*

MacMicking, J., Xie, Q. W. & Nathan, C. (1997). Nitric Oxide and macrophage function. *Annu Rev Immunol*, Vol. 15, (April 1997), pp. 323-350 ISSN 0732-0582

Mastromarino, P., Brigidi, P., Macchia, S., Maggi, L., Pirovano, F., Trinchieri, V., Conte, U. & Matteuzz,i D. (2002). Characterization and selection of vaginal Lactobacillus strains for the preparation of vaginal tablets. *J Appl Microbiol*, Vol. 93, No. 5, (October 2002), pp.884-893 ISSN 1365-2672

Mills, S. & Bone. K. (2000). Buchu. In: *Principles and Practice phytotherapy: Mordern herbal medicine*. Churchill Livingstone, pp. 310-312 ISBN 0443060169

Najar, M. S., Saldanha, C. L. & Banday, K. A. (2009). Approach to urinary tract infections. *Indian J Nephrol*, Vol. 19, No. 4, (October 2009), pp. 129-139 ISSN 0971-4065

Nickel, J. C. (2005a). Practical management of recurrent urinary tract infections in premenopausal women. *Rev Urol*, Vol. 7, No. 1, (Winter), pp. 11-17 ISSN 1523-6161

Nickel, J. C. (2005b). Management of urinary tract infections: historical perspective and current strategies: part 1 - before antibiotics. *The Journal of Urology*, Vol. 173, No. 1, (January 2005), pp. 21-26 ISSN 0022-5347

Nickel, J. C. (2005c). Management of urinary tract infections: historical perspective and current strategies: part 2 - modern management. *The Journal of Urology*, Vol. 173, No. 1, (January 2005), pp. 27-32 ISSN 0022-5347

Nicolle, L. E. (2002). Urinary tract infection: traditional pharmacologic therapies. *Am J Med*, Vol. 113, No. 1A, (July 2002), pp. 35s-44s ISSN 0002-9343

Ochoa-Brust, G. J., Fernandez, A. R., Villanueva-Ruiz, G. J., Velasco, R., Trujillo-Hernández, B. & Vásquez, C. (2007). Daily intake of 100 mg ascorbic acid as urinary tract infection prophylactic agent during pregnancy. *Acta Obstet Gynecol Scand*, Vol. 86, No. 7, (July 2007), pp.783-787 ISSN 0300-8835

Ofek, I. & Beachey, E. H. (1978). Mannose binding and epithelial cell adherence of Escherichia coli. *Infect Immun*, Vol. 22, No. 1, (October 1978), 247-254 ISSN 0019-9567

Ofek, I., Godhar, J., Zafriri, D., Lis, H., Adar, R. & Sharon, N. (1991). Anti-*Escherichia coli* adhesion activity of cranberry and blueberry juices. *N Engl J Med*, Vol. 324, No. 22, (May 1991), pp. 1599 ISSN 0028-4793

Ofek, I., Goldhar, J. & Sharon, N. (1996). Anti-*Escherichia coli* adhesin activity of cranberry and blueberry juices. *Adv Exp Med Biol*, Vol. 408, pp.179-83 ISSN 0065-2598

Ohnishi, R., Ito, H., Kasajima, N., Kaneda, M., Kariyama, R., Kumon, H., Hatano, T. & Yoshida, T. (2006). Urinary excretion of anthocyanins in humans after cranberry juice ingestion. *Biosci Biotechnol Biochem*, Vol. 70, No. 7, (July 2006), pp. 1681-1687 ISSN 0916-8451

Ohno, T., Kita, M., Yamaoka, Y., Imamura, S., Yamamoto, T., Mitsufuji, S., Kodama, T., Kashima, K. & Imanishi, J. (2003). Antimicrobial activity of essential oils against *Helicobacter pylori*. *Helicobacter*, Vol. 8, No. 3, (June 2003), pp. 207-215 ISSN 1083-4389

Osset, J., Bartolomé, R. M., García, E. & Andreu, A. (2001). Assessment of the capacity of Lactobacillus to inhibit the growth of uropathogens and block their adhesion to vaginal epithelial cells. *J Infect Dis*, Vol. 183, No. 3, (February 2001), pp.485-491 ISSN 1553-6203

Pereira, R. S., Sumita, T. C., Furlan, M. R., Jorge, A. O. & Ueno, M. (2004). Antibacterial activity of essential oils on microorganisms isolated from urinary tract infection. *Rev Saude Publica*, Vol. 38, No. 2, (April 2004), pp.326-328 ISSN 0034-8910

Pérez-López, F. R., Haya, J. & Chedraui, P. (2009). Vaccinium macrocarpon: an interesting option for women with recurrent urinary tract infections and other health benefits. *J Obstet Gynaecol Res*, Vol. 35, No. 4, (August 2009), pp. 630-639 ISSN 1341-8076

Rabbani, G. H., Butler, T., Knight, J., Sanyal, S. C. & Alam, K. (1987). Randomized controlled trial of berberine sulfate therapy for diarrhea due to enterotoxigenic *Escherichia coli* and *Vibrio cholerae*. *J Infect Dis*, Vol. 155, No. 5, (May 1987), pp.979-984 ISSN 0022-1899

Raz, R. & Stamm, W. E. (1993). A controlled trial of intravaginal estriol in postmenopausal women with recurrent urinary tract infections. *N Engl J Med*, Vol. 329, No. 11, (September 1993), pp.753-756 ISSN 0028-4793

Raz, R., Chazan, B. & Dan, M. (2004). Cranberry juice and urinary tract infection. *Clin Infect Dis*, Vol. 38, No. 10, (May 2004), pp. 1413-1419 ISSN 1058-4838

Reid, G., Bruce, A. W. & Taylor, M. (1992). Influence of three-day antimicrobial therapy and Lactobacillus vaginal suppositories on recurrence of urinary tract infections. *Clin Ther*, VOl. 14, No. 1, (January-February 1992), pp.11-16 ISSN 0149-2918

Reid, G., Bruce, A. W. & Taylor, M. (1995). Instillation of Lactobacillus and stimulation of indigenous organisms to prevent recurrence of urinary tract infections. *Microecol Ther*, Vol. 23, pp.32-45 ISSN 0720-0536

Reid, G., Beuerman, D., Heinemann, C. & Bruce, A. W. (2001). Probiotic Lactobacillus dose required to restore and maintain a normal vaginal flora. *FEMS Immunol Med Microbiol*, Vol. 32, No. 1, (December 2001), pp.37-41 ISSN 0928-8244

Ronald, A. (2003). The etiology of urinary tract infection: traditional and emerging pathogens. *Dis Mon*, Vol. 49, No. 2, (February 2003), pp. 71-82 ISSN 0011-5029

Ross, S. M. (2006). Clinical applications of cranberry in urinary tract infections. *Holist Nurs Pract*. Vol. 20, No. 4, (July-August 2006), pp.213-214 ISSN 0887-9311

Sack, R. B. & Froehlich, J. L. (1982). Berberine inhibits intestinal secretory response of *Vibrio cholerae* and *Escherichia coli* enterotoxins. *Infect Immun*, Vol. 35, No. 2, (February 1982), pp.471-475 ISSN 0019-9567

Scazzocchio, F., Cometa, M. F., Tomassini, L. & Palmery, M. (2001). Antibacterial activity of *Hydrastis canadensis* extract and its major isolated alkaloids. *Planta Med*, Vol. 67, No. 6, (August 2001), pp.561-564 ISSN 0032-0943

Schaeffer, A. J., Amundsen, S. K. & Jones, J. M. (1980). Effect of carbohydrates on adherence of *Escherichia coli* to human urinary tract epithelial cells. *Infect Immun*, Vol. 30, No. 2, (November 1980), pp.531-537 ISSN 0019-9567

Schaeffer, A. J., Chmiel, J. S., Duncan, J. L. & Falkowski, W. S. (1984). Mannose-sensitive adherence of *Escherichia coli* to epithelial cells from women with recurrent urinary tract infections. *J Urol*, Vol. 131, No. 5, (May 1984), pp.906-910 ISSN 0022-5347

Schaeffer, A. J. & Stuppy, B. A. (1999). Efficacy and safety of self-start therapy in women with recurrent urinary tract infection. *J. Urol.*, Vol. 161, No. 1, (January 1999), pp. 207-211 ISSN 0022-5347

Schindler, G., Patzak, U., Brinkhaus, B., von Niecieck, A., Wittig, J., Krähmer, N., Glöckl, I. & Veit, M. (2002). Urinary excretion and metabolism of arbutin after oral administration of *Arctostaphylos uva ursi* extract as film-coated tablets and aqueous solution in healthy humans. *J Clin Pharmacol*, Vol. 42, No. 8, (August 2002), pp.920-927 ISSN 1198-581X

Seeram, N. P. (2008). Berry fruits for cancer prevention: current status and future prospects. *J Agric Food Chem*, Vol. 56, No. 3, (February 2008), pp. 630-635 ISSN *0021-8561*

Siciliano, A. A. (1996). Cranberry. *HerbalGram,* Vol. 38, (September 1996), pp. 51-54 ISSN *0899-5648*

Sikkema, J., De Bont, J. A. M. & Poolman, B. (1994). Interactions of cyclic hydrocarbons with biological membranes. *J Biol Chem*, Vol. 269, pp. 8022-8028 ISSN 0021-9258

Simpson, D. (1998). Buchu – South Africa's amazing herbal remedy. *Scott Med J*, Vol. 43, No. 6, (December 1998), pp. 189-191 ISSN 0036-9330

Smith, R. D., Yago, M., Millar, M. & Coast, J. (2006). A macroeconomic approach to evaluating policies to contain antimicrobial resistance: A case study of methicillin-resistant *staphylococcus aureus* (MRSA). *Appl Health Econ Health Policy*, Vol. 5, No. 1, (January 2006), pp. 55-65 ISSN 1175-5652

Smith-Palmer, A., Stewartt, J &, Fyfe, L. (2002). Inhibition of listeriolysin O and phosphatidylcholine-specific production in *Listeria monocytogenes* by subinhibitory concentrations of plant essential oils. *J Med Microbiol*, Vol. 51, No. 7, pp.567-574 ISSN 0022-2615

Smith-Palmer, A., Stewart, J. & Fyfe, L. (2004). Influence of subinhibitory concentrations of plant essential oils on the production of enterotoxins A and B and alpha-toxin by *Staphylococcus aureus*. *J Med Microbiol*, Vol. 53, No. 10, pp.1023-1027 ISSN 0022-2615

Spooner, J. B. (1984). Alkalinisation in the management of cystitis. *J Int Med Res*, Vol. 12, No.1 , (January 1984), pp.30-34 ISSN 0300-0605

Stamm, W. E., & Hooton, T. M. (1993). Management of urinary tract infections in adults. *N Engl J Med*, Vol. 329, No. 18, (October 1993), pp. 1328-1334 ISSN 0028-4793

Strassner, C. & Friesen, A. (1995). Therapy of candiduria by alkalinization of the urine. Oral treatment with potassium-sodium-hydrogen citrate. *Fortschr Med*, Vol. 113, No. 25, (September 1995), pp.359-362 ISSN 0015-8178

Sun, D., Abraham, S. N. & Beachey, E. H. (1988a). Influence of berberine sulfate on synthesis and expression of Pap fimbrial adhesin in uropathogenic *Escherichia coli*. *Antimicrob Agents Chemother*, Vol. 32, No. 8, (August 1988), pp.1274-1277 ISSN 1098-6596

Sun, D., Courtney, H. S. & Beachey, E. H. (1988b). Berberine sulfate blocks adherence of *Streptococcus pyogenes* to epithelial cells, fibronectin, and hexadecane. *Antimicrob Agents Chemother*, Vol. 32, No. 9, (September 1988), pp.1370-1374 ISSN 1098-6596

Tabibian, J. H., Gornbein, J., Heidari, A., Dien, S. L., Lau, V. H., Chahal, P., Churchill, B. M. & Haake, D. A. (2008). Uropathogens and host characteristics. *J Clin Microbiol*, Vol. 46, No. 12, (December 2008), pp. 3980-3986 ISSN 0095-1137

Türi, M., Türi, E., Kõljalg, S. & Mikelsaar, M. (1997). Influence of aqueous extracts of medicinal plants on surface hydrophobicity of *Escherichia coli* strains of different origin. *APMIS*, Vol. 105, No. 12, (December, 1997), pp.956-962 ISSN 1600-0463

Uva ursi. (2004). In: LaGow, B, chief editor. *PDR for Herbal Medicines*. 3rd ed. Montvale, NJ: Thomson; pp. 847-851 ISBN 1563635127

Vaughan, V. (2007). *C. difficile* endemic in health service. *Health Serv J*, Vol. 117, No. 6038, (January 2007), pp. 6 ISSN 0020-7314

Velraeds, M. M., van der Mei, H. C., Reid, G. & Busscher, H. J. (1996). Inhibition of initial adhesion of uropathogenic *Enterococcus faecalis* by biosurfactants from Lactobacillus isolates. *Appl Environ Microbiol*, Vol. 62, No. 6, (June 1996), pp.1958-1963 ISSN 0099-2240

Weiss, E. L., Lev-Dor, R., Sharon, N. & Ofek, I. *(2002)*. Inhibitory effect of a high-molecular-weight constituent of cranberry on adhesion of oral bacteria. *Crit Rev Food Sci Nutr*, Vol. 42, No. 3, pp.285-292 ISSN 1040-8398

Wellens, A., Garofalo, C., Nguyen, A. M., Van Gerven, N., Slättegård, R., Hernalsteens, J. P., Wyns, L., Oscarson, S., De Greve, H., Hultgren, S. & Bouckaert, J. (2008). Intervening with urinary tract infections using anti-adhesives based on the crystal structure of the FimH-oligomannose-3 complex. *PLoS One*, Vol. 3, No. 4, (April 2008), pp.e2040 ISSN *1932-6203*

Wendakoon, C. N. & Sakaguchi, M. (1995). Inhibition of amino acid decarboxylase activity of *Enterobacter aerogenes* by active components in spices. *J Food Prot*, Vol. 58, pp.280-283 ISSN 0362-028X

Wieser, A., Romann, E., Magistro, G., Hoffmann, C., Nörenberg, D., Weinert, K. & Schubert, S. (2010). A multiepitope subunit vaccine conveys protection against extraintestinal pathogenic *Escherichia coli* in mice. *Infect Immun*, Vol. 78, No. 8, (August 2010), pp.3432-3442 ISSN 0019-9567

Wollenweber, E. (1988). Occurrence of flavonoid aglycones in medicinal plants. *Prog Clin Biol Res*, Vol. 280, pp. 45-55 ISSN 0361-7742

Yan, D., Jin, C., Xiao, X. H. & Dong, X. P. (2008). Antimicrobial properties of berberines alkaloids in Coptis chinensis Franch by microcalorimetry. *J Biochem Biophys Methods*, Vol. 70, No. 6, (April 2008), pp.845-849 ISSN 0165-022X

Yilmaz, A., Bahat, E., Yilmaz, G. G., Hasanoglu, A., Akman, S. & Guven, A. G. (2007). Adjuvant effect of vitamin A on recurrent lower urinary tract infections. *Pediatr Int*, Vol. 49, No. 3, (June 2007), pp.310-313 ISSN 1442-200X

# 14

# Prevention Strategy of Urogenital Infections by Using Lactobacilli with Probiotic Properties

Liliana Pascual and Lucila Barberis
*National University of Río Cuarto Department of Microbiology,*
*Faculty of Exact, Physical-Chemical and Natural Sciences,*
*Río Cuarto, Córdoba,*
*Argentina*

## 1. Introduction

Lactic acid bacteria (LAB) constitute a group of Gram-positive nonsporing nonrespiring bacteria, cocci or rods, that produce lactic acid as the major end product during the fermentation of carbohydrates. The term LAB is associated with bacteria involved in food fermentation and bacteria normally associated with the mucosal surfaces of human and animals. The classification of lactic acid bacteria into different genera is based on morphology, mode of glucose fermentation, growth at different temperatures, configuration of the lactic acid produced, ability to grow at high salt concentrations, and acid or alkaline tolerance (Pascual, 2004).

Bacteria belonging to the genus *Lactobacillus* are considered to be the main LAB and the predominant microorganisms in the gastrointestinal and urogenital tracts of humans as well as homeotermic animals. They are also used for elaborating different fermented foods categorized as GRAS (generally considered as safe).

Although there are data on simultaneous colonization of the human vagina by two different species of *Lactobacillus*, which can be homofermentative, heterofermentative or a combination of both (Kaewsrichan et al., 2006; Pascual et al, 2006), only one species has been isolated from the vaginal tract. Also, there are evidences of their effectivity in the prevention of urogenital infections (Pascual, 2004; Axelsson, 2004).

The urogenital microbiota of a healthy woman comprises approximately 50 species of organisms, witch differ in composition according to reproductive stages and exposure to several factors, including antibiotics and spermicides (Pascual, 2004).

In the complex vaginal environment, bacteria of the lactobacilli group ($10^7$–$10^8$ CFU $g^{-1}$ of vaginal fluid) are the dominant microorganisms in healthy pre-menopausal women, and play an important protective role by limiting growth of pathogenic microorganisms. When lactobacilli are reduced, eliminated, or replaced by pathogenic species, the host has an increased susceptibility to urinary tract infections (UTIs), genital tract infections (GTIs), bacterial vaginosis (BV), vulvovaginal candidiasis (VVC), and infection by *Neisseria gonorrhoeae* or *Trichomonas vaginalis*. Worldwide studies of UTIs or GTIs have revealed increasing antibiotic resistance among pathogenic microorganisms. Our research group has isolated human vaginal lactobacilli, selecting those with beneficial or probiotic properties (Czaja et al., 2007).

Urogenital infections are a major reason for women to visit their family's physician and are generally derived to gastroenterology, gynecology, urology, and infectious diseases specialists. The association between abnormal vaginal microbiota and increased risk for sexually transmitted infections, bladder and vaginal infections, and a higher rate of preterm labor indicate the need to better understand and manage urogenital health (Reid et al., 2004). Urogenital infections, defined here to include those that affect the bladder, kidneys, vagina, urethra, periurethra, and cervix, constitute a worldwide problem (Roos et al., 2006). The majority of UTI's occur in sexually active women (Howes et al., 2008). Risk increases by 3-5 times when diaphragms are used for contraception. Risk also slightly increases with not voiding after sexual intercourse and use of spermicides such as nonoxynol-9, which have been shown to be toxic to lactobacilli. Depletion of disturbances of vaginal lactobacilli biota has been associated with establishment of opportunistic infections like BV (bacterial vaginosis) and an increased risk of acquiring type 1 HIV. Nonoxynol-9 is the active compound in many spermicidal formulas. It is a nonionic detergent that reduces the superficial tension of the human spermatozoon membrane, causing loss of motility, decrease of its glucolytic power and alteration in permeability. It also affects the lipidic content of the human spermatozoon membrane. Nonoxynol-9 is generally used at concentrations of 5% in creams. It is possible that the presence of N-9 affects the ecological balance of the vagina through the inhibition of protective lactobacilli, especially those that produce $H_2O_2$. Nonoxynol-9 is a spermicide that has antimicrobial activity. Some studies have shown that lactobacilli present resistance or sensitivity to this compound (Pascual et al., 2006).

Increased risk has not been demonstrated with oral contraceptives, not voiding before intercourse, non-cotton underwear, and use of condoms. The prevalence and incidence of urinary tract infection is higher in women than in men, which is likely the result of several clinical factors including anatomic differences, hormonal effects, and behavior patterns (Standiford et al., 2005).

Historical data indicate that the vast majority of urinary tract infections (UTI) in a suburban, nonhospitalized community is caused by *Escherichia coli*, followed by other *Enterobacteriaciae* and *Staphylococcus saprophyticus*. The most frequent bacterial cause of UTI in adult women is *Escherichia coli*, which is part of the normal gut microbiota. This organism accounts for approximately 85% of community-acquired UTIs and 50% of hospital acquired UTIs (Talan et al., 2008).

However, a recent study reported that by infections *E. coli* were less common and that *Enterococcus faecalis* was the second most prevalent uropathogen. The latter result was also found in hospitalized patients. UTI affect millions of women each year, with an annual societal cost of billions of dollars. More than one quarter of women with a UTI will have a recurrent infection within six months. There are few established options for prevention of UTI other than the use of prophylactic antibiotics. Most uncomplicated UTI cases are resolved within 1 to 7 d of antibiotic therapy (Talan et al., 2008). However, drug resistance to commonly used antibiotics (eg, trimethoprim/sulfamethoxazole) is increasing among uropathogens and patients are experimenting more and more with alternative natural medicines, which appear to contain antiadhesive compounds that are active against uropathogens and can help prevent UTI (Pascual, 2004). The phenological characteristics of the lactobacilli strains including adhesive ability and production of acids, bacteriocins, hydrogen peroxide, and biosurfactants appear to be important in conferring protection to the host. Therefore, effective nonantibiotic methods of prevention are needed. One potential alternative may bee probiotic lactobacilli (Reid et al., 2005; Pascual et al, 2008a). The rationale for the use of probiotics is based on the genitourinary regulatory role played by the commensal microbiota and the need for restoration of this microbial ecosystem after insult. Health care providers who are interested in the therapeutic potential of probiotics require evidence of efficacy from randomized controlled assays, including data on successful local colonization and strain-specific outcomes, and information on product integrity and stability. This article reviews available information on the efficacy and tolerability of probiotics in the treatment and prophylaxis of bacterial vaginosis (BV) and the prophylaxis of UTI (Barrons and Tassone, 2008).

The administration of lactobacilli does not produce adverse effects in the urogenital tract; thus, it effectively prevents urinary tract infections. Several clinical assays have demonstrated that certain *Lactobacillus* species can be given orally or vaginally with resulting colonization of the vagina, reduction in vaginal coliform counts, and even reduction in UTI recurrence (Reid et al.,2004).

## 2. Probiotics

### 2.1 The history of probiotics

The first observation of the positive role of some bacteria can be credited to the work of Metchinkoff (1908); who reported on the potential health benefits of probiotics after he observed that Bulgarian peasants that consumed fermented milk products showed long, healthy lives (Sanders, 1999; Senok *et al.*, 2005). At the same time Henry Tissier (1906), a French pediatrician, observed that children with diarrhea had in their stools a low number of bacteria characterized by a peculiar morphology. These bacteria were, on the contrary, abundant in healthy children. He suggested that these bacteria could be administered to patients with diarrhea to help restore a healthy gut biota (WHO/ FAO, 2006).

The application of ''health promoting'' bacteria for therapeutic purposes has a long tradition in medicine; however, this so-called ''bacteriotherapy'' has long been considered to be a nonstandard procedure whose efficacy has not yet been proved or is at most based on observation but not on clinical studies (Suvarna and Body; 2005). The successful introduction of probiotics to the market has helped and inspired research in this area to a huge extent. In recent years, there has been a great increase in the number of clinical studies in which the prevention, alleviation, or therapy of diseases has been scientifically investigated not only to find evidence for a health claim for a target group of ''healthy consumers'' but also to test the medicinal (preventive and therapeutic) application of probiotics (Reid et al., 2006).

The term "Probiotic" derives from the Greek meaning "for life". It was first introduced in 1965 by Lilly and Stillwell for describing substances secreted by one organism which stimulate the growth of another (Reid *et al.*, 2003). In 1974, Parker referred to "Probiotic" as organisms and substances which contribute to the intestinal microbial balance. However, this term was subsequently redefined by Fuller (1989) as a live microbial feed supplement which beneficially affects the host animal by improving its intestinal microbial balance (Desai, A., 2008). This definition was broadened by Havenaar and Huis in't Veld (1992) to a mono or mixed culture of live microorganisms which benefits man or animals by improving the properties of the indigenous microbiota (Klaenhammer, 2000; Ranadheera et al., 2010).

At present is defined, by FAO/OMS, as "Live microorganisms which, when administered in adequate amounts, confer a health benefit on the host" (WHO / FAO, 2001). In a healthy host, a balance exists between members of the microbiota, such that potential pathogenic and non-pathogenic microorganisms can be found in apparent harmony. During infection, this balance can become disturbed, leading to often dramatic changes in the composition of the microbiota. The most important genus of Gram positive bacteria used extensively as probiotics are *Lactobacillus* and *Bifidobacterium* (Table 1).

| *Lactobacillus* spp. | ***Bifidobacterium*** **spp.** | **Others** |
|---|---|---|
| *L. acidophilus* | *B. bifidum* | *Enterococcus faecalis* |
| *L. rhamnosus* | *B. breve* | *E. faecium* |
| *L. gasseri* | *B. infantis* | *Streptococcus salivarus subsp. thermophilus* |
| *L. casei* | *B. longum* | *S. termophilus* |
| *L. reuteri* | *B. lactis* | *Lactococcus lactis subsp. lactis* |
| *L. delbrueckii subsp. bulgaricus* | *B. adolescentis* | *L. lactis subsp. cremoris* |
| *L. crispatus* | *B.essensis* | *Propionibacterium freudenreichii* |
| *L. plantarum* | *B.laterosporum* | *Pediococcus acidilactici* |
| *L. salivarus* | | *Leuconostoc mesenteroides* |
| *L. johnsonii* | | |
| *L. gallinarum* | | |
| *L.plantarum* | | |
| *L. fermentum* | | |
| *L. helveticus* | | |
| *L. paracasei* | | |
| *L. lactis* | | |

Table 1. Microorganisms applied as probiotics. Ranadheera *et al.*, 2010 and Gupta and Garg, 2009.

More than 20 years ago, the production of substances that inhibited pathogen growth on agar plates or the ability to reduce adherence of pathogens *in vitro* defined a probiotic (Chan et al., 1985). Now, the bar has been raised significantly higher, and use of the term 'probiotic' needs bacteria to be properly speciated, shown in appropriate formulations to be safe and effective at conferring health benefits on mammalian hosts, and manufactured and sold in a way that accurately reflects what benefits a consumer can obtain (Reid, 2005; Corcionivoschi et al., 2010). Sadly, governments and industry have not yet taken these requirements to heart, and whereas many so-called probiotic products are available, relatively few true probiotic products exist (Table 2).

### 2.2 Mechanisms of action

Mechanisms by which probiotics exert healthy effects are incompletely understood. Some authors include competitive inhibition with pathogenic bacteria, effects on barrier function, antagonism through the production of antimicrobial substances (acids, hydrogen peroxide and bacteriocins) and modulation of the immune system (Cabana *et al.*, 2006; Almeghaiseeb, 2007). These mechanisms vary according to the specific strain or combination of strains used, the presence of prebiotics [a non-digestible food ingredient which beneficially affects the host by selectively stimulating the growth and/or activity of one or a limited number of bacteria in the colon having the potential to improve host health (Gupta and Garg, 2009)] and the condition that is being treated the patient (Devine and Marsh, 2009).

Probiotics microorganisms compete with pathogens for nutrients and physical space (Fuller, 1991; Johannsen, 2003).

| | |
|---|---|
| Appropriateness | |
| i. | Accurate taxonomic identification |
| ii. | Normal inhabitant of the species targeted: human origin for human probiotics |
| iii. | Nontoxic, nonpathogenic, GRAS status |
| Technological suitability | |
| iv. | Amenable to mass production and storage: adequate growth, recovery, concentration, freezing, dehydration, storage, and distribution |
| v. | Viability at high populations (preferred at $10^6$–$10^8$) |
| vi. | Stability of desired characteristics during culture preparation, storage, and delivery |
| vii. | Provides desirable organoleptic qualities (or no undesirable qualities) when included in foods or fermentation processes |
| viii. | Genetically stable |
| ix. | Genetically amenable |
| Competitiveness | |
| x. | Capable of survival, proliferation, and metabolic activity at the target site in vivo |
| xi. | Resistant to bile |
| xii. | Resistant to acid |
| xiii. | Able to compete with the normal microflora, including the same or closely related species; potentially resistant to bacteriocins, acid, and other antimicrobials produced by residing microflora |
| xiv. | Adherence and colonization potential preferred |
| Performance and functionality | |
| xv. | Able to exert one or more clinically documented health benefits (e.g. lactose tolerance) |
| xvi. | Antagonistic toward pathogenic/cariogenic bacteria |
| xvii. | Production of antimicrobial substances (bacteriocins, hydrogen peroxide, organic acids, or other inhibitory compounds) |
| xviii. | Immunostimulatory |
| xix. | Antimutagenic |
| xx. | Anticarcinogenic |
| xxi. | Production of bioactive compounds (enzymes, vaccines, peptides) |

Table 2. Criteria for selection of probiotic strains. Adapted from Klahenhammer (2007).

Some bacteria can inhibit and prevent the colonization by pathogenic microorganisms by means of a mechanism of steric obstruction or blocking of specific receptors (Amores *et al.*, 2004). LGG and *L. plantarum* have been shown to competitively inhibit the attachment of enteropathogenic *E. coli* 0157H7 to HT-29 human colonic cancer cells (Michail *et al.*, 1997; Alvarez-Olmos and Oberhelman. 2001).

The effect of probiotics may be classified in three modes of action: (i) Probiotics have a direct effect on other microorganisms, commensal and/or pathogenic ones. This principle is in many cases of importance for the prevention and therapy of infections and restoration of the microbial equilibrium. (ii) Probiotics also might be able to modulate the host's defenses including the innate as well as the acquired immune system. This mode of action is most likely important for the prevention and therapy of infectious diseases but also for the treatment of chronic inflammation. (iii) Probiotic effects may be based on actions affecting microbial products like toxins, host products e.g.bile salts and food ingredients (Oeslschaeger, 2010).

## 3. Probiotics: effects on other microorganisms

### 3.1 Production of antimicrobial compounds

Lactobacilli produce a variety of compounds that are inhibitory to both Gram-positive and Gram-negative bacteria. These inhibitory substances include organic acids, bacteriocins, hydrogen peroxide and biosurfactants (Rolfe, 2000).

### 3.1.1 Organic acids

Lactic and acetic acids are the main products of carbohydrates fermentation by LAB. These acids diffuse through the membrane of the target organisms, in their hydrophobic undissociated form. Inside of the bacterial cytoplasm they are exposed to a pH value near to neutrality; subsequently, they dissociate (anion and $H^+$), reduce cytoplasmic pH and reduce metabolic activities (Kotikalapudi, 2009; Dalié *et al.*, 2010). This lower cytoplasmic pH inhibits glycolysis, prevents active transport and interferes with signal transduction. Furthermore, the anionic part of the acid cannot diffuse freely through the cell wall and accumulates inside the bacterial cell. Accumulation of anions leads to internal osmotic disorders for the bacteria (Kotikalapudi, 2009).

Among the antimicrobial compounds synthesized by the two human lactobacilli strains used in our work, *L. fermentum* L23 and *L. rhamnosus* L60, we have only researched the antimicrobial activity attributed to the bacteriocins and not necessarily to $H_20_2$ and lactic acid production. In previous reports, our group has shown the probiotic properties and the production of metabolites with biological activity against a wide spectrum of other microorganisms of these lactobacilli strains (Pascual et al., 2008a; Ruiz et al., 2009).

Juarez Tomás *et al.* (2003) tested the antimicrobial activity of lactobacilli strains *in vitro* (*Lactobacillus brevis* CRL 1335 and *L. acidophilus* strains CRL 1259, CRL 1307, CRL 1320 and CRL 1324). They found that these strains were able to inhibit the growth of *E. coli, S. aureus, S. agalactiae, E. faecalis, Klebsiella* sp., *N. gonorrhoeae* and *G. vaginalis*. Inhibition was shown to be produced by the low pH of the lactobacilli supernatants, as it disappeared when the supernatants were neutralized.

### 3.2 Bacteriocins

Bacteriocins are antimicrobial substances of protein nature, some of which may contain an associated lipid or carbohydrate, that inhibit growth of related or unrelated bacterial species and are potentially useful for prevention or treatment of bacterial infectious diseases ( Riley and Chavan, 2007; Pascual et al., 2008b).

Bacteriocins produced by lactic acid bacteria are divided into five classes based on primary structure, molecular mass, heat stability, and molecular organization : class I, lantibiotics; class II, nonlantibiotic peptides (subclass IIa, pediocin-like bacteriocins with strong antilisterial activity; subclass IIb, bacteriocins whose activity depends on complementary action of two peptides; subclass IIc, secdependent secreted bacteriocins); class III, large, heat labile protein bacteriocins; class IV, bacteriocins consisting of an undefined mixture of protein(s), lipid(s), and carbohydrate(s); and class V, bacteriocins with circular, unmodified posttransductional structure (including AS-48, gasericine A, enterocin) (Kemperman et al., 2003; Gutiérrez Merino J, 2005).

Lactobacilli bacteriocins are of interest because of their potential application for inhibition of pathogenic bacteria that affect humans. Two *Lactobacillus* strains from human vagina, *L. fermentum* L23 and *L. rhamnosus* L60, were previously identified and characterized as probiotics and producers of bacteriocins.

In a study carried out by our research group (Pascual et al. 2008a,b), we described the isolation, purification, and partial characterization of bacteriocins from *L. fermentum* L23 and *L. rhamnosus* L60. The inhibitory spectrum of these strains was quite broad, including Gram-negative and Gram-positive pathogenic strains and *Candida* species. To evaluate the proteinaceous nature of the antibacterial substances, the effect of proteolytic enzymes (trypsin, protease VI) was tested. Incubation of samples for 1 h at 37 °C with these enzymes completely inhibited the antibacterial activity. The bacteriocin produced by *L. fermentum* strain L23 was sensitive to several proteases, indicating that the inhibitory material was proteinaceous. Catalase and urease had no effect on its activity. Bacteriocin activity was most stable at acid or neutral pH. At alkaline pH, the bacteriocin became progressively inactivated. The partially purified bacteriocin was further purified by chromatography gel filtration (Sephadex G25). The sample was concentrated by evaporation and diluted in a small volume of phosphate buffer at pH 6.5. Fractions of 2.0 ml were collected, and their activity towards the indicator strain was tested. Fractions F15, F16, F17, and F18 displayed inhibitory activity against *E. coli*. They were pooled and concentrated.

The fraction collected after C18 reversed-phase HPLC exhibited activity against the indicator strain *E. coli*. The corresponding elution profile from reversed-phase HPLC, recorded at 220 nm, revealed one peak collected in the fraction eluted at 30 min. When an aliquot of the 30-min fraction was subjected to agar well diffusion assay, a zone of inhibition was produced in the agar. The fractions with antibacterial activity (F15, F16, F17, F18) obtained by chromatography assays were analyzed by TLC on silica gel plates.

The bacteriocin L23 produced by *L. fermentum* strain 23 showed a wide inhibitory spectrum, including some lactobacilli. A noteworthy observation was the inhibition of the pathogenic Gram-negative bacteria *E. coli*, *Proteus vulgaris*, *P. mirabilis*, *Klebsiella pneumoniae*, and *Neisseria gonorrhoeae*. In general, bacteriocins from lactic acid bacteria are active only towards Gram-positive bacteria. A wide inhibitory spectrum, as observed here for *L. fermentum* and *L. rhamnosus* L60, seems to be common among bacteriocin-producing isolates from the genus *Lactobacillus* (group III). Bacteriocin L23 did not show inhibitory activity against species of vaginal microbiota, including lactobacilli. Strain L23 secretes an antibacterial substance other than lactic acid, which is heat stable and only moderately sensitive to enzyme treatment. Several characteristics of the component responsible for the antibacterial activity suggest that it contains an unusual acidic amino acid present in a novel peptidic agent (Ruiz et al., 2009).

### 3.1.3 Interactions of bacteriocins

Also, the interactions between pairs of bacteriocins that inhibit the growth of urogenital pathogens were studied. To evaluate types of interaction between L23 and L60 bacteriocins, 207 isolates were considered. Synergistic interaction between these two bacteriocins was found in 68.6% of the cases (Fig. 1). Interactions were interpreted based on the shape of the inhibition zone, as follows: (1) lack of interaction (indifference) is indicated by growth at a right angle; (2) a synergistic effect results in concave growth between the two inhibition zones; (3) an antagonistic effect results in a junction in which growth covers the angle formed by the inhibition zones. A synergistic effect was observed with inhibition zones > 2mm compared with each antimicrobial activity of L60 or L23. Bacteriocin interactions were also determined using the checkerboard assay as previously described by Petersen et al. (2006). The initial concentrations of bacteriocins used in this experiment were at least the double of that of MIC. Serial dilutions of bacteriocins of L23 and L60 along the ordinate and abscissa were made, respectively, in MRS broth. The fractional inhibitory concentration (FIC) indexes (ΣFICs) were calculated as follows: ΣFIC= FIC A + FIC B, where FIC A is the MIC of A in the combination/MIC of A alone, and FIC B is the MIC B in the combination / MIC of B alone. The FIC was interpreted as follows: synergy, FIC≤0.5; indifference,

0.5<FIC<2; antagonism >2. There was neither an indifferent nor an antagonistic interaction between the substances evaluated either by qualitative or semi-quantitative method.

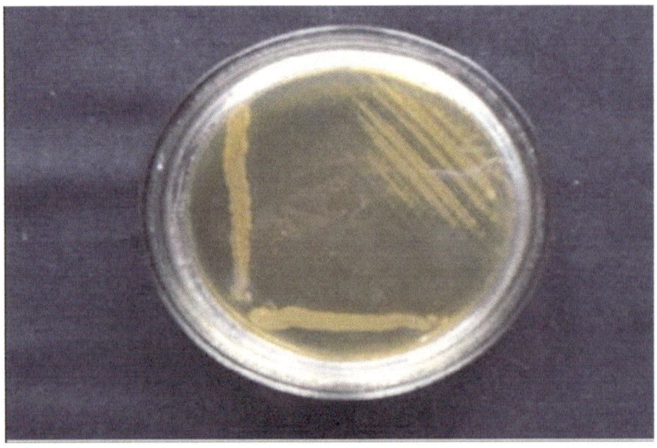

Fig. 1. Synergistic interaction between bacteriocins from L23 and L60 strains against *E. cloacae*

| Indicator strains | Number of strains | Indifferent interaction (%) | Antagonistic interaction (%) | Synergistic interaction (% |
|---|---|---|---|---|
| *Escherichia coli* | 100 | 45 (45) | - | 55 (55) |
| *Klebsiella pneumoniae* | 8 | 2 (25) | - | 6 (75) |
| *Klebsiella oxytoca* | 10 | 1 (10) | - | 9 (90) |
| *Proteus mirabilis* | 14 | 9 (64.28) | - | 5 (35.71) |
| *Proteus vulgaris* | 2 | - | - | 2 (100) |
| *Enterobacter cloacae* | 14 | 1 (7.14) | - | 13 (92.85) |
| *Citrobacter freundii* | 5 | 2 (40) | - | 3 (60) |
| *Serratia marcescens* | 4 | 1 (25) | - | 3 (75) |
| *Acinetobacter baumanii* | 5 | - | - | 5 (100) |
| *Pseudomonas aeruginosa* | 3 | - | - | 3 (100) |
| *Staphylococcus epidermidis* | 6 | - | - | 6 (100) |
| *Staphylococcus saprophyticus* | 15 | 3 (20) | - | 12 (80) |
| *Staphylococcus aureus* | 4 | - | - | 4 (100) |
| *Streptococcus agalactiae* | 2 | - | - | 2 (100) |
| *Enterococcus faecalis* | 7 | - | - | 7 (100) |
| *Neisseria gonorrhoeae* | 8 | - | - | 8 (100) |
| Total % of interactions observed | | 31.40 | 0 | 68.59 |

Table 3. Percentage of interactions between bacteriocins produced by *Lactobacillus fermentum* strain L23 and *Lactobacillus rhamnosus* strain L60.

Sensitive species that showed synergistic interaction in 100% of cases were: *A. baumanii, P. aeruginosa, S. epidermidis, S. aureus, S. agalactiae, E. faecalis, P. vulgaris*, and *N. gonorrhoeae*. Smaller percentages of synergistic interactions were found for *E. cloacae, K. oxytoca, S. saprophyticus, K. pneumoniae, C. freundii*, and *S. marcescens*. Indifferent interaction between L23 and L60 bacteriocins was found in 31.4% of the total cases. In addition, the highest percentages of indifferent interaction were observed for *P. mirabilis* and *E. coli*. Antagonistic interaction between L23 and L60 bacteriocins was not observed (Table 3).

Mulet-Powell et al. (1998) were the first to describe interactions between bacteriocins from lactic acid bacteria
(LAB). Here, we report rates of inhibitory activity and interactions between two bacteriocins produced by two potential probiotics from lactobacilli of human vagina. Mulet-Powell et al. showed antagonistic interaction between LAB bacteriocins, whereas we found no antagonistic interaction between L23 and L60 from cell-free supernatants (Ruiz et al., 2009).

### 3.1.4 Hydrogen peroxide

Hydrogen peroxide ($H_2O_2$) is produced by most LAB in the presence of oxygen. LAB are unable to produce catalase; therefore, they can not degrade hydrogen peroxide that, after accumulation, develops its oxidative properties with the production of powerful oxidants such as singlet oxygen, superoxide radicals, and the hydroxyl radical. Reactive oxygen species can cause irreversible damage to a number of cell components such as enzymes, membrane constituents and DNA (Schurman, 2001; Dalié *et al.*, 2010).
$H_2O_2$ is produced by many *Lactobacillus* strains in different amounts. There are techniques for measuring these compounds. In a qualitative method that was carried out by Eschenbach *et al.* (1989), a LAB strain was plated onto MRS agar containing 5 mg 3,3',5,5'-tetramethylbenzidine (TMB) and 0,2 mg horseradish peroxidase (HRPO). Peroxidase generates $O_2$ from $H_2O_2$ and TMB dyes the colonies with a blue color when oxidation occurs in the presence of $O_2$ (Pascual et al., 2008a). Pick and Mizel's phenol red solution method was used for testing $H_2O_2$ production by macrophages. This quatitative method is modified when working with BAL strains. A 50 µl aliquot of centrifuged microorganisms is placed onto a 96-well plate. Then, 50 ml of reagent 1 (2 ml of phenol red, 2 ml of HRPO, 46 ml DPBS buffer and 10 ml 1N sodium hydroxide) is added. $H_2O_2$ was measured indirectly by the 600nm absorbance of phenol red (Strus *et al.*, 2005). As was described in previous studies by our group, a number of cultured lactobacilli generate hydrogen peroxide at inhibitory levels on many pathogenic genitourinary microorganisms. Production of $H_2O_2$ by the *Lactobacillus* species is considered to represent a nonspecific antimicrobial defense mechanism of the normal vaginal ecosystem. Eschenbach et al. (1989) detected 96% $H_2O_2$-producing (LB+) strains. In the present study, we found 62% LB+ and 38% non- $H_2O_2$-producing strains (LB-). Species with the largest number of LB+ strains were *L. acidophilus* and *L. fermentum*.

### 3.1.5 Biosurfactants

Biosurfactants are microbial amphiphilic polymers and polyphilic polymers that tend to interact with the boundary between two phases in a heterogeneous system, defined as the interface (Rivardo *et al.*, 2009; Gudin *et al.*, 2010). They comprise a wide range of chemical structures, such as glycolipids, lipopeptides, polysaccharide-protein complexes, phospholipids, fatty acids and neutral lipids. Several biosurfactants exhibit antibacterial, antifungal and antiviral activities (Gudin *et al.*, 2010). These molecules alter surface hydrophobicity and therefore inhibit the adhesion of pathogenic microorganisms to infection sites. The release of biosurfactants by probiotic bacteria *in vivo* can be considered as a defence mechanism against other colonizing strains in the urogenital tract (Rodrigues *et al.*, 2006; Gudin *et al.*, 2010). Reid and Bruce (2001c) found that *L. fermentum* RC-14 produces large amounts of biosurfactants. These compounds inhibit the adhesion of a broad spectrum of urogenital pathogens.

### 3.2 Immune modulation

Recent studies have clarified the importance of the immunoregulatory ability of probiotics for exertion of their preventive and therapeutic effects on several diseases. The epithelial barrier consists of a dense mucous layer containing secretory IgA and antimicrobial peptides as well as dynamic functional complexes that regulate permeability between cells (Ohland and MacNaughton, 2010). When barrier function is interrupted due to several factors such as chronic psychological stress, epithelial ion secretion and permeability is enhanced, binding of luminal bacteria to surface epithelia increases, the uptake of luminal antigens through follicle associated epithelium increases and mucosal inflammation initiates (Zareie *et al.*, 2006). There is evidence that consumption of probiotic strains can improves the integrity of the intestinal barrier and the upregulation of mucin production (Devine and Marsh, 2009).

Stimulation and modulation of the mucosal immune system by probiotics reduces production of pro-inflammatory cytokines through activity on NFkB pathways, increase in production of anti-inflammatory cytokines, such as IL-10 and host defence peptides such as b-defensin 2, enhancement in IgA defences and influence on dendritic cell maturation (Devine and Marsh, 2009). It has also been shown that probiotics are able to regulate linfocite cell proliferation *in vitro*, as well as the production of specific and nonspecific antibodies (Amores *et al.*, 2004).

The immune system is roughly divided into the acquired immune system, consisting mainly of B lymphocytes and sensitized T lymphocytes, and the innate immune system, consisting mainly of macrophages and NK cells. The ratio of involvement of the systems varies depending on conditions of infection such as species of microorganisms and the amount and site of infection. Mouse studies have clarified that direct activation of macrophages by probiotics increased the bactericidal effect of macrophages on pathogenic bacteria. Probiotics strains have also been reported to promote proliferation of phagocytes such as macrophages and neutrophils in the bone marrow and spleen (hematopoietic tissues). Thus, activation of the innate immune system may be important in the infection preventing effect of probiotics. However, probiotics are also able to protect the integrity of the mucosal barrier against the destructive action of pathogenic microorganisms (Oelschlaeger T, 2010).

### 3.3 Probiotic effects on microbial toxins

One of the most important groups of bacterial virulence factors are toxins. The effectiveness of certain probiotics in suppressing diarrhoea is most likely based on their ability to protect the host against toxins. This protection can result from inhibition of toxin expression in pathogens. Certain probiotics are even able to protect against cyanobacterial and fungal toxins. The basis of the observed protective effect is rather a physicochemical interaction between toxin and a probiotic than a metabolic inactivation (Musa et al., 2009; Oelschlaeger, 2010). This mechanism of action of probiotics is not considered in this chapter.

## 4. Benefical properties of probiotics

Lactobacilli are able to interfere with genitourinary pathogens by several mechanisms. Other functions of lactobacilli include competitive exclusion of pathogens from the cell surface, co-aggregation with certain pathogenic bacteria, adherence to epithelial cells and biofilm formation based on autoaggregation and surface hydrophobicity (Dunne et al., 2001). Previous studies indicated that autoaggregation of probiotic strains is necessary for adherence to vaginal epithelial cells, and that co-aggregation leads to formation of a barrier that prevents colonization by pathogens (Boris et al., 1998; Zhou et al., 2004). These are some of the desired characteristics by which specific vaginal lactobacilli strains were selected as potential probiotic agents.

### 4.1 Autoaggregation assay

The aggregation ability could be described as the clumping of cells of the same strain, known as autoaggregation or self-aggregation (Nikolic *et al.*, 2010).

In a study performed by our research group, autoaggregation was described as the ability to form aggregates within 2 min. (Andreu et al., 1995). Necessary characteristics for *Lactobacillus* strains to serve as effective prophylactic agents include avid adherence to vaginal epithelial cells, interference with the adherence of other bacteria, production of bacteriocins, and production of hydrogen peroxide capable of inhibiting the growth of pathogens (Zhou et al., 2004).

### 4.2 Surface hydrophobicity

The surface hydrophobicity of lactobacilli was studied by the salt-aggregation test (SAT). The lowest final concentration of ammonium sulfate causing the bacteria to aggregate was defined as the SAT value. Strains were classified into three groups: high surface hydrophobicity (SAT< 0.9 mol/L), intermediate hydrophobicity (SAT 0.9-1.5 mol/L), and hydrophilic (SAT> 1.5 mol/L) (Andreu et al., 1995). Two lactobacilli strains studied by our group showed high hydrophobicity. Thus, we conclude that hydrophobicity is an important mechanism in bacterial adherence.

### 4.3 Co-aggregation assays

Co-aggregation of probiotic bacterial strains has been suggested to enable them to form a physical-chemical barrier that prevents colonization by pathogenic bacteria. Lactobacilli have been found to co-aggregate with some uropathogenic bacteria and inhibit their growth. A co-aggregation assay is positive when lactobacilli produce aggregates with other strain (Reid et al., 1990). *Lactobacillus fermentum* L23 and *L. rhamnosus* L60 showed co-aggregation with *E. coli*, *G. vaginalis*, and *Candida albicans*, but not with *C. glabrata* (Pascual *et al.*, 2008a). Such co-aggregation could be an important factor in maintaining vaginal health because it produces an area around the pathogen where the concentration of antimicrobial substances produced by these lactobacilli is increased. This would constitute an important host defense mechanism against infection (Kotikalapudi, 2009; Taheri *et al.*, 2009).

### 4.4 Bacterial adherence

The ability to adhere to epithelial surfaces is considered an indispensable pre-requisite of probiotic strains in order to colonise and then to exert health promoting effects. Bacterial adhesion is initially based on non-specific physical interactions between two surfaces (like hydrophobic interaction), which then enable specific interactions between adhesins (usually proteins) and complementary receptors (Kos *et al.*, 2003; Canzi *et al.*, 2005). To identify bacterial traits related to adhesion ability, potential probiotics strains could be assayed for adherence to cell lines or more frequently, to individual epithelial cells isolated from tissue surfaces by mechanical scraping, brushing or by freezing followed by a rapid thawing (Sillanpää, 2001). Some microorganisms are able to bind to epithelial cells of the gastrointestinal tract through lectins present in their surface structures. Lectins are carbohydrate-binding proteins or glycoproteins from non-immune origin which agglutinate cells with receptors (Gusilis, *et al.* 2002). Several authors observed a good correlation between adhesion ability and cell surface hydrophobicity (Canzi *et al.*, 2005). Adherence was assessed by counting the number of bacteria adhered to the intact epithelial cells. The number of adhering lactobacilli in the present study was comparable. Such adherence may promote colonization of the vaginal epithelium through formation of a bacterial "film" that tends to exclude pathogens from the mucosa ( Reid and Burton , 2002; Pascual et al., 2008a).

### 4.5 Competitive exclusion

Several studies reported that adhesive probiotic bacteria can prevent the attachment of pathogens and remove them from the urogenital tract. Studies showed that indigenous bacteria isolated from cervical, vaginal, and urethral surfaces of healthy women are able to adhere to human uroepithelial cells *in vitro*. These microorganisms were found to block the adherence of uropathogenic bacteria to uroepithelial cells from women with and without a history of urinary tract infections. Competitive exclusion was most effective with whole viable cells and less effective with cell wall fragments. Analysis of the *Lactobacillus* cell wall preparations suggested that lipoteichoic acid was responsible for the adherence of the *Lactobacillus* cells to uroepithelial cells but that steric hindrance was the major factor in preventing the adherence of uropathogens. Microbiota from the urinary tract may be used as protection against the attachment of uropathogens to the surfaces of uroepithelial cells (Revolledo *et al.*, 2006; Kotikalapudi, 2009).

## 5. Applications and beneficial effect of probiotics

There is preliminary evidence that probiotic microorganisms may antagonize the growth of nosocomial pathogens on inanimate surfaces. Among the several health benefits attributed to probiotic bacteria, the modulation of the intestinal microbiota of the host and the capacity to interact with the immune system directly or mediated by the autochthonous microbiota are basic mechanisms. Well-recognized probiotic effects are: 1. Prevention of rotavirus-induced or antibiotic-associated diarrhea as well as alleviation of lactose intolerance symptoms. 2. Reduction of the concentration of cancer-promoting enzymes. 3. Prevention and alleviation of gastrointestinal tract problems in healthy people. 4. Beneficial effects on inflammatory diseases of the gastrointestinal tract (*Helicobacter pylori* infection). 5. Normalization of stool passage in subjects with obstipation or an irritable colon. 6. Prevention of allergies and atopic diseases in infants. 7. Prevention of respiratory tract infections. 8. Prevention as well as treatment of urogenital infections and 9. Hypocholesterolemic effect. Evidence suggests that probiotic microorganisms may have a role in lowering the incidence of vaginal candidiasis, bacterial vaginosis and recurrent lower urinary tract infections (de Vrese and Schrezenmeir, 2008). Certain microorganisms, like *S. aureus* and *E. coli*, are able to adhere to inanimate surfaces by forming biofilms, which consist of an extracellular matrix of polysaccharides. Biofilm formation provides these microorganisms with a survival advantage against their planktonic competitors, and is an optimal environment for proliferation, gene transfer, and quorum sensing within the bacterial population. In this sense, it has been shown that probiotic microorganisms, such as *Lactobacillus* spp., can produce multifunctional molecules, known as biosurfactants, which have antagonistic antiadhesive properties against microbial pathogens. Biosurfactants, which are amphipathic molecules, have so far found limited application in biomedical sciences; however, indications of their potential clinical applicability are increasing (Falagas and Makris , 2009).

The probiotic concept has focused on two principal areas: Health and human nutrition, and health and animal production. In this chapter we will approach to the study of probiotics in human health.

### 5.1 Probiotics in human health

Several studies have shown the positive use of probiotics in diverse human health problems. They are considered to offer potential therapeutic applications in the prevention and treatment of different diseases (Anuradha et al., 2006; Harish and Varghese, 2006; Rao *et al.*, 2009).

### 5.2 Urogenital tract infections

Among women producing estrogen or receiving estrogen supplementation, the largest part of the vaginal flora consists of lactobacilli, which possesses antimicrobial properties that regulate urogenital microbiota. Genitourinary infections in women are often characterized by an alteration in the local flora from a predominance of lactobacilli to coliform uropathogens as a result of hormone deficiency, sexual activity, contraceptive measures, and other factors (Forsum et al., 2005).

In the complex vaginal environment, bacteria of the lactobacilli group ($10^7$–$10^8$ CFU $g^{-1}$ of vaginal fluid) are the predominant microorganisms in healthy pre-menopausal women and play an important protective role by limiting growth of pathogenic microorganisms (Reid, 2005; Anukam et al., 2006; Pascual *et al.*, 2008a). When lactobacilli are reduced, eliminated or replaced by pathogenic species, the host has an increased susceptibility to urinary tract infections (UTIs), genital tract infections (GTIs), bacterial vaginosis (BV), vulvovaginal candidiasis (VVC), and infection by *N. gonorrhoeae* or *Trichomonas vaginalis* (Reid et al, 2003; Klebanoff *et al.*, 2004, Ruíz *et al.*, 2009)

The use of probiotics *per se* and mainly lactobacilli has received greater attention as an alternative, inexpensive and natural remedy to restore and maintain the genitourinary health (Reid, 2001a,c).

Reid *et al.* (2001b) reported the first clinical evidence that probiotic lactobacilli can be delivered to the vagina following oral intake, strain *L. rhamnosus* GR-1 and *L. fermentum* RC-14 were suspended in skim milk and given twice daily for 14 days to 10 women with a history of recurrent yeast vaginitis, bacterial vaginosis and urinary tract infections. Six cases of asymptomatic BV or intermediate BV were resolved within 1 week of treatment. Also, a recent clinical trial showed that oral administration of capsules containing *L. fermentum* RC-14 and *L. rhamnosus* GR-1 was effective as adjuvant in the treatment of patients diagnosed with VVC (Gil *et al.*, 2010).

Pascual *et al.* (2010) found that *L. fermentum* L23 isolated from vaginal swabs of healthy, non-pregnant, pre-menopausal woman was able to prevent and cure *Escherichia coli* infection in a murine vaginal tract model. The study of vaginal colonization by lactobacilli showed that the human *L. fermentum* L23 strain had the ability to colonize the vaginal tract. A single inoculation was sufficient to establish the probiotic lactobacilli into that niche. Vaginal tract levels of *L. fermentum* L23 remained fairly high for 4 days, with bacterial levels ranging from

4.6 to 3.8 log10 c.f.u. $ml^{-1}$. On day 5, values decreased to 2.6 $log_{10}$ c.f.u.$ml^{-1}$. No growth of L23 strain was observed thereafter (Fig. 2). Infection with the pathogen was maintained in the vaginal tract for more than 7 days (Fig. 3), and this human *E. coli* uropathogenic strain was able to produce a strong infection when inoculated at this concentration, producing significant morphological alterations of the mucosal structure, mainly due to infiltration of polymorphonuclear cells.

The test on the preventive effect produced by strain L23 showed that a single administration of *Lactobacillus (*$1x10^8$ u.f.c. $ml^{-1}$) inhibited *E. coli* growth and, on the third post-infection day, the *E. coli* growth was not detected, showing that the pathogen was eliminated by the probiotic strain (Fig. 4). The curative effect produced by L23 showed complete inhibition of pathogen's growth after 5 days of treatment (Fig. 5). Thus, *L. Fermentum*, at that concentration, effectively eliminated *E. coli* from the vagina and had no negative effect on the host.

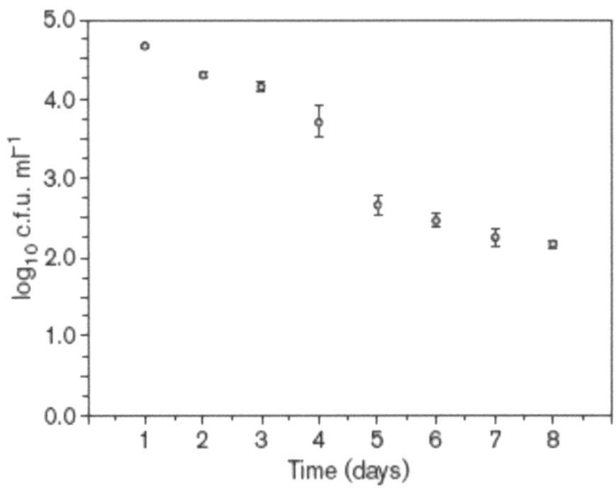


Fig. 2. BALB/c mice vaginal colonization by *L. fermentum* L23. Results are shown as means±SD.

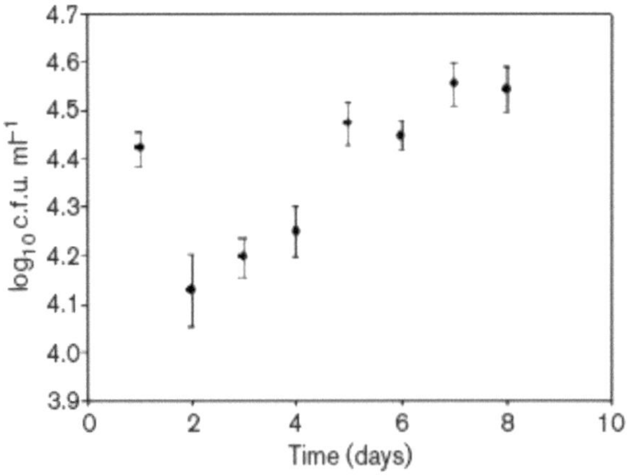


Fig. 3. Vaginal infection of *E. coli* in female mice. Results are shown as means±SD.

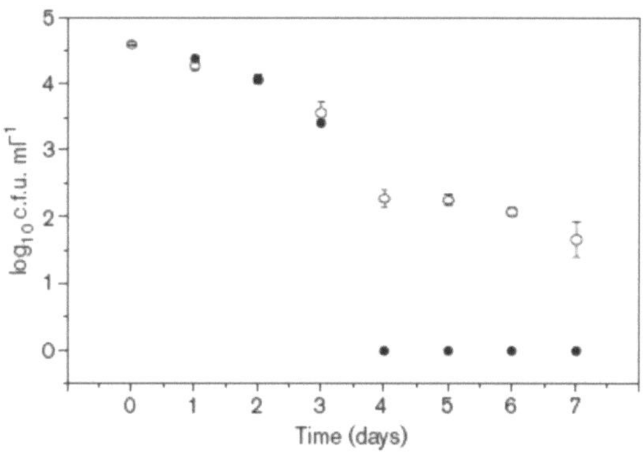


Fig. 4. Preventative effect of *L. fermentum* L23 (o) on *E. coli* (•) in BALB/c mice. Results are shown as means±SD. Significant differences between the untreated control (Fig. 3) and the treated group were found ($P<0.05$).

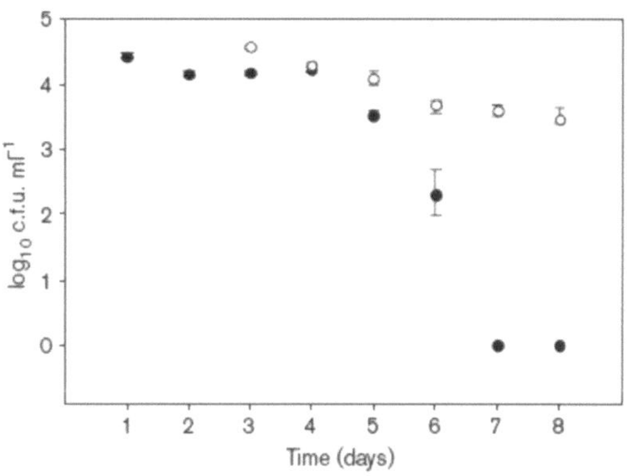


Fig. 5. Curative effect of *L. fermentum* L23(o) on *E. coli*(•) in female BALB/c mice. Results are shown as means±SD.

## 6. Safety considerations

Probiotics are viable microorganisms, and therefore it is feasible that they could infect the host. First selection criteria mentioned that a probiotic supplement have to be generally regarded as safe microorganisms (Reid *et al.*, 2003; Cabana *et al.*, 2006). Species of *Lactobacillus* or *Bifidobacterium* are normal residents of the gastrointestinal and/or vaginal microbiota and do not display infectivity or toxicity. The risk of infection with these microorganisms is lower (World Gastroenterology Organization Practice Guideline, 2008; Gupta and Garg, 2009).

Probiotics are safe for using in healthy people, but should be used with caution in high risk cases such as: People with immune compromise and premature infants. Current WHO/FAO guidelines (2001) recommend that, before using probiotic strains, a number of parameters should be evaluated to prevent health damages, including antibiotic susceptibility patterns, toxin production, metabolic and haemolytic activities, infectivity in immunocompromised animal models, side-effects and adverse incidents in humans (Senok *et al.*, 2005).

## 7. Conclusion

This chapter focuses on a group of lactobacilli, which may protect the vaginal epithelium through a series of barrier mechanisms (adherence), interference mechanisms (co-aggregation with potential pathogens), and production of antimicrobial substances. They appear to be excellent candidates for development as prophylactic agents. The *L. fermentum* L23 and *L. rhamnosus* L60 strains were selected for further studies of possible therapeutic application in the vaginal tract. Further studies are needed to evaluate their immunomodulatory capabilities.The bacteriocins produced by these lactobacilli are strong candidates for treatment or prevention of urogenital disorders in women.
Probiotics do not represent a magic result, but evidence is accumulating that the use of probiotic strains and manipulation of the host's own vaginal/urethral microbiota will provide valuable options to help restore and maintain urogenital health. Once appropriate product formulations with supporting clinical data become available, it will be up to the physician to determine their place in patient management.

## 8. Acknowledgment

Pascual L and Barberis L declare that they own the intellectual property rights associated with *Lactobacillus fermentum* L23 and *Lactobacillus rhamnosus* L60 strains. This work was supported by Secretaría de Ciencia y Técnica, Universidad Nacional de Río Cuarto.

## 9. References

Almeghaiseeb, E. S. (2007). Probiotics: an overview and their role in inflammatory bowel disease. Saudi J. Gastroenterol. 13 (3): 150-152.
Alvarez-Olmos, M. I. and Oberhelman, R. A. (2001). Probiotic Agents and Infectious Diseases: A Modern Perspective on a Traditional Therapy. Clin. Infect. Dis. 32: 1567-1576.
Amores, R.; Calvo, A.; Maestre, J. R. and Martínez-Hernández, D. (2004). Probióticos. Rev. Esp. Quimioterap. 17(2): 131-139.
Andreu, A., Stapleton, A., Fennell, C., Hillier, S. and Stamm, E. (1995) Hemagglutination, adherence and surface properties of vaginal *Lactobacillus* species. *J. Infect. Dis.*, 171, 1237-1243.
Anukam, K.C.; Osazuwa, E. O.; Ahonkhai, I. and Reid, G. (2006). *Lactobacillus* vaginal microbiota of women attending a reproductive health care service in Benin city, Nigeria. Sex. Trans. Dis. 33: 59–62.
Anuradha, S. and Rajeshwari, K. (2005). Probiotics in health and disease. JIACM. 6: 67-72.
Axelsson L. (2004). Lactic acid bacteria: classification and physiology. *Lactic acid bacteria.* (edition). Editorial Board, Marcel Deckker Inc. ISBN: 0-8247-5332-1.
Barrons R ; and Tassone D. (2008). Use of *Lactobacillus* Probiotics for Bacterial Genitourinary
Boris S, Suárez JE, Vázquez F, Barbés C.(1998). Adherence of human vaginal lactobacilli to vaginal epithelial cells and interaction with uropathogens. Infect Immun. May;66(5):1985-9.
Cabana, M. D.; Shane, A. L.; Chao, C. and Hemker, M. O. (2006). Probiotics in primary care pediatrics. Clin. Pediatr. 45: 405-410.
Canzi, E.; Guglielmetti, S.; Mora, D.; Tamagnini, I. and Parini C. (2005). Conditions affecting cell surface properties of human intestinal bifidobacteria. Anton. Van Lee. 88: 207–219.
Chan RC, Reid G, Irvin RT, Bruce AW & Costerton JW (1985). Competitive exclusion of uropathogens from human uroepithelial cells by Lactobacillus whole cells and cell wall fragments. Infect Immun 47: 84–89.

Corcionivoschi, N.; Drinceanu, D.; Steff, L.; Luca, I.; Julean, C. And Mingyart, O. 2010. Probiotics-Identification and ways of action. Innovative Romanian Food Biotechnology. 6: 1-11.

Czaja C, Stapleton A, Yarrova-Yarovaya Y and Stamm W. (2007). Phase I trial of a *Lactobacillus crispatus* vaginal suppository for prevention of recurrent urinary tract infection in women.

Dalié, D. K. D.; Deschamps, A. M. and Richard-Forget, F. (2010). Lactic acid bacteria - Potencial for control of mould growth and mycotoxins: A review. Food control. 21: 370-380.

de Vrese M, Schrezenmeir J.(2008). Probiotics, prebiotics, and synbiotics. Adv Biochem Eng Biotechnol ;111:1-66.

Desai, A. (2008). Strain identification, viability and probiotics properties of *Lactobacillus casei*. Doctoral thesis. Victoria University. Australia.

Devine, D. A. and Marsh, P. D. (2009). Prospects for the development of probiotics and prebiotics for oral applications. J. Oral Microbiol. DOI: 10.3402/jom.v1i0.1949.

Dunne, C.; O'mahony, L.; Thornton, G.; Feeney, M.; Daly, C.; O'Sullivan, G. and Collins, J. K. (2001). *In vitro* selection criteria for probiotic bacteria of human origin: Correlation with *in vivo* findings. Am. J. Clin. Nutr. 73: 386-392.

Eschenbach, D. A.; Davick, P. R. and Williams, B. L. (1989). Prevalence of hydrogen peroxide-producing *Lactobacillus* species in normal women and women with bacterial vaginosis. J. Clin. Microbiol. 27: 251-256.

Falagas M. and Makris G. (2009). Probiotic bacteria and biosurfactants for nosocomial infection control: a hypothesis. J Hosp Infect; 71:301-306.

Forsum U, Holst E, Larsson PG (2005). Bacterial vaginosis a microbiological and immunological enigma. ;113:81-90.

Fuller, R. (1991). Probiotics in human medicine. Gut. 32: 439-442.

Gil, N. F.; Martinez, R. C. R.; Gomes, B. C.; Nomizo, A. and De Martinis, E. C. P. (2010). Vaginal Lactobacilli as potencial probiotics against *Candida* spp. Braz. J. Microbiol. 41: 6-14.

Gudin, E. J.; Rocha, V.; Texeira, J. A. and Rodrigues, L. R. (2010). Antimicrobial and antiadhesive properties of a biosurfactant isolated from *Lactobacillus paracasei* ssp. *paracasei* A20. Lett. Appl. Microbiol. 50: 419-424.

Gupta, V. and Garg, R. (2009). Probiotics. Indian J. Med. Microbiol. 27 (3): 202-209.

Gusilis, C.; Bujazha, M. and González, S. (2002). Preliminary Studies to desing a probiotic for use in swine feed. Interciencia. 27: 409-413.

Gutiérrez Merino J. (2005). Caracterización inmunoquímica de la enterocina p y evaluación de su clonación, producción y expresión funcional en *Escherichia coli, Methylobacterium extorquens, Lactococcus lactis* y *Pichia pastoris.* Tesis doctoral Universidad Complutense de Madrid. Facultad de Veterinaria. España.

Harish, K. and Varghese. (2006). T. Probiotics in humans - evidence based review. Calicut Med. J. 4: e3.

Havenaar, R. and Huis in't Veld, J. H. J. (1992). Probiotics: a general view. In: The Lactic Acid Bacteria, Vol. 1: The Lactic Acid Bacteria in Health and Disease (Wood, B.J.B., ed.), pp. 209-224. Chapman & Hall, New York, NY.

Howes DS, Bogner MP. (2008).Urinary tract infections. In: Tintinalli JE, et al, eds. *Emergency Medicine: A Comprehensive Study Guide.* 7th ed. New York, NY: McGraw-Hill .

Johannsen, E. (2003). Probiotic bacteria: their properties and mode of action. SA Fam. Pract. 45 (3): 36-38.

Juárez Tomás, M. S.; Ocaña, V.; Wiese, B. and Nader- Macías, M. E. (2003). Growth and lactic acid production by vaginal *Lactobacillus acidophilus* CRL 1259, and inhibition of uropathogenic *Escherichia coli.* J. Med. Microbiol. 52: 1117-1124.

Kaewsrichan, J.; Peeyananjarassri, K. and Kongprasertkit, J. (2006). Selection and identification of anaerobic lactobacilli producing inhibitory compounds against vaginal pathogens. FEMS Immunol. Med. Microbiol.48(1): 75-83.

Kemperman R, Jonker M, Kuipers O, Kok J (2003) Functional analysis of the gene cluster involved in production of the bacteriocin circularin A by *Clostridium beijerinckii* ATCC 25752. Appl Environ Microbiol 69:5839–5848

Klaenhammer, T. R. (2000). Probiotic Bacteria: Today and Tomorrow. J. Nutr. 130: 415S–416S.

Klaenhammer, T. R. Probiotics and Prebiotics (2007). Chapter 39 of Food Microbiology. Amer society for microbiology. pp 802.

Klebanoff, M. A.; Schwebke, J. R.; Zhang, J.; Nansel, T. R.; Yu, K.F. and Andrews W. W. (2004). Vulvovaginal symptoms in women with bacterial vaginosis. Obstet. Gynecol. 104: 267–272.

Kos, B.; Suscovic, J.; Vucovic, S.; Simpraga, M.; Frece, J. and Matosic, S. (2003). Adhesion and aggregation ability of probiotic strain *Lactobacillus acidophilus* M92. J. Appl. Microbiol. 94: 981–987.

Kotikalapudi, B. L. (2009). Characterization and encapsulation of probiotic bacteria using a pea-protein alginate matrix. Master thesis. University of Saskatchewan. Canada.

Lilly, D. M. and Stillwell. (1965). Probiotics:growth promoting factors produced by microorganisms. Science. 147: 747-748.

Metchnikoff, E. (1908). The propagation of life. Optimistic studies New York: Putman's sons. pp 161-183.

Michail, S.; Wei, S. and Mack, D. R. (1997). *Escherichia coli* strain E2348/69 in vitro adhesion is reduced in the presence of a *Lactobacillus* species. Gastroenterology 1997; 112:A1042.

Mulet-Powell N, Lacoste-Armynoty AM, Vinas M, Simeon de Buochberg M (1998). Interaction between pairs of bacteriocins from Lactic Bacteria. J Food Protect 61:1210–1212

Musa, H. H.; Wu, S. L.; Zhu, C. H.; Seri, H. I. and Zhu, G. Q. (2009). The Potential Benefits of probiotics in animal production and health. J. Anim. Vet. Adv. 8 (2): 313-321.

Nikolic, M. Jovcic, B.; Kojic, M. and Topisirovic, L. (2010). Surface properties of *Lactobacillus* and *Leuconostoc* isolates from homemade cheeses showing auto-aggregation ability. Eur Food Res Technol . 231: 925–931.

Oelschlaeger T. (2010). Mechanisms of probiotic actions–A review. International Journal of Medical Microbiology 300: 57–62.

Ohland, C. L. and MacNaughton, W. K. (2010). Probiotic bacteria and intestinal epithelial barrier function. Am. J. Physiol. Gastrointest. Liver. Physiol. 298: G807–G819.

Parker, R. B. (1974). Probiotics, the other half of the antibiotics story. Anim. Nutr. Health. 29: 4–8

Pascual LM, Daniele MB, Pajaro C, Barberis L (2006). *Lactobacillus* species isolated from the vagina; identification, hydrogen peroxide production and nonoxynol-9 resistance. Contraception 73:78-81.

Pascual, L. M. (2004). Bacteriocinogenia en el género Lactobacillus: características benéficas de lactobacilos de vagina humana. Doctoral thesis, Universidad Nacional de Río Cuarto, Argentina.

Pascual, L. M.; Daniele, M. B.; Giordano, W.; Pájaro, M. C. and Baberis, I. L. (2008b). Purification and parcial characterization of novel bacteriocin L23 produced by *Lactobacillus fermentum* L23. Curr. Microbiol. 56: 397-402.

Pascual, L. M.; Daniele, M. B.; Ruiz, F.; Giordano, W.; Pajaro, C. and Barberis, L. (2008a). *Lactobacillus rhamnosus* L60 a potential probiotic isolated from human vagina. J. Gen. and Appl. Microbiol. 54:141–148.

Pascual, L. M.; Ruiz, F.; Giordano, W. and Barberis, L. (2010). Vaginal colonization and activity of the probiotic bacterium *Lactobacillus fermentum* L23 in a murine model of vaginal tract infection. J. Med. Microbiol. 59: 360-364.

Ranadheera, R. D. C. S.; Banes, S. K.; Adams, M. C. 2010. Importance of food in probiotic efficacy. Food Res. Int. 43: 1-7.

Rao, R. K.; Polk, D. B.; Seth, A. and Yan, F. (2009). Probiotics the good Neighbor: guarding the gut mucosal barrier. Am. J. Infect. Dis. 5 (3): 188-192.

Reid G (2005). Colonization of the vagina and urethral mucosa. Colonization ofMucosal Surfaces (Nataro JP, Cohen PS,Mobley HLT & Weiser JN, eds) pp. 431–448. ASM Press, Washington,DC.

Reid G, Burton J, Devillard E (2004) The rationale for probiotics in female urogenital healthcare. Med Gen Med 6(1):49–62.

Reid G; Kim S &. Kohler G. (2006). Selecting, testingand understanding probioticmicroorganisms. FEMS Immunol Med Microbiol 46 :149–157

Reid, G. (2001a). Probiotic agents to protect the urogenital tract against infection. Am. J. Clin. Nutr.73: 437–43.

Reid, G. and Bruce A. W. (2001c). Selection of *Lactobacillus* strains for urogenital probiotic applications. J. Infect. Dis. 183: 77-80.

Reid, G. and Burton, J. (2002) Use of *Lactobacillus* to prevent infection by pathogenic bacteria. *Microbes Infect.*, 4, 319-324.

Reid, G., Anand, S., Bingham, M., Wadstrom, T., Fuller, R., Anukam, K. & Katsivo, M. (2005). Probiotics for the developing world. J Clin Gastroenterol 39, 485–488.

Reid, G., Jass, J., Sebulsky, M. T. & McCormick, J. K. (2003). Potential uses of probiotics in clinical practice. Clin Microbiol Rev 16, 658–672.

Reid, G., Mac Groarty, J., Chow, A., Bruce, A., Eisen, A. and Costerton, W. (1990). Coaggregation of urogenital bacteria in vitro and in vivo. *Curr. Microbiol.* 20, 47-52.

Reid, G.; Bruce, A. W.; Fraser,N.; Heinemann, C.; Owen, J. and Henning, B. (2001b). Oral probiotics can resolve urogenital infections. FEMS Immunol. Med. Mic. 30: 49-52.

Reid, G.; Jass, J; Sebulsky, M. T. and Mc Cormick, J. K. (2003). Potential uses of probiotics in clinical practice. Clin. Microbiol. Rev. 16: 658-672.

Revolledo, L.; Ferreira, A. J. P. and Mead, G. C. (2006). Prospects in *Salmonella* control: competitive exclusion, probiotics, and enhancement of avian intestinal immunity. J. Appl. Poult. Res. 15: 341–351.

Riley, M. A. and Chavan, M. A. (2007). Book: Bacteriocins ecology and evolution. Chapter 4: the diversity of bacteriocins in Gram positive bacteria. Pp 45-46.

Rivardo, F.; Turner, R. J.; Allegrone, G.; Ceri, H. and Martinotti, M. G. ( 2009). Anti-adhesion activity of two biosurfactants produced by *Bacillus* spp. prevents biofilm formation of human bacterial pathogens. Appl. Microbiol. Biotechnol. 83: 541–553

Rodrigues, L. R.; Banat, I. M.; Texeira, J. A. and Oliveira, R. (2006). Biosurfactants: potential applications in medicine. J. Antimicrob. Chemoth. 57: 609–618.

Rolfe, R. D. (2000). The role of probiotic cultures in the control of gastrointestinal health. J. Nutr. 130: 396S–402S.

Roos, V., Ulett, G., Schembri, M. & Klemm, P. (2006). The asymptomatic bacteriuria Escherichia coli strain 83972 outcompetes uropathogenic E. coli strains in human urine. Infect Immun 74, 615–624.

Ruiz, O. F.; Gerbaldo, G.; Asurmendi, P.; Pascual, L. M.; Giordano, W. and Barberis, I. L. (2009). Antimicrobial activity, inhibition of urogenital pathogens, and synergistic interactions between *Lactobacillus* strains. Curr. Microbiol. DOI 10.1007/s00284-009-9465-0.

Sanders, M. E. (1999). Probiotics. Food technol. 53: 67-77.

Schurman, J. J. (2001). Antibacterial activity of hydrogen peroxide against *Escherichia coli* O157:H7 ans *Salmonella* spp. in fruit juices, both alone and in combination with organic acids. Master thesis. Faculty of the Virginia Polytechnic Institute and State University. United States.

Senok, A. C.; Ismaeel, A. Y. and Botta, G. A. (2005). Probiotics: facts and myths. Clin. Microbiol. Infect. 11: 958-966.

Sillanpää, J. (2001). Tissue-adherence in lactic acid bacteria: Identification and characterization of the collagen-binding S-Layer protein of *Lactobacillus crispatus.* Academic Dissertation in General Microbiology. Faculty of Science of the University of Helsinki. Finland.

Standiford C, Green L,. Van Harrison R.(2005). Urinary Tract Infection Guideline Team. Taubman Medical Library. 1-9.

Strus, M.; Kucharska, A.; Kukla, G.; Brzychczy- Wloch, M.; Maresz, K and Heczko, P. B. (2005). The in vitro activity of vaginal *Lactobacillus* with probiotic properties against *Candida.* Infectious Diseases in Obstetrics and Gynecology. 13(2): 69–75.

Suvarna, V. C. and Boby, V.U. (2005). Probiotics in human health: A current assessment. Curr. Sci. 88: 1744-1748.

Taheri, H. R.; Moravej, H., Tabandeh, F.; Zaghari, M. and Shivazad, M. (2009). Screening of lactic acid bacteria toward their selection as a source of chicken probiotic. Poultry Sci. 88: 1586–1593.

Talan DA, Krishnadasan A, Abrahamian FM, Stamm WE, Moran GJ. (2008). Prevalence and risk factor analysis of trimethoprim-sulfamethoxazole- and fluoroquinolone-resistant Escherichia coli infection among emergency department patients with pyelonephritis. *Clin Infect Dis.* Nov 1 ;47(9):1150-8.

Tissier, H . (1906). Traitement des infections intestinales par la méthode de la flore bactérienne de l'intestin. CR.Soc. Biol. 60 : 359-361.

World Gastroenterology Organization Practice Guideline. (2008). Probiotics and prebiotics. www.worldgastroenterology.org

World Health Organization and Food and agriculture Organization of the United Nations (WHO/FAO). (2001). Health and nutritional properties of probiotics in food including powder milk with live lactic acid bacteria - Joint Food and Agricultural Organization of the United Nations and World Health Organization Expert Consultation Report, Córdoba, Argentina. <http://www.who.int /foodsafety/publications/fs_management/probiotics/en/index.html>.

World Health Organization and Food and agriculture Organization of the United Nations (WHO/FAO). (2006). Probiotics of food: Health and nutritional properties and guidelines for evaluation. pp 3.

Zareie, M.; Johnson-Henry, K.; Jury, J.; Yang, P. C.; Ngan, B. Y.; McKay, D. M.; Soderholm, J. D.; Perdue, M. H.; Sherman, P. M. (2006). Probiotics prevent bacterial translocation and improve intestinal barrier function in rats following chronic psychological stress. Gut. 55:1553–1560.

Zhou JS, Pillidge CJ, Gopal PK, Gill HS (2005) Antibiotic susceptibility profiles of new probiotic Lactobacillus and *Bifidobacterium* strains. J Food Microbiol 98:211–217.

Zhou, X., S.J. Bent, M.G. Schneider, C.C. Davis, M.R. Islam, L.J. Forney. (2004). Characterization of vaginal microbial communities in adult healthy women as determined by sequencing clones and terminal restriction fragment length polymorphism (T-RFLP) analyses. Microbiology 150: 2565–2573.

# Part 3

## Urinary Tract Infections in Children

# 15

# Current Management of Urinary Tract Infection in Children

Yusuf Kibar
*Gulhane Military Medical Academy, Department of Urology,
Section of Pediatric Urology,
Ankara,
Turkey*

## 1. Introduction

Urinary tract infection (UTI) is the most commonly diagnosed bacterial infection of childhood, and has a significant healthcare impact. Renal parenchymal infection and scarring are well-established complications of UTI in children and can lead to renal insufficiency, hypertension and renal failure. Although frequently encountered and well researched, diagnosis and management of UTI continue to be a controversial issue with many challenges for the clinician.

The evolving state of knowledge about pediatric UTI leaves many questions and controversies. The goal of this chapter is to provide an up-to-date summary of the literature with particular attention to practical questions about diagnosis and management for the clinician. This chapter reviews also recent evidence regarding the epidemiology and evaluation of children with UTI.

## 2. Definitions

UTI is defined as the presence of bacteria in urine along with symptoms of infection. However, since asymptomatic colonization of the urinary tract can occur, other features such as the presence of inflammatory markers or follow-up cultures may be needed to definitively diagnose a UTI.

UTIs have been classified in many ways: upper versus lower urinary tract, complicated versus uncomplicated, first episode versus recurrent, symptomatic versus asymptomatic, and according to severity simple versus severe infection.

Pediatric UTIs are most simply categorized into two types: first infections and recurrent infections. Recurrent UTI is defined as two or more UTIs over a six-month period (Ditchfield et al., 1994). Recurrent UTI increases the risk of subsequent renal scarring. Recurrent UTI may be subclassified into three groups (Ma & Shortliffe, 2004):

1. *Unresolved infection*: due to subtherapeutic level of antimicrobial (because of poor renal concentrating ability or gastrointestinal malabsorption), non-compliance with treatment, and resistant pathogens. Most unresolved infections are treated succesfully when proper culture and antimicrobial sensitivity patterns are available.

2. *Bacterial persistence*: may be due to a nidus in the urinary tract (Shortliffe, 1995). Surgical correction or medical treatment for urinary dysfunction may be needed. The surgically correctable sources of bacterial persistence are infection stones, infected nonfunctioning or poorly functioning kidneys or renal segments, infected ureteral stumps after nephrectomy, fistulas with bowels, infected necrotic papillae, and infected urachal cyst.
3. *Reinfection*: each episode is a new infection acquired from periurethral, perineal or rectal flora.

First childhood UTIs are considered *complicated* because of the evaluation and management implications. Lower UTI's include bladder infections (cystitis), whereas upper UTI's include pyelonephritis and perinephric and renal abscess. Ascending infection of the urinary tract is a complex process that has been associated with bacterial adhesion, virulence, and motility properties as well as host anatomic, humoral, and genetic factors (Svanborg & Godaly, 1997). The presence of fever, chills, and flank pain has usually been considered clinical evidence of upper tract infection.

From the clinical point of view, UTI could also be classified as *simple* or *severe UTI*. Severe UTI is related to the presence of fever of > 39ºC, the feeling of being ill, persistent vomiting, and moderate or severe dehydration. A child with a simple UTI may have only mild pyrexia, but is able to take fluids and oral medication. The child is only slightly or not dehydrated and has a good expected level of compliance. When a low level of compliance is expected, such a child should be managed as one with a severe UTI.

*Breakthrough UTI* may be caused by a change in the resistance pattern of organisms colonizing the urethra, noncompliance, vesicoureteral reflux (VUR) or dysfunctional voiding. Recognizing and addressing these associated factors are essential in treating breakthrough UTI.

It is certainly possible to have bacteria within the urinary tract and be asymptomatic without having clinical infection or renal scarring. The prevalence of *asymptomatic bacteriuria* has been documented to be approximately 0.9% among young schoolgirls. Of these patients, 10% were found to have VUR without any renal scarring. Controversy continues regarding the need for antibiotic treatment of asymptomatic bacteriuria (Schoen, 1990; Ahmed, 1996). If recurrent bacteriuria is truly asymptomatic, no antimicrobial treatment may be the best option, as some studies have shown that asymptomatic children are at very low risk of renal scarring, and prophylactic treatment did not decrease the risk of UTI recurrence (Shortliffe, 1995).

## 3. Epidemiology

The epidemiology of UTI during childhood varies by age, gender, and other factors. The incidence of UTI in infants ranges from approximately 0.1 to 1.0 percent in all newborn infants to as high as 10 percent in low-birth-weight infants (Klein & Long, 1995). It represents the most common bacterial infection in children less than 2 years of age. It is the most common cause of fever of unknown origin in boys less than 3 years (Jodal, 1987). In the first year of life, mostly the first 3 months, UTI is more common in boys (3.7%) than in girls (2%), after which the incidence changes, being 3% in girls and 1.1% in boys (Foxman, 2002).

Two studies of the prevalence of UTI among children presenting to an emergency department with fever found rates ranging from 3.5 to 5.5% (Hoberman et al., 1993; Shaw et al., 1998). Girls were more than twice as likely as boys to have UTI, and among boys, uncircumcised infants had an eightfold higher risk. This finding compares well with population-based studies of UTI which document a 4- to 10-fold increase in risk of UTI among uncircumcised males during the first year of life, likely due to colonization of the mucosal surface of the foreskin with bacteria (To et al., 1998). White children were significantly more likely to have UTI than black children in both prevalence studies, with rates as high as 16 to 17% among white girls (Shaw et al., 1998). The reason for this increase associated with race is unclear, and referral bias may be a factor for these emergency department-based studies. However, some studies of white females suggest that there may be genetic tendencies for UTI, such as lack of secretion of carbohydrates that protect against bacterial adherence in the urinary tract (Jantausch et al., 1994; Sheinfeld et al., 1989).

## 4. Importance of UTI

The clinical significance of UTI has been controversial. In the preantibiotic era, UTI had a mortality rate as high as 20%, although acute complications in healthy children are now uncommon except in young infants, who may progress to systemic infection (Dayan et al., 2004; Hansson et al., 1997). Long-term complications of UTI have been associated with renal scarring and include hypertension, chronic renal failure, and toxemia in pregnancy. Long-term follow-up data are limited, although one Swedish study found that children diagnosed with renal scarring due to pyelonephritis during the 1950s and 1960s developed high rates of hypertension (23%) and end-stage renal disease (10%)(Jacobson et al., 1989). More recent studies question the association between pyelonephritis and end-stage renal disease (Esbjorner et al., 1997; Sreenarasimhaiah & Hellerstein, 1998). Although the individual risks associated with UTI remain unclear, the high prevalence of UTI and potential morbidity associated with complications require careful attention to diagnosis and management.

## 5. Etiology

Clinically important infections usually occur due to bacteria, although viruses, fungi, and parasites can also cause infection. Common bacterial pathogens include gram-negative species such as *Escherichia coli, Klebsiella, Proteus, Enterobacter, Pseudomonas,* and *Serratia* spp. and gram-positive organisms, including group B streptococci, *Enterococcus* sp., and *Staphylococcus aureus. Escherichia coli* is the most common infecting pathogen in children, accounting for up to 90 percent of UTIs (Shapiro, 1992). Gram-positive organisms represent 5-7% of cases. Groups A and B streptococci are relatively common in the newborn (Richards et al., 1999). There is an increasing trend towards the isolation of *Staphylococcus saprophyticus* in UTIs in children, although the role of this organism is still debatable (Abrahamsson et al., 1993). The virulence of the invading bacteria and the susceptibility of the host are of primary importance in the development of UTI (Feld, 1991).

Fungi can cause cystitis in certain settings and with associated risk factors. Fungi are the second most common cause of nosocomial UTI in children, and can spread systemically and can be life-threatening. Risk factors for fungal UTI's include the use of invasive devices (drains and catheters), previous broad-spectrum antibiotic exposure, and systemic immunosuppression. A true candidurial infection can be difficult to diagnose, since it can represent colonization, contamination, or infection, and may or may not have associated symptoms. The potential for candiduria to develop into invasive candidiasis in the neonatal intensive care unit is significant. Risk factors for this progression include prematurity, congenital urinary tract abnormalities, parenteral nutrition, respiratory intubation, and

umbilical artery or intravenous catheterization. Furthermore, the kidney is the most commonly affected organ in candidiasis, with "fungus balls" representing a life-threatening infection. As such, renal and bladder sonography is important in the evaluation of neonates with candiduria.
Viral cystitis represents another form of non-bacterial UTI affecting children. *Adenovirus types 11 and 21, Influenza A, polyomavirus BK,* and *Herpes simplex* viruses can cause irritative voiding symptoms, hemorrhagic cystitis and even VUR or urinary retention. In non-immunized or immunosuppressed children, *Herpes zoster* cystitis presents similarly. Fortunately, these forms of cystitis are self-limited. Immunosuppressed children undergoing kidney or bone marrow transplantation, or those receiving chemotherapy are especially susceptible to viral cystitis, including those caused by *Cytomegalovirus* and *Adenoviruses 7, 21* and *35*. Antivirals such as ribavirin and vidarabine may be helpful when viral cystitis is diagnosed.

## 6. Pathogenesis and risk factors

In neonates, the usual route of infection is presumed to be hematogenous. Later in life, infection is usually caused by ascension of bacteria into the urinary tract. Retrograde ascent is the most common mechanism of infection. Any condition that leads to urinary stasis (renal calculi, obstructive uropathy, VUR and dysfunctional voiding) may predispose to the development of UTI in children (Batisky, 1996). Obstruction and dysfunctional voiding are among the most common causes of UTI (Ma & Shortliffe, 2004). A wide variety of congenital urinary tract abnormalities can cause UTIs through obstruction, e.g. urethral valves, ureteropelvic and ureterovesical junctions' obstructions, ureteroceles, ectopic ureters, bladder extrophy, or non-obstructive urinary stasis (e.g. prune belly syndrome, VUR). More mundane but significant causes of UTIs include labial adhesion and chronic constipation (Abrahamsson et al., 1993).
Phimosis is the inability to retract the foreskin, and is a anormal physiologic occurrence in newborn boys. Phimosis can predispose to UTI (Craig et al., 1996; To et al., 1998). The prepuce can serve as a reservoir for potentially uropathogenic bacteria. Enterobacteria derived from intestinal flora colonize the preputial sac, glandular surface and the distal urethra. Among these organisms are strains of *E. coli* expressing P fimbriae which adhere to the inner layer of the preputial skin and to uroepithelial cells (Fussel et al., 1988). Neuropathic bladder dysfunction (spina bifida, sphincter dyssynergia, etc) may also lead to postvoid residual urine and secondary VUR (Schulman, 2004).
Dysfunctional voiding refers to dysfunction of the lower urinary tract in the absence of any apparent organic cause. The child with dysfunctional voiding habitually contracts the urethral sphincter during voiding. The term cannot be applied unless repeated urofow measurements have shown curves with a staccato pattern or if verified by invasive urodynamic investigation. Dysfunctional voiding may result in infrequent bladder emptying aided by delaying manoeuvres, e.g. crossing legs, sitting on heels (Wan et al., 1995). It is often associated with daytime enuresis and constipation (Smith & Elder, 1994). Dysfunctional voiding can lead to secondary VUR, and may be exacerbated by chronic constipation because of alterations in pelvic floor activity caused by impacted stool. Normally, any bacteria that enter the bladder are flushed out of the bladder with complete and frequent voiding. Infrequent voiding and residual urine residual urine in the bladder allows bacteria that enter the bladder to grow and multiply enough to cause enfection.

Incomlete relaxation of the pelvic flor during voiding can couse poor compliance and/or incomplete emptying, both of which are thought to contribute to bacteriuria and UTI. Girls with recurrent UTIs have a particularly high incidence of voiding dysfunction (Chen et al., 2004; Mingin et al., 2004) and should be screened with a thorough history, voiding diary, and appropriate clinical evaluation to rule out constipation. In children who demonstrate a high likelihood for this diagnosis, it may be appropriate to address these issues before proceeding to more invasive tests such as a VCUG. Treatment of voiding dysfunction includes timed voiding, treatment of constipation, prophylactic antibiotics and, in some cases, use of anticholinergic medication (e.g., oxybutynin) or biofeedback (Kibar et al., 2009, 2007a, 2007b; Yagci et al., 2005).

VUR is the abnormal retrograde flow of bladder urine into the upper urinary tract through an incompetent ureterovesical junction. Reflux in itself that is without bacterial contamination and low in pressure has not been documented to be deleterious. Reflux in the presence of bacteria as a risk factor for upper UTIs or pyelonephritis. In children without urologic symptoms or history of infection, the insidence of reflux is likely less than 1%. In children with a history of symptomatic UTI, the insidence of reflux has been estimated to range from 20% to 50%. Untreated upper UTIs have been shown to lead to acquired renal scarring or reflux nephropathy in children (Yeung et al., 1997). Controversy continues regarding the association of VUR with the pathogenesis of renal scarring, reflux nephropathy and pyelonephritis (Ditchfield et al., 1994; Eggli & Tulchinsky, 1993). Studies reporting on investigation during a febrile UTI document initial defect and subsequent scarring in 34 to 70% and 9.5 to 38%, respectively (Benador et al., 1997; Ditchfield & Nadel, 1998; Hoberman et al., 2003; Majd & Rushton, 1992). Unfortunately, many studies do not have complete enough follow-up to determine the true incidence of scarring, as it has been shown that defects will change up to 6 months later (Ditchfield et al., 2002; Wallin et al., 2001). There is also the potential for interobserver variability in renal scans, with differences ranging from small to notable (Gacinovic et al., 1996)). Children less than one year of age with a UTI are at much greater risk for renal scarring than older children; children over five years of age uncommonly have new renal scarring with UTI (Andrich & Majd, 1992). While some researchers emphasize the risk of renal scarring from recurrent UTI without reflux (Gordon, 1995), others are just as adamant regarding the risk of scarring from reflux in the absence of infection (Blumenthal, 1995). The fact that renal scarring develops in only a minority of patients with pyelonephritis and/or VUR suggests that the development of renal scarring likely involves the interplay of several factors and cannot simply be attributed to the presence of infection or reflux alone.

## 7. Clinical presentation

The presenting symptoms of UTI depend on the anatomic site of the infection and the age of the patient. Regardless of UTI location, infants and many young children cannot describe their symptoms; hence it is critical to understand the observable signs and symptoms of infection to make the diagnosis. In a child with so-called "asymptomatic" bacteriuria, only subtle clues, such as enuresis or squatting, may be present. Alternatively, a systemically ill neonate may be lethargic and hypotensive.

Cystitis is second in frequency only to respiratory infection as a reason for pediatric medical visits. Classic symptoms of cystitis include urinary frequency, urgency, dysuria, hematuria, suprapubic pain, sensation of incomplete emptying, and even incontinence. Non-specific

symptoms can include poor feeding, irritability, lethargy, vomiting, diarrhea, ill appearance, and abdominal distension. Fever and flank pain are unusual symptoms for lower UTI.
Pyelonephritis, and to a lesser degree renal abscesses, typically begin as a lower UTI that proceeds to an upper UTI as the infections ascends. However, pyelonephritis and renal abscesses can also result from hematogenous spread of infection (e.g., bacteremia). Symptoms that occur with upper UTI's overlap those for cystitis, in part because cystitis is common in both. In upper UTI's, flank pain and fevers (classically intermittent and >39°C) are more pronounced and important

## 8. Diagnosis

A thorough history from parents, and the child if possible, and a physical examination are essential in the evaluation of pediatric UTI. There are no signs spesific for UTI in the infant. If there is a gross genitourinary anatomic abnormality, a renal mass may be palpable, as found in children with xanthogranulomatous pyelonephritis or infected severe hydronephrosis. Palpation in the suprapubic and flank areas may cause pain in the older child, but generelized abdominal or upper quadrant pain may also be present. Perineal examination rarely shows an ectopic ureteral opening, ureterocele, or ureteral discharge in girls. It is mandatory to look for phimosis and labial adhesion. Signs such as back scars, sacral fat pads, or sacral dimples or pits may suggest neurogenic bladder and may require further investigation. On boys, the testes are abnormal if affected by epididymitis or epididymo-orchitis. The absence of fever does not exclude the presence of an infective process. The presence of irritative urinary symptoms in the absence of bacteria suggests a non-UTI cause such as vaginitis, urethritis, pinworms, or the use of bubble baths (Zelikovic, 1992).
The question of when to screen for UTI has been evaluated in a number of studies. The presence of specific symptoms for UTI, including dysuria, frequency, urgency, suprapubic discomfort, and flank pain, should lead to screening. However, young children with UTI may present ith nonspecific symptoms, such as poor feeding, vomiting, irritability, jaundice (in newborns), or fever alone may be appropriate.
Dipstick urinalysis is the most common initial laboratory testing, and may be the most cost-effective screen for infant UTI. Urine cultures and blood cultures (if sepsis is suspected) are the mainstays of diagnosis. However, diagnosis is complicated by contamination from fecal bacteria that colonize the perineal area and distal urethra. The guideline issued by the American Academy of Pediatrics (AAP) for the evaluation of fever (39.0°C [102.2°F] or higher) of unknown origin suggests urinalysis in all cases and a urine culture in all boys younger than six months of age and all girls younger than two years of age (Baraff et al., 1993).
The definitive diagnosis of infection in children requires a positive urine culture (Ma & Shortliffe, 2004). Urine must be obtained under bacteriologically reliable conditions when undertaking a urine specimen culture (Zorc et al., 2005). A positive urine culture is defined as the presence of more than 100,000 cfu/mL of one pathogen. Most UTIs are caused by a single organism; the presence of two or more organisms usually suggests contamination. The urine specimen may be difficult to obtain in a child less than 4 years old and different methods are advised since there is a high risk of contamination (Watson, 2004).
The final concentration of bacteria in urine is directly related to the method of collection, diuresis, and method of storage and transport of the specimen. In order to obtain a urine

sample in the best condition in children under 2 years of age (girls and uncircumcised boys without sphincteric control), it is better to use suprapubic bladder aspiration or bladder catheterization. In older children with sphincteric control, clean-voided midstream specimen is possible and reliable (Ma & Shortliffe, 2004). Voided specimen should be obtained after cleansing of the urethral meatus. Girls should be positioned backwards on the toilet seat to help spread the labia. Suprapubic bladder aspiration is the most sensitive method, but has a low rate of success unless aided by ultrasound visualization of urine in the bladder. Urine may be obtained in 23-99% of cases (Ma & Shortliffe, 2004). Bladder catheterization is also a sensitive method, even though there is the risk of introduction of nosocomial pathogens (Hellerstein, 2002). Urine from bagged and voided specimens are easier for the child, but have significant false positive rates, ranging from 85-99% (Ma & Shortliffe, 2004). It is helpful when the culture is negative and has a positive predictive value of 15% (Cavagnaro, 2005). Any number of colonies from a suprapubic bladder aspiration, more than $10^3$ colonies from an intermittent catheterization, and more than $10^5$ colonies from a midstream clean-catch urine collection indicate UTI (Batisky, 1996).

Although urine culture is the gold standard for diagnosis of UTI, results are not available for 24 to 48 h. Rapid techniques to predict UTI include urine dipstick tests for leukocyte esterase and nitrites and various forms of urinalysis, including standard microscopy on a centrifuged specimen, high-powered microscopy with a hemacytometer, and Gram stain of unspun urine for organisms.

Nitrite is the degradation product of the nitrates of bacterial metabolism, particularly of Gram-negative bacteria. When an infection is caused by Gram-positive bacteria, the test may be negative (Ma & Shortliffe, 2004; Cavagnaro, 2005). Limitations of the nitrite test include: not all uropathogens reduce nitrate to nitrite (e.g. *Pseudomonas aeruginosa*, enterococci), even nitrite-producing pathogens may show a negative test result (due to the short transit time in the bladder in cases of high diuresis and urine dilution, e.g. neonates). The nitrite test has a sensitivity of only 45-60%, but a very good specificity of 85-98% (Ma & Shortliffe, 2004; Watson, 2004; Deville et al., 2004).

Leucocyte esterase is produced by the activity of leucocytes. The test for leucocyte esterase has a sensitivity of 48-86% and a specificity of 17-93% (Ma and Shortliffe, 2004; Watson, 2004; Hoberman & Wald, 1997; Deville et al., 2004). A combination of nitrite and leucocyte esterase testing improves sensitivity and specificity, but carries the risk of false-positive results (Deville et al., 2004). Back-up urine culture should be sent to detect the approximately 12% of UTIs that will be missed by the dipstick test (Huicho et al., 2002).The dipstick test has become useful to exclude rapidly and reliably the presence of a UTI, provided both nitrite and leucocyte esterase tests are negative. If the tests are positive, it is better to confirm the results in combination with the clinical symptoms and other tests (Watson, 2004; Deville et al., 2004).

The presence or absence of pyuria on urinalysis, along with a urine culture, help make the diagnosis of pediatric UTI. Pyuria with a negative urine culture suggests viral infection, infection with fastidious organisms such as mycobacterium or haemophilus, or noninfectious cystitis. The lack of pyuria and a negative urine culture suggests a non-infectious etiology for cystitis. A positive urine culture along with pyuria likely represents bacterial or fungal infection. A positive urine culture without pyuria may indicate contamination or an immunosuppressed host.

## 9. Evaluation after UTI

After establishing the diagnosis of UTI, certain children require additional testing to determine possible causes for their infection. This is important as eradication of UTI with antibiotics may not be possible without correction of underlying structural abnormalities. In addition, the early diagnosis of anatomically based UTI's can prevent or ameliorate long-term sequelae of persistent or recurrent infections. The evaluation of children after a UTI was once thought to be quite straightforward and focused primarily on detecting and treating VUR in order to prevent end-stage renal disease from reflux nephropathy. Hutch and Hodson were among the first to describe a relationship between reflux and renal scarring. Subsequently, a relationship was established between reflux and chronic pyelonephritis (Smellie et al., 1964; Williams & Eckstein, 1965). Until recently, further evaluation of UTI has centered on the search for reflux with anatomic studies. AAP has suggested guidelines for radiologic imaging of children with UTIs. Urinary tract imaging is recommended in a febrile infant or young child between the ages of 2 months and 2 years with a first documented UTI. Typically this involves a renal and bladder ultrasound and a voiding cystourethrogram (VCUG) (AAP, 1999).

## 10. Standard radiological studies

There is more controversy than consensus regarding the appropriateness of different diagnostic imaging modalities in the evaluation of UTI in children (Slovis, 1995). A "Gold Standard" imaging technique has to be cost-effective, painless, safe, with minimal or no radiation, and an ability to detect any significant structural anomaly. Current techniques do not fulfil all such requirements. Imaging is indicated if patients have known anatomic structural abnormalities, unusual uropathogens such as *Proteus* or *Mycobacterium tuberculosis*, fail to improve with appropriate antimicrobial therapy, or have an unclear source of infection. VCUG should be performed as soon as a child is infection-free and bladder irritability has passed, since delaying the VCUG is associated with losing patients to follow-up. Other radiologic studies are computerized tomography (CT), magnetic resonance imaging (MRI), intravenous urography (IVU), and technetium-99m labeled dimercapto-succinic acid (DMSA) and technetium-99m labeled mercaptoacetyl triglyceride (MAG-3) scans. The most commonly used imaging techniques are discussed in the following sections.

IVU provides a precise anatomic image of the kidneys and can readily identify some urinary tract abnormalities (e.g., cysts, hydronephrosis) (Smellie, 1995a). The major disadvantages of IVU include decreased sensitivity compared with renal scintigraphy in the detection of both pyelonephritis and renal scarring (Smellie, 1995a). Higher dosage of radiation and risk of reaction to contrast medium are also reasons for concern. Given these disadvantages, IVU appears to have little role in the work-up of UTI in children, and the role of IVU is declining with the increasing technical superiority of CT (Huang et al., 1992) and MRI. However, the indication for their use is still limited in UTI.

Although IVU has been a time-honored examination in the initial radiologic evaluation of UTI in children, ultrasonography (US) has largely replaced IVU as the initial screening examination (Rushton et al., 1992). US has become very useful in children because of its safety, speed and high accuracy in identifying the anatomy and size of the renal parenchyma and collecting system (Pickworth et al., 1995). Most physicians believe that it is an appropriate screening test to rule out major abnormalities. US alone is not generally adequate for investigation of UTI in children, as it is unreliable in detecting VUR, renal scarring or inflammatory changes (Smellie, 1995a). It is subjective and therefore operator-dependent, and gives no information on renal function. However, scars can be identified, although not as well as with DMSA scanning (Pickworth et al., 1995).

VCUG is considered mandatory in the evaluation of UTIs in children less than 1 year of age. Typically, the contrast study is chosen for the first study due to its greater anatomic detail, although the radionuclide cystography has been shown in some studies to have a higher sensitivity (Polito et al., 2000). Radionuclide cystography is performed by prolonging the period of scanning after the injection of DTPA or MAG-3 as part of a dynamic renography. It represents an attractive alternative to conventional cystography, especially when following patients with reflux, because of its lower dose of radiation. Radiation dose used for this technique is only 1 percent of that used for standart VCUG (Batisky, 1996). Its continuous monitoring is also more sensitive for identifying reflux than the intermittent flouroscopic monitoring of VCUG. Disadvantages are a poor image resolution and difficulty in detecting lower urinary tract abnormalities (De Sadeleer et al., 1994; Piaggio et al., 2003). While debate exists regarding the timing of a VCUG study, it is generally accepted that it can be performed once the child is afebrile and has a negative urine culture, because VUR may be the transient effect of infection (Mahant et al., 2001). Compliance also appears to be better when the VCUG is performed early after a UTI (McDonald et al., 2000). However, because of low sensitivity and specificity, and because VCUG involves gonadal irradiation and catheterization, its use in diagnosing VUR has been questioned (Ditchfield et al., 1994; Haycock, 1991). In recent years, tailored low-dose fluoroscopic VCUG has been used for the evaluation of VUR in girls in order to minimize radiological exposure (Kleinman et al., 1994). VCUG is mandatory in the assessment of febrile childhood UTI, even in the presence of normal ultrasonography. Up to 23% of these patients may reveal VUR (Kass et al., 2000). It can be performed as a standard contrast study or with a radionuclide.

Renal cortical scintigraphy has replaced IVU as the standard technique for the detection of renal inflammation and scarring (Eggli & Tulchinsky, 1993). Technetium-99m labeled DMSA is a radiopharmaceutical that is bound to the basement membrane of proximal renal tubular cells. This technique is highly sensitive and specific. This technique ensures an accurate diagnosis of cortical scarring by showing areas of hypoactivity indicating lack of function. DMSA scanning offers the advantages of earlier detection of acute inflammatory changes and permanent scars compared with US or IVU (Bircan et al., 1995; MacKenzie et al., 1994). It is also useful in neonates and patients with poor renal function. UTI interferes with the uptake of this radiotracer by the proximal renal tubular cells, and may show areas of focal defect in the renal parenchyma. A star-shaped defect in the renal parenchyma may indicate an acute episode of pyelonephritis. A focal defect in the renal cortex usually indicates a chronic lesion or a renal scar (Kass, 1994; Britton, 1998). A focal scarring or a smooth uniform loss of renal substance has generally been regarded as being associated with VUR (reflux nephropathy) (Rosenberg et al., 1992). The use of Tc-99m DMSA scans can be helpful in the early diagnosis of acute pyelonephritis. About 50-85% of children will show positive findings in the first week. Minimal parenchymal defects, when characterized by a slight area of hypoactivity, can resolve with antimicrobial therapy (Risdon et al., 1994). However, defects lasting longer than 5 months are considered to be renal scarring (Jakobsson & Svensson, 1997). CT is sensitive and specific for the detection of acute pyelonephritis, but CT is more expensive than scintigraphy and exposes the patient to higher levels of radiation, and its use is not supported by evidence.

Contrast material-enhanced voiding ultrasonography has been introduced for the diagnoses of VUR without irradiation (Westwood et al., 2005; Piaggio et al., 2003). Further studies are necessary to determine the role of this new imaging modality in UTI.
When voiding dysfunction is suspected, e.g. incontinence, increased residual urine, increased bladder wall thickness, urodynamic evaluation with uroflowmetry and electromyography should be considered.

## 11. Schedule of investigation

Screening of infants for asymptomatic bacteriuria is unlikely to prevent pyelonephritic scar formation, as these usually develop very early in infancy. Only a minority of children with a UTI have an underlying urological disorder, but when present such a disorder can cause considerable morbidity. Thus, after a maximum of two UTI episodes in a girl and one episode in a boy, investigations should be, but not in the case of asymptomatic bacteriuria (Piaggio et al., 2003; Melis et al., 1992; Smellie 1995b). The need for DTPA/MAG-3 scanning is determined by the ultrasound findings, particularly if there is suspicion of an obstructive lesion.

## 12. Treatment

Therapeutic trials in children with UTI are rare and poorly controlled (Helwig, 1994). Thus, controversy regarding dosage or length of therapy with antimicrobials continues. Treatment's goals are elimination of symptoms and eradication of bacteriuria in the acute episode, prevention of a recurrent UTI, prevention of renal scarring, and correction of associated urological lesions. Initial antibiotic therapy should be based on age, clinical severity, location of infection, presence of structural abnormalities, and allergy to certain antibiotics.
Hospitalization is suggested for symptomatic young infants (less than three months of age) and all children with clinical evidence of acute severe pyelonephritis (high fever, toxic appearance, severe flank pain) (Berman, 1991). Parenteral fluid replacement and appropriate antimicrobial treatment, preferably with cephalosporins (third generation) should be given. In patients with an allergy to cephalosporins, aztreonam or gentamicin may be used. If a Gram-positive UTI is suspected by Gram stain, it is useful to administer aminoglycosides in combination with ampicillin or amoxycillin/clavulanate (Smellie, 1995b). Treatment generally begins with a broad-spectrum antibiotic, but it may need to be changed based on the results of urine culture and sensitivity testing.
When the child becomes afebrile and is able to take fluids, he/she may be given an oral agent to complete the 10-14 days of treatment, which may be continued on an outpatient basis (Hoberman & Wald, 1997). The preferred oral antimicrobials are: trimethoprim (TMP), TMP plus sulphamethoxazole (co-trimoxazole), an oral cephalosporin, or amoxicillin/clavulanate. In children less than 3 years of age, who have difficulty taking oral medications, parenteral treatment for 7-10 days seems advisable, with similar results to those with oral treatment (Bloomfield et al., 2005).
The choice of antibiotic may be affected by local resistance patterns and other considerations. Amoxicillin was traditionally the first-line therapy for outpatient treatment of UTI in children. However, increased rates of *Escherichia coli* resistance have made amoxicillin a less acceptable choice, and studies have found higher cure rates for co-

trimoxazole (AAP, 1999). Fluoroquinolones are widely used in adult patients, although concerns about potential effects on musculoskeletal joint development based on animal data have restricted their use in young children. A recent review of the use of for pediatric UTI noted a high rate of efficacy among patients with complex medical conditions or multidrug resistance, although data on the safety of these agents are limited (Koyle et al., 2003). Fluoroquinolones may be used as second-line therapy in the treatment of serious infections (Grady, 2003). Chloramphenicol, sulphonamides, tetracyclines, rifampicin and amphotericin B should be avoided. The use of ceftriaxone must also be avoided due to its undesired side effect of jaundice.

The duration of outpatient treatment for patients with a less toxic appearance and uncomplicated UTI (no systemic signs of infection) is also controversial (Zelikovic et al., 1992) Evidence is lacking for the use of short-course therapy in children with UTI (Hellerstein, 1994). Oral empirical treatment with TMP, an oral cephalosporin or amoxycillin/clavulanate is recommended, according to the local resistance pattern. The duration of treatment in uncomplicated UTIs treated orally should be 5-7 days (Michael et al., 2003; Tran et al., 2001). A single parenteral dose may be used in cases of doubtful compliance and with a normal urinary tract (Khan, 1994). If the response is poor or complications develop, the child must be admitted to hospital for parenteral treatment (Hellerstein, 1995).

There is no consensus regarding the treatment of pediatric candiduria. Measures include stopping antibiotics, removing or changing indwelling catheters, and antifungal therapy. Commonly used antifungal agents include oral fluconazole and parenteral or intravesical amphotericin B. In patients with obstruction or failure to improve with medical management, urgent percutaneous nephrostomy tube placement to drain the kidney may be needed. Additional measures include amphotericin B irrigation of the nephrostomy tube, or even nephrectomy in severe cases.

## 13. Prophylaxis

If there is an increased risk of pyelonephritis, e.g. VUR, and recurrent UTI, low-dose antibiotic prophylaxis is recommended (Smellie et al., 1988; Arant, 2001). It may also be used after an acute episode of UTI until the diagnostic work-up is completed. The most effective antimicrobial agents are: nitrofurantoin, TMP, cephalexin and cefaclor (Smellie et al., 1988).

## 14. Conclusions

UTI is a common pediatric problem with the potential to produce long-term morbidity. Renal parenchymal infection and scarring are well-established complications of UTI in children and can lead to renal insufficiency, hypertension and renal failure. The clinical presentation of UTI is variable. Young children presenting with fever may have nonspecific symptoms of UTI, and a high index of suspicion is appropriate in this setting. Although culture of the urine remains the gold standard for diagnosing and treating UTIs, technical considerations including method of collection of the urine as well as the time necessary for culture results remain problematic. The appropriate treatment of UTI is controversial and becomes more complex with the emergence of resistance to commonly used antibiotics. The length of antibiotic therapy for UTI in children is also an area of controversy. Therapeutic trials in children with UTI are rare and poorly controlled. Thus, controversy regarding dosage or length of therapy with antimicrobials continues. The diagnostic work-up should be tailored to uncover functional and structural abnormalities such as dysfunctional voiding, VUR and obstructive uropathy. A more aggressive work-up, including renal cortical scintigraphy, ultrasound and voiding cystourethrography, is recommended for patients at greater risk for pyelonephritis and renal scarring, including infants less than one year of age and all children who have systemic signs of infection concomitant with a UTI. Antibiotic prophylaxis is used in patients with reflux or recurrent UTI who are at greater risk for subsequent infections and complications.

## 15. References

AAP. (1999). Practice parameter: the diagnosis, treatment, and evaluation of the initial urinary tract infection in febrile infants and young children. American Academy of Pediatrics. Committee on Quality Improvement. Subcommittee on Urinary Tract Infection. *Pediatrics,* Vol. 103, pp. 843-52, ISSN 0031-4005.

Abrahamsson, K., Hansson, S., Jodal, U. & Lincoln, K. (1993). Staphylococcus saprophyticus urinary tract infections in children. *Eur J Pediatr,* Vol. 152, No. 1, pp. 69-71, ISSN 1432-1076.

Ahmed, SM. (1996). Acute urinary tract infection in children, In: *Manual of Medical Therapeutics,* Rakel, RE. (Ed.), 547-9, Saunders, ISSN 0021-972X, Philadelphia, USA

Andrich, MP., & Majd, M. (1992). Diagnostic imaging in the evaluation of the first urinary tract infection in infants and young children. *Pediatrics,* Vol. 90, No. 3, pp. 436-41, ISSN 0031-4005.

Arant, BS Jr. (2001). Vesicoureteral reflux and evidence-based management. *J Pediatr, Vol.* 139, No. 5, pp. 620-1, ISSN 0022-3476.

Baraff, LJ., Bass, JW., Fleisher, GR., Klein, JO., McCracken, GH., Powell, KR. & Schriger, DL. (1993). Practice guideline for the management of infants and children 0 to 36 months of age with fever without source. *Pediatrics,* Vol. 92, pp. 1-12, ISSN 0031-4005.

Batisky, D. (1996). Pediatric urinary tract infections. *Pediatr Ann,* Vol. 25, No. 266, pp. 269-76, ISSN 0090-4481.

Benador, D., Benador, N., Slosman, D., Mermillod, B., & Girardin, E. (1997). Are younger children at highest risk of renal sequelae after pyelonephritis? *Lancet* Vol. 349, pp. 17-19, ISSN 0140-6736.

Berman, S. (1991). Urinary tract infection, In: *Pediatric Decision Making*, Berman, S. (Ed.), 204-7, Decker, ISBN 1556641419, Philadelphia, USA

Bircan, ZE., Buyan, N., Hasanoglu, E., Ozturk, E., Bayhan, HI. & Sik, S. (1995). Radiologic evaluation of urinary tract infection. *Int Urol Nephrol,* Vol. 27, No. 1, pp. 27-32, ISSN 0301-1623.

Bloomfield, P., Hodson, EM. & Craig, JC. (2005). Antibiotics for acute pyelonephritis in children. *Cohrane Database Syst Rev,* Vol. 25, No. 1, pp. CD003772, ISSN 1469-493X.

Blumenthal, I. (1995). Vesico-ureteric reflux, urinary-tract infection, and renal damage in children. *Lancet,* Vol. 346, pp. 900, ISSN 0140-6736.

Britton, KE. (1998). Renal radionuclide studies, In: *Textbook of Genitourinary Surgery,* Whitfield, HN., Hendry, WF., Kirby, RS., Duckett, W. (Eds), 76-103, Blackwell Science, ISSN 0042-1138, Oxford.

Cavagnaro, F. (2005). Urinary tract infection in childhood. *Rev Chilena Infectol, Vol.* 22, No. 2, pp. 161-8, ISSN 0716-1018.

Chen, JJ., Mao, W., Homayoon, K., & Steinhardt, GF. (2004). A multivariate analysis of dysfunctional elimination syndrome, and its relationships with gender, urinary tract infection and vesicoureteral reflux in children. *J Urol,* Vol. 171, pp. 1907-10, ISSN 0022-5347.

Craig, JC., Knight, JF., Sureshkuman, P., Mantz, E. & Roy, LP. (1996). Effect of circumcision on incidence of urinary tract infection in preschool boys. *J Pediatr,* Vol. 128, no. 1, pp. 23-7, ISSN 0022-3476.

Dayan, P S., Hanson, E., Bennett, JE., Langsam, D. & Miller, SZ. (2004). Clinical course of urinary tract infections in infants younger than 60 days of age. Pediatr Emerg Care, Vol. 20, pp. 85-88, ISSN 1535-1815.

De Sadeleer, C., De Boe, V., Keuppens, F., Desprechins, B., Verboven, M. & Piepsz, A. (1994). How good is technetium-99m mercaptoacetyltriglycine indirect cystography? *Eur J Nucl Med,* Vol. 21, No. 3, pp. 223-7, ISSN 1619-7089.

Deville, WL., Yzermans, JC., van Duijn, NP., Bezemer, PD., van der Windt, DA. & Bouter, LM. (2004). The urine dipstick test useful to rule out infections. A meta-analysis of the accuracy. *BMC Urol* Vol. 4, pp. 4, ISSN 1471-2490.

Ditchfield, MR., de Campo, JF., Nolan, TM., Cook, DJ., Grimwood, K., Powell, HR., Sloane, R., Grimwood, K. & Cahill S.(1994). Risk factors in the development of early renal cortical defects in children with urinary tract infection. AJR *Am J Roentgenol,* Vol. 162, pp. 1393-7, ISSN 1546-3141.

Ditchfield, MR. & Nadel, HR. (1998). The DMSA scan in paediatric urinary tract infection. Australasian Radiol, Vol. 42, pp. 318-20, ISSN 1440-1673.

Ditchfield, M R., Grimwood, K., Cook, DJ., Powell, HR., Sloane, R., Nolan, TM. & de Campo, JF. (2002). Time course of transient cortical scintigraphic defects associated with acute pyelonephritis. *Pediatr Radiol,* Vol. 32, pp. 849-852, ISSN 1432-1998.

Eggli, DF. & Tulchinsky, M. (1993). Scintigraphic evaluation of pediatric urinary tract infection. *Semin Nucl Med,* Vol. 23, pp. 199-218, ISSN 0001-2998.

Esbjorner, E., Berg, U. & Hansson, S. (1997). Epidemiology of chronic renal failure in children: a report from Sweden 1986-1994. Swedish Pediatric Nephrology Association. *Pediatr Nephrol,* Vol. 11, pp. 438-442, ISSN 0931-041X.

Feld, LG. (1991). Urinary tract infections in childhood: definition, pathogenesis, diagnosis, and management. *Pharmacotherapy,* Vol. 11, pp. 326-35, ISSN 1492-2525.

Foxman, B. (2002). Epidemiology of urinary infections: incidence, morbidity, and economic costs. *Am J Med,* Vol. 8, No. 113 (Suppl), pp. 1A:5S-13S, ISSN 0002-9343.

Fussell, EN., Kaack, MB., Cherry, R. & Roberts, JA. (1998). Adherence of bacteria to human foreskins. *J Urol,* Vol. 140. No. 5, pp. 997-1001, ISSN 0022-5347.

Gacinovic, S., Buscombe, J., Costa, DC., Hilson, A., Bomanji, J. & Ell PJ. (1996). Interobserver agreement in the reporting of 99Tcm-DMSA renal studies. *Nuclear Med Commun,* Vol. 17, pp. 596-602, ISSN 1473-5628.

Gordon, I. (1995). Vesico-ureteric reflux, urinary-tract infection, and renal damage in children. *Lancet,* Vol. 346, pp. 489-90, ISSN 0140-6736.

Grady, R. (2003). Safety profile of quinolone antibiotics in the pediatric population. *Pediatr Infect Dis J,* Vol. 22, No. 12, pp. 1128-32, ISSN 1532-0987.

Hansson, S., Martinell, J., Stokland, E. & Jodal, U. (1997). The natural history of bacteriuria in childhood. *Infect Dis Clin North Am*, Vol. 11, pp. 499-512, ISSN 0002-9343.

Haycock, GB. (1991). A practical approach to evaluating urinary tract infection in children. *Pediatr Nephrol*, vol. 5, No. 4, pp. 401-2, ISSN 0931-041X.

Hellerstein, S. (1994). Evolving concepts in the evaluation of the child with a urinary tract infection. *J Pediatr*, Vol. 124, pp. 589-92, ISSN 0022-3476.

Hellerstein, S. (1995). Urinary tract infections. Old and new concepts. *Pediatr Clin North Am*, Vol. 42, No. 6, pp. 1433-57, ISSN 0031-4005.

Hellerstein, S. (2002). Urinary tract infection in children: pathophysiology, risk factors and management. *Infect Med*, Vol. 19, pp. 554-60, ISSN 0749-6524.

Helwig, H. (1994). Therapeutic strategies for urinary tract infections in children. Infection, Vol. 22(Suppl 1), pp. S12-3, ISSN 0300-8126.

Hoberman, A., Chao, HP, Keller, DM, Hickey, R, Davis, HW. & Ellis, D. (1993). Prevalence of urinary tract infection in febrile infants. *J Pediatr*, Vol. 123, pp.:7-23, ISSN 0022-3476.

Hoberman, A. & Wald, ER. (1997). Urinary tract infections in young febrile children. *Pediatr Infect Dis J*, Vol. 16, No. 1, pp. 11-7, ISSN 1532-0987.

Hoberman, A., Charron, M., Hickey, RW., Baskin, M., Kearney, DH. & Wald, ER. (2003). Imaging studies after a first febrile urinary tract infection in young children. *N Engl J Med*, Vol. 348, pp. 195-202, ISSN 0028-4793.

Huang, JJ., Sung, JM., Chen, KW., Ruaan, MK., Shu, GH. & Chuang, YC. (1992). Acute bacterial nephritis: a clinicoradiologic correlation based on computer tomography. *Am J Med*, Vol. 93, No. 3, pp. 289-98, ISSN 0002-9343.

Huicho, L., Campos-Sanchez, M. & Alamo, C. (2002). Metaanalysis of urine screening tests for determining the risk of urinary tract infection in children. *Pediatr Infect Dis J*, Vol. 21, pp. 1-88, ISSN 1532-0987.

Jacobson, SH., Eklof, O., Eriksson, CG., Lins, LE, Tidgren, B. & Winberg, J. (1989). Development of hypertension and uraemia after pyelonephritis in childhood: 27 year follow up. *Br Med J*, Vol. 299, pp. 703-706, ISSN 09598138.

Jakobsson, B. & Svensson, L. (1997). Transient pyelonephritic changes on 99mTechnetium-dimercaptosuccinic acid scan for at least five months after infection. *Acta Paediatr*, Vol. 86, No. 8, pp. 803-7, ISSN 0803-5253.

Jantausch, B. A., V. R. Criss, R. O'Donnell, B. L. Wiedermann, M. Majd, H. G. Rushton, R. S. Shirey, and N. L. Luban. 1994. Association of Lewis blood group phenotypes with urinary tract infection in children. J. Pediatr. 124:863-868.

Jodal, U. (1987). The natural history of bacteriuria in childhood. *Infect Dis Clin North Am*, Vol. 1, No. 4, pp. 713-29, ISSN 0002-9343.

Kass, EJ. (1994). Imaging in acute pyelonephritis. *Curr Opin Urol*, Vol. 4, pp. 39-44, ISSN 0963-0643.

Kass, EJ., Kernen, KM. & Carey, JM. (2000). Paediatric urinary tract infection and the necessity of complete urological imaging. *BJU Int*, Vol. 86, No. 1, pp. 94-6, ISSN 1464-410X.

Khan, AJ. (1994). Efficacy of single-dose therapy of urinary tract infection in infants and children: a review. *J Nalt Med Assoc*, Vol. 86, No. 9, pp. 690-6, ISSN 0027- 9684.

Kibar, Y., Demir, E., Irkilata, HC., Ors, O., Gok, F. & Dayanc, M. (2007). Effect of biofeedback treatment on spinning top urethra in children with voiding dysfunction. *Urology*, Vol. 70, No. 4, pp. 781-4, ISSN 0090-4295.

Kibar, Y., Ors, O., Demir, E., Kalman, S., Sakallioglu, O. & Dayanc. M. (2007). Results of biofeedback treatment on reflux resolution rates in children with dysfunctional voiding and vesicoureteral reflux. *Urology*, Vol. 70, No. 3, pp. 563-6, ISSN 0090-4295.

Kibar, Y., Piskin, M., Irkılata, HC., Aydur, E., Gok, F. & Dayanc, M. (2009). Management of abnormal postvoid residual urine in children with dysfunctional voiding. *Urology*, Vol. 75, No. 6, pp. 1472-5, ISSN 0090-4295.

Klein, JO. & Long, SS. (1995). Bacterial infections of the urinary tract, In: *Infectious Diseases of the Fetus and Newborn Infant*, Remington, JS., Klein, JO. (Eds.), 925-34, Saunders, ISSN 1058-4838, Philadelphia, USA

Kleinman, PK., Diamond, BA., Karellas, A., Spevak, MR., Nimkin, K. & Belanger, P. (1994). Tailored low-dose fluoroscopic voiding cystourethrography for the reevaluation of vesicoureteral reflux in girls. AJR *Am J Roentgenol*, Vol. 162, No. 5, pp. 1151-6, ISSN 1546-3141.

Koyle, MA., Barqawi, A., Wild, J., Passamaneck, M. & Furness, PD. (2003). Pediatric urinary tract infections: the role of fluoroquinolones. *Pediatr Infect Dis J*, Vol. 22, pp. 1133-37, ISSN 1532-0987.

Ma, JF. & Shortliffe, LM. (2004). Urinary tract infection in children: etiology and epidemiology. *Urol Clin North Am*, Vol. 31, No. 3, pp. 517-26, ISSN 1063-5777.

MacKenzie, JR., Fowler, K., Hollman, AS., Tappin, D., Murphy, AV., Beattie, TJ. & Azmy, AF. (1994). The value of ultrasound in the child with an acute urinary tract infection. *BJU Int*, Vol. 74, No. 2, pp. 240-4, ISSN 1464-410X.

Mahant, S., To, T. & Friedman, J. (2001). Timing of voiding cystourethrogram in the investigation of urinary tract infections in children. *J Pediatr*, Vol. 139, pp. 568-71, ISSN 0022-3476.

Majd, M. & Rushton, HG. (1992). Renal cortical scintigraphy in the diagnosis of acute pyelonephritis. *Semin Nuclear Med*, Vol. 22, pp. 98-111, ISSN 0001-2998.

McDonald, A., Scranton, M., Gillespie, R., Mahajan, V. & Edwards, GA. (2000). Voiding cystourethrograms and urinary tract infections: how long to wait? *Pediatrics*, Vol. 105, No. 4, pp. E50, ISSN 0031-4005.

Melis, K., Vandevivere, J., Hoskens, C., Vervaet, A., Sand, A. & Van Acker, KJ. Involvement of the renal parenchyma in acute urinary tract infection: the contribution of 99mTc dimercaptosuccinic acid scan. *Eur J Pediatr*, Vol. 151, No. 7, pp. 536-9, ISSN 1432-1076.

Michael, M., Hodson, EM., Craig, JC., Martin, S. & Moyer, VA. (2003). Short versus standard duration oral antibiotic therapy for acute urinary tract infection in children. *Cochrane Database Syst Rev*, Vol. 1, pp. CD003966, ISSN 1469-493X.

Mingin, GC., Hinds, A., Nguyen, HT. & Baskin, LS. (2004). Children with a febrile urinary tract infection and a negative radiologic workup: factors predictive of recurrence. *Urology*, Vol. 63, pp. 562-65, ISSN 0090-4295.

Piaggio, G., Degl' Innocenti, ML., Toma, P., Calevo, MG. & Perfumo, F. (2003). Cystosonography and voiding cystourethrography in the diagnosis of vesicoureteral reflux. *Pediatr Nephrol*, Vol. 18, No. 1, pp. 18-22, ISSN 0931-041X.

Pickworth, FE., Carlin, JB., Ditchfield, MR., de Campo, MP., de Campo, JF., Cook, DJ., Nolan,

T., Powell, HR., Sloane, R. & Grimwood, K. (1995). Sonographic measurement of renal enlargement in children with acute pyelonephritis and time needed for resolution: implications for renal growth assessment. *AJR Am J Roentgenol*, Vol. 165, No. 2, pp. 405-8, ISSN 1546-3141.

Polito, C., Rambaldi, PF., La Manna, A., Mansi, L. & Di Toro R. (2000). Enhanced detection of vesicoureteric reflux with isotopic cystography. *Pediatr Nephrol*, Vol. 14, pp. 827-830, ISSN 0931-041X.

Richards, MJ., Edwards, JR., Culver, DH. & Gaynes, RP. (1999). Nosocomial infections in pediatric intensive care units in the United States. National Nosocomial Infections Surveillance System. *Pediatrics*, Vol. 103, No. 4, pp. e39, ISSN 0031-4005.

Risdon, RA., Godley, ML., Parkhouse, HF., Gordon, I. & Ransley, PG. (1994). Renal pathology and the 99mTc-DMSA image during the evolution of the early pyelonephritic scar: an experimental study. *J Urol*, Vol. 151, No. 3, pp. 767-73, ISSN 0022-5347.

Rushton, HG., Majd, M., Jantausch, B., Wiedermann, BL. & Belman, AB. (1992). Renal scarring following reflux and nonreflux pyelonephritis in children: evaluation with a 99m technetium-dimercaptosuccinic acid scintigraphy. *J Urol*, Vol. 147, pp. 1327-32, ISSN 0022-5347.

Rosenberg, AR., Rossleigh, MA., Brydon, MP., Bass, SJ., Leighton, DM. & Farnsworth, RH. Evaluation of acute urinary tract infection in children by dimercaptosuccinic acid scintigraphy: a prospective study. *J Urol*, Vol. 148, No. 5 Pt 2, pp. 1746-49, ISSN 0022-5347.

Schoen, EJ. (1990). The status of circumcision of newborns. *N Engl J Med*, Vol, 322, pp. 1308-12, ISSN 0028-4793.

Schulman, SL. (2004). Voiding dysfunction in children. *Urol Clin North Am*, Vol. 31, No. 3, pp. 481-90, ISSN 1063-5777.

Shapiro, ED. (1992). Infections of the urinary tract. *Pediatr Infect Dis J*, Vol. 11, No. 2, pp. 165-8, ISSN 1532-0987.

Shaw, KN., Gorelick, M., McGowan, K L., Yakscoe, NM. & Schwartz, JS. (1998). Prevalence of urinary tract infection in febrile young children in the emergency department. *Pediatrics*, Vol. 102, pp. e16, ISSN 0031-4005.

Sheinfeld, J., A. J. Schaeffer, C. Cordon-Cardo, A. Rogatko, and W. R. Fair. 1989. Association of the Lewis blood-group phenotype with recurrent urinary tract infections in women. N. Engl. J. Med. 320:773-777.

Shortliffe, LM. (1995). The management of urinary tract infections in children without urinary tract abnormalities. *Urol Clin North Am*, Vol. 22, pp. 67-73, ISSN 1063-5777.

Slovis, TL. (1995). Is there a single most appropriate imaging workup of a child with an acute febrile urinary tract infection? *Pediatr Radiol*, Vol. 25 (Suppl 1), pp. S46-9, ISSN 1432-1998.

Smellie, JM., Hodson, CJ., Edwards, D. & Normand, IC. (1964). Clinical and radiological features of urinary infection in childhood. *Br Med J*, Vol. 1, pp. 1222-26, ISSN 09598138.

Smellie, JM., Gruneberg, RN., Bantock, HM. & Prescod, N. (1988). Prophylactic co-trimoxazole and trimethoprim in the management of urinary tract infection in children. *Pediatr Nephrol*, Vol. 2, No. 1, pp. 12-7, ISSN 0931-041X.

Smellie, JM. (1995). The intravenous urogram in the detection and evaluation of renal damage following urinary tract infection. *Pediatr Nephrol*, Vol. 9, pp. 213-20, ISSN 0931-041X.

Smellie, JM., Rigden, SP. & Prescod, NP. (1995). Urinary tract infection: a comparison of four methods of investigation. *Arch Dis Child*, Vol. 72, No. 3, pp. 247-50, ISSN 1743-0585.

Smith, EM. & Elder, JS. (1994). Double antimicrobial prophylaxis in girls with breakthrough urinary tract infections. *Urology*, Vol. 43, pp. 708-13, ISSN 0090-4295.

Sreenarasimhaiah, S. & Hellerstein, S. (1998). Urinary tract infections per se do not cause end-stage kidney disease. *Pediatr Nephrol*, Vol. 12, pp. 210-13, ISSN 0931-041X.

Svanborg, C. & Godaly, G. (1997). Bacterial virulence in urinary tract infection. *Infect Dis Clin North Am*, Vol, 11, pp. 513-29, ISSN 0002-9343.

To, T., Agha, M., Dick, PT. & Feldman, W. (1998). Cohort study on circumcision of newborn boys and subsequent risk of urinary-tract infection. *Lancet*, Vol. 352, No. 9143, pp. 1813-6, ISSN 0140-6736.

Tran, D., Muchant, DG. & Aronoff, SC. (2001). Short-course versus conventional length antimicrobial therapy for uncomplicated lower urinary tract infections in children: a meta-analysis of 1279 patients. *J Pediatr*, Vol. 139, No. 1, pp. 93-9, ISSN 0022-3476.

Wallin, L., Helin, I. & Bajc, M. (2001). Follow-up of acute pyelonephritis in children by Tc-99m DMSA scintigraphy: quantitative and qualitative assessment. *Clin Nuclear Med*, Vol. 26, pp. 423-32, ISSN 0363-9762.

Wan, J., Kaplinsky, R. & Greenfield, S. (1995). Toilet habits of children evaluated for urinary tract infection. *J Urol*, Vol. 154, No. 2 Pt 2, pp. 797-9, ISSN 0022-5347.

Watson, AR. (2004). Pediatric urinary tract infection. *EAU Update Series 2*, pp. 94-100, ISSN 1570-1924.

Westwood, ME., Whiting, PF., Cooper, J., Watt, IS. & Kleijnen, J. (2005). Further investigation of confirmed urinary tract infection (UTI) in children under five years: a systematic review. *BMC Pediatr*, Vol. 5, No. 1, pp. 2, ISSN 1471-2431.

Williams, DI. & Eckstein, HB. (1965). Surgical treatment of reflux in children. *BJU Int*, Vol. 37, pp. 13-24, ISSN 1464-410X.

Yagci, S., Kibar, Y., Akay, O., Kilic, S., Erdemir, F., Gok, F. & Dayanc, M. (2005). The effect of biofeedback treatment on voiding and urodynamic parameters in children with voiding dysfunction. J Urol, Vol. 174, No. 5, pp. 1994-97, ISSN 0022-5347.

Yeung, CK., Godley, ML., Dhillon, HK., Gordon, I., Duffy, PG. & Ransley, PG. (1997). The characteristics of primary vesico-ureteric reflux in male and female infants with pre-natal hydronephrosis. BJU In, Vol. 80, No. 2, pp. 319-27, ISSN 1464-410X.

Zelikovic, I., Adelman, RD. & Nancarrow, PA. (1992). Urinary tract infections in children. An update. *West J Med*, Vol. 157, pp. 554-61, ISSN 0093-0415.

Zorc, JJ., Kiddoo, DA. & Shaw, KN. (2005). Diagnosis and management of pediatric urinary tract infections. *Clin Microbiol Rev*, Vol. 18, No. 2, pp. 417-22, ISSN 0893-8512.

# 16

# Urinary Tract Infection in Children – Onset of a New Era?

Tanja Kersnik Levart and Rajko B Kenda
*University Medical Center Ljubljana*
*Division of Paediatrics, Department of Nephrology*
*Ljubljana*
*Slovenia*

## 1. Introduction

The prevalence of urinary tract infection (UTI) in febrile infants, young children and older children with urinary symptoms and/or fever is 7 to 8 percent and varies by age, race, sex, and circumcision status (1, 2, 3). White children have a two- to four-fold higher prevalence of UTI than black children. The same proportion can be found among girls and circumcised boys.

## 2. Microbiology

Eighty-five percent of UTI in children is caused by Escherichia coli (E. coli). Other gram-negative bacteria include Klebsiella, Proteus, Pseudomonas, Enterobacter, and Citrobacter. Gram-positive bacteria include Staphylococcus saprophyticus, Enterococcus, and, rarely, Staphylococcus aureus. Non-E. coli UTI is more often associated with urinary tract anomalies, younger age, and previous antibiotic treatment (4). Viruses and fungi are uncommon causes of UTI in children (5, 6).

## 3. Pathogenesis

Most UTIs beyond the newborn period are the result of ascending infection, while only a minority of them result from bacteremia (7, 8). Bacterial–host interactions are major factors in UTI taking place, and occur when bacterial factors prevail over the hosts.

Bacterial factors that interact with the host and can cause UTI include the ability to colonize the periurethral area, the ability to ascend into the bladder and kidneys, and the ability to generate inflammatory response. Colonization of the periurethral area by uropathogenic enteric pathogens is the first step in the development of UTI. The bacteria ascend into the bladder and kidneys by a variety of virulence factors. The best-studied virulence factors in E. coli are pili, hair-like appendages on the cell surface. Bacteria possessing pili can adhere effectively to the uroepithelium and ascend into the kidneys, even in children without vesicoureteric reflux (VUR). In the kidneys, the bacterial inoculum generates an intense inflammatory response, which may ultimately lead to renal scarring (9, 10).

Young age (males younger than one year and females younger than four years), phymosis, female sex, white race, genetic factors, urinary tract obstruction, dysfunctional voiding,

VUR, sexual activity, and duration of bladder catheterization are some host factors influencing the predisposition to UTI in children (1-3, 11-18).

## 4. Clinical presentation

Children with UTI can present with various symptoms and signs, depending largely on the site of infection (lower or upper urinary tract) and the age of the child. Infants and young children can present with very nonspecific symptoms ranging from life-threatening urosepsis to asymptomatic bacteriuria, whereas the clinical presentation of UTI in older children can be very similar to that of adults. Fever, poor feeding, irritability, failure to thrive, conjugated hyperbilirubinemia, gastrointestinal symptoms, convulsions, hypotension, pallor and cyanosis are some nonspecific symptoms of UTI in infants. The symptoms of UTI in older children may include fever, urinary symptoms (dysuria, urgency, frequency, incontinence, macroscopic hematuria), and abdominal pain (19-21). The constellation of fever, chills, and flank pain is suggestive of pyelonephritis in older children (22).

### 4.1 Clinical and laboratory evaluation

The evaluation of a child with suspected UTI should include a history of the acute illness and relevant information from his/her past medical history about chronic urinary symptoms, chronic constipation, previous UTI, VUR, previous undiagnosed febrile illnesses, family history of frequent UTIs, VURs and other genitourinary abnormalities, antenatally diagnosed renal abnormality, elevated blood pressure, poor growth and, in sexually active girls, whether barrier contraception with spermicidal agents is used (23).

Following the detailed history evaluation, a child should have a physical examination concentrating on his/her general well-being, including failure to thrive, body temperature, blood pressure, abdominal examination for tenderness and mass, assessment of suprapubic and costovertebral tenderness, examination of external genitalia for anatomic abnormalities, evaluation of the lower back for signs of occult myelodysplasia, and evaluation for other sources of fever.

The laboratory evaluation of a child with suspected UTI should obligatorily include the collection of a urine sample for dip-stick and microscopic analysis and urine culture, the last being necessary to make the diagnosis of UTI.

Obtaining a proper urine sample is of prime importance for the proper diagnosis of UTI in children. In general, there are invasive in noninvasive ways of obtaining urine samples in children. *Suprapubic aspiration of the bladder and bladder catheterization* are invasive procedures. Although the first is not without danger for the patient, it is the most accurate way of obtaining a urine sample. The second method is used only when a catheter is inserted into the bladder for other reasons, such as performing a cystography. We believe that both invasive procedures are not suitable for use in outpatient clinics, and should be strictly reserved for use in hospitals whenever needed. In toilet-trained children, the most widely used and preferred method of collecting urine is the noninvasive **clean-catch**. In infants and young children who are not toilet-trained, urine can be obtained in a **urine bag**. However, up to 85 percent of positive cultures from bag specimens give false-positive results, and therefore the results of urine cultures from bag specimens are useful only if they are negative (24). A better alternative to the urine bag is the **urine collector** designed by Kenda in 1993, which is actually a plastic, sterile, disposable urine collector that highly resembles the urine bag, except for the plastic tube in which the final portion of urine is caught (25-27). The collector is attached via a self-adhesive strip in the same way as the urine bag. During micturition, urine flows through a funnel extending into a tube, which is encircled by a test tube, and flows further into a second chamber (urine bag). Urine is finally collected in the bag, except for the very last portion, which is caught in the test tube, free of contaminants from the urethra. The test tube is separated from the collector, sealed with a lid and sent to the laboratory (Figure 1).

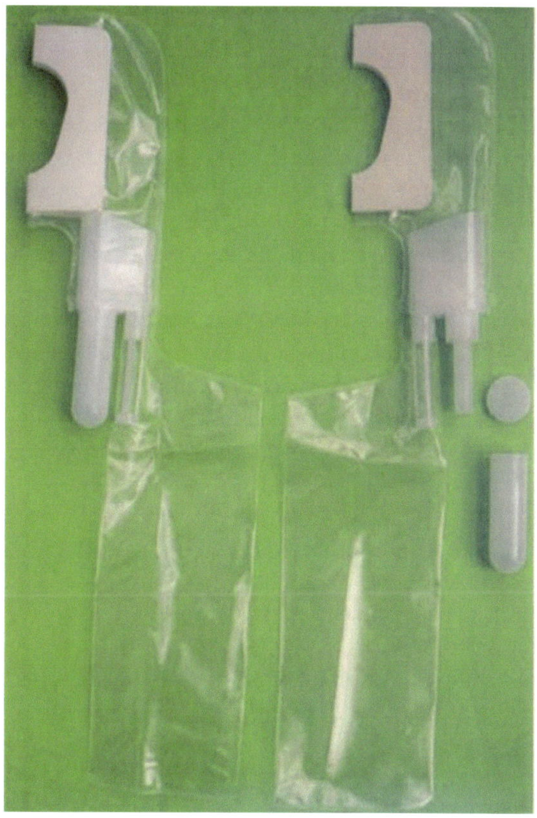

Fig. 1. The paediatric midstream urine collector.

When a proper urine sample is obtained, it can be tested for significant bacteriuria with the following more or less reliable tests:

- **Dipstick analysis** – Dipstick tests are convenient, inexpensive, require little training for proper usage, and may be the only test available in some settings. However, they do not have a sufficiently high specificity and sensitivity for detecting UTI to replace the urine culture (28). The most suggestive for UTI on dipstick analysis is the presence of leukocyte esterase and nitrite. The presence of leukocyte esterase is suggestive of UTI, but does not always signal a true UTI. A child with a positive nitrite test is likely to have UTI, since the nitrite test is highly specific and has a low false-positive rate. However, false-negative results are common, because urine needs to remain in the bladder for at least four hours to accumulate a detectable amount of nitrite. Thus, the negative nitrite test does not exclude UTI.

- **Microscopic exam** - A microscopic examination requires more equipment and training than dipstick tests. In standard microscopy, a centrifuged sample of unstained urine is examined for white blood cells (WBC) and bacteria. When performed in this way, pyuria is defined as ≥5 WBC/high power field (hpf) and bacteriuria as the presence of any bacteria per hpf. The sensitivity of the standard microscopic examination conducted using a centrifuged urine specimen is at best 81 percent.
- **Urine culture** - Quantitative urine culture is the gold standard for diagnosing UTI, and should be performed in any child with suspected UTI before antibiotic treatment is started.

There are other laboratory tests that can help to diagnose UTI in children, but are not particularly helpful. These include:

- **Markers of inflammation** - Elevated peripheral white blood cell (WBC), erythrocyte sedimentation rate (ESR), C-reactive protein (CRP), and procalcitonin (PCT) are indicators of an acute inflammatory process. These markers are associated with upper urinary tract infection. Even though they do not always reliably differentiate between children with cystitis and children with pyelonephritis, we believe that a febrile child with elevated markers of inflammation and culture proven UTI does not need a dimercaptosuccinic acid renal scan (DMSA) to prove acute pyelonephritis.
- **Serum creatinine** — Measurement of serum creatinine is not routinely necessary in children with suspected UTI. However, it should be measured in children with a history of multiple UTI and suspected renal involvement.
- **Blood culture** — Bacteremia occurs in 4 to 9 percent of infants with UTI (29, 30). Fever in bacteremic infants with UTI persists, on average, one day longer than in non-bacteremic infants with UTI (31). However, a positive blood culture does not alter management, except for the length of treatment, in the vast majority of children because the organisms isolated from the blood and urine are usually identical. Blood culture should be routinely performed in the neonatal period, and thereafter it should be taken on the basis of clinical judgment.
- **Lumbar puncture** — Infants under 1 month of age with fever and a positive urinalysis should have a lumbar puncture performed; approximately 1 percent of infants with UTI also have bacterial meningitis (32).

## 5. Diagnosis

In a child with suspected UTI, a urine sample should be taken. The methods of obtaining a proper urinary sample are described in the previous section (Clinical and laboratory evaluation). The urine sample should be cultured, since a urinary culture of properly collected urine sample is the standard test for UTI diagnosis. A positive urinary culture or significant bacteriuria is defined as 100,000 or more colony-forming units (CFU)/ml of urine taken with a clean-catch, urine bag, or urine collector. The number may be lower in small children, who empty the bladder more frequently, and any bacterial growth in urine taken by suprapubic aspiration of the bladder signifies a significant bacteriuria. When culturing urine samples, one may encounter logistic problems. Not all doctors have the possibility of sending a urine sample to the microbiology laboratory at any time of the day. Urine samples can be stored at 4 degrees Celsius up to 24 hours and sent to the laboratory once daily, while on the other hand many logistic problems can be solved with the use of semi-quantitative dip-slide urine cultures. These are cheap accessories of different manufacturers, composed of a sterile pot containing a bar covered with an agar for bacterial growth. All bacteria can grow on one side of the agar (agar CLED), while the other side is designed for the growth of gram negative bacteria (agar MacConkey). In addition to agar CLED and MacConkey, there is a special agar for Echerichia coli in a semi-quantitative dip-slide urine culture named Uricult-trio (Figure 2). Due to their many advantages, semi-quantitative urine cultures are very useful in private medical examinations, as well as in welfare centers and hospitals. Compared to quantitative urine cultures, they are several folds cheaper, do not require transport to the microbiology laboratory, are easy to handle, and the results can easily be interpreted and read in 18 to 24 hours. If these are positive, the bar can be sent to a microbiology laboratory for exact isolation and identification of bacteria with an antibiogram.

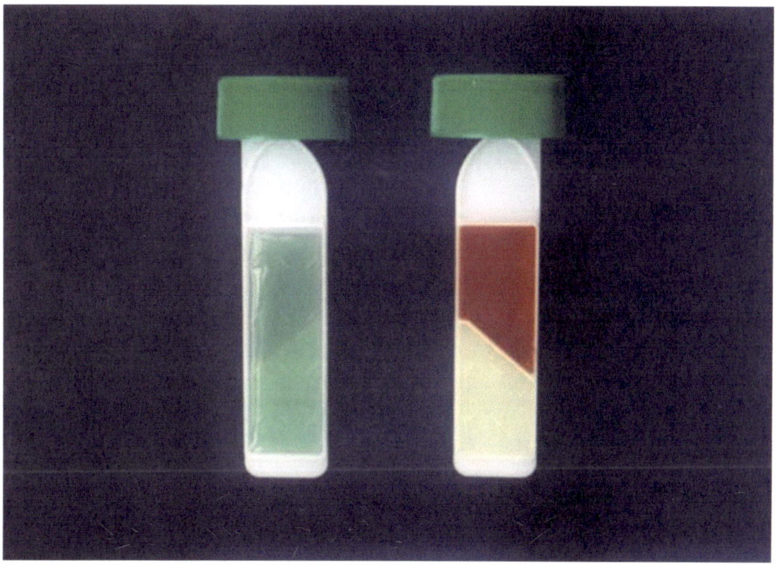

Fig. 2. Uricult-trio.

## 6. Diferential diagnosis

A differential diagnosis in a child with suspected UTI includes all diseases that present with fever, failure to thrive, abdominal pain, or urinary symptoms (urgency, frequency, dysuria). The older the child, the easier it is to differentiate between upper and lower UTI.

## 7. Treatment

Prompt recognition and treatment of UTI are important factors in the prevention of renal scarring. The site of UTI (upper or lower), general welfare of a child and his/her age are major factors that dictate management. There is, however, no doubt that in young children who are at increased risk for UTI on the basis of demographic and clinical factors, as well as in children with underlying urologic abnormalities, treatment should be started immediately after urine was taken for culture and before the results are obtained. Treatment can be postponed only in cases when the child is well, has little or no symptoms of UTI, and the urine results (dipsticks analysis, microscopic examination) are uncertain. In such cases, the results of urine culture are awaited before treating the child, and the urine culture is repeated. Children with asymptomatic bacteriuria should be treated as long urinary tract anomalies are not excluded with an appropriate history, clinical evaluation and urinary tract imaging; thereafter they are treated only if they are symptomatic.

Antibiotics are given as a specific treatment to eliminate infection and prevent urosepsis, while supportive treatment with fluids and antipyretics is also of great importance in relieving acute symptoms. Immediately after urine is taken for culture, the type of antibiotic and the mode of its administration are chosen on the grounds of empirical assumptions about causative bacteria, a knowledge of its resistance, a knowledge of preceding treatment and, above all, on the basis of the child's clinical condition and his/her laboratory results. When the results of urine culture are available, antibiotic treatment is adapted accordingly.

In general, most UTIs in children can be treated successfully in 7 to 14 days (33). Shorter treatment is appropriate only in children older than 5 years with proven lower UTI, provided they do not have any urinary tract anomalies.

The decision to hospitalize a child with UTI depends largely on the child's age, the site of UTI (upper or lower), and the child's general well-being. Infants should always be treated in hospital, since many of them are bacteremic and septic (7, 8). The same is true of all other children with acute pyelonephritis if they are very ill and show clinical signs of urosepsis, immunocompromised patients, patients who vomit or are unable to tolerate oral medication, and patients who fail to respond to outpatient therapy or if there is a lack of adequate outpatient follow-up (34, 35). When these children get better, the antibiotic treatment can be continued and finished orally at home.

Empiric antibiotic therapy for UTI in children should include an antibiotic that provides adequate coverage for E. coli. The agent of choice should, however, be guided by local resistance patterns. Second- and third-generation cephalosporins (eg, cefprozil, cefpodoxime, cefixime, cefotaxime, ceftriaxone) and aminoglycosides (eg, gentamicin, amikacin) are appropriate first-line agents for the empiric treatment of UTI in children. However, these drugs are not effective in treating Enterococcus and should not be used for patients in whom enterococcal UTI is suspected (eg, those with a urinary catheter in place, instrumentation of the urinary tract, or an anatomical abnormality). In such patients, amoxicillin or ampicillin should be added.

There is no firm consensus on the usage of the antibiotic prophylaxis and its duration. The available proof does not justify its broad usage. Moreover, a growing number of reports advise against it, and recommend its usage only in selected groups of patients in whom there is no proof of its inefficacy. In such cases, it seems wise to use it until the condition for which it was taken subsides. Taking into account the above mentioned, prophylaxis is still prescribed to the following groups of children (36):

- children after their first UTI until urinary tract imaging is performed,
- children who are at risk for renal scarring and/or urosepsis (these include children with VUR, especially if it is high-grade, children who are very young or already have scars; other risk factors are also recidivated UTI or obstructive uropathy),
- children with infected kidney stones,
- children without urinary tract anomalies, but with very disturbing, recidivated lower UTI.

The antibiotics used in small doses once daily (in the evening) for long-term prophylaxis are: trimetoprim-sulfomethoxason, nitrofurantoin and, rarely, cefaclor or amoxicillin with clavulanic acid (in infants) (37).

## 8. Management of children after urinary tract infection

Children with UTI should be investigated after their first UTI for possible urinary tract anomalies. The extent of investigations depends largely upon the age of the child, micturation habits and history of possible voiding dysfunction.

In recent decades, a significant change in the management of children after UTI has occurred. It was long believed that vesicoureteric reflux (VUR) of infected urine or even sterile VUR of high grade per se can lead to renal scarring and progressive chronic kidney disease (38-40). Lately, however, such a role of VUR has been questioned by many authors (41-50). It is no wonder that the diagnostic algorithm for children after UTI has changed, and it is hard to expect that a unified approach can be unanimously agreed upon. Those who believe that VUR as such is an important risk factor for renal scarring still favor its detection in all children after proven UTI (51). On the other hand, there is a growing number of pediatric nephrologists who prefer screening for scars (mostly using a 99mTc-dimercaptosuccinic acid renal scan (DMSA)), and recommend cystography (preferably X-ray voiding cystourethrography (VCUG)) only in those cases where renal scarring has been confirmed (41-50). Regardless which approach one finds closer to one's opinion, there should nevertheless be general agreement that the ongoing search for patient-friendly investigations should be an imperative in taking care of the children in question. In addition, when in doubt whether a child benefits from our knowledge of an existing problem, the decision to perform the procedure in question seems more justified when it is simple, painless, radiation-free and noninvasive.

There is really no data to support the assertion that all children after UTI require investigation; however, there is also no convincing data to support the assertion that they do not. Until this dilemma is solved, we believe that all children after UTI still deserve investigation where, in a growing number of cases, ultrasonography (US) and investigations using US techniques appear to be sufficient.

## 9. Management of children after urinary tract infection with emphasis on detection of vesicoureteric reflux

The chronological development of techniques for VUR detection is schematically presented in Figure 3.

Twenty years ago, X-ray voiding cystourethrography (VCUG) was the only method for VUR detection and until not long ago it was considered a gold standard method. In order to diminish the radiation burden on patients, radionuclide voiding cystography (RVC) was introduced some 15 years ago. Unfortunately, in spite of its lower radiation burden and confirmed better sensitivity, it has not replaced VCUG in all justified cases. It was only with the development of new echo contrast agents that echo-enhanced voiding urosonography (VUS) was offered as an alternative. So far, numerous studies have confirmed that its sensitivity and specificity are high enough to allow it to be introduced as a routine method (52-56). It should be noted that this was the first method with no radiation at all, while the fact that catheterization is still necessary, as in VCUG and RVC, posed a drawback to those who strongly opposed catheterization as such. It was therefore not surprising that various investigators were vigorously searching for a noninvasive (catheter-free) method that would still provide all the necessary information regarding VUR. Till now, a number of such methods for VUR detection have been described, i.e. noninvasive radionuclide voiding cystography, noninvasive voiding urosonography, measurement of midline to orifice distance, Color Flow Doppler ultrasonography, and Ureteric jet Doppler Waveform (UJDW) measurement.

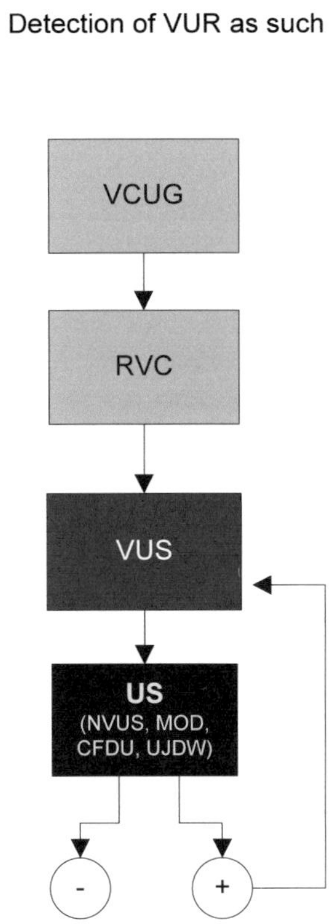


VUR - vesicoureteric reflux, VCUG - X-ray voiding cystourethrography, RVC - radionuclide voiding cystography, VUS - echo-enhanced voiding urosonography, NVUS - noninvasive voiding urosonography, MOD - midline to orifice distance measurement, CFDU - Color Flow Doppler ultrasonography, UJDW - Ureteric jet Doppler Waveform measurement, US - ultrasonography

Fig. 3. Schematic presentation of the chronological development of techniques for vesicoureteric reflux detection.

*Noninvasive radionuclide voiding cystography.* This method is based on the use of dynamic renography, and is performed following a dynamic renogram when the child voids spontaneously; a contrast appearing in the kidney suggests VUR (57). Although this is a catheter-free method for VUR detection, it still poses a certain radiation burden to the patient, has relatively low sensitivity, requires venepuncture with intravenous application of a contrast medium, and is more or less a »side-product« of dynamic renography, which does not appear to be the first line investigation when looking for VUR.

All other noninvasive methods for VUR detection are based on the use of US and are therefore radiation-free.

*Noninvasive voiding urosonography.* An increase in the antero-posterior diameter of the collecting system during and/or after voiding is suggested to be an indirect sign of VUR in noninvasive voiding urosonography. This method was shown to be sensitive enough only in detecting high grade VUR. It could probably be used for detecting VUR in toilet-trained children, but at this point there is not sufficient data to recommend it as a routine method for this purpose (58-61).

*Measurement of midline to orifice distance.* It was suggested that this method be used as an indirect predictor of VUR due to the well-known fact that ureters with more laterally placed ureteric orifices are more likely to be affected by VUR than ureters with orifices that are placed more medially. In spite of being the simplest and the quickest method for VUR detection, data are unfortunately lacking to define a reliable cut-off point suggesting VUR (62, 63).

*Color Flow Doppler ultrasonography.* This method detects any reversal flow from the bladder into the distal ureter as a change in color on the monitor. It was shown to have a relatively high overall sensitivity, while the fact that it must be performed during voiding renders the procedure applicable only in toilet-trained children (63-67).

*Ureteric jet Doppler Waveform measurement.* In this method, the shape of UJDW is used to predict VUR. At this point, it seems to be the most promising of the above-mentioned methods, especially as a screening method in a two-stage protocol in detecting VUR. If one were to proceed from UJDW measurement to VUS only in those cases where UJDW measurement was indicative for VUR, a considerable number of children over 3 years of age would be spared from one of the invasive micturating cystographies (68-71).

The replacement of VCUG with RVC and finally with VUS presents a significant improvement in diminishing the radiation burden on patients, while the catheter-free procedures presenting a "final solution" remain to be validated. From here on, more studies are needed to define the exact role of each of the latest noninvasive (catheter-free) methods for VUR detection.

## 10. Management of children after urinary tract infection with emphasis on the detection of vesicoureteric reflux through its consequences (renal scarring)

The chronological development of techniques for VUR detection through its consequences (renal scarring) is schematically presented in Figure 4.

In the eighties, intravenous urography was considered the gold standard for renal scar detection, and it was recommended that it be performed in every child together with VCUG after UTI (72). Later on, it was almost completely substituted by DMSA, and is nowadays recognized as an obsolete method for this purpose due to the radiation hazard and side effects caused by the contrast medium. At the same time, the role of VUR as a predisposing factor for renal scarring has been questioned by many pediatric nephrologists. It was therefore suggested that VUR should be looked for (mostly using VCUG) only in those cases where renal scars had been confirmed by DMSA. The latter is recognized as the most sensitive method for renal scar detection (73-75), but it unfortunately involves a relatively high radiation load for the patient and can only be performed in nuclear medicine departments. However, even when following this protocol, which differs significantly from the one described above, a less invasive and user friendly approach can be achieved. There are reports confirming that US, a harmless and widely available method, can be used as a safe and efficient substitute for DMSA in the detection and follow-up of children with renal scars (76, 77). These papers are based on the assumption that although US is less sensitive than DMSA in detecting renal scars, it might well be the other way around, namely, that DMSA is too sensitive and detects scars that are too small to be clinically significant, while

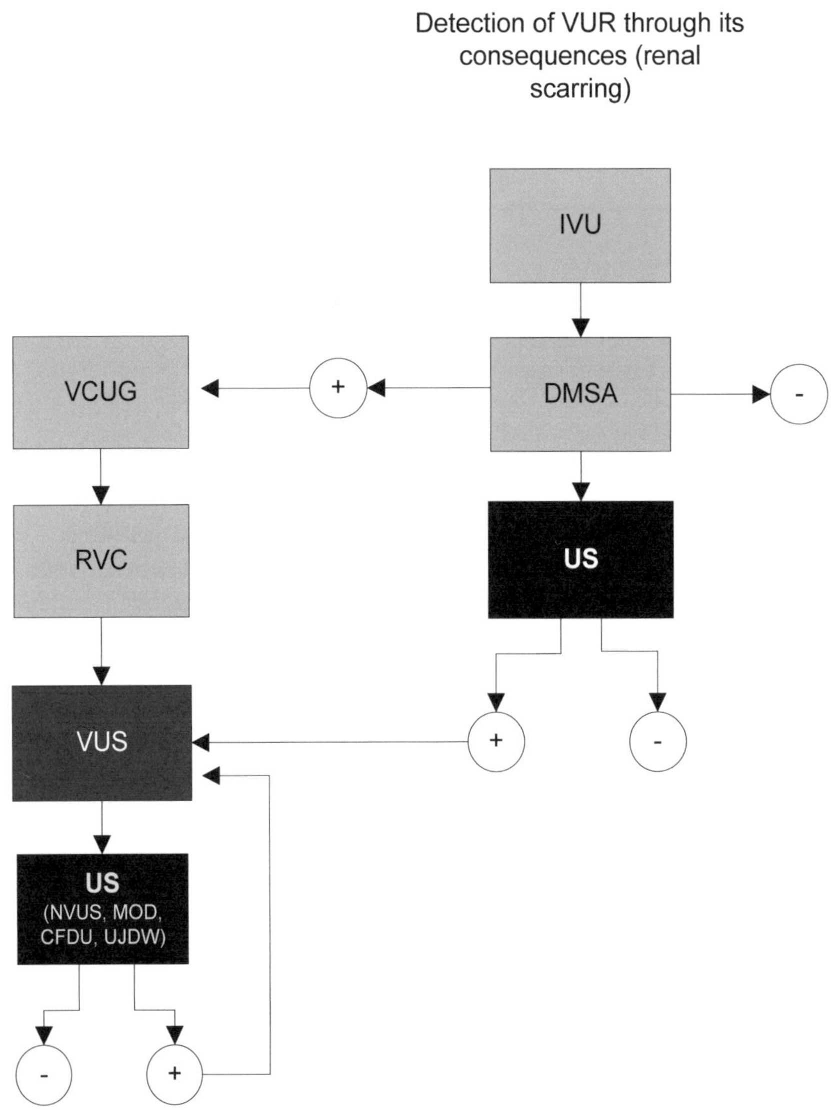


VUR – vesicoureteric reflux, VCUG – X-ray voiding cystourethrography, RVC – radionuclide voiding cystography, VUS – echo-enhanced voiding urosonography, NVUS – nonivasive voiding urosonography, MOD – midline to orifice distance measurement, CFDU – Color Flow Doppler ultrasonography, UJDW – Ureteric jet Doppler Waveform measurement, IVU – intravenous urography, DMSA - 99mTc-dimercaptosuccinic acid renal scan, US – ultrasonography

Fig. 4. Schematic presentation of chronological development techniques for vesicoureteric reflux detection through its consequences (renal scarring).

US is sensitive enough to detect clinically significant scars. This assumption was proved by stratifying DMSA results according to the extent of renal scarring, and correlating them to clinical parameters suggestive of renal impairment in our latest studies (76, 77). Furthermore, when one follows this protocol, which suggests VCUG only in those children with proven scars, we believe there is enough evidence supporting the statement that the sensitivity and specificity of VUS is high enough for it to replace VCUG (52, 56). In other words, DMSA could be replaced by US and VCUG by VUS, while the role of new, catheter-free US techniques for VUR detection, as already described, has yet to be validated.

## 11. Conclusions

Urinary tract infections (UTI) are common and still an important clinical problem in children. Most UTIs beyond the newborn period are the result of ascending infection, while only a minority of them result from bacteremia. Bacterial-host interactions are major factors in the pathogenesis of UTI.

Children with UTI can present with various symptoms and signs that may be very nonspecific, especially in infants and young children, depending largely on the site of infection (lower or upper urinary tract) and the age of the child.

Prompt recognition and treatment of UTI are important factors in the prevention of renal scarring. The gold standard method of proving UTI is a positive urine culture of a properly obtained urine sample. Antibiotics are given as a specific treatment, while fluids and antipyretics are given as a supportive treatment.

Children with UTI should be investigated after their first UTI for possible urinary tract anomalies. The extent of investigations depends largely on the age of the child, his/her micturation habits and history of possible voiding dysfunction. In recent decades, a significant change in the management of children after UTI has occurred. There is no data to support the assertion that all children after UTI require investigation; however, there is also no convincing data to support the assertion that they do not. Until this dilemma is solved, we believe that all children after UTI still deserve investigation, where, in a growing number of cases, ultrasonography (US) and investigations using US techniques appear to be sufficient.

## 12. References

[1] Hoberman A, Chao HP, Keller DM, Hickey R, Davis HW, Ellis D. Prevalence of urinary tract infection in febrile infants. J Pediatr. 1993;123(1):17.

[2] Shaw KN, Gorelick M, McGowan KL, Yakscoe NM, Schwartz JS. Prevalence of urinary tract infection in febrile young children in the emergency department. Pediatrics. 1998;102(2):e16.

[3] Shaikh N, Morone NE, Bost JE, Farrell MH. Prevalence of urinary tract infection in childhood: a meta-analysis. Pediatr Infect Dis J. 2008;27(4):302.

[4] Friedman S, Reif S, Assia A, Mishaal R, Levy I. Clinical and laboratory characteristics of non-E. coli urinary tract infections. Arch Dis Child. 2006;91(10):845.

[5] Wald, ER. Cystitis and pyelonephritis. In: Textbook of Pediatric Infectious Diseases, 6th ed, Feigin, RD, Cherry, JD, Demmler-Harrison, GJ, Kaplan, SL (Eds), Saunders, Philadelphia, 2009. p. 554.

[6] Sobel JD, Vazquez JA. Fungal infections of the urinary tract. World J Urol. 1999;17(6): 410.

[7] Zorc JJ, Kiddoo DA, Shaw KN. Diagnosis and management of pediatric urinary tract infections. Clin Microbiol Rev. 2005;18(2):417.

[8] Struthers S, Scanlon J, Parker K, Goddard J, Hallett R. Parental reporting of smelly urine and urinary tract infection. Arch Dis Child. 2003;88(3):250.

[9] Godaly G, Bergsten G, Hang L, Fischer H, Frendéus B, Lundstedt AC, Samuelsson M, Samuelsson P, Svanborg C. Neutrophil recruitment, chemokine receptors, and resistance to mucosal infection. J Leukoc Biol. 2001;69(6):899.

[10] Svanborg C, Bergsten G, Fischer H, Godaly G, Gustafsson M, Karpman D, Lundstedt AC, Ragnarsdottir B, Svensson M, Wullt B. Uropathogenic Escherichia coli as a model of host-parasite interaction. Curr Opin Microbiol. 2006;9(1):33.

[11] Mårild S, Jodal U. Incidence rate of first-time symptomatic urinary tract infection in children under 6 years of age. Acta Paediatr. 1998;87(5):549.

[12] Singh-Grewal D, Macdessi J, Craig J. Circumcision for the prevention of urinary tract infection in boys: a systematic review of randomised trials and observational studies. Arch Dis Child. 2005;90(8):853.

[13] Mårild S, Wettergren B, Hellström M, Jodal U, Lincoln K, Orskov I, Orskov F, Svanborg Edén C. Bacterial virulence and inflammatory response in infants with febrile urinary tract infection or screening bacteriuria. J Pediatr. 1988; 112(3):348.

[14] Lundstedt AC, Leijonhufvud I, Ragnarsdottir B, Karpman D, Andersson B, Svanborg C. Inherited susceptibility to acute pyelonephritis: a family study of urinary tract infection. J Infect Dis. 2007;195(8):1227.

[15] Jantausch BA, Criss VR, O'Donnell R, Wiedermann BL, Majd M, Rushton HG, Shirey RS, Luban NL. Association of Lewis blood group phenotypes with urinary tract infection in children. J Pediatr. 1994;124(6):863.

[16] Sheinfeld J, Schaeffer AJ, Cordon-Cardo C, Rogatko A, Fair WR. Association of the Lewis blood-group phenotype with recurrent urinary tract infections in women. N Engl J Med. 1989;320(12):773.

[17] Ragnarsdóttir B, Samuelsson M, Gustafsson MC, Leijonhufvud I, Karpman D, Svanborg C. Reduced toll-like receptor 4 expression in children with asymptomatic bacteriuria. J Infect Dis. 2007;196(3):475.

[18] Haraoka M, Hang L, Frendéus B, Godaly G, Burdick M, Strieter R, Svanborg C. Neutrophil recruitment and resistance to urinary tract infection. J Infect Dis. 1999;180(4):1220.

[19] Winberg J, Andersen HJ, Bergström T, Jacobsson B, Larson H, Lincoln K. Epidemiology of symptomatic urinary tract infection in childhood. Acta Paediatr Scand Suppl. 1974;(252):1.

[20] Majd M, Rushton HG, Jantausch B, Wiedermann BL. Relationship among vesicoureteral reflux, P-fimbriated Escherichia coli, and acute pyelonephritis in children with febrile urinary tract infection. J Pediatr. 1991;119(4):578.

[21] Smellie JM, Hodson CJ, Edwards D, Normand IC. Clinical and radiological features of urinary infection in childhood. Br Med J. 1964;2(5419):1222.

[22] Zorc JJ, Kiddoo DA, Shaw KN. Diagnosis and management of pediatric urinary tract infections. Clin Microbiol Rev. 2005;18(2):417.
[23] Hooton TM, Scholes D, Stapleton AE, Roberts PL, Winter C, Gupta K, Samadpour M, Stamm WE. A prospective study of asymptomatic bacteriuria in sexually active young women. N Engl J Med. 2000;343(14):992.
[24] Downs SM. Technical report: urinary tract infections in febrile infants and young children. The Urinary Tract Subcommittee of the American Academy of Pediatrics Committee on Quality Improvement. Pediatrics. 1999;103(4):e54.
[25] Kenda RB, Trebše R. New paediatric urine collector. Acta Paediatr. 1998;87(1):98.
[26] Kenda RB. Intercepting apparatus sampling urine for examination purposes. US Patent 1993;5:255 689.
[27] Kenda RB. Urine sampling apparatus. European Patent 1995;0:510 536 B1.
[28] Gorelick MH, Shaw KN. Screening tests for urinary tract infection in children: A meta-analysis. Pediatrics. 1999;104(5):e54.
[29] Smellie JM, Poulton A, Prescod NP. Retrospective study of children with renal scarring associated with reflux and urinary infection. BMJ. 1994;308(6938):1193.
[30] Hoberman A, Wald ER, Hickey RW, Baskin M, Charron M, Majd M, Kearney DH, Reynolds EA, Ruley J, Janosky JE. Oral versus initial intravenous therapy for urinary tract infections in young febrile children. Pediatrics. 1999;104(1 Pt 1):79
[31] Honkinen O, Jahnukainen T, Mertsola J, Eskola J, Ruuskanen O. Bacteremic urinary tract infection in children. Pediatr Infect Dis J. 2000;19(7):630.
[32] Bachur R, Caputo GL. Bacteremia and meningitis among infants with urinary tract infections. Pediatr Emerg Care. 1995;11(5):280.
[33] Čižman M, Beović B, Marolt Gomiščček M. Priporočila za uporabo protimikrobnih zdravil. Ljubljana: Tiskarna Povše; 2006.
[34] Chang SL, Shortliffe LD. Pediatric urinary tract infections. Pediatr Clin North Am. 2006;53(3):379.
[35] Practice parameter: the diagnosis, treatment, and evaluation of the initial urinary tract infection in febrile infants and young children. American Academy of Pediatrics. Committee on Quality Improvement. Subcommittee on Urinary Tract Infection. Pediatrics. 1999;103(4 Pt 1):843.
[36] Beetz R. May we go on with antibacterial prophylaxis for urinary tract infections? Pediatr Nephrol 2006;21(1):5.
[37] Hansson S, Jodal U. Urinary Tract Infection. In: Avner ED, Harmon WE, Niaudet P, eds. Pediatric Nephrology. 5th ed. Lippincott Williams & Wilkins; 2003. p. 1007.
[38] Arat BS: Vesicoureteric reflux and renal injury. Am J Kidney Dis 1991;17(5):491.
[39] Smellie JM, Normand IC: Bacteriuria, reflux, and renal scarring. Arch Dis Child 1975;50(8):581.
[40] Mannhardt W, Schofer O, Schulte-Wissermann H: Pathogenic factors in recurrent urinary tract infections and renal scar formation in children. Eur J Paediatr 1986; 145(5):330.
[41] Jodal U, Smellie JM, Lax H, Hoyer PF: Ten-year results of randomized treatment of children with severe vesicoureteral reflux. Final report of the International Reflux Study in Children. Pediatr Nephrol 2006;21(6):785.

[42] Tamminen-Möbius T, Brunier E, Ebel KD et al: Cessation of vesicoureteral reflux for 5 years in infants and children allocated to medical treatment. International Reflux Study in Children. J Urol 1992;148(5 Pt 2):1662.
[43] Wheeler D, Vimalachandra D, Hodson EM, Roy LP, Smith G, Craig JC: Antibiotics and surgery for vesicoureteral reflux: a meta-analysis of randomized controlled trials. Arch Dis Child 2003;88(8):688.
[44] O'Donnell B. Reflections on reflux. J Urol 2004;172 (4 Pt 2):1635.
[45] Marra G, Oppezzo C, Ardissino G, Dacco V, Testa S, Avolio L et al: Severe vesicoureteral reflux and chronic renal failure: a condition peculiar to male gender? Data from the ItalKid Project. J Pediatr 2004;144(5):677.
[46] Craig JC, Irwig LM, Knight JF, Roy LP: Does treatment of vesicoureteric reflux in childhood prevent end-stage renal disease attributable to reflux nephropathy? Pediatrics 2000;105(6):1236.
[47] Moorthy I, Easty M, McHugh K, Ridout D, Biassoni L, Gordon I: The presence of vesicoureteric reflux does not identify a population risk for renal scarring following a first urinary tract infection. Arch Dis Child 2005;90(7):733.
[48] Gordon I, Barkovics M, Pindoria S, Cole T, Woolf AS: Primary vesicoureteral reflux as a predictor of renal damage in children hospitalized with urinary tract infection: a systemic review and meta-analysis. J Am Soc Nephrol 2003;14:739.
[49] National Institute for Health and Clinical Excellence (NICE): Urinary tract infection in children. http://guidance.nice.org.uk/CG054 2007.
[50] Venhola M, Uhari M: Vesicoureteral reflux, a benign condition. Pediatri Nephrol 2009;24(2):223.
[51] Coulthard MG: Vesicoureteric reflux is not a benign condition. Pediatri Nephrol 2009;24(2):227.
[52] Bosio M: Cystosonography with echocontrast: a new imaging modality to detect vesicoureteric reflux in children. Pediatr Radiol 1998;28(4):250.
[53] Darge K, Duetting T, Zieger B, Mohring K, Roschneider W, Troeger J: Diagnosis of vesicoureteral reflux with echo-enhanced micturation urosonography. Radiology 1998;38(5):405.
[54] Darge K, Troeger J, Duetting T et al: Reflux in young patients: comparison of voiding US of the bladder and retrovesical space with echo enhancement versus voiding cystourethrography for diagnosis. Radiology 1999;210(1):201.
[55] Mentzel HJ, Vogt S, Patzer L et al: Contrast-enhanced sonography of vesicoureteral reflux in children: preliminary results. AJR 1999;173(3):737.
[56] Kenda RB, Novljan G, Kenig A, Hojker S, Fettich JJ: Echo-enhanced ultrasound voiding cystography in children: a new approach. Pediatr Nephrol 2000;14(4):297.
[57] Gordon I, Colarinha P, Fettich JJ et al: Guidelines for indirect radionuclide cystography. Eur J Nucl Med 2001;28(3):BP16.
[58] Hiraoka M, Hori C, Tsukahara H et al: Vesicoureteral reflux in male and female neonates as detected by voiding ultrasonography. Kidney Inter 1999;55(4):1486.
[59] Hiraoka M, Kasuga K, Hori C, Sudo M: Ultrasonic indicators of ureteric reflux in the newborn. Lancet 1994;343(8896):519.

[60] Hiraoka M, Hashimoto G, Hori C, Tsukahara H, Konishi Y, Sudo M: Use of ultrasonography in the detection of ureteric reflux in children suspected of having urinary tract infection. J Clin Ultrasound 1997;25(4):195.
[61] Kopač M, Kenig A, Ključevšek D, Kenda RB: Indirect voiding urosonography for detecting vesicoureteral reflux in children. Pediatr Nephrol 2005;20(9):1285.
[62] Marshall JL, Johnson ND, De Campo MP: Vesicoureteric reflux in children: prediction with color Doppler imaging. Radiology 1990;175(2):355.
[63] Oak SN, Kulkarni B, Chaubal N: Color flow Doppler sonography: a reliable alternative to voiding cystourethrogram in the diagnosis of vesicoureteral reflux in children. Urology 1999;53(6):1211.
[64] Nishizawa O, Ishida H, Sugaya K, Kohama T, Harada T, Tsuchida S: Application of Doppler color flow imaging method on the detection of vesicoureteric reflux. Tohoku J Exp Med 1989;159(2):163.
[65] Salih M, Baltaci S, Kiliç S, Anafarta K, Bedük Y: Color flow Doppler sonography in the diagnosis of vesicoureteric reflux. Eur Urol 1994;26(1):93.
[66] Koşar A, Yeşiladağ A, Oyar O, Perk H, Gülsoy U: Detection of vesico-ureteric reflux in children by colour-flow Doppler ultrasonography. BJU International 2003; 91(9):856.
[67] Heberlik A: Detection of low-grade vesicoureteric reflux in children by color Doppler imaging mode. Pediatr Surg Int 1997;12(1):38.
[68] Leung VY, Chu W, Yeung CK, Metreweli C: Doppler waveforms of the ureteric jet: an overview and implications for the presence of a functional sphincter at the vesicoureteric junction. Pediatr Radiol 2007;37(5):417.
[69] Leung VY, Metreweli C, Yeung CK: The ureteric jet Doppler waveform as an indicator of vesicoureteric sphincter function in adults and children. An observational study. Ultrasound in Med. & Biol 2002;28(7):865.
[70] Leung VY, Metreweli C, Yeung CK: Immature ureteric jet Doppler patterns and urinary tract infection and vesicoureteric reflux in children. Ultrasound in Med & Biol 2002;28(7):873.
[71] Ključevšek D, Ključevšek T, Kersnik Levart T, Kenda RB: Ureteric jet Doppler waveform: is it a reliable predictor of vesicouretric reflux in children? Pediatr Nephrol 2009;24(2):313.
[72] Royal College of Physicians Research Unit Working Group: Guidelines for the management of acute urinary tract infection in childhood. J R Coll Physicians Lond 1991;
25(1):36.
[73] Mackenzie JR: A reveiw of renal scarring in children. Nuclear Medicine Communications 1996;17(3):176.
[74] Moorthy I, Wheat D, Gordon I: Ultrasonography in the evaluation of renal scarring using DMSA scan as the gold standard. Pediatr Nephrol 2004;19(2):153.
[75] Monsour M, Azmy AF, MacKenzie JR: Renal scarring secondary to vesicoureteric reflux. Clinical assessment and new grading. Br J Urol 1987;60(4):320.

[76] Kersnik Levart T, Kenig A, Fettich JJ, Ključevšek D, Novljan G, Kenda RB: Sensitivity of ultrasonography in detecting renal parenchyma defects in children. Pediatr Nephrol 2002;17(12):1059.

[77] Kersnik Levart T, Ključevšek D, Kenig A, Kenda RB: Sensitivity of ultrasonography in detecting renal parenchyma defects: six years follow-up. Pediatr Nephrol 2009;24(6):1193.

# 17

# UTI in Children

Samileh Noorbakhsh and Vida Zarabi
*Research Center of Pediatric Infectious Diseases, Tehran University of Medical Sciences, Tehran, Iran*

## 1. Introduction

Urinary tract infection is common in children. Before the age of 6 months; boys are more susceptible to UTI than girls thereafter, the incidence is substantially higher in girls than in boys .Up to 11.3% of girls and 3.6% of boys studied in UK will have had an UTI by age 16years .UTI is usually caused by gram-negative organisms, especially Escherichia coli which accounts for about 80% of all pathogens. Proteus is more common in boys. (1, 2)
In childhood, upper UTI with 5.3% prevalence rate, are one of the most important causes of hospitalization. Although acute pyelonephritis might presents with fever, lethargy, anorexia, and vomiting but there are no certain specific diagnostic laboratory tests and clinical symptoms for diagnosis of UTI (1, 2)
Untreated upper UTI can produce severe renal damages. Delay in treatment of acute pyelonephritis increases the risk of kidney damage. Complications of acute pyelonephritis include intra renal and peri renal abscess. Early diagnosis and treatment of urinary tract infection in children is important (3, 4)
Recurrent UTI is defined as a further infection by a new organism. Relapsing UTI is defined as a further infection with the same organism. (1-5)
Uncomplicated UTI infection requires no imaging and often shows no imaging abnormalities. Children who fail to respond to treatment or are severely ill need imaging evaluation (11) Obstructive anomalies are found in up to 4%, and vesico ureteral reflux in 8% to 40% of those with first urinary tract infection. Acute pyelonephritis and reflux are two synergistic factors in the destruction of kidneys of children (1-5)
In children, vesico ureteral reflux of infected urine is the most common cause of chronic pyelonephritis and chronic interstitial nephritis. Intra renal reflux induces reflux nephropathy, progressive renal injury and cortical scarring. Reflux nephropathy usually observed as a focal cortical scar that overlies a blunted calyx in the upper pole of kidney (11)
Imaging findings in children with reflux nephropathy is similar to chronic pyelonephritis in adults. Both type of nephropathy are best demonstrated on IVP or US and CT as classically lobar, with normal lobes with normal calyces interposed between diseased lobes. (11-17) CT is more sensitive than Ultrasound in demonstrating subtle changes in the renal parenchyma associated with uncomplicated pyelonephritis. CT is normal in some patients with mild uncomplicated pyelonephritis. Complications such as renal or peri renal abscess are well demonstrated by CT or US (17)
Although imaging studies have been considered after the diagnosis of a first urinary tract infection, the effect of such studies on outcome has been unclear. Recently, low radiation procedures recommended for diagnosis of VUR (18)

Urinary tract infections accounting for a considerable percentage of antibiotic prescriptions in some countries (18-30)
The prevalence of resistant gram negative organisms is increased during last decade (19, 20)
The first febrile uncomplicated UTI in children is caused by E coli in 70% to 90% of cases. In recent studies a high rates of resistant uropathogens (other than E coli) to various antimicrobial agents in children received prophylactic antibiotics prophylaxis (21-24). So a high level of diagnostic accuracy is essential in view of the increasing prevalence of antibiotic resistance.

## 2. UTI diagnosis

The normal urinary tract is sterile. UTI is defined by pure growth of more than 10 5 colony forming units of bacteria per ml of urine.Urine culture is the gold standard for the diagnosis of UTI ,but negative urine culture reported in up to 60 to 80% of UTI cases and urine culture is time-consuming (4, 5) In urine sample obtained by suprapubic aspiration any growth of urinary pathogens is clinically important. (6)
Upon Schmiemann et al opinion differentiating UTI from asymptomatic bacteriuria, which usually requires no treatment, can lower the frequency of unnecessary antibiotic prescriptions (7) Rapid urine tests, such as microscopy with Gram stain, for bacteria and white cells, and dipsticks, for leucocyte esterase and nitrites often used for diagnosis (6-7)
In recent years, fast screening methods that can reduce the necessity for urine cultures studied by some authors .The Sysmex UF-1000i is a urine flow cytometer that uses two separate channels for counting blood cells and bacteria such as microscopic examination and culture. (8-11)
Broeren et al reported the high percentage of false-negative results in screened negative urine samples with the sysmex UF-1000i urine flow cytometer. Broeren et al did not warrant the UF-1000i as a screening analyzer. (8)Indeed van der Zwet et al did not recommend urine flow cytometer for use in complicated patient populations, such as neutropenic patients and patients in whom yeast infection is suspected (9) Manoni et al studied 214 untreated urine samples using the Sysmex UF-1000i and compared with results obtained from quantitative manual microscopy using the Fuchs-Rosenthal counting chamber. They concluded automated urine particle analysis is sufficiently precise and improves the workflow in a routine laboratory (10) Williams et al determined that accuracy of microscopy for white cells is no better than that of dipstick. Up to 10% of children with a urinary tract infection had negative rapid tests. Rapid test cannot replace urine culture (11)

### 2.1 Diagnostic imaging studies

Acute pyelonephritis and reflux diagnosed by several imaging methods; ultrasonography, IVP, VCUG , CT , Doppler , DMSC scintigraphy and MRU. Danger of exposure to radiation is important in patients.Renal ultrasonography and renal scanning at the time of the acute illness are of limited value, because they do not provide information that modifies management (12-18)

## 3. Renal ultrasonography

Ultrasonography is a noninvasive test which routinely performed after the diagnosis of a first UTI.US has replaced IVP for evaluating the size and shape of the kidneys but is not sensitive enough to detect the presence of hydronephrosis, hydroureter, acute pyelonephritis, or renal scarring (11) VUR which affects approximately 30 to 40 percent of young children cannot be consistently detected by US has been an important consideration in ultrasonography.

### 3.1 IVP (IV pyelography)

Excretory urography, the traditional method of imaging the kidneys replaced by non invasive and safe methods in last decades. However, US, CT, MR all provide better images of the renal parenchyma.

### 3.2 VCUG

VCUG is used to identify children with vesicoureteral reflux currently performed any time after three to four days of therapy.

Vesicoureteral reflux was graded according to the classification system of the international reflux international study committee. Prophylactic therapy recommended in children with at least grade ii VUR.

Otokesh et al compared voiding urosonography or cystosonography with radio nucleotide cystography for evaluation of VUR (12). Sensitivity and specifity of voiding urosonography was 87% and 88%, respectively, with a 94% positive predictive value and a 77% negative predictive value. It concluded that voiding urosonography is a highly accurate, safe and inexpensive tool for the screening, diagnosis and follow-up of VUR.

### 3.3 Renal DMSA scans

Acute pyelonephritis was defined by the presence of focal or diffuse areas of decreased uptake of labeled DMSA without evidence of cortical loss or by the presence of diffusely decreased uptake in an enlarged kidney (15).

DMSA scans obtained at presentation and six months later identify children with acute pyelonephritis and renal scarring. The degree of scarring was assessed quantitatively by outlining the scarred area (15).

The accuracy of renal artery resistive index (RI) in doppler ultrasonography with DMSA scan and VCUG for diagnosis of APN and reflux in pediatrics patients were assessed and compared. There is a significant relationship between increased RI and the severity of renal involvement.

### 3.4 MRU

In recent years, Dynamic gadolinium -MRU as a new alternative imaging method with free of radiation hazards presented by some authors. (16-18).

Dynamic gadolinium DTPA-enhanced MR urography has been shown to give high-quality views of the morphology of the obstructed urinary tract and an accurate evaluation of urinary excretion (17).

Zarabi et al observed good agreement between MRU and DMSA scan in results of IVP&VCUG. No agreement presented between MRU and DMSA scan with ultra sonographic studies. So, dynamic MRU might be a valuable method in diagnosis of urinary tract anomalies like as hydronephrosis, obstractive uropathy, congenital malformation, pyelonephritis, renal scar (18).

The contrast medium used in MRU is also less toxic and with fewer adverse effects than the radiographic contrast medium used in conventional IVP .Although the economic aspect is still problematic and needing for sedation, it is obvious that MR urography will continue to increase its role in clinical uro radiology. MR imaging offers a potential to reduce the need for invasive retrograde pyelography. (16-18)

## 4. UTI Treatment

UTI is caused by E. coli in over 80% of cases and treatment is a course of antibiotics. The uro pathogens other than E coli in the gastrointestinal tract were selected while children were receiving antibiotic prophylaxis (1-4).

Due to acute illness caused by UTI and the risk of pyelonephritis-induced permanent kidney damage, many children are given long-term antibiotics for reducing the recurrence (5-7) The risk of delayed versus early treatment of acute pyelonephritis in children is not well defined and renal scarring would be investigated (8) The prophylactic antibiotic was not effective in reducing bacterial colonization of the prepuce. Some uro pathogens might have come from the external genitalia (19-20).

### 4.1 Modes of antibiotic administration

The optimal route for antibiotic therapy oral (PO) or intravenous (IV) versus intramuscular administration is not clear. Consensus guidelines from the 1990s still recommend IV antibiotics. (1-5)

The American Academy of Pediatrics recommended early antibiotic treatment, given parenterally if necessary in febrile infants and young children suspected of having a UTI (1-4).

Treatment failure for generally healthy young infants hospitalized with utis is uncommon and is not associated with the duration of intravenous antibiotic treatment. Severity of illness and the presence of known abnormalities of the genitourinary tract, but not young age, were associated with increased risk for treatment failure. (3, 4)

As intravenous antibiotic therapy is associated with side effects, toxicity, high cost, and long hospitalization period in treatment of UTIs (4,5) Switch therapy (intravenous-to-oral antibiotic) has been considered . Clinicians should consider PO antibiotics for these children who are nontoxic and have close parental and follow-up care. Treating more infants with short-course intravenous antibiotic therapy would decrease the length of hospitalization for children and families without affecting the readmission rate. (5, 6)

Recently, the national institute for health and clinical excellence published treatment guidelines advocating PO antibiotics in uncomplicated patients as young as three months of age controlled trials for choice of antibiotics in children with acute pyelonephritis. There are no data on PO antibiotics for UTIs in infants younger than one month of age due to higher risks of bacteremia, meningitis and nonspecific findings, these children would benefit from conservative IV antibiotics. (1-5)

Some authors reported no different results for renal scarring and serious adverse events between IV and PO antibiotic groups. PO antibiotic therapy for children with UTIs has the advantages of ease and cost over IV therapy. (24-30)

The lack of association between the length of intravenous antibiotic therapy and subsequent treatment failure reported in recent years. In a prospective, randomized trial the incidence of renal scars was similar in patients who received 3 days compared 8 days of intravenous

ceftriaxone. Increased renal height at initial ultrasound examination and grade 3 VUR were significant risk factors for renal scars. (28-30)
Hodson et al identified po antibiotics appear to be as effective as initial IV antibiotics for UTIs in children older than one month of age with no known structural urological abnormality. (24)
Perri et al reported the oral antibiotics equivalent to intravenous antibiotics for the initial management of pyelonephritis in children .Two nuclear radiologists interpreted the renal scans independently and resolved any discrepancies by consensus. (27)
VUR rather than antibiotic choices might affect renal scarring. There was no risk difference in renal scarring between treatment groups, despite the presence of VUR. However, these children have a higher risk of renal scarring than children without VUR. (28-30)
The standard antibiotic therapy was sequential IV cefotaxime or ceftriaxone for three days, followed by cefixime , amoxi -clavulanate or ceftibutin for either seven days or 11 days versus the same total duration with po antibiotics alone. (25-30)
Noorbakhsh et al (2004) compared the efficacy and safety of ceftriaxone with switch to cefixime, 8 mg/kg once a day with aminoglycoside therapy in urinary tract infections. Response rate in cases with switch therapy was higher than children treated with intravenous aminoglycoside (88% vs. 80%; p value = 0.82). Most of those patients had a favorable clinical/microbiologic response assessment at the 7 days post therapy. (25)
Mertz et al (26) reported the acceptable rate of response both clinically and microbiologically in children, who received ceftriaxone with switch to cefixime.
Cefixime, ceftibuten and amoxicillin / clavulanic acid recommended for oral antibiotics, or with short courses (2 to 4 days) of IV therapy followed by oral therapy. If IV therapy is chosen, single daily dosing with aminoglycosides is safe and effective. (25-30)
Cefixime is a third-generation oral cephalosporin that is highly active against a broad range of gram-negative and some gram-positive aerobic bacteria, and has a low rate of side effects. On the basis of the literature data, cefixime could be indicated in the treatment of UTIs in children either as monotherapy or as switch therapy. (25, 26)
Resistance to common PO antibiotics may be greater in UTI cases with prophylactic drugs (21-30) Several risk factors explained for the emergence of resistant organisms, including underlying genitourinary tract abnormalities, in-hospital treatment of UTI (19,20) previous antibiotic exposure, history of previous UTI. (21-23 )

## 5. UTI management

The prevention of renal scars by early and appropriate antibiotics is essential. (1, 2)APN can induce irreversible renal scars, with a risk for hypertension or chronic renal failure at long-term follow-up. (3, 4)
In all children with a previous febrile urinary tract infection, the routine performance of urinalysis, urine culture, or both during subsequent febrile illnesses is needed. (4-10) However, different approaches to management considered on age of children: children under 1 year; young children (1–4, 5, or 7 years, depending on the information source); and older children (up to 12–16 years). [12-18]
Approximately 60 to 65 percent of imaging studies will be abnormal in children younger than 2 years who have a first febrile UTI (12-14).Currently DMSA scans, is the best way to detect renal scars, the percentage of residual renal scars after first APN episode has been

shown to vary between 25% and 60%(15) Parenchymal defects on DMSA reported in 36% of all involved kidneys and at least one scarred kidney in 59% of children with VUR. VUR was a weak predictor of renal damage in children admitted to hospital. Local or systemic immune problems are factors in the development of UTI. (14)
VUR runs in families. The incidence of reflux ranged from 26% in asymptomatic siblings to 86% in symptomatic (UTI) siblings in compare with a rate of less than 1% in the general population. No clear link has yet been established between specific genes and an adverse outcome. (14, 15)

### 5.1 Prophylactic treatment

A widespread practice has been to initiate long-term prophylactic antimicrobial therapy in children found to have VUR (1, 2) The currently recommended antibiotics, including co - trimoxazole, nitrofurantoin, and nalidixic acid or amoxicillin- clavulanate (5-7). Greater antimicrobial resistance observed in patients receiving antibiotic prophylaxis (21-23) Except in 1 study, with co- trimoxazole prophylaxis , decreased antimicrobial susceptibilities were as prominent as those in children receiving cephalexin or cefaclor prophylaxis. (19-23)
Although concerns have existed that VUR may be a risk factor for recurrent UTIs, recent findings had not showed an increased risk of treatment failure (eg recurrence of fever or positive urine culture) in children with VUR. (21-30)
Attitudes toward the use of prophylactic antibiotics had changed during last decade. Previous empirical approach, which has recently been questioned, was based on an international study conducted in the 1980s that compared medical management (i.e prophylactic antimicrobial therapy) with surgical management of VUR and did not include an observation group as a control. A meta - analyses in prevention and treatment of UTI had done. The useful ness of empirical prophylactic antimicrobial therapy had not confirmed by Masson et al study. (22)

## 6. References

[1] James larcombe. Urinary tract infection in children.Clinical evidence .Cochrane Data base syst Rev 2009
[2] Sudhir K. Anand .urinary tract infections. Pediatrics, 2005, pages 738-742 Arc Int Med 2010: 8 ; 170 (5):489-90.
[3] Gabrielle J. Williams, petra macaskill ,siew f chan. et al. absolute and relative accuracy of rapid urine tests for urinary tract infection in children: a meta-analysis. The Lancet Inf Dis :2010( 10) 4:240 - 250
[4] Drekonja DM, Okoye NC, Kuskowski MA, Johnson JR. Appropriateness of urinary tract infection diagnosis and treatment duration. Arch Intern Med 2010 :8; 170 (5):489-90.
[5] F Bouissou, C Munzer, S Decramer, B Roussel Prospective, randomized trial comparing short and long intravenous antibiotic treatment of acute pyelonephritis in children: dimercaptosuccinic acid scintigraphic ...... - Pediatrics, 2008 - Am Acad Pediatrics
[6] Westwood ME, Whiting PF, Cooper J, Watt IS, Kleijnen J. Further investigation of confirmed urinary tract infection (UTI) in children under five years: a systematic review. C Pediatrics 2005 15; 5(1):2.
[7] Schmiemann G, Kniehl E, Gebhardt K, Matejczyk MM, Hummers-Pradier E. Dtsch Arztebl Int. 2010 May;107(21):361-7. Epub 2010 May 28. The diagnosis of urinary tract infection: a systematic review.

[8] MAC Broeren, S Bahceci, HL Vader. Screening for urinary tract infection with the sysmex UF-1000i urine flow cytometer.J of Clinical Mic, Volume 49, Issue 3, March 2011, Pages 1025-1029

[9] Will C. van der Zwet, Jan Hessels, Fatih Canbolat, Martine M.L. Deckers. Clinical Evaluation of the Sysmex UF-1000i® urine flow cytometer in the diagnostic work-up of suspected urinary tract infection in a Dutch general hospital. Chem and Lab Med. Volume 48, Issue 12, Pages 1765–1771

[10] Fabio Manoni, Agostino Tinello, Lucia Fornasiero, Paolo Hoffer, Valeria Temporin, Sara Valverde, Gianluca Gessoni. Urine particle evaluation: a comparison between the UF-1000i and quantitative microscopy. Clinical Chemistry and Laboratory Medicine Aug 2010, Vol. 48, No. 8, Pages 1107–1111

[11] Malcolm G Coulthard, Andrew Nelson,Terry Smith. Point-of-care diagnostic tests for childhood urinary-tract infection: phase-contrast microscopy for bacteria, stick testing, and counting white blood cells. Clini Pat 2010 ( 63):823- 829.

[12] Hang Luk, Yip Hin Woo drea Wai San Au-Yeung , James Chi Sang Chan .Imaging in Pediatric Urinary Tract Infection: A 9-Year Local Experience. Wing AnAJR: 192, May 2009

[13] Otukesh H, Hoseini R, Behzadi AH, et al .Accuracy of cystosonography in the diagnosis of vesico urethral reflux in children. Saudi J Kidney Dis Transpl . 2011 May; 22(3):488-91.

[14] N Ataei,F Sayari-Fard ،A Madani ،S T Esfahani ،M Khorasani ,F Ataei . Scintigraphic screening in the detection of renal scarring in siblings of children with primary reflux .Act Med Iranica 2007;45(3): 219-226.

[15] Chroustová D, Palyzova D, Urbanova I, Kolska M. Results of a five-year study of (99m)Tc DMSA renal scintigraphy in children and adolescents following acute pyelonephritis. Nuc Med Rev Cent East Eur. 2006; 9 (1):46 –50

[16] Riccabona M.Pediatric MRU-its potential and its role in the diagnostic work-up of upper urinary tract dilatation in infants and children. World J Urol. 2004 Jun; 22(2):79-87

[17] Vivier PH, Blondiaux E, Dolores M, Marouteau-Pasquier N, Brasseur M, Petitjean C, Dacher JN.Functional MR urography in children.J Radiol : 2009 ; 90(1 Pt 1):11-9.

[18] V zarabi ,S Noorbakhsh *,N Rahim Zadeh. K Samimi ,M Ghafori ,A Jafarian,A Tabatabaei .Diagnostic value of dynamic Magnetic Resonance Urogram imaging in children with Urinary Tract Infection TUMJ 2011, 69( 2): 872-877

[19] Chi-Hui Cheng, Ming-Horng Tsai, Yhu-Chering Huang, Lin-Hui Su , Yong-Kwei Tsau, Chi-Jen Lin, MD, Cheng-Hsun Chiu, Tzou-Yien Lin. Antibiotic Resistance Patterns of Community-Acquired Urinary Tract Infections in Children With Vesicoureteral Reflux Receiving Prophylactic Antibiotic Therapy. PED 2008,122 ( 6):1212-1217

[20] S Noorbakhsh, M Farhadi, A Tabatabaei. Determination of the MIC of antibiotics for gram negative microorganisms isolated from the sterile sites of children hospitalized in Rasool Akram hospital.Iranian Journal of Pediatrics,2006;16(4) : 419-425 20.

[21] Williams G, Craig JC. Long-term antibiotics for preventing recurrent urinary tract infection in children.Update of Cochrane Database Sys Rev. 2006;3: CD001534

[22] P. Masson, S. Matheson, A. Webster, J. Craig.Meta-analyses in Prevention and Treatment of Urinary Tract Infections. INFECTIOUS DISEASE CLINICS OF NORTH AMERICA, Volume 23, Issue 2, Pages 355-385.
[23] W Gabrielle; Craig, Jonathan, Prevention of recurrent urinary tract infection in children. Current Opinion in Inf Dis: 2009 - Volume 22 - Issue 1 - p 72-76
[24] Hodson EM, Willis NS, Craig JC. Antibiotics for acute pyelonephritis in children .Cochrane Database Syst Rev. 2007 Oct 17; (4): CD003772.
[25] Noorbakhsh S, Lari AR, Masjedian F, Mostafavi H, Alaghehbandan R. Comparison of intravenous aminoglycoside therapy with switch therapy of cefixime in urinary tract infections. Saudi Med J. 2004 Oct; 25(10):1513-519.
[26] Mertz et al. Outcomes of early switching from intravenous to oral antibiotics on medical wards. J ANTIMICROB CHEMOTHER 2009; 64:188-199.
[27] John D Perry, J Hom .Are oral antibiotics equivalent to intravenous antibiotics for the initial management of pyelonephritis in children? Ped Child Health: 2010 15(3): 150–152.
[28] RA Santucci .New Concepts in Antimicrobial Treatment for Complicated Urinary Tract Infections: Single Daily Aminoglycoside Dosing and SwitchTherapy. Drug treatment in urology, 2006 - books.google.com
[26] A Pohl .Modes of administration for antibiotics for symptomatic severe urinary tract infections' Evidence-Based Child Health: A Cochrane; 2009
[30] TJ Neuhaus, C Berger, K Buechner .Randomised trial of oral versus sequential intravenous/oral cephalosporins in children with pyelonephritis. Eur J of Ped 2008; 167(9):1037-1047.

# 18

# Post-Inflammatory Nephropathy

Beata Bieniaś, Małgorzata Zajączkowska, Halina Borzęcka,
Przemysław Sikora, Marek Majewski,
Ewelina Książek and Andrzej Borzęcki
*Medical University of Lublin*
*Poland*

## 1. Introduction

Post-inflammatory nephropathy is a progressive renal scarring which may be a consequence of one or more episodes of acute pyelonephritis.

Macroscopically, post-inflammatory nephropathy leads to gradual decrease in kidney size and deformity and dilation of pelvicalyceal system. These alternations are due to tubulointerstitial fibrosis and glomerular sclerosis followed by renal parenchymal atrophy and kidney cirrhosis development (Bernstein, 1994). It was demonstrated that there was positive correlation between severity of renal scarring and loss of renal function (Eddy et al., 2000; Eddy, 2000).

Post-inflammatory nephropathy is the leading cause of end-stage renal failure. In Europe, children with end-stage renal failure due to post-inflammatory nephropathy constitutes 10-24% of those on renal replacement therapy (Broyer et al., 1993).

The development of post-inflammatory nephropathy is influenced by age and gender of patient, the number of acute pyelonephritis episodes, the presence of anatomical and/or functional urinary system abnormalities, the virulence of invading pathogen, the time of appropriate treatment initiation and genetic predisposition.

The majority of studies demonstrated that the risk of renal scarring decreases with age and is highest in children in the first year of life (Hansson et al., 1999; Vernon et al., 1997; Arant, 1991; Benador et al., 1997; Smellie et al.,1998; Sheu et al., 2009). This may be related to the correction of anatomical and/or functional urinary system abnormalities and the decrease in susceptibility of renal parenchyma to infection due to defense mechanisms maturation (Benador et al., 1997; Rushton et al.,1992). Dissimilar results were obtained by Pecile et al. (2009). The authors showed that the lowest risk of renal scarring after first episode of febrile urinary tract infection was in children in the first year of life and the highest one - in children aged 5 -14 years.

It was also demonstrated that the male gender is an independent risk factor for renal scarring (Silva et al., 2009; Mohanan et al., 2008).

The risk of post-inflammatory nephropathy development increases with the number of acute pyelonephritis episodes. Renal scarring develops in 15% of children after the first episode of acute pyelonephritis. After two episodes of acute pyelonephritis renal scarring occurs in 35% of children and after three or more episodes - in 60% of children. The study by Orellana et al. (2004) showed that one episode of pyelonephritis caused permanent renal parenchymal injury in 55.9% of children whereas recurrent urinary tract infection - in 72.6% of children.

Anatomical and functional abnormalities of urinary system particularly predispose to post-inflammatory nephropathy development, although renal scarring may occur after acute pyelonephritis in children without these abnormalities (Gordon et al., 1987; Vanderfaeillie et al., 1998).
Numerous studies emphasized the significance of invading pathogen virulence for post-inflammatory nephropathy development. P, I and F1C fimbriae of *Escherichia coli* give rise to secretion of interleukins 6 and 8 by uroepithelial cells (Backhed et al., 2001; Hedlund et al., 1996, 2001). In addition, lipopolysaccharides of Gram-negative bacteria stimulate the release of cytotoxic nitric oxide and proinflammatory cytokines (Backhed et al., 2001; De Man et al., 1989; Traylor & Mayeux, 1997) whereas lipid A stimulates synthesis of nitric oxide (Traylor & Mayeux, 1997). Alfa-hemolysins of *Escherichia coli* give rise to cytolysis (Uhlen et al., 2000) and induce apoptosis of tubular cells (Chen et al., 2003, 2004].
Immediate initiation of appropriate therapy is of utmost importance in prevention of renal scarring development. Antibacterial treatment initiated within 24 hours prevents migration of neutrophils to inflammatory foci (Ransley & Risdon, 1981). A delay in initiation of therapy increases the risk of renal scarring from 5% to over 15%.
In numerous studies, the importance of genetic predisposition to renal scarring was emphasized. An association between polymorphism of angiotensin-converting enzyme gene and renal scarring was demonstrated (Haszon et al., 2002; Hohenfellner et al., 1999; Ohtomo et al., 2001; Ozen et al., 1999; Pardo et al., 2003). Similarly, polymorphism of transforming growth factor β gene (Kowalewska-Pietrzak et al., 2008; Hussein et al., 2010) and polymorphism of vascular endothelium growth factor gene (Hussein et al., 2010) had impact on severity of renal scarring.
Post-inflammatory nephropathy may be classified into reflux nephropathy due to vesico-ureteral reflux and obstructive nephropathy due to urinary tract obstruction (Marra et al., 2004; Orikasa et al., 1995; Smellie et al., 1981).

## 2. Pathogenesis of post-inflammatory nephropathy

Pathogenesis of post-inflammatory nephropathy is complex and not fully understood (Fig.1). In the last years, the investigators paid particular attention to the role of molecular factors in initiation and progression of post-inflammatory nephropathy. Numerous studies concerning molecular mechanisms leading to renal scarring were published (Eddy, 2000; Eddy et al., 2000; Guroze et al., 2005; Jahnukainen et al., 2005; Lane et al., 2002, Nath, 1998; Solari et al., 2004; Strutz et al., 1995,1996,1999, 2003; Weiss et al., 1994). The process of renal scarring may be divided into four phases: induction, fibrogenic signaling, fibrogenic, and destructive phases (Eddy, 2000). Induction phase is also known as cellular activation and injury phase. The interstitial space is infiltrated by both neutrophils and monocytes. In acute inflammation, the migration of neutrophils is primarily observed whereas in chronic inflammation monocytes predominate.
Neutrophils release numerous cytokines, lysosomal enzymes and free oxygen radicals. In addition, neutrophils may activate fibroblasts directly or indirectly via release of elastase and thus they participate in fibrogenic process (Bailey, 1973; Kishimoto & Harano, 1988).
Monocytes transform into macrophages which also participate in fibrogenic process (Lane et al., 2002; Nath, 1998). Solari et al. (2004) demonstrated that in reflux nephropathy, an increase in number of mastocytes was observed. Mastocytes produce numerous cytokines among others profibrogenic transforming growth factor β (TGF-β) and basic fibroblast

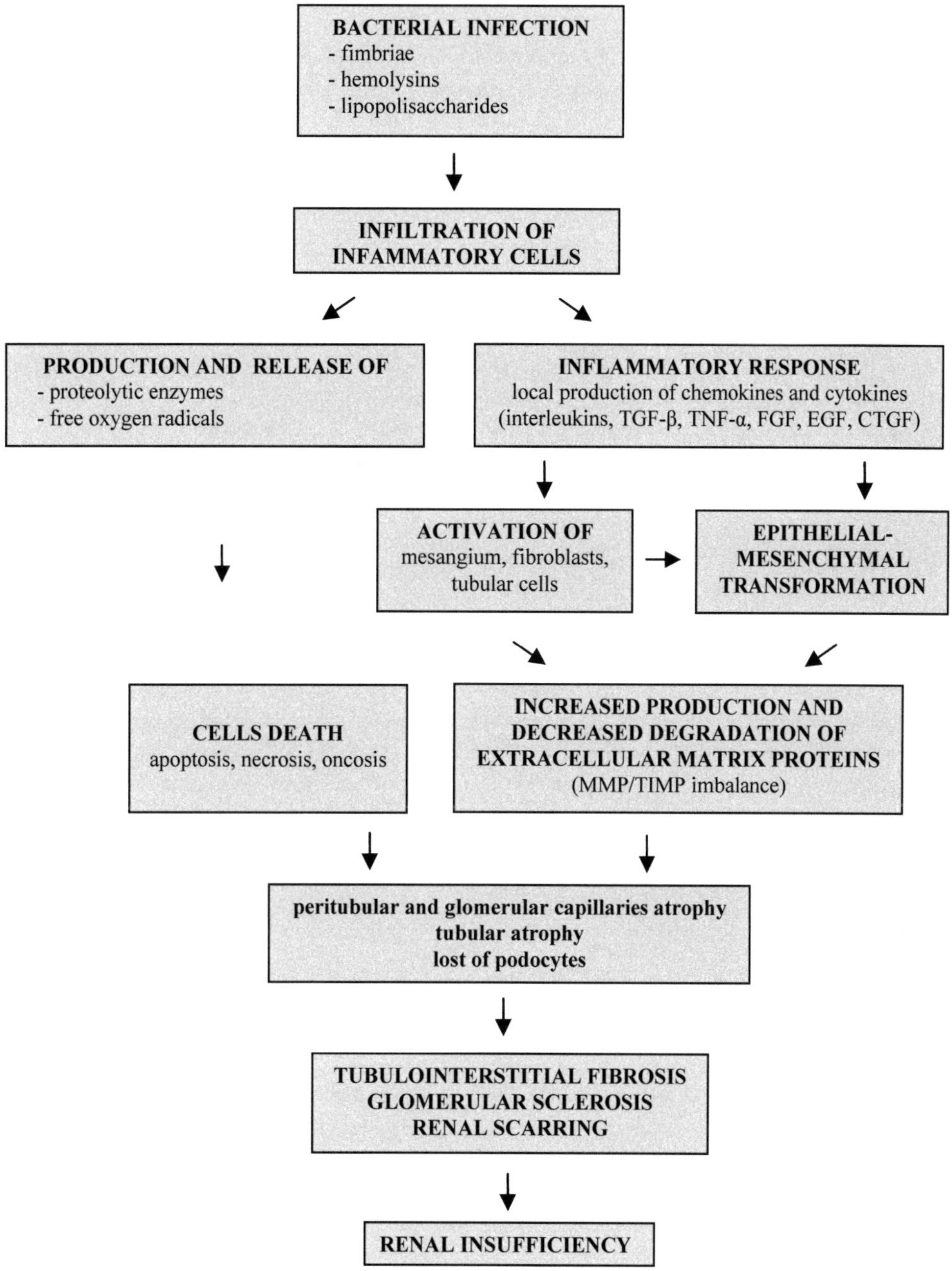


Fig. 1. Pathogenesis of post-inflammatory nephropathy.

growth factor (bFGF). In addition, mastocytes produce enzymes - tryptase and chymase. Tryptase stimulates type I collagen production by fibroblasts whereas chymase releases TGF-β from inactive complexes and converts angiotensin I to angiotensin II. This suggests participation of mastocytes in fibrogenic process.

Inflammatory infiltration cells produce other cytokines such as interleukins 1, 6, 8 (IL-1, IL-6, IL-8) and tumor necrosis factor α (TNF-α).
The study by Wolfs et al. (2002) demonstrated that Toll-like receptors-2,-4 (TLR-2, TLR-4) were responsible for defense response during acute pyelonephritis. Activated by endogenous danger signals TLR-2 expression is also of significance in induction of inflammation during progressive renal injury (Leemans et al., 2009).
During acute interstitial inflammation activated tubular cells directly participate in activation of myofibroblasts and fibroblasts (Abbate et al., 2002; Alpers et al., 1994; Roberts et al., 1997) and produce monocyte chemoattractant protein-1 (MCP-1) (Okada et al., 2000), endothelin-1 (ET-1) (Bruzzi et al., 1997), angiotensin II causing vasoconstriction, and transferrin (Chen et al., 1998) activating free oxygen radicals (Chertin et al., 2002).
As a result of acute interstitial inflammation expression of novel antigens on tubular cells occurs and these new antigens stimulate an immune response of lymphocyte T which enhances inflammation and progression of nephropathy (Szeto et al., 2005).
In addition, tubular cells and fibroblasts transform into myofibroblasts. This process is called epithelial-mesenchymal transformation or transition (EMT). Numerous authors confirmed the possibility of EMT (Oldfield et al., 2001; Rastaldi et al., 2002; Strutz et al., 1995; Zeisberg et al., 2001). Myofibroblast, unlike typical interstitial fibroblasts, are characterized by their expression of the myocyte protein α-smooth muscle actin. These cells are considerably more profibrotic than interstitial fibroblasts.
During acute interstitial inflammation activation of complement system via classic and alternative pathway is also observed. C3a and C5a component are known to be chemotactic for monocytes. There is evidence for participation of complement system in inflammatory infiltration formation, tubular atrophy and tubulointerstitial fibrosis (Nangaku et al., 1999).
In pathogenesis of chronic interstitial inflammation leukocyte adhesion molecules such as integrins, selectins and members of the immunoglobulin superfamily (intercellular adhesion molecules - ICAMs and vascular cell adhesion molecules - VCAMs) seem to play a crucial role but details remain unclear. ICAMs, VCAMs and osteopontin are chemoattractant for monocytes (Okada et al., 2000; Ricardo et al., 1996).
An early phase of acute interstitial inflammation is reversible provided that nociceptive factor is eliminated (Eddy, 2000; Eddy et al., 2000).
In fibrogenic signaling phase, numerous fibrogenic factors are released, including TGF-β1, tissue growth factor (TGF), angiotensin II, ET-1, platelet growth factor (PDGF-BB), bFGF, TNF-α, and IL-1. Fibrogenic factors activate their cognate receptors expressed by tubulointerstitial cells and subsequent extracellular matrix accumulation along tubular basement membranes and within the interstitial space occurs.
In fibrogenic phase, fibrogenic factors activate a new group of genes that lead to excessive accumulation of extracellular matrix proteins and polysaccharides within the interstitial space (Beck-Schimmer et al., 1998; Pichler et al., 1996). In this phase, disequilibrium between extracellular matrix production and its degradation is observed.
A main cause of impairment of extracellular matrix remodeling and degradation is a decrease in activity of metalloproteinases (MMP) due to induction of tissue inhibitors of metalloproteinases (TIMP). Four major TIMP have been identified (TIMP-1, TIMP-2, TIMP-3, and TIMP-4). In the majority of progressive renal diseases, marked induction of TIMP-1 is observed (Chromek et al., 2003,2004; Eddy et al., 2000; Kim et al., 2001). Within kidney, TIMP-1 is produced by tubular cells, fibroblasts and macrophages. Production of TIMP-1 is stimulated by growth factors (TGF-β1, TGF-α, epithelial growth factor (EGF), PDGF, TNF-

α), interleukins (IL-1, IL-6, IL-10), oncostatin M, endotoxin and thrombin. Recently, the induction of plasminogen activator inhibitor-1 (PAI-1) in progressive renal diseases was documented. This may suggest its participation in tubulointerstitial fibrosis. PAI-1 is produced by tubular cells, fibroblasts and myofibroblasts. Its expression is induced by TGF-β, EGF, PDGF, TNF-α and bFGF (as cited in Eddy, 2000).

In destructive phase, a gradual loss of functioning nephrons occurs as a result of excessive accumulation of extracellular matrix. Glomerular sclerosis, peritubular capillaries and tubular atrophy lead to progressive renal failure (Orphanides et al., 1997; Seron et al., 1990). TGF-β, TNF-α, IL-1β, IL-6 and IL-8 seem to play a major role in renal scarring.

Transforming growth factor β (TGF-β)

TGF-β is released primarily by macrophages, neutrophils, lymphocytes and platelets. TGF-β is produced as an inactive complex with LAP (*latent associated protein*) and LTBP (*latent TGF-β binding protein*) which are components of extracellular matrix. These proteins have potential to store and release of TGF-β. Five isoforms of TGF-β (TGF-β 1-5) have been identified. In mammalians, only TGF-β 1-3 are found. Active TGF-β is a homodimeric 25kD protein. Within kidneys numerous factors increase TGF-β expression, including angiotensin II, endothelin I, interleukin 1β, platelet activating factor (PAF), thromboxane, thrombospondin, glucose, insulin, atrial natriuretic peptide (ANP), secreted protein acidic and rich in cysteine (SPARC), and hypoxia (Pichler et al., 1996). Increased TGF-β expression in kidneys is also caused by TNF-α and connective tissue growth factor (CTGF) (Zhang et.al., 2004). In addition, proteoglycans accumulated within the interstitial space may be a reservoir of TGF-β.

TGF-β stimulates production of proinflammatory cytokines (IL-1, IL-6, IL-8 and TNF-α). It is known to be chemotactic for monocytes, neutrophils, and fibroblasts. TGF-β stimulates production of extracellular matrix proteins such as fibronectin, collagen and proteoglycans. In addition, it increases expression of TIMPs. This contributes to depressed activity of MMP and stabilization of extracellular matrix (Boettinger & Bitzer, 2002; Boettinger et al., 1997; Broder et al., 1994; Cotton et al., 2002; Deng et al., 2006; Fan et al., 1999; Goumneos et al., 2002; Guo et al., 1997; Jahnukainen et al., 2005; Korzon et al., 2004; Lane et al., 2002; Liapis, 2003). Poncelet & Schnaper (1998) documented that TGF-β stimulates production of collagen I, III and IV by mesangial cells. Experimental studies on transgenic mice showed that overexpression of TGF-β resulted in glomerular and interstitial fibrosis (Kelly et al., 1999). In experimental model of ureteral obstruction (Shinozaki et al., 1998) and in proteinuric state (Jernigan et al., 1996), overexpression of the type II receptor for TGF-β gave rise to increased accumulation of collagen within the interstitial space.

TGF-β induces EMT (Fan et al., 1999; Ng et al., 1998) and inhibits apoptosis of myofibroblasts (Zhang & Phan,1999; Fan et al., 1999; Frazier et al., 2000). In addition, TGF-β induces apoptosis of endothelial cells. This results in peritubular and glomerular capillaries atrophy followed by fibrosis (Choi & Ballermann, 1995; Kang et al., 2002; Ohashi et al., 2000). TGF-β is also known to induce apoptosis of tubular cells leading to tubular atrophy with subsequent fibrosis (Dai et al.,2003; Gobe & Axelsen,1987; Kopp et al., 1996; Lane et al., 2002; Ortiz et al., 1997; Sanderson et al., 1995).

Experimental studies demonstrated increased TGF-β mRNA expression during infection with *Escherichia coli* (Khalil et al., 2000). Increased urinary TGF-β excretion was showed in children with urinary tract infection (Farmaki et al., 2005).

An association between TGF-β gene polymorphism and susceptibility to renal scarring was observed. Solari et al. (2005) documented that the risk of reflux nephropathy was higher in patients with -509CT and Leu10Pro genotypes. Khalil et al. (2005) showed that homozygosity for -509T and Arg25 resulted in more rapid progression of renal failure whereas patients with -800GA genotype were less susceptible to renal scarring (Cotton et al., 2002).

Numerous studies confirmed a significant participation of TGF-β in pathogenesis of obstructive nephropathy (Blom et al., 2001; Chevalier, 2004; Duncan et al., 1999; Kaneto et al., 1999; Klahr & Morrissey, 1998, 2002, 2003; Sato et al., 2003; Schnaper et al., 2003). In this type of nephropathy, increased angiotensin II production is observed and angiotensin II enhances TGF-β expression. Thus angiotensin II plays a key role in initiating of tubulointerstitial fibrosis in obstructive nephropathy. Recently, in patients with ureteropelvic junction obstruction, increased urinary TGF-β excretion was observed (Almodhen et al., 2009, Sager et al., 2009).

Tumor necrosis factor α (TNF-α)

TNF-α also known as cachectin is produced by several cells within kidneys, including proximal tubular cells, mesangial cells, interstitial fibroblasts and macrophages. The most potent stimulus for TNF-α production is lipopolysaccharides of Gram-negative bacteria. TNF-α stimulates production of proinflammatory cytokines (IL-1 and Il-6) by macrophages and increases macrophages cytotoxicity. In addition, it is known to be chemotactic for fibroblasts and stimulates their proliferation. TNF-α has also antifibrotic effects because it enhances collagenase activity and inhibits collagen gene expression. In addition, TNF-α diminishes activity of TIMP and increases production of latent MMP-9 (Nee et al., 2004).

Profibrogenic effects of TNF-α was confirmed in study by Guo et al. (1999). The authors demonstrated less severe renal scarring in mice genetically deficient of receptors specific for TNF-α. In addition, TNF-α contributes to renal scarring by releasing IL-1β and TGF-β from inflammatory infiltration cells (Jahnukainen et al., 2005). Recently, experimental study demonstrated less severe renal scarring in rats with nephritis when monoclonal antibodies against TNF-α were administered (Khan et al., 2005). Wolfs et al. (2002) showed that TNF-α induced overexpression of TLR-2 and -4. TNF-α contributes to the development of obstructive nephropathy. Overexpression of TNF-α is due to increased angiotensin II secretion observed in upper urinary tract obstruction.

Interleukin 1 (IL-1)

IL-1 is one of the major regulator inflammatory and immune reactions. It may be produced by several cells within the kidney, including macrophages, mesangial cells, endothelial cells and macrophages. It is also known to be chemotactic for neutrophils and monocytes. Other activities of IL-1 include: - stimulation of production of IL-1, IL-6, IL-8 and TNF-α by macrophages, - stimulation of production of IL-6 and collagenase by fibroblasts, - stimulation of fibroblast proliferation and possibly of extracellular matrix production, - activation of endothelial cells, - induction of smooth muscle cells lysis. Fibrosis-promoting effects of IL-1 were also demonstrated (Ichino et al., 2008, Mittal et al., 2009). It also inhibits MMP-9 activity which degrades type IV collagen of extracellular matrix and diminishes activity of IL-1 receptor antagonist (IL-1Ra).

Vesey et al. (2002, 2002) demonstrated that IL-1β stimulated proliferation of interstital fibroblast and enhanced production of type I collagen, fibronectin, TGF-β and nitric oxide.

Study by Zang et al. (2005) showed that IL-1β induced transformation of tubular cells into myofibroblasts. In addition, IL-1β stimulates production of IL-6 and IL-8. This intensifies inflammation and promotes interstitial fibrosis (Lonnemann et al., 1995).

Kassem et al. (2005) demonstrated increased urinary IL-1β excretion in children with acute pyelonephritis. The authors also revealed positive correlation between urinary IL-1β and IL-8 excretion. The survey by Wetmore et al. (2005) showed an association between IL-1 gene polymorphism and occurrence of chronic renal diseases which resulted in impairment of renal function. Elevated urinary IL-1β excretion was demonstrated in patients with chronic renal failure. The highest urinary IL-1β excretion was observed in pre-dialysis patients. In those patients, considerably higher plasma IL-1Ra level as compared to controls was disclosed (Pereira et al., 1994).

Interleukin 6 (IL-6)

IL-6 is produced by several cells within kidney, including macrophages, interstitial fibroblasts and endothelial cells. The study by Patel et al. (2005) demonstrated that IL-6 intensified inflammation and impaired renal function. Increased urinary IL-6 excretion in children with urinary tract infection and positive correlation between urinary IL-6 excretion and severity of proteinuria, hematuria and pyuria were also observed (Benson et al., 1996; Gendrel et al., 1998; Jantausch et al., 2000; Nicolle et al, 1993; Otto et al., 1999; Mizuano et al., 2001). Experimental studies revealed increased expression of renal IL-6 in mice with acute pyelonephritis due to ureteral obstruction (Kabore et al., 1999; Rugo et al., 1992) and increased serum IL-6 level in the majority of mice with acute pyelonephritis (Rugo et al., 1992). Khalil et al. (2000) demonstrated increased mortality in mice with acute pyelonephritis and IL-6 deficiency. The authors also disclosed more severe histopathological changes in kidneys of IL-6 deficient mice. Numerous studies demonstrated that urinary IL-6 excretion was higher in patients with acute pyelonephritis than in those with asymptomatic bacteriuria (Benson et al., 1994; Hedges et al., 1992; Kassem et al., 2005; Ko et al., 1993; Ohta et al., 1992; Otto et al., 1999; Roilides et al., 1999). Positive correlation between urinary IL-6 excretion and the risk of renal scarring was also disclosed (Benson et al., 1996; Jacobson et al., 1998; ; Roilides et al., 1999; Tullus et al., 1994). Wang et al. (2001) observed significant correlation between urinary IL-6 excretion and renal scars diagnosed by static renoscintigraphy in children with vesicoureteral reflux. In those children, there were positive correlations between urinary IL-6 excretion and serum α1- microglobulin, β2-microglobulin, creatinine levels and urinary albumin excretion. These authors (Wang et al., 2001) also performed immunohistochemical evaluation of specimens obtained from removed scarred kidneys. Overexpression of IL-6 in renal tubules and scars was observed. Data on serum IL-6 level in patients with urinary tract infection and post-inflammatory nephropathy are scarce and conflicting. Smółko et al. (2004) revealed higher serum IL-6 level in children with vesicoureteral reflux of high grade as compared to controls. The study by Gokce et al. (2010) showed the similar results. Increased serum IL-6 level was observed primarily in patients with febrile urinary tract infection (Benson et al., 1994; Hedges et al., 1991,1992; Jacobson et al., 1994, 1998).

IL-6 gene polymorphism influenced susceptibility to urinary tract infections but had no effect on renal parenchymal scarring (Cotton et al., 2000).

Interleukin 8 (IL-8)

Within kidney IL-8 is produced primarily by macrophages, interstitial fibroblasts, tubular and endothelial cells. It has bactericidal and pro-inflammatory activity because it causes chemotaxis and degranulation of neutrophils. In patients with acute urinary tract infection and post-inflammatory nephropathy, increased serum IL-8 level and increased urinary IL-8 excretion were observed (Kassem et al., 2005; Tikhonov et al., 1997; Haraoka et al., 1996). Increased urinary IL-8 excretion is thought to be a marker of vesicoureteral reflux and post-inflammatory nephropathy (Galanakis et al., 2006; Gokce et al., 2010; Haraoka et al., 1996; Smółko et al., 2004). Taha et al. (2003) demonstrated increased urinary IL-8 excretion in patients with acute and chronic urinary tract infections. The authors also disclosed higher urinary IL-8 excretion in females as compared to males and positive correlation between urinary IL-8 excretion and markers of inflammation, including leukocytosis and serum C-reactive protein level.

In patients with urinary tract infection, increased urinary IL-8 excretion was observed in numerous studies (Jacobson et al., 1994; Kassem et al., 2005; Nicolle et al., 1993; Olszyna et al., 2000; Otto et al., 1999; Rao et al., 2001; Sheu et al., 2009; Tullus et al., 1994). Roilides et al. (1999) and Ko et al. (1993) revealed increased urinary IL-8 excretion in newborns with abnormal static renoscintigraphy result. Increased urinary IL-8 excretion was also revealed in patients with chronic pyelonephritis (Rebenok et al., 1999; Tikhonov et al., 1997). Experimental studies in mice and rabbits with urinary tract infection and without or mutated IL-8 receptor disclosed more severe course of infection, massive renal scarring and considerable impairment of renal function (Frendeus et al., 2001; Hang et al., 2000). The authors suggested that overproduction of IL-8 promoted clearance of bacteria from kidneys and thus diminished the risk of renal scarring. There is an opinion that overproduction of IL-8 in response to urinary tract infection results in univocal and distinct symptoms leading to prompt diagnosis and early initiation of appropriate treatment and thus diminishes the risk of renal scarring (Jahnukainen et al., 2005).

### 2.1 Reflux nephropathy

Reflux nephropathy (RN) refers to renal scarring due to vesicoureteral reflux. Chronic renal failure as a result of RN is observed in 5%-40% of children aged below 16 years and in 5%-20% of adults (Kenda et al., 1997; Noe, 1992; Wan &Greenfield, 1996). RN is also a frequent cause of end-stage renal failure.

Vesicoureteral reflux is a back-flow of urine from the bladder into the ureter and pelvicalyceal system. The back-flow of urine from pelvicalyceal system into collecting ducts is called intrarenal reflux. When urine is infected, intrarenal reflux results in renal infection. The prevalence of intrarenal reflux is particularly high in children aged below 5 years. In 1960, Hodson and Edwards (as cited in Sieniawska & Wyszyńska, 2003) first demonstrated that there was association between vesicoureteral reflux and chronic pyelonephritis. Antenatal renal damage due to vesicoureteral reflux may also develop (Arant, 1991; Bailey, 1973; Lerner, 1994; Smellie, 1975; Peters & Rushton, 2010).

Classification of grades of vesicoureteral reflux according to International Reflux study Committee, (1981) is showed on Fig. 2.

Vesicoureteral reflux may be primary or secondary. Primary vesicoureteral reflux is due to congenital abnormal lateralization of ureteral orifice. Secondary vesicoureteral reflux is a result of anatomical and/or functional abnormalities of lower urinary tract.

Primary vesicoureteral reflux is the most common congenital abnormality of urinary system and is diagnosed in 20% - 60% of children with urinary tract infection (Ataei et al., 2004; Zajaczkowska et al., 2001; Alvarez et al., 2009). In the noninfected general population, the prevalence of vesicoureteral reflux is 1% -2% and in siblings of children with vesicoureteral reflux and urinary tract infection – 5% -50% (Noe, 1992).

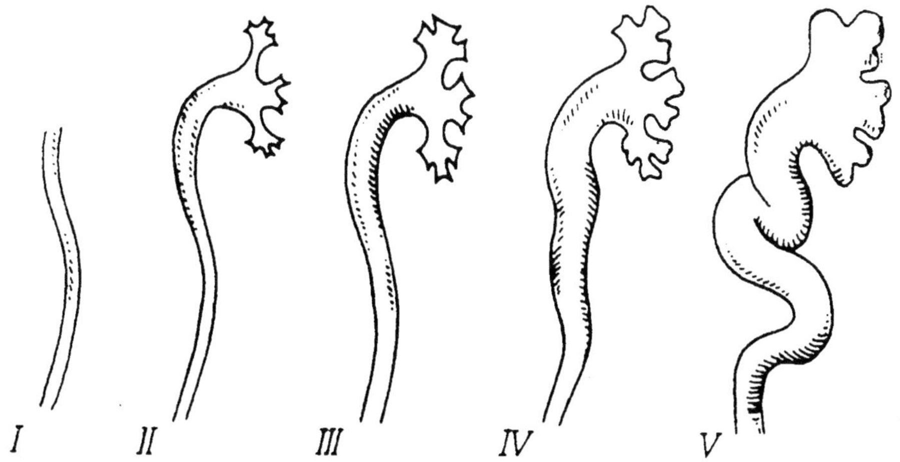


Fig. 2. The International Reflux Study classifies reflux grades as follows: I) reflux into ureter only; II) reflux into ureter, pelvis, and calyces, no dilation, normal calyceal fornices; III) mild or moderate dilation and/or tortuosity of the ureter and mild or moderate dilation of renal pelvis but no or little blunting of the fornices; IV) moderate dilation and/or tortuosity of the ureter and moderate dilation of the renal pelvis and calyces V) gross dilation and tortuosity of the ureter and gross dilation of the renal pelvis and calyces. Papillary impressions are no longer visible in the majority of calyces. There is complete obliteration of the sharp angle of the fornices, but maintenance of papillary impressions in major calyces.

Relation between urinary tract infection, vesicoureteral reflux and renal scarring has been known since a long time (Bailey, 1973; ; Kincaid-Smith,1975; Smellie et al., 1975; Van den Abbeele et al., 1987). In the early 1970s, Bailey (1973) coined the term "reflux nephropathy" to describe renal scarring in patients with vesicoureteral reflux. The study by Sheikh et al. (2010) confirmed higher risk of renal scarring in patients with vesicoureteral reflux. Orellana et al. (2004) demonstrated that prevalence of renal scarring is higher in children with vesicoureteral reflux than in those without that anomaly (72% versus 52%). In addition, it was revealed significant association between vesicoureteral reflux diagnosed after first episode of urinary tract infection and chronic renal failure (Marra et al., 2004).
Previously, vesicoureteral reflux was thought to be an independent risk factor for renal scarring. Nowadays, this hypothesis is questioned. However, an association between urinary tract infection in children with vesicoureteral reflux and renal scarring remains unquestionable (Faust et al., 2009; Jahnukainen et al., 2005; Muinuddin et al., 2008). This was confirmed by recent studies that demonstrated an increase in the risk of renal scarring after acute pyelonephritis in patients with vesicoureteral reflux (Kanellopoulos et al., 2006; Lee et al., 2006; Polito et al., 2006; Oh et al., 2008). Studies by Svensson et al. (2005) and Mohanan et al. (2008) disclosed that renal scarring was detected less frequently in infants with vesicoureteral reflux and without urinary tract infection than in those with vesicoureteral reflux and urinary tract infection. In study by Ylinen et al. (2003) renal scarring was found more frequently in infants in whom vesicoureteral reflux was diagnosed after the first episode of urinary tract infection than in those in whom vesicoureteral reflux was detected antenatally. The risk of acute pyelonephritis and thus renal scarring increases along with grade of vesicoureteral reflux (Arant, 1991; Oh et al., 2008, Shaikh et al., 2010, Silva et al.,

2010) because vesicoureteral reflux of high grade occurs throughout micturition in contrast to vesicoureteral reflux of low grade which occurs only at the peak of micturition (Jacobsson et al., 1992).

In the last years, an association between ACE gene polymorphism and development/progression of RN was demonstrated. The D allele of ACE gene polymorphism was associated with higher converting enzyme activity and thus higher concentration of angiotensin II in plasma and tissues. This resulted in more rapid development and progression of RN (Haszon et al., 2002; Hohenfellner et al., 1999; Ohtomo et al., 2001; Ozen et al., 1999). Some studies questioned the significance of ACE gene polymorphism as an independent risk factor for the development and progression of RN (Dudley et al., 2002; Pardo et al., 2003). An association between TGF-β1 gene polymorphism and the risk of renal scarring in patients with vesicoureteral reflux was also disclosed Kowalewska-Pietrzak et al. (2008), whereas Hussein et al. (2010) demonstrated an association between vascular endothelium growth factor (VEGF) gene polymorphism and the risk of the development of RN.

## 2.2 Obstructive nephropathy

Obstructive nephropathy (ON) refers to renal scarring due to mechanical obstruction to urine flow (Liapis, 2002).

Obstruction to urine flow may be congenital or acquired. It can occur at any level of urinary tract, including renal tubules, renal pelvis, ureters, bladder and urethra. Obstruction to urine flow most commonly occurs at ureteropelvic junction (Koff, 1990; Norbeck et al., 1993). The severity of obstructive nephropathy depends on severity of obstruction, its location and duration, age of occurrence and concomitant infection.

Complete or severe obstruction to urine flow leads to obstructive nephropathy more rapidly than incomplete one. In addition, the higher the obstruction is located the more severe obstructive nephropathy develops. Age of patient is of great significance. Fetal and neonatal kidneys are at greatest risk for damage. Antenatal urinary tract obstruction disturbs kidney development and results in polycystic dysplasia or hypodysplasia (Chevalier, 2004).

Re-expression of Pax-2 (Li et al., 2010) gene and decreased expression of Bcl-1 gene (Zhang et al. 2001) enhance susceptibility to the development of obstructive nephropathy.

In the development and progression of obstructive nephropathy, primarily cytokines and vasoactive substances are implicated (Chevalier, 2004; Chevalier et al., 2009; Chiou et al., 2004; Grande et al.,2010; Klahr, 2001; Klahr & Marrissey, 1998, 2002, 2003; Rice et al., 2004). Nowadays, TGF-β1 and TNF-α are thought to play a crucial role in renal damage. Obstruction to urine flow and alternations in intra- renal hemodynamics result in increased secretion of angiotensin II which in turn enhances TGF-β1 and TNF-α expression (Grande et al., 2010; Leonova et al., 2007; Manucha, 2007; Padillo et al., 2007; Pimentel et al., 1995; Sager et al., 2009; Wang et al.,2010). Due to urine stasis urinary tract infection may develop. Infection is an additional factor which causes renal damage.

Bilateral complete or severe urinary tract obstruction are the most dangerous anomalies. In this clinical settings, even early surgery does not always protect kidneys from permanent damage leading to end stage renal failure during childhood (Chevalier et al., 2000). Patients after surgical correction of urinary tract obstructions requires careful monitoring in order to early detect of obstructive nephropathy symptoms and initiation of nephroprotective therapy.

## 3. History and clinical manifestations of post-inflammatory nephropathy

The clinician needs to obtain a detailed history about the type and duration of symptoms. Most often there is a history of recurrent urinary tract infections which cease or occur less frequently after surgical correction of anatomical anomaly, appropriate therapy of functional disturbances of lower urinary tract and/or antibacterial prophylaxis. Severe and developed early in life post-inflammatory nephropathy leads to dwarfism and body weight deficit (Polito et al., 1999; Seidel et al., 1993). The patient may complain of loin or abdominal pain which may be a result of urinary tract infection, dilation of urinary tract due to obstruction or urolithiasis secondary to urine stasis. The patient should be asked questions about difficulty initiating urination, decreases in the force of urine stream, posturination dribbling, and incomplete emptying. In addition, the patient should be questioned about nocturia as chronic renal failure is characterized by the lack of ability to concentrate urine during the night. Post-inflammatory nephropathy may also be asymptomatic.

20% of children with post-inflammatory nephropathy develop end-stage renal failure before $18^{th}$ year of age and approximately 50% of them - in the fourth decade of life .

Post-inflammatory nephropathy may lead to arterial hypertension due to ischemia of renal scars and resultant increase in renin production (Wyszynska & Litwin, 2000). Arterial hypertension develops most commonly in patients with diffuse bilateral renal scarring (Hamed et al., 1992; Kohler et al., 1997, 2003). According to Rushton (1997) it may occur at any age but its beginning is most commonly observed in the third decade of life. Arant (1991) diagnosed arterial hypertension in 20% of children with post-inflammatory nephropathy and the majority of them was over 5 years of age. In Polish children aged 7 -10 years with post-inflammatory nephropathy, the prevalence of arterial hypertension was approximately 50% (Wyszynska & Litwin, 2000). In children with obstructive nephropathy, arterial hypertension seems to be sodium-dependent and occurs more commonly when urinary tract obstruction is bilateral.

A late consequence of post-inflammatory nephropathy may be urolithiasis which was observed in 18% patients with renal scarring (Kohler et al., 2003; Vachvanichsanong, 2007).

In pregnants with reflux nephropathy, recurrent urinary tract infections, arterial hypertension, gestosis and/or renal failure may occur (Vachvanichsanong, 2007) therefore they are at risk for spontaneous abortion and premature delivery. Increased mortality of newborns from these mothers was observed.

## 4. Diagnosis of post-inflammatory nephropathy

Diagnostics of post-inflammatory nephropathy include laboratory and imaging studies. Initially, urinalysis may be normal or may show sparse proteinuria and/or microhematuria. Proteinuria may gradually increase with time. Slightly decreased ability to concentrate and acidify urine may also be observed (Polito et al., 1999; Seidel et al., 1993).

An acetyl-beta-D-glucose aminidase and β2-microglobulin are a widely used markers of tubulointerstitial fibrosis. Recently, early and more specific markers of tubulointerstitial fibrosis have been introduced such as neutrophil gelatinase-associated lipocalin (NGAL) (Ichnio et al., 2010; Wasilewska et al., 2011), kidney injury molecule-1 (KIM-1) (Wasilewska et al., 2011], type IV collagen and gluthatione S-transferases alpha and pi (GST-α and GST-π) (Cawood et al., 2010, Branten et al., 2000). GST-α is a marker of proximal tubular injury whereas GST-π -distal tubular injury. Chromek et al. (2003, 2004) recommended ratios of MMP-1, MMP-2 and MMP-9 to their tissue inhibitors TIMP-1 and TIMP-2 as markers of tubulointerstitial fibrosis.

Valuable diagnostic clues are provided by radiologic evaluation, including ultrasonography, static renoscintigraphy (99mTc DMSA) and dynamic renoscintigraphy (99mTcDTPA, 99mTcEC, 99mTcMAG-3). Urography and voiding cystourethrography (VCUG) are also helpful.

Kersnik et al. (2002) evaluated ultrasonography efficacy in detection of renal scarring. They demonstrated that sensitivity of ultrasonography in detection of benign, moderate and severe renal scarring was 34.1%, 79.2% and 100%, respectively. The study by Moorthy et al. (2004) revealed that in detection of renal scarring, ultrasonography was characterized by higher specificity (91.8%) and lower sensitivity (47.2%) as compared to static renoscintigraphy. At present, ultrasonography still remains an important tool in evaluation of renal scarring.

The advent of static renoscitigraphy using dimercaptosuccinic acid labeled by 99m technetium (99mTcDMSA) was a turning-point in diagnostic evaluation of post-inflammatory nephropathy. 99mTcDMSA is thought to be the gold standard for detection and monitoring of renal scarring. 99mTcDMSA undoubtedly contributes to expansion of our knowledge concerning pathogenesis of post-inflammatory nephropathy (Gordon, 1987; Orleana et al., 2004; Rushton, 1997; Shapiro et al., 1988; Smellie, 1985; Stokland et al., 1996). On the basis of 99mTcDMSA, the classification of severity of renal scarring was made (Fig. 3.) (Goldraich et al., 1983).

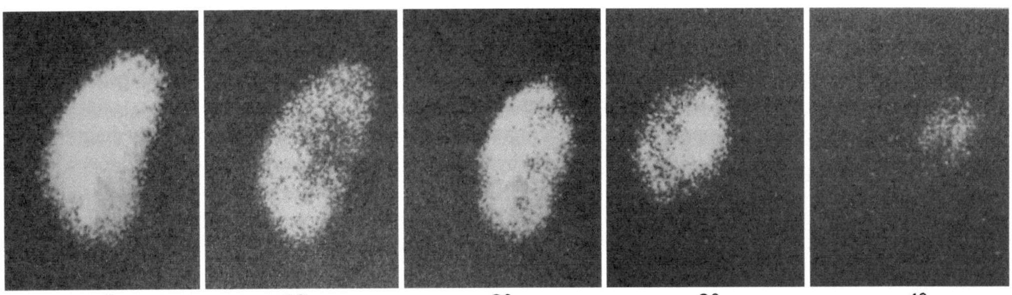


Fig. 3. Classification of renal scarring according to findings at 99mTcDMSA renal scan: 0 – normal, 1° - no more than 2 scarred areas, 2° - more than 2 scars with some areas of normal parenchyma, 3° - generalized damage to the whole kidney, 4° - cirrhotic kidney with little or no uptake of DMSA.

Dynamic renoscintigraphy also has potential to detect renal scarring reliably (Gad et al., 2004; Narayana et al., 2004). In addition, it evaluates renal function as well as status of pelvicalyceal systems and ureters. In dynamic renoscintigraphy, diethylene triaminepentaacetic acid (DTPA), ethylenodicysteine (EC), and mercaptoacetyltriglycerin (MAG-3) labeled by 99m technetium are used.

Nowadays, urography is performed less commonly because there are more effective methods of urinary system visualization. In addition, urography is viewed as more harmful than beneficial for patients. Urography enables to evaluate renal size and margins. It also visualizes pelvicalyceal systems and ureters and thus has potential to detect anatomical obstruction location.

VCUG is performed in order to detect vesicoureteral reflux and anatomical anomalies of the bladder and urethra. In the presence of vesicoureteral reflux, VCUG may demonstrate dilation and deformity of renal calyces and occasionally intrarenal refluxes. VCUG may give only a suspicion of post-inflammatory nephropathy. VCUG visualizes the bladder and urethra and thus has potential to detect anatomical obstruction to urine flow. Instead of VCUG videocystometry is more and more commonly performed because it is able to detect both vesicoureteral reflux and anatomical/functional abnormalities of lower urinary tract.

## 5. Management of post-inflammatory nephropathy

Management of post-inflammatory nephropathy include therapy and prophylaxis of urinary tract infection, correction of anatomical and functional abnormalities of urinary tract and nephroprotection based primarily on inhibition of production or activity of TGF-β. Nowadays, a proven nephroprotective activity is displayed by angiotensin-converting enzyme inhibitors, angiotensin II receptor blockers (Khalil et al., 2000, Wang et al., 2005), aldosterone antagonists (eplerenone), renin inhibitors (aliskiren) and anti-oxidants (α-tocopherol) (Chan et al., 2001; Cojocel et al., 2005; Saborio et al., 2000).

Novel drugs which inhibit tubulointerstitial fibrosis include low-molecular leucine-rich proteoglycans, decorin, and biglycan. They have potential to permanent bond with TGF-β and thus they inhibit its activity (Solari et al., 2005). Inhibition of tubulointerstitial fibrosis was also observed after blockade of type II TGF-β receptor (Jernigan et al., 1996; Kasuga et al., 2001; Kushibiki et al., 2005) and as a result of therapy with antibodies against TGF-β (Gagliardini & Benigni, 2006). Inhibition of activity of tissue transglutaminases which participate in activation of TGF-β may be a therapeutic option in patients with post-inflammatory nephropathy in future (Shweke et al., 2008). Other factors which are likely to inhibit tubulointerstitial fibrosis are hepatocyte growth factor (HGF) (Mizuno et al., 2001) and bone morphogenic protein 7 (BMP-7) (Kopp, 2002). The latest studies demonstrated nephroprotective activity of Lefty-A which inhibits and even reverses transformation of tubular cells into myofibroblasts (Li et al., 2010, Yao et al., 2011).

## 6. Serum concentrations of selected cytokines in children with reflux and obstructive nephropathy – original studies

The purposes of the study were - to assess serum TGF-$\beta_1$, TNF-α, IL-1 β, IL-6 and IL-8 levels in children with post-inflammatory nephropathy (reflux and obstructive nephropathy), - to compare serum TGF-$\beta_1$, TNF-α, IL-1 β, IL-6 and IL-8 levels between children with unilateral and bilateral vesicoureteral reflux, and between those with vesicoureteral reflux of high and low grade, - to compare serum TGF-$\beta_1$, TNF-α, IL-1 β, IL-6 and IL-8 levels between children with and without hypertension, and between those with and without proteinuria.

Patients and methods: The study comprised 70 children (24 boys and 46 girls) aged 1-17 years with renal scarring diagnosed scintigraphically. All children had a history of recurrent urinary tract infections including at least one episode of acute pyelonephritis. Vesicoureteral reflux and unilateral ureteropelvic/vesicoureteric junction obstruction were detected in 85.7% (60/70) and 14.3% (10/70) of children, respectively. Arterial hypertension was diagnosed in 17.2% (12/70) of patients. Proteinuria was observed in 25.7% (18/70) of children. Renal insufficiency developed in 5,7% (4/70) of patients. Serum TGF-$\beta_1$, TNF-α, IL-1 β, IL-6 and IL-8 concentrations were measured by ELISA.

Results: In children with reflux/obstructive nephropathy, the mean serum TGF-$\beta_1$ and IL-1$\beta$ concentrations were significantly lower than in controls. Similarly, serum IL-8 concentrations were lower in both studied groups than in controls but the differences were not statistically significant. There were no statistically significant differences in the mean serum TNF-$\alpha$ and IL-6 concentrations between children with reflux/obstructive nephropathy and controls.

There were no statistically significant differences in the mean serum TGF-$\beta_1$, TNF-$\alpha$, IL-1 $\beta$, IL-6 and IL-8 levels between children with unilateral vesicoureteral reflux and those with bilateral vesicoureteral reflux. There were also no statistically significant differences in the mean serum TGF-$\beta_1$, TNF-$\alpha$, IL-1 $\beta$, IL-6 and IL-8 levels between children with vesicoureteral reflux of high grade and those with vesicoureteral reflux of low grade.

Statistically significant differences in the mean serum TGF-$\beta_1$, TNF-$\alpha$, IL-1 $\beta$, IL-6 and IL-8 levels between children with arterial hypertension and the remaining patients were not observed.

In children with proteinuria, the mean serum TGF-$\beta_1$ level was significantly lower than in the remaining patients. There were no statistically significant differences in the mean serum TNF-$\alpha$, IL-1 $\beta$, IL-6 and IL-8 levels between children with proteinuria and the remaining patients.

## 7. Conclusions

1. The low serum TGF-$\beta_1$ and IL-1$\beta$ concentrations in patients with reflux and obstructive nephropathy seems to be a result of increased influx of this cytokines into renal parenchyma and/or increased urinary TGF-$\beta_1$ and IL-1$\beta$ excretion due to tubular damage associated with nephropathy.
2. The lower serum concentration of TGF-$\beta_1$ in patients with proteinuria secondary to post-inflammatory nephropathy may confirm participation of this factor in progression of nephropathy

## 8. Refferences

Abbate M., Zoja C., Rottoli D., Corna D., Tomasowi S. & Remuzzi G. (2002). Proxima tubular cells promot fibrogenesis by TGF-beta1-mediated induction of peritublar myofibroblast, *Kidney Int* 62:2066-2077.

Almodhen F, Loutochin O, Capolicchio JP, Jednak R & El-Sherbiny M. (2009). The role of bladder urine transforming growth factor-beta1 concentrations in diagnosis and management of unilateral prenatal hydronephrosis, *J Urol.* 182(1):292-298.

Alpers C.E., Hudkins K.L., Floege J. & Johnson R.J. (1994). Human renal cortical interstitial cells with some features of smooth muscle cells participate in tubulointerstitial and crescentic glomerular injury, *J Am Soc Nephrol* 5:201-209.

Alvarez MD, Batista BA, Córdova RP, Arias MI & Marrero BD. (2009). Prevalence and characteristics of the vesicoureteral reflux in infants who suffered neonatal urinary tract infection, *Arch Argent Pediatr* 107(4):329-334.

Arant B.S. (1991). Vesicoureteric reflux and renal injury, *Am J Kidney Dis* 17:491-511.

Ataei N., Madani A., Esfahani S.T., Kejbafzadeh A., Ghaderi O., Jalili S. & Sharafi B. (2004). Screening for vesicoureteral reflux and renal scars in siblings of children with known reflux, *Pediatr Nephrol* 19: 1127-1131.

Backhed F., Soderhall M., Ekman P., Normark S. & Richter-Dahlfors A. (2001). Induction of innate immune responses by Escherichia coli and purified lipopolysaccharide correlate with organ- and cell-specific expression of Toll-like receptors within the human urinary tract, *Cell Microbiol* 3:153-158.

Bailey R.R. (1973). The relationship of vesicoureteric reflux and chronic pyelonephritis-reflux nephropathy, *Clin Nephrol* 1:132-141.

Beck-Schimmer B., Oertli B., Pasch T. & Wuthrich R.P. (1998). Hyaluronan induces monocyte chemoattractant protein-1 expression in renal tubular epithelial cells, *J Am Soc Nephrol* 9:2283-2290.

Benador D., Benador N., Slosman D., Mermillod B. & Girardin E.R. (1997). Are younger children at highest risk of renal sequelae after pyelonephritis?, *Lancet* 349:17-19.

Benson M., Jodal U., Agace W., Hellstrom M., Marild S., Rosberg S., Sjostrom M., Wettergren B., Jonsson S. & Svanborg C. (1996). Interleukin (IL)-6 and IL-8 in children with febrile urinary tract infection and asymptomatic bacteriuria, *J Infect Dis* 174:1080-1084.

Benson M., Jodal U., Andreasson A., Karlsson A., Rydberg J. & Svanborg C. (1994). Interleukin 6 response to urinary tract infection in childhood, *Pediatr Infect Dis J* 13:612-616.

Bernstein J. (1994). Interstitial injury with vescoureteral reflux, *Pediatr Nephrol* 8:633-635.

Blom I.E., van Dijk A.J., Wieten L., Duran K., Ito Y., Kleij L., deNichilo M., Rabelink T.J., Weening J.J., Aten J. & Goldschmeding R. (2001). In vitro evidence for differential involvement of CTGF, TGFbeta, and PDGF-BB in mesangial response to injury, *Nephrol Dial Transplant* 16:1139-1148

Boettinger E.P. & Bitzer M. TGF-β signaling in renal disease, (2002). *J Am Soc Nephrol* 13:2600-2610.

Boettinger E.P., Letterio J.J. & Roberts A.R. (1997). Biology of TGF- β in knockout and transgenic mouse models, *Kidney Int* 51:1355-1360.

Branten AJ, Mulder TP, Peters WH, Assmann KJ & Wetzels JF. (2000). Urinary excretion of glutathione S transferases alpha and pi in patients with proteinuria: reflection of the site of tubular injury, *Nephron* 85(2):120-126.

Broder W.A. & Noble N.A. (1994). Transforming growth factor beta in tissue fibrosis, *N Eng J Med* 331:1286-1292.

Broyer M., Chantler C., Donckerwolcke R., Ehrich J.H., Rizzoni G. & Scharer K. (1993). The paediatric registry of the European Dialysis and Transplant Association: 20 years' experience, *Pediatr Nephrol* 7:758-768.

Bruzzi I., Corna D., Zoja C., Orisio S., Schiffrin E.L., Cavallotti D., Remuzzi G. & Benigni A. (1997). Time course and localization of endothelin-1 gene expression in a model of renal disease progression, *Am J Pathol* 151:1241-1247.

Cawood T.J., Bashir M., Brady J., Murray B.,. Murray P.T. & O'SheaD. (2010). Urinary Collagen IV and πGST: Potential Biomarkers for Detecting Localized Kidney Injury in Diabetes - A Pilot, *Am J Nephrol* 32:219-225

Chan W., Krieg R.J., Ward K., Santos F., Lin K. & Chan J.C.M. (2001). Progression after release of obstructive nephropathy, *Pediatr Nephrol* 16:238-244.

Chen L., Boadle R.A. & Harris D.C. (1998). Toxicity of holotransferrin but not albumin in proximal tubule cells in primary culture, *J Am Soc Nephrol* 9:77-84.

Chen M., Bao W., Aizman R., Huang P., Aspevall O., Gustafsson L.E., Ceccatelli S. & Celsi G. (2004). Activation of extracellular signal-regulated kinase mediates apoptosis induced by uropathogenic Escherichia coli toxins via nitric oxide synthase: protective role of heme oxygenase-1, *J Infect Dis* 190:127-135.

Chen M., Jahnukainen T., Bao W., Dare E., Ceccatelli S. & Celsi G. (2003). Uropathogenic Escherichia coli toxins induce caspase-independent apoptosis in renal proximal tubular cells via ERK signaling, *Am J Nephrol* 23:140-151.

Chertin B., Rolle U., Farkas A. & Puri P. (2002). The role of nitric oxide in reflux nephropathy, *Pediatr Surg Int* 18:630-634.

Chevalier R.L. (2004). Biomarkers of congential obstructive nephropathy: past, present and future, *J Urol* 172:852-857.

Chevalier R.L., Goyal S., Wolstenholme J.T. & Thornhill B.A. (1998). Obstructive nephropathy in the neonatal rat is attenuated by epidermal growth factor, *Kidney Int* 54:38-47.

Chevalier R.L., Thornhill B.A. & Chang A.Y. (2000). Unilateral ureteral obstruction in neonatal rats leads to renal insufficiency in adulthood, *Kidney Int* 58:1987-1995.

Chevalier RL, Forbes MS & Thornhill BA. (2009). Ureteral obstruction as a model of renal interstitial fibrosis and obstructive nephropathy, *Kidney Int* 75(11):1145-52.

Chiou Y.Y., Chiu N.T., Wang S.T., Cheng H.L. & Tang M.J. (2004). Factors associated with outcomes of children with unilateral uretropelvic junction obstruction, *J Urol* 171:397-402.

Choi M.E. & Ballermann B.J. (1995). Inhibition of capillary morphogenesis and associated apoptosis by dominant negative mutant transforming growth factor-beta receptors, *J Biol Chem* 270:21144-21150.

Chromek M., Tullus K., Hertting O., Jaremko G., Khalil A., Li Y.H. & Brauner A. (2003). Matrix metalloproteinase-9 and tissue inhibitor of metalloproteinases-1 in acute pyelonephritis and renal scarring, *Pediatr Res* 53:698-705.

Chromek M., Tullus K., Lundahl J. & Brauner A. (2004). Tissue inhibitor of metalloproteinase 1 activates normal human granulocytes, protects them from apoptosis, and blocks their transmigration during inflammation, *Infect Immun* 72:82-88.

Cojocel C., Al-Maghrebi M., Thomson M.S., Rawoot P. & Raghupathy R. (2005). Modulation of the transforming growth factor beta1 by vitamin E in early nephropathy, *Med Princ Pact* 14:422-429.

Cotton S.A., Gbadegesin R.A. Watson C.J., Brenchley P.E.C. & Webb N.S.A. (2000). Association between pro-inflammatory cytokines IL-6, IL-1beta, IL-1RA and TNF-α gene polymorphisms and acute pyelonephritis following child hood urinary tract infection, *J Am Soc Nephrol* 11:558A-566A.

Cotton S.A., Gbadegesin R.A., Williams S., Brenchley P.E. & Webb N.J. (2002). Role of TGF beta-1 in renal parenchymal scarring following childhood urinary tract infection, *Kidney Int* 61, 1, 61-67.

Dai C., Yang J. & Liu Y. (2003). Transforming growth factor-beta 1 potentiates renal tubular epithelial cell death by a mechanism independent signaling, *J Biol Chem* 278:12537-12545.

De Man P., van Kooten C., Aarden L., Engberg I., Linder H. & Svanborg Eden C. (1989). Interleukin-6 induced at mucosal surfaces by gram-negative bacterial infection, *Infect Immun* 57:3383-3388.

Deng C.L., Song X.W., Liang H.J., Feng C., Sheng Y.J. & Wang M.Y. (2006). Chronic hepatitis B serum promotes apoptotic damage in human rental tubular cells, *Word J Gastroenterol* 12:1752-1756.

Dudley J., Johnston A., Gardner A. & McGraw M. (2002). The deletion polymorphism of ACE gene is not an independent risk factor of renal scarring in children with vesico-ureteric reflux, *Nephrol Dial Transplant* 17:652-654.

Duncan M.R., Frazier K.S., Abramson S., Williams S., Klapper H., Huang X. & Grotendorst G.R. (1999). Connective tissue growth factor mediates transforming growth factor beta-induced collagen synthesis, down-regulation by cAMP, *FASEB J* 13:1774-1786.

Eddy A.A., Kim H., Lopez-Guisa J., Oda T. & Soloway P.D. (2000) Interstitial fibrosis in mice with overload proteinuria: deficiency of TIMP-1 is not protective, *Kidney Int* 58:618-628.

Eddy A.A. (2000): Molecular basis of renal fibrosis, *Pediatr Nephrol* 15:290-301.

Fan J.M., Ng Y.Y., Hill P.A., Nikolic-Paterson D.J., Mu W., Atkins R.C. & Lan H.Y. (1999). Transforming growth factor-beta regulates tubular epithelial-myofibroblast transdifferentiation in vitro, *Kidney Int* 56:1455-1467.

Farmaki E., Papachristou F., Winn R.M., Karatzas N., Sotiriou J. & Roilides E. (2005). Transforming growth factor-$\beta$1 in the urine of young children with urinary tract infection, *Pediatr Nephrol* 20:180-183.

Faust W.C., Diaz M. & Pohl H.G. (2009). Incidence of post-pyelonephritic renal scarring: a meta-analysis of the dimercapto-succinic acid literature, *J Urol* 181(1):290-298.

Frazier K.S., Paredes A., Dube P. & Styer E. (2000). Connective tissue growth factor expression in the rat remnant kidney model and association with tubular epithelial cells undergoing transdifferentiation, *Vet Pathol* 37:328-335.

Frendéus B., Godaly G., Hang L., Karpman D. & Svanborg C. (2001). Interleukin-8 receptor deficiency confers susceptibility to acute pyelonephritis, *J Infect Dis*, 183: 56-60.

Gad H.M., Shokeir A.A. & Mohy El-Din M.S. (2004). $^{99m}$TC-MAG3 dynamic imaging in diagnosis of pyelonephritic changes and renal scarring : a comparative study with $^{99m}$TC-DMSA, Abstract, *Alasbimn Journal*, 6.

Gagliardini E. & Benigni A (2006): Role of anti-TGF-beta antibodies in the treatment of renal injury, *Cytokine Growth Factor Rev* 17:89-96.

Galanakis E., Bitsori M., Dimitriou H., Giannakopoulou Ch., Karkavitsas N.S. & Kalmanti M. (2006). Urine interleukin -8 as a marker of vesicoureteral reflux in infants, *Pediatrics* 117:863-867.

Gendrel D. (1998). Urinary tract infecton and biologigal markers: C-reactive protein, interleukins and procalcitonin, *Arch Pediatr* 5:269-273.

Gobe G.C. & Axelsen R.A. (1987). Genesis of renal tubular atrophy in experimental hydronephrosis in the rat. Role of apoptosis, *Lab Invest* 56:273-281.

Gokce I., Alpay H., Biyikli N., Unluguzel G., Dede F. & Topuzoglu A. (2010). Urinary levels of interleukin-6 and interleukin-8 in patients with vesicoureteral reflux and renal parenchymal scar, *Pediatr Nephrol* 25(5):905-912.

Goldraich I.H., Goldraich N.P. & Ramos O.L. (1983). Classification of reflux nephropathy according to findings at DMSA renal scan, *Eur J Pediatr* 140:212-218.

Goldraich N.P. & Goldraich I.H. (1992). Follow up of conservatively treated children with high and low grade vesicoureteral reflux. A prospective study, *J Urol* 148:1688-1692.

Goldraich N.P., Ramos O.L. & Goldraich I.H. (1989). Urography versus DMSA scan in children with vesicoureteric reflux, *Pediatr Nephrol* 3:1-5.

Gordon I. (1987). Indications for 99mtechnetium dimercapto-succinic acid scan in children, *J Urol* 137:464-467.

Goumenos D.S., Tsakas S., El Nahas A.M., Alexandri S., Oldroyd S., Kalliakmani P. & Vlachojannis J.G. (2002). Transforming growth factor-beta(1) in the kidney and urine of patients with glomerular disease and proteinuria, *Nephrol Dial Transplant* 17: 2145-2152.

Grande M.T., Pérez-Barriocanal F. & López-Novoa J.M. (2010). Role of inflammation in tubulo-interstitial damage associated to obstructive nephropathy, *J Inflamm* 22;7:19

Guo G., Morrissey J., McCracken R., Tolley T. & Klahr S. (1999). Role of TNFR1 and TNFR2 receptors in tubulointerstitial fibrosis of obstructive nephropathy, *Am J Physiol* 277:F766-772.

Guo N., Krutzsch H.C., Inman J.K. & Roberts D.D. (1997). Thrombospondin 1 and type I repeat peptides of thrombospondin 1 specifically induce apoptosis of endothelial cells, *Cancer Res* 57:1735-1742.

Guroze M.K., Akarsu S., Yilmaz E., Godekmerdan A., Akca Z., Ciftei I. & Avgun A.D. (2005). Proinflammatory cytokines and procalcitonin in children with acute pyelonephritis, *Pediatr Nephrol* 20:1445-1448.

Hamed R.M., Ellis G., Levy M., McLorie G.A. & Balfe J.W. (1992). Captopril test in children with reflux nephropathy, *Pediatr Nephrol* 6:33-37.

Hang L., Frendéus B., Godaly G. & Svanborg C. (2000). Interleukin-8 receptor knockout mice have subepithelial neutrophil entrapment and renal scarring following acute pyelonephritis, *J Infect Dis* 182:1738-1748.

Hansson S., Bollgren I., Esbjorner E., Jakobsson B. & Marild S.R. (1999). Urinary tract infections in children below two years of age: a quality assurance project in Sweden. The Swedish Pediatric Nephrology Association, *Acta Paediatr* 88:270-274.

Haraoka M., Senoh K., Ogata N., Furukawa M., Matsumoto T. & Kumazawa J. (1996). Elevated interleukin-8 levels In the urine of children with renal scarring and/or vesicoureteral reflux, *J Urol* 155:678-680.

Haszon I., Friedman A.L., Papp F., Bereczki C., Baji S., Bodrogi T., Karoly E., Endreffy E. & Turi S. (2002). ACE gene polymorphism and renal scarring in primary vesicoureteric reflux, *Pediatr Nephrol* 17:1027-1031.

Hedges S., Anderson P., Lidin-Janson G., de Man P. & Svanborg C. (1991). Interleukin-6 response to deliberate colonization of the human urinary tract with gram-negative bacteria, *Infect Immun* 59:421-427.

Hedges S., Stenqvist K., Lidin-Janson G., Martinell J., Sandberg T. & Svanborg C. (1992). Comparison of urine and serum concentrations of interleukin-6 in women with acute pyelonephritis or asymptomatic bacteriuria, *J Infect Dis* 166:653-656.

Hedlund M., Frendeus B., Wachtler C., Hang L., Fischer H. & Svanborg C. (2001). Type 1 fimbriae deliver an LPS- and TLR4-dependent activation signal to CD14-negative cells, *Mol Microbiol* 39:542-552.

Hedlund M., Svensson M., Nilsson A., Duan R.D. & Svanborg C. (1996). Role of the ceramide-signaling pathway in cytokine responses to P-fimbriated Escherichia coli, *J Exp Med* 183:1037-1044.

Hohenfellner K., Hunley T.E., Brezinska R., Brodhag P., Shyr Y., Brenner W., Habermehl P. & Kon V. (1999). ACE I/D gene polymorphism predicts renal damage in congenital uropathies, *Pediatr Nephrol* 13:514-518.

Hussein A., Askar E., Elsaeid M.& Schaefer F. (2010). Functional polymorphisms in transforming growth factor-beta-1 (TGFbeta-1) and vascular endothelial growth factor (VEGF) genes modify risk of renal parenchymal scarring following childhood urinary tract infection, *Nephrol Dial Transplant* 25(3):779-85.

Ichino M., Kusaka M., Kuroyanagi Y., Mori T., Morooka M., Sasaki H., Shiroki R., Shishido S., Kurahashi H. & Hoshinaga K. (2010) Urinary neutrophil-gelatinase associated lipocalin is a potential noninvasive marker for renal scarring in patients with vesicoureteral reflux, *J Urol* 183(5):2001-2007.

Ichino M., Mori T., Kusaka M., Kuroyanagi Y., Ishikawa K., Shiroki R., Kowa H., Kurahashi H. & Hoshinaga K. (2008). Global gene expression profiling of renal scarring in a rat model of pyelonephritis, *Pediatr Nephrol* 23(7):1059-71.

Ingraham S.E., Saha M., Carpenter A.R., Robinson M., Ismail I., Singh S., Hains D., Robinson M.L., Hirselj D.A., Koff S.A., Bates C.M. & McHugh K.M. 2010 Pathogenesis of Renal Injury in the Megabladder Mouse: A Genetic Model of Congenital Obstructive Nephropathy, *Pediatr Res* 68:500-507.

International Reflux Study Committee (1981). Medical versus surgical treatment of primary vesicoureteral reflux: report of the, *Pediatrics* 67:392-400.

Jacobson S.H., Hylander B., Wretlind B. & Brauner A. (1994). Interleukin-6 and interleukin-8 in serum and urine in patients with acute pyelonephritis in relation to bacterial-virulence-associated traits and renal function, *Nephron* 67:172-179.

Jacobson S.H., Lu Y. & Brauner A. (1998) Soluble interleukin-6 receptor, interleukin-10 and granulocyte colony-stimulating factor in acute pyelonephritis: relationship to marcers of bacterial virulence and renal function, *Nephron* 80:401-407.

Jahnukainen T., Chen M. & Celsi G. (2005). Mechanisms of renal damage owing to infection, *Pediatr Nephrol* 20:1043-1053.

Jakobsson B., Nolstedt L., Svensson L., Soderlundh S. & Berg U. (1992). 99mTechnetium-dimercaptosuccinic acid scan in the diagnosis of acute pyelonephritis in children: relation to clinical and radiological findings, *Pediatr Nephrol* 6:328-334.

Jantausch B.A., O'Donnell R. & Wiedermann B.L. (2000). Urinary interleukin-6 and interleukin-8 in children with urinary tract infection, *Pediatr Nephrol* 15:236-240.

Jernigan S., Wing D., Schnaper H.W., Poncelet A.C., Lopez-Guisa J., Ueno H. & Eddy A.A. (1996). Effects of chronic blockade with soluble TGF-β II receptor in rads with overload proteinuria. Abstract, *J Am Soc Nephrol* 10:573.

Kabore A.F., Simard M. & Bergeron M.G. (1999). Local production of inflammatory mediators in an experimental model of acute obstructive pyelonephritis, *J Infect Dis* 179:1162-1172.

Kanellopoulos T.A., Salakos C., Spiliopoulou I., Ellina A., Nikolakopoulou N.M. & Papanastasiou D.A. (2006). First urinary tract infection in neonates, infants and young children: a comparative study, *Pediatr Nephrol* 21:1131-1137.

Kaneto H., Ohtani H., Fukuzaki A., Ishidoya S., Takeda A., Ogata Y., Nagura H. & Orikasa S. (1999). Increased expression of TGF-β1 but not of its receptors contributes to human obstructive nephropathy, *Kidney Int* 56:2137-2146.

Kang D.H., Kanellis J., Hugo C., Truong L., Anderson S., Kerjaschki D., Schreiner G.F. & Johnson R.J. (2002). Role of the microvascular endothelium in progressive renal disease, *J Am Soc Nephrol* 13:806-816.

Kapoor R., Reddy K., Liatsikos E.N., Smith A.D. & Singhal P.C. (2001). Escherichia coli-human uroepithelial cell interaction products enhance fibroblast migration and matrix accumulation, *J Endourol* 15:155-159.

Kassem J.A., Wasilewska A.M. & Zoch-Zwierz W.M. (2005). Urinary concentration of proinflamatory cytokines with regard to infected urinary tract region, *Wiad Lek* 58:14-19.

Kasuga H., Ito Y., Sakamoto S., Kawachi H., Shimizu F., Yuzawa Y. & Matsuo S. (2001). Effects of anti-TGF-beta type II receptor antibody on experimental glomerulonephritis, *Kidney Int* 60:1745-1755.

Kelly F.J., Anderson S., Thompson M.M., Oyama T.T., Kennefick T.M., Corless C.L., Roman R.J., Kurtzberg L., Pratt B.M. & Ledbetter S.R. (1999). Acute and chronic renal effects of recombinant human TGF-beta2 in the rat, *J Am Soc Nephrol* 106:1264-1273.

Kenda R.B., Zupancic Z., Fettich J.J. & Meglic A. (1997). A follow-up study of vesico-ureteric reflux and renal scars in asymptomatic siblings of children with reflux, *Nucl Med Commun* 18:827-831.

Kersnik Levart T., Kenig A., Fettich J.J., Ključevšek D., Novljan G. & Kenda R. (2002). Sensitivity of ultrasonography in detecting renal parenchymal defects in children, *Pediatr Nephrol* 17:1059-1062.

Khalil A., Tullus K., Bakhiet M., Burman L.G. Jaremko G. & Brauner A. (2000). Angiotensin II type 1 receptor antagonist (losatran) down-regulates transforming growth factor-beta in experimental acute pyelonephritis, *J Urol* 164:186-191.

Khalil A., Tullus K., Bartfai T., Bakhiet M., Jaremko G. & Brauner A. (2000). Renal cytokine responses in acute escherichia coli pyelonephritis in IL-6-deficient mice, *Clin Exp Immunol* 122:200-206.

Khalil M.S., El Nahas A.M. & Blakemore A.I.F. (2005). Transforming growth factor-$\beta_1$ SNPs, genetic and phenotypic correlations in progressive kidney insufficiency, *Nephron Exp Nephrol* 101:31-41.

Khan S.B., Cook H.T., Bhangal G., Smith J., Tam F.W.K. & Pusey C.D. (2005). Antibody blockade of TNF-α reduces inflammation and scarring in experimental crescentic glomerulonephritis, *Kidney Int* 67:1812-1820.

Kim H., Oda T., Lopez-Guisa J., Wing D., Edwards D.R., Soloway P.D. & Eddy A.A. (2001). TIMP-1 deficiency does not attenuate interstitial fibrosis in obstructive nephropathy, *J Am Soc Nephrol* 12(4):736-748.

Kincaid-Smith P. (1975). Glomerular lesions in atrophic pyelonephritis and reflux nephropathy, *Kidney Int* 4:81-83.

Kishimoto T. & T. Harano. (1988). Molecular regulation of B lymphocyte response, *Annu Rev Immunol* 6:485-512.

Klahr S. (2001). Urinary tract obstruction, *Semin Nephrol* 21:133-145.

Klahr S. & Morrissey J. (2002). Obstructive nephropathy and renal fibrosis, *Am J Renal Physiol* 283:861-875.

Klahr S. & Morrissey J.J. (2003). Obstructive nephropathy and renal fibrosis: The role of bone morphogenic protein-7 and hepatocyte growth factor, *Kidney Int Suppl* 87:S105-112.

Klahr S. & Morrissey J.J. (1998). The role of growth factors, cytokines, and vasoactive compounds in obstructive nephropathy, *Semin Nephrol* 18:622-632.

Ko Y.C., Mukaida N., Ishiyama S., Tokue A., Kawai T., Matsushima K. & Kasahara T. (1993). Elevated interleukin-8 levels in the urine of patients with urinary tract infections, *Infect Immun* 61:1307-1314.

Koff S.A. (1990). Pathophysiology of ureteropelvic junction obstruction. Clinical and experimental observations, *Urol Clin North Am* 17:263-272.

Kohler J., Tencer J., Thysell H. & Forsberg L. (1997). Vesicoureteral reflux diagnosed in adulthood. Incidence of urinary tract infections, hypertension, proteinuria, back pain and renal calculi, *Nephrol Dial Transplant* 12:2580-2587.

Kohler J.R., Tencer J., Thysell H., Forsberg L. &Hellstrom M. (2003). Long-term effects of reflux nephropathy on blood pressure and renal function in adults, *Nephron Clin Pract* 93:C35-C46.

Kopp J.B., Factor V.M., Mozes M., Nagy P., Sanderson N., Bottinger E.P., Klotman P.E. & Thorgeirsson S.S. (1996). Transgenic mice with increased plasma levels of TGF- beta 1 develop progressive renal disease, *Lab Incest* 74:991-1003.

Kopp JB. (2002). BMP-7 and the proximal tubule, *Kidney Int* 61: 351–352

Korzon M., Liberek A., Marek A. Szlagatys-Sidorkiewicz A. & Marek K. (2004). Rola transformującego czynnika wzrostu beta 1 (TGF-β1) i jego polimorfizmu genowego w etiopatogenezie i przebiegu klinicznym niektórych stanów chorobowych u ludzi, *Ped Pol* 79:963-970.

Kowalewska-Pietrzak M., Klich I. & Mlynarski W. (2008). TGF-beta1 gene polymorphisms and primary vesicoureteral reflux in childhood, *Pediatr Nephrol* 23(12):2195-2200.

Kushibiki T., Nagata-Nakajima N., Sugai M., Shimizu A. & Tabata Y. (2005). Delivery of plazmid DNA expressing small interferencje RNA for TGF-beta type II receptor by cationized gelatin to prezent interstitial renal fibrosis, *J Control Release* 105:318-331.

Lane A., Johnson D.W., Pat B., Winterford C., Endre Z., Wei M. & Gobe G.C. (2002). Interacting roles of myofibroblasts, apoptosis and fibrogenic growth factors in the pathogenesis of renal tubulo-interstitial fibrosis, *Growth Factors* 20:109-119.

Lee J.H., Son C.H., Lee M.S. & Park Y.S. (2006). Vesicoureteral reflux increases the risk of renal scars: a study of unilateral reflux, *Pediatr Nephrol* 21:1281-1284.

Leemans J.C., Butter L.M., Pulskens W.P., Teske G.J., Claessen N., van der Poll T. & Florquin S. (2009). The role of Toll-like receptor 2 in inflammation and fibrosis during progressive renal injury, *PLoS One* 27;4(5):e5704.

Leonova L.V., Severgina E.S., Popova O.P., Konovalov D.M., Petruchina Iu.V. & Simonova N.A. (2007). Transforming growth factor as a marker beta of nephrogenetic disturbance in congenital obstructive uropathies, *Arkh Pato* 69(4):35-8.

Lerner G.R. (1994). Urinary tract infections in children, *Pediatr Ann* 23:463, 466-473.

Li L., Wu Y. & Zhang W. (2010). PAX2 re-expression in renal tubular epithelial cells and correlation with renal interstitial fibrosis of rats with obstructive nephropathy, *Ren Fail* 32(5):603-611.

Li Y., Zhang J., Fang L., Luo P., Peng J. & Du X. (2010). Lefty A attenuates the TGF-beta1-induced epithelial to mesenchymal transition of human renal proximal epithelial tubular cells, *Mol Cell Biochem* 39(1-2):263-270.

Liapis H. (2003). Biology of congenital obstructive nephropathy, *Nephron Exp Nephrol* 93:e87-91.

Lonnemann G., Engler-Blum G., Muler G.A., Koch K.M. & Dinarello C.A. (1995). Cytokines in human renal interstitial fibrosis. II. Intrinsic interleukin (IL)-1 synthesis and IL-1-dependent production of IL-6 and IL-8 by calculated kidney fibroblasts, *Kidney Int* 47:845-854.

Manucha W. (2007). Biochemical-molecular markers in unilateral ureteral obstruction, *Biocell* 31(1):1-12.

Marra G., Oppezzo C., Ardissino G., Dacco V., Testa S., Avolio L., Taioli E. & Sereni F. (2004). ItalKid Project. Severe vesicoureteral reflux and chronic renal failure: a condition peculiar to male gender?, *J Pediatr* 144:677-681.

Mittal R., Sharma S., Chhibber S. & Harjai K. (2009). Evaluation of tumour necrosis factor-alpha and interleukin-1beta in an experimental pyelonephritis model induced with planktonic and biofilms cells of Pseudomonas aeruginosa, *Can J Infect Dis Med Microbiol* 20(3):e35-42.

Mizuno S., Matsumoto K. & Nakamura T. (2001). Hepatocyte growth factor suppresses interstitial fibrosis in a mouse of obstructive nephropathy, *Kidney Int* 59:1304-1314.

Mohanan N., Colhoun E. & Puri P. (2008). Renal parenchymal damage in intermediate and high grade infantile vesicoureteral reflux, *J Urol* 180:1635-1638.

Moorthy I., Wheat D. & Gordon I. (2004). Ultrasonography in the evaluation of renal scarring using DMSA scan as the gold standard, *Pediatr Nephrol* 19:153-156.

Muinuddin G., Rahman H., Hossain M.M., Jahan S. & Begum A. (2008). Urinary tract infection and vesicoureteric reflux in children, *Mymensingh Med J* 17:S28-31.

Nangaku M., Pippin J. & Couser W.G. (1999). Complement membrane attack complex (C5b-9) mediates interstitial disease in experimental nephrotic syndrome, *J Am Soc Nephrol* 10:2323-2331.

Narayana C., Tripathi M., Kumar A., Gowda N.K., Phom H., Chandra P., Bandopadhyaya G. &vBal C. ( 2004). Technetium-99m-L,L-ethylenedicysteine renal scan as a single-modality investigation for the evaluation of renal morphology and function: a comparative study with technetium-99m-dimercaptosuccinic acid, *Nucl Med Commun* 25:743-747.

Nath K.A. (1998). The tubulointerstitium in progressive renal disease, *Kidney Int* 54:992-994.

Nee L.E., Mc Morrow T., Campbell E., Slattery C. & Ryan M.P. (2004). TNF-alpha and IL-1beta-mediated regulation of MMP-9 and TIMP-1 in renal proximal tubular cells, *Kidney Int* 66:1376-1386.

Ng Y.Y., Huang T.P., Yang W.C., Chen Z.P., Yang A.H., Mu W., Nikolic-Paterson D.J., Atkins R.C. & Lan H.Y. (1998). Tubular epithelialmyofibroblast transdifferentiation in progressive tubulointerstitial fibrosis in 5/6 nephrectomized rats. *Kidney Int* 54: 864-876.

Nicolle L.E., Brunka J., Orr P., Wilkins J. & Harding G.K. (1993). Urinary immunoreactive interleukin-1 alpha and interleukin-6 in bacteriuric institutionalized elderly subjects, *J Urol* 149:1049-1053.

Noe H.N. (1992) The long-term results of prospective sibling reflux screening, *J Urol* 148:1739-1742.

Norbeck J.C., Ritchey M.R. & Bloom D.A. (1993). Labial fusion causing upper urinary tract obstruction, *Urology* 42:209-211.

Oh M.M., Jin M.H., Bae J.H., Park H.S., Lee J.G. & Moon du G. (2008). The role of vesicoureteral reflux in acute renal cortical scintigraphic lesion and ultimate scar formation, *J Urol* 180(5):2167-2170.

Ohashi R., Kitamura H. & Yamanaka N. (2000). Peritubular capillary injury during the progression of experimental glomerulonephritis in rats, *J Am Soc Nephrol* 11: 47-56.

Ohta K., Takano N., Seno A., Yachie A., Miyawaki T., Yokoyama H., Tomosugi N., Kato E. & Taniguchi N. (1992). Detection and clinical usefulness of urinary interleukin-6 in the diseases of the kidney and the urinary tract, *Clin Nephrol* 38:185-189.

Ohtomo Y., Nagaoka R., Kaneko K., Fukuda Y., Miyano T. & Yamashiro Y. (2001). Angiotensin converting enzyme gene polymorphism in primary vesicoureteral reflux, *Pediatr Nephrol* 16:648-652.

Okada H, Moriwaki K., Kalluri R., Imai H., Ban S., Takahama M. & Suzuki H. (2000). Inhibition of monocyte chemoattractant protein-1 expression in tubular epithelium attenuates tubulointerstitial alteration in rat Goodpasture syndrome, *Kidney Int* 57:927-936.

Okada H., Moriwaki K., Kalluri R., Takenaka T., Imai H., Ban S., Takahama M. & Suzuki H. (2000). Osteopontin expressed by renal tubular epithelium mediates interstitial monocyte infiltration in rats, *Am J Physiol Renal Physiol* 278:F110-121.

Oldfield M.D., Bach L.A., Forbes J.M., Nikolic-Paterson D., McRobert A., Thallas V., Atkins R.C., Osicka T., Jerums G. & Cooper M.E. (2001). Advanced glycation end products cause epithelial-myofibroblast transdifferentiation via the receptor for advanced glycation end products (RAGE), *J Clin Invest* 108:1853-1863.

Olszyna D.P., Opal S.M., Prins J.M., Horn D.L., Speelman P., van Deventer S.J.H. & van der Poll T. (2000). Chemotatic activity of CXC chemokines interleukin-8, growth-related oncogene-α, and epithelial cell-derived neutrophil-activating protein-78 in urine of patients with urosepsis, *J Infect Dis* 182:1731-1737.

Orikasa S., Fukuzaki A. & Konda R. (1995). Obstructive and reflux nephropathy. Abstract, *Nippon Rinsho* 53:2019-2026.

Orleana P., Baguedano P., Rangarajan V., Zhao J.H., Chee Eng N.D., Fettich J., Chaiwatanarat T., Sonmezoglu K., Kumar D., Park Y.H., Samuel A.M., Sixt R., Bhtnagar V. & Padhy A.K. (2004). Relation ship between acute pyelonephritis, renal scarring, and vesicoureteral reflux, *Pediatr Nefrol* 19:1122-1126.

Orphanides C., Fine L.G. & Norman J.T. (1997). Hypoxia stimulates proximal tubular cell matrix production via a TGF-beta1-independent mechanism, *Kidney Int* 52:637-647.

Ortiz A., Ziyadeh F.N. & Neilson E.G. (1997). Expression of apoptosis regulatory genes in renal proximal tubular epithelial cells exposed to high ambient glucose and in diabetic kidneys, *J Investig Med* 45:50-56.

Otto G., Braconier J., Andreasson A. & Svanborg C. (1999). Interleukin-6 and disease severity in patients with bacteremic and nonbacteremic febrile urinary tract infection,
*J Infect Dis* 179:172-179.

Ozen S., Alikasifoglu M., Saatci U., Bakkaloglu A., Besbas N., Kara N., Kocak H., Erbas B., Unsal I. & Tuncbilek E. (1999). Implications of certain genetic polymorphisms in scarring in vesicoureteric reflux: importance of ACE polymorphism, *Am J Kidney Dis* 34:140-145.

Padillo F.J., Cruz A., Segura-Jiménez I., Ruiz-Rabelo J., Vázquez-Ezquerra M.R., Perea-Alvarez M.D., Peña J., Briceño J. & Muntané J. (2007). Anti-TNF-alpha treatment and bile duct drainage restore cellular immunity and prevent tissue injury in experimental obstructive jaundice, *Int J Immunopathol Pharmacol* 20(4):855-60.

Pardo R.., Malaga S., Coto E., Navarro M., Alvarez V., Espinosa L., Alvarez R., Vallo A., Loris C. & Branga S. (2003). Renin-angiotensin system polymorphisms and renal scarring, *Pediatr Nephrol* 18:110-114.

Patel N.S., Chatterjee P.K., Di Paola R., Mazzon E., Brotti D., De Sarro A., Cuzzocrea S. & Thiemermann C. (2005). Endogenous interleukin-6 enhances the renal injury, dysfunction, and inflammation caused by ischemia/reperfusion, *J Pharmacol Exp Ther* 312:1170-1178.

Pecile P., Miorin E., Romanello C., Vidal E., Contardo M., Valent F. & Tenore A. (2009). Age-related renal parenchymal lesions in children with first febrile urinary tract infections, *Pediatrics* 124(1):23-9.

Pereira B.J., Shapiro L., King A.J., Falagas M.E., Strom J.A. & Dinarello C.A. (1994). Plasma levels of IL-1beta, TNF-alfa and their specific inhibitors in undialyzed chronic renal failure, CAPD and hemodialysis patients, *Kidney Int* 45:890-896.

Peters C. & Rushton H.G. (2010). Vesicoureteral reflux associated renal damage: congenital reflux nephropathy and acquired renal scarring, *J Urol* 184(1):265-273.

Pichler R.H., Hugo C., Shankland S.J., Reed M.J., Bassuk J.A., Andoh T.F., Lombardi D.M., Schwartz S.M., Bennett W.M., Alpers C.E., Sage E.H., Johnson R.J. & Couser W.G. (1996). SPARC is expressed in renal interstitial fibrosis and in renal vascular injury, *Kidney Int* 50:1978-1989.

Pimentel J.L. (1995). Role of angiotensin II in the expression and regulation of transforming growth factor-beta in obstructive nephropathy, *Kidney Int* 48:1233-1246.

Polito C., La Manna A., Mansi L., Rambaldi P.F., Papale M.R., Marte A. & Di Toro R. (1999). Body growth in early diagnosed vesicoureteric reflux, *Pediatr Nephrol* 13:876-879.

Polito C., Rambaldi P.F, Signoriello G., Mansi L. & La Manna A. (2006). Permanent renal parenchymal defects after febrile UTI are closely associated with vesicoureteric reflux, *Pediatr Nephrol* 21:521-526.

Poncelet A.C. & Schnaper H.W. (1998). Regulation of human mesangial cell collagen expression by transforming growth factor-β1, *Am J Physiol* 275:458-466.

Ransley P.G. & Risdon R.A. (1981). Reflux nephropathy: effects of antimicrobial therapy on the evolution of the early pyelonephritic scar, *Kidney Int* 20:733-742.

Rao W.H., Evans G.S. & Finn A.(2001). The significance of interleukin 8 in urine, *Arch Dis Child* 85:256-262.

Rastaldi M.P., Ferrario F., Giardino L., Dell'Antonio G., Grillo C., Grillo P., Strutz F., Muller G.A., Colasanti G. & D'Amico G. (2002). Epithelial-mesenchymal transition of tubular epithelial cells in human renal biopsies, *Kidney Int* 62:137-146.

Rebenok A.Z., Tikhonov I.I. & Chizh A.S. (1999). Role of IL-8 defensins in pathogenesis of chronic glomerulonephritis and pyelonephritis, *Ter Arkh* 71:62-67.

Ricardo S.D., Levinson M.E., DeJoseph M.R. & Diamond J.R. (1996) Expression of adhesion molecules in rat renal cortex during experimental hydronephrosis, *Kidney Int* 50:2002-2010.

Rice E.K., Nikolic-Paterson D.J., David J.R., Bucala R., Metz Ch.N., Atkins R.C. & Tesch G.H. (2004). Macrophage accumulation and rental fibrosis are independent of macrophage migration inhibitory factor in mouse obstructive nephropathy, *Nephrology* 9:278-287.

Roberts A.B. & Sporn M.B. (1987). Transforming growth factor-beta: potential common mechanisms mediating its effects on embryogenesis, inflammation-repair, and carcinogenesis, *Int J Rad Appl Instrum B* 14:435-439.

Roberts I.S., Burrows C., Shanks J.H., Venning M. & McWilliam L.J. (1997). Interstitial myofibroblasts: predictors of progression in membranous nephropathy, *J Clin Pathol* 50:123-127.

Roilides E., Papachristou F., Gioulekas E., Tsaparidou S., Karatzas N., Sotiriou J. & Tsiouris J. (1999). Increased urine interleukin-6 concentrations correlate with pyelonephritic changes on $^{99m}$Tc-dimercaptosuccinic acid scans in neonates with urinary tract infections, *J Infect Dis* 180:904-907.

Rugo H.S., O'Hanley P., Bishop A.G., Pearce M.K., Abrams J.S., Howard M. & O'Gara A. (1992). Local cytokine production in a murine model of Escherichia coli pyelonephritis, *J Clin Invest* 89:1032-1039.

Rushton H.G. (1997). Urinary tract infections in children. Epidemiology, evaluation, and management, *Pediatr Clin North Am* 44:1133-1169.

Rushton H.G., Majd M., Jantausch B., Wiedermann B.L. & Belman A.B. (1992). Renal scarring following reflux and nonreflux pyelonephritis children: evaluation with 99mtechnetium dimercaptosuccinic acid scintigraphy, *J Urol* 147:1327-1332.

Rushton H.G. (1997). The evaluation of acute pyelonephritis and renal scarring with technetium 99m-dimercaptosuccinic acid renal scintigraphy: evolving concepts and future directions, *Pediatr Nephrol* 11:108-120.

Saborio P., Krieg R.J., Kuemmerle N.B., Norokus E.P., Schwartz Ch.C. & Chan J.C.M. (2000). α-Tocopherol modulates lipoprotein cytotoxicity in obstructive nephropathy, *Pediatr Nephrol* 14:740-746.

Sager C., Lopez J.C., Duran V., Burek C. & Perazzo E. (2009) Transforming growth factor-beta1 in congenital ureteropelvic junction obstruction: diagnosis and follow-up. *Int Braz J Urol* 35(3):315-323.

Sanderson N., Factor V., Nagy P., Kopp J., Kondaiah P., Wakefield L., Roberts A.B., Sporn M.B. & Thorgeirsson S.S. (1995). Hepatic expression of mature transforming growth factor beta 1 in transgenic mice results in multiple tissue lesions, *Proc Natl Acad Sci USA* 92:2572-2576.

Sato M., Muragaki Y., Saika S., Roberts A.B. & Ooshima A. (2003). Targeted disruption of TGF-β1/Smad3 signaling protects against renal tubulointerstitial fibrosis induced by unilateral ureteral obstruction, *J Clin Invest* 112:1486-1494.

Schnaper H.W., Hayashida T., Hubchak S.C. & Poncelet A.C. (2003). TGF-beta signal transduction and mesangial cell fibrogenesis, *Am J Physiol Renal Physiol* 284:243-252.

Seidel C., Schaefer F. & Scharer K. (1993). Body growth in urinary tract malformations, *Pediatr Nephrol* 7:151-155.

Seron D., Alexopoulos E., Raftery M.J., Hartley B. & Cameron J.S. (1990). Number of interstitial capillary cross-sections assessed by monoclonal antibodies: relation to interstitial damage, *Nephrol Dial Transplant* 5:889-893.

Shaikh N., Ewing A.L., Bhatnagar S. & Hoberman A. (2010). Risk of renal scarring in children with a first urinary tract infection: a systematic review, *Pediatrics* 126(6):1084-1091.

Shapiro E., Slovis T.L., Perlmutter A.D. & Kuhns L.R. (1988). Optimal use 99mtechnetium-glucoheptonate scintigraphy in the detection of pyelonephritic scarring in children: a preliminary report, *J Urol* 149:1175-1177.

Sheu J.N., Chen S.M., Meng M.H. & Lue K.H. (2009). The role of serum and urine interleukin-8 on acute pyelonephritis and subsequent renal scarring in children, *Pediatr Infect Dis J* 28(10):885-90.

Shinozaki M., Ueno H., Ando T., Kashiwagi M., Fukusa K., Hirakata H., Okuda S. & Fujishima M. (1998). Marked suppression of interstitial fibrosis with adenovirus-mediated In vivo gene transfer of soluble TGF-β II receptor in experimental hydronephrosis. Abstract, *J Am Soc Nephrol* 9:527A.

Shweke N., Boulos N., Jouanneau C., Vandermeersch S., Melino G., Dussaule J.C., Chatziantoniou C., Ronco P. & Boffa J.J. (2008). Tissue transglutaminase contributes to interstitial renal fibrosis by favoring accumulation of fibrillar collagen through TGF-beta activation and cell infiltration, *Am J Pathol* 173(3):631-642.

Sieniawska M. &Wyszyńska T. (2003). Nefrologia dziecięca, t.2. Ośrodek Informacji Naukowej „Polfa" Sp. z o.o. Warszawa.

Silva J.M., Diniz J.S., Lima E.M., Pinheiro S.V., Marino V.P., Cardoso L.S., Colosimo E.A., Silva A.C. & Oliveira E.A. (2009). Independent risk factors for renal damage in a series of primary vesicoureteral reflux: a multivariate analysis, *Nephrology* (Carlton) 14(2):198-204.

Smellie J.M., Edwards D., Hunter N., Normand I.C.S. & Prescod N. (1975). Vesico-ureteric reflux and renal scarring, *Kidney Int* 4:62-72.

Smellie J.M., Normand I.C. & Katz G. (1981). Children with urinary tract infection: a comparision of those with and those without vesicoureteral reflux, *Kidney Int*, 20:717-722.

Smellie J.M., Prescod N.P., Shaw P.J., Risdon R.A. & Bryant T.N. (1998). Childhood reflux and urinary infection: a follow-up of 10-41 years in 226 adults, *Pediatr Nephrol* 12: 727-736.

Smellie J.M., Ransley P.G., Normand I.C., Prescod N. & Edwards D. (1985). Development of new renal scars: a collaborative study, *Br Med J* 29:1957-1960.

Smółko M., Zoch-Zwierz W. & Wasilewska A. (2004). Ocena stężenia interleukiny 6 i 8 w moczu i surowicy dzieci z odpływami pęcherzowo-moczowodowymi, *Prob Lek* 43:22.

Smółko M., Zoch-Zwierz W., Wasilewska A. & Kassem J.A.D. (2004). Ocena stężenia TGF- $\beta_1$ w moczu u dzieci z odpływami pęcherzowo-moczowodowymi, *Ped Pol*, 79:115-119.

Solari V., Owen D. & Puri P. (2005). Association of transforming growth factor-beta1 gene polymorphism with reflux nephropathy, *J Urol* 174:1609-1611.

Solari V., Unemoto K., Piaseczna-Piotrowska A. & Puri P. (2004). Increased expression of mast cells in reflux nephropathy, *Pediatr Nephrol* 19:157-163.

Stokland E., Hellstrom M., Jacobsson B. & Jodal U. (1996). Renal damage one year after first urinary tract infection: role of dimercaptosuccinic acid scintigraphy, *J Pediatr* 129:815-820.

Strutz F. & Muller G.A. (1999). Interstitial pathomechanisms underlying progressive tubulointerstitial damage, *Kidney Blood Press Res* 22:71-80.

Strutz F., Muller G.A. & Neilson E.G. (1996). Transdifferentiation, a new angle on renal fibrosis, *Experimental Nephrol* 4:267-270.

Strutz F. & Neilson E.G. (2003). New insights into mechanisms of fibrosis in immune renal injury, *Springer Semin Immunopathol* 24:459-476.

Strutz F., Okada H., Lo C.W., Danoff T., Carone R.L., Tomaszewski J.E. & Neilson E.G. (1995). Identification and characterization of a fibroblast marker: FSP1, *J Cell Biol* 130:393-405.

Svensson M., Irjala H., Alam P., Holmqvist B., Lundstedt A.C. & Svanborg C. (2005). Natural history of renal scarring in susceptible mIL-8Rh-/- mice, *Kidney Int* 67: 103-110.

Szeto C.C., Chan R.W.Y., Lai K.B., Szeto C.Y.K., Chow K.m., Li P.K.T. & Lai F.M.M. (2005). Messenger RNA Expression of target genes in the urinary sediment of patients with chronic kidney diseases, *Nephrol Dial Transplant* 20:105-113.

Taha A.S., Grant V. & Kelly R.W. (2003). Urinalysis for interleukin-8 in the non-invasive diagnosis of acute and chronic inflammatory diseases, *Postgrad Med J* 79:159-163.

Tikhonov I., Rebenok A. & Chyzh A. (1997). A study of interleukin-8 and defenses in urine and plasma of patients with pyelonephritis and glomerulonephritis, *Nephrol Dial Transplant* 12:2557-2561.

Traylor L.A. & Mayeux P.R. (1997). Nitric oxide generation mediates lipid A-induced oxidant injury in renal proximal tubules, *Arch Biochem Biophys* 338:129-135.

Tullus K., Fituri O., Linne T., Escobar-Billing R., Wikstad I., Karlsson A., Burman L.G., Wretlind B. & Brauner A. (1994). Urine interleukin-6 and interleukin-8 in children with acute pyelonephritis, in relation to DMSA scintigraphy in the acute phase and at 1-year follow-up, *Pediatr Radiol* 24:513-515.

Uhlen P., Laestadius A., Jahnukainen T., Soderblom T., Backhed F., Celsi G., Brismar H., Normark S., Aperia A. & Richter-Dahlfors A. (2000). Alpha-haemolysin of uropathogenic E. coli induces Ca2+ oscillations in renal epithelial cells, *Nature* 405:694-697.

Vachvanichsanong P. (2007). Urinary tract infection: one lingering effect of childhood kidney diseases--review of the literature, *J Nephrol* 20(1):21-8.

Van den Abbeele A.D., Treves S.T., Lebowits R.L., Bauers Davis R.T., Retik A. & Colodny A. (1987). Vesicoureteral reflux in asymptomatic siblings of patients with known reflux: radionuclide cystography, *Pediatrics* 79:147-153.

Vanderfaeillie A., Flamen P., Wilikens A., Desprechins B. & Piepsz A. (1998). Technetium-99m-dimercaptosuccinic acid renal scintigraphy in children over 5 years, *Pediatr Nephrol* 12:295-297.

Vernon S.J., Coulthard M.G., Lambert H.J., Keir M.J. & Matthews J.N. (1997). New renal scarring in children who at age 3 and 4 years had had normal scans with dimercaptosuccinic acid: follow up study, *BMJ* 315:905-908.

Vesey D.A, Cheung K.W.Y., Cuttle L., Endre Z.A., Gobe G. & Johnson D.W. (2002). Interleukin -1β induces human proximal tubule cell injury, α-smooth muscle actin expression and fibronectin production, *Kidney Int* 62:31.

Vesey D.A., Cheung C., Cuttle., Endre Z., Gobe G. & Johnson D.W. (2002). Interleukin-1β stimulates human renal fibroblast proliferation and matrix protein production by means of a transforming growth factor-β-dependent mechanism, *J Lab Clin Med* 140: 342-350.

Wan J., Greenfield SP., Ng M., Zerin M., Ritchey M.L. & Bloom D. (1996). Sibling reflux: a dual center retrospective study, *J Urol* 156:677-679.

Wang J., Konda R., Sato H., Sakai K., Ito S. & Orikasa S. (2001). Clinical significance of urinary interleukin-6 in children with reflux nephropathy, *J Urol* 165:210-214.

Wang P.X., Fan M.Q., Huang C.B., Feng J.Y., Xiao Y., Fang Z.Q. & Zhang Y.P. (2005). Effect of losartan on slowing progression of chronic allograft nephropathy, *Chin Med Sci J* 20:231-236.

Wang S., Wilkes M.C., Leof E.B. & Hirschberg R . (2010). Noncanonical TGF-beta pathways, mTORC1 and Abl, in renal interstitial fibrogenesis, *Am J Physiol Renal Physiol* 298:F142-F149.

Wasilewska A., Taranta-Janusz K., Dębek W., Zoch-Zwierz W. & Kuroczycka-Saniutycz E. (2011). KIM-1 and NGAL: new markers of obstructive nephropathy, *Pediatr Nephrol* 26(4):579-586.

Weiss R.A., Madaio M.P., Tomaszewski J.E. & Kelly C.J. (1994). T cells reactive to an inducible heat shock protein induce disease in toxin-induced interstitial nephritis, *J Exp Med* 180:2239-2250.

Wetmore J.B., Hung A.M., Lovett B.H., Sen S., Quershy O., Johansen K.L. (2005). Interleukin-1 gene cluster polymorphisms predict risk of ESRD, *Kidney Int* 68: 278-284.

Wolfs T.G.A.M., Buurman W.A., Van Schadewijk A., De Vries B., Daemen M.A.R.C., Hiemstra P.S. & Van't Veer C. (2002). In vivo expression of toll-like receptor 2 and 4 by renal epithelial cells: INF-gamma and TNF-alpha mediated up-regulation during inflammation, *J Immun* 168:1286-1293.

Wyszyńska T. & Litwin M. (2000). Nadciśnienie tętnicze u dzieci i młodzieży, *PZWL* Warszawa.

Yao Y., Zhang J., Ye D.F., Tan D.Q., Peng J.P., Xie M. & Fang L. (2011). Left-right determination factor is down-regulated in fibrotic renal tissue of human hydronephrosis, *BJU Int* 107(6):1002-1008.

Ylinen E., Ala-Houhala M. & Wikstrom S. (2003). Risk of renal scarring in vesicoureteral reflux detected either antenatally or during the neonatal period, *Urology* 61:1238-1242.

Zajączkowska M., Zinkiewicz Z., Duda B., Kołacz A. & Szajner-Milart I. (2001). Zaburzenia anatomiczne i czynnościowe dróg moczowych u dzieci z zakażeniem układu moczowego, *Pol Merk Lek* 58:213-215.

Zeisberg M., Bonner G., Maeshima Y., Colorado P., Müller G.A., Strutz F. & Kaluri R. (2001). Collagen composition ans assemby regulates epithelial-mesenchymal transdifferntiation, *AJP* 159:1313-1321.

Zhang C., Meng X., Zhu Z., Liu J. &, Deng A. (2004). Connective tissue growth factor regulates the key events in tubular epithelial to myofibroblast transition in vitro, *Cell Bio Int* 28:863-873.

Zhang G., Oldroyd S.D., Huang L.H., Yang B., Li Y., Ye R. & El Nahas AM. (2001) . Role of apoptosis and Bcl-2/Bax in the development of tubulointerstitial fibrosis during experimental obstructive nephropathy, *Exp Nephrol* 9(2):71-80

Zhang H. & Phan S. (1999). Inhibition of myofibroblast apoptosis by transforming growth factor $\beta_1$, *Am J Respir Cell Mol Biol* 21:658-665.

Zhang M., Tang J., Li X. Interleukin-1β-induced Transdifferentiation of renal proximal tubular cells is mediated by activation of JNK and p38 MAPK. Nephron Experimental Nephrol 2005, 99:68-76.

# 19

# Studies on Clinical Characteristics, Urovirulence Factor and Host Susceptibility Gene in Pediatric Acute Lobar Nephronia

Chi-Hui Cheng[1, 3], Yong-Kwei Tsau[4] and Tzou-Yien Lin[2, 3]
*[1]Division of Pediatric Nephrology and*
*[2]Division of Pediatric Infectious Diseases, Department of Pediatrics,*
*Chang Gung Children's Hospital, Chang Gung Memorial Hospital, Taoyuan,*
*[3]College of Medicine, Chang Gung University, Taoyuan,*
*[4]Division of Pediatric Nephrology, Department of Pediatrics,*
*National Taiwan University Hospital, Taipei,*
*Taiwan*

## 1. Introduction

Urinary tract infections (UTIs) have been described as one of the most common serious bacterial diseases affecting infants and young children. Approximately 3% of prepubertal girls and 1% of prepubertal boys are diagnosed with UTIs (Riccabona 2003; Ma and Shortliffe 2004). The clinical severity of acute renal bacterial infection spans continuously from an uncomplicated lower urinary tract infection (i.e. cystitis) to frank abscess formation (Soulen et al., 1989). Among these UTIs, renal parenchymal infections, including uncomplicated acute pyelonephritis (APN), acute lobar nephronia (ALN), and intrarenal abscess, are considered to be more serious forms of UTI.

Acute lobar nephronia (ALN), also known as acute focal bacterial nephritis, is an acute localized bacterial renal infection presenting as an inflammatory mass without liquefaction (Rosenfield *et al.*, 1979; Zaontz *et al.*, 1985; Kline *et al.*, 1988; Klar *et al.*, 1996, Uehling *et al.*, 2000). The typical clinical presentations include fever, flank pain, leukocytosis, pyuria and bacteriuria, similar to presentations of patients with renal abscess or acute pyelonephritis (Zaontz *et al.*, 1985; Soulen *et al.*, 1989). It has previously been indicated as a complicated form of acute renal infection, representing the progression of the inflammatory process of APN (Nosher *et al.*, 1988). ALN may also represent a relatively early stage of the development of renal abscess (Shimizu *et al.*, 2005). The management of these renal parenchymal infections differs widely. Most patients with renal abscess require intensive medical therapy with or without surgical intervention, whereas treatment of those with ALN, like uncomplicated APN, entails only intravenous and oral antibiotics (Zaontz *et al.*, 1985; Rathore *et al.*, 1991; Klar *et al.*, 1996). Hence it is important to differentiate these renal parenchymal infections. In this Chapter, we would like to review the diagnosis scheme, treatment modality, bacterial urovirulence factors, host susceptibility gene and the renal scar outcome of ALN.

## 2. Effective ultrasonographic predictor for the diagnosis of acute lobar nephronia

Sonographically, ALN generally presents as severe nephromegaly or a poorly defined, irregularly margined focal mass with hyper-, iso- or hypoechogenicity, depending on the temporal sequence of the lesions and the resolution of the disease (Rathore *et al.*, 1991; Boam and Miser, 1995). Although renal ultrasonography (US) has been considered as the best and most-effective screening method, various false positive and false negative findings have been reported previously (Rosenfield *et al.*, 1979; Soulen *et al.*, 1989). Computed tomography (CT), instead, has been currently recognized as the most-sensitive and -specific imaging modality for diagnosing ALN (Kline *et al.*, 1988; Soulen *et al.*, 1989; Rathore *et al.*, 1991; Klar *et al.*, 1996; Uehling *et al.*, 2000). CT images of the ALN-infected areas typically appear as wedge-shaped, poorly defined regions of decreased nephrogenic density after contrast medium administration (Figure 2.1) (Kline *et al.*, 1988; Soulen *et al.*, 1989; Rathore *et al.*, 1991; Cheng *et al.*, 2004), and mass-like hypodense lesions in the more-severe form (Lee *et al.*, 1980). CT, however, is costly and requires the sedation of a young patient.

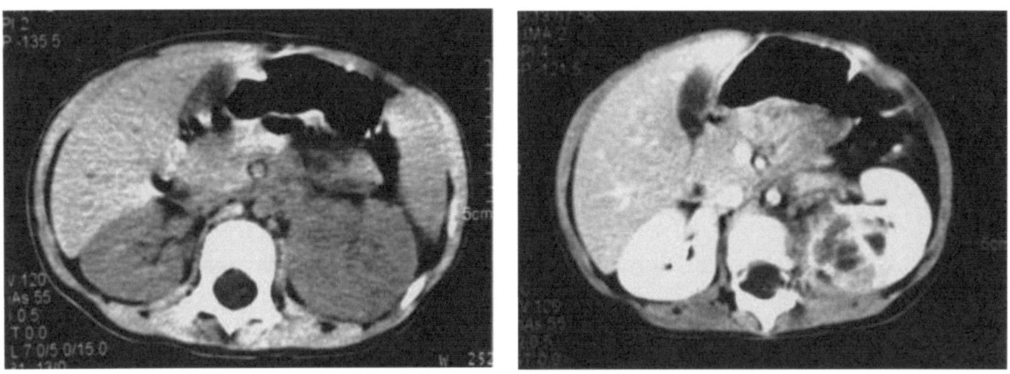

(a) (b)

Fig. 2.1. The characteristic non-enhanced (a) and contrast-enhanced (b) CT scans for a 2-year-old patient with acute lobar nephronia, who presented with severe left nephromegaly while without a focal mass sonographically. Note no attenuation area seen in the kidney before enhancement (Cheng *et al.*, 2004).

A new systemic radiologic imaging evaluation scheme, the combination of renal US and CT scanning, was proposed to assist ALN diagnosis in pediatric patients. Enlarged kidneys and/or focal masses were utilized to be the sonographic preselection features for subsequent CT evaluation. CT scan is used when the patient shows (1) a markedly enlarged kidney or focal mass on the initial US scan; or (2) poor response to the initial 72 hours antibiotic treatment while his/her kidneys appear borderline nephromegaly sonographically (Cheng *et al.*, 2004).

From our results (Cheng *et al.*, 2004), severe nephromegaly (i.e. renal length greater than mean +3 SD for age) on at least one side of the kidneys is very sensitive for the diagnosis of ALN. A higher sensitivity was achieved when US focal mass findings were included with severe nephromegaly as the diagnosing criteria. In terms of the kidneys, focal masses on US scans correlated much better with the final ALN diagnosis than other US characteristics evaluated. The use of focal mass findings as an effective predictor for ALN was limited since its sensitivity was only 25% despite a specificity of 100%. Severe nephromegaly was a very useful sonographic diagnostic criterion for kidneys affected with ALN with a sensitivity of 90.0%. Sensitivity increased to 95% when severe nephromegaly together with focal mass was used as the sonographic predictor.

In summary, pediatric ALN was effectively predicted using sonographic findings of severe nephromegaly and/or focal mass prior to CT scanning.

## 3. Effective duration of antimicrobial therapy for the treatment of acute lobar nephronia

Treatment for patients with ALN generally requires intravenous and oral antibiotic medication as does treatment for uncomplicated APN (Zaontz *et al.*, 1985; Rathore *et al.*, 1991; Klar *et al.*, 1996). Surgical intervention is rarely needed for ALN patients, except for those with concomitant urological abnormalities which may increase the risks of occurrence of acute bacterial infection (Uehling *et al.*, 2000). Although it has been suggested that the treatment duration for ALN needs to be at least the same as that for uncomplicated APN, recommendations for the duration of antibiotic treatment still remains somewhat inconclusive, and to the best of our knowledge, for neither condition, has a rigorous therapeutic efficacy comparison of relevant medication been performed (Rathore *et al.*, 1991).

We have performed a study sought to determine the appropriate duration of effective antibiotic therapy for the management of pediatric ALN patients (Cheng *et al.*, 2006). Patients who first presented as febrile UTI and who later were diagnosed with positive CT findings of ALN were entered into this study for receiving either a two-week or a three-week intravenous and oral antibiotic therapeutic program. The demographic data and clinical results of these patients were compared. In addition, the identification of any clinical or laboratory factors that are likely associated with treatment failure was also attempted.

These two treatment groups had similar demographic data and clinical results (Table 3.1). Most of the patients had been febrile for around three-to-four days, ranging from one day to two weeks or so, prior to admission. Once patients had been admitted, all responded well to the initial antibiotic treatment regimen and the fever generally subsided within about a week. CT scans indicated that 18 patients had left ALN, 12 right ALN, and 11 bilateral ALN in the two-week treatment group. Corresponding figures for the three-week treatment group were 16, 12 and 11 patients respectively. The distribution of these ALN diagnoses was quite similar between the two treatment groups.

Among the 80 patients participating in this study, *Escherichia coli* was the most-common pathogen cultured from the patient urine samples (59/61) such a finding being consistent with the results of previous studies (Kline *et al.*, 1988; Nosher *et al.*, 1988; Rathore *et al.*, 1991; Boam and Miser, 1995; Uehling *et al.*, 2000). Interestingly, the proportion (percentage) of *Escherichia coli* cultured in cases of ALN appears to be much greater than the corresponding figure reported for first-time UTIs (Hoberman and Wald, 1999).

Sixty-nine ALN patients, 40 from the two-week treatment group and 29 from the three-week treatment group, underwent VCUG evaluation. Sixteen patients in the two-week treatment group (40%) and eleven in the three-week treatment group (38%) had vesicoureteral reflux (VUR). Among the patients with VUR, a grade-III or greater was noted in eight and nine patients respectively, treated by the two-week and the three-week antibiotic courses. For patients who underwent VCUG, no difference as regards the presence of VUR in either frequency or severity was found between the two treatment groups.

| | Two-week treatment group (n=41) | Three-week treatment group (n=39) | P |
|---|---|---|---|
| Age, years | 3.72 ± 4.14 | 4.16 ± 4.22 | NS |
| Range | 4 mo - 16 yr | 4 mo - 14yr 8mo | |
| Girls | 24 (58.5%) | 23 (59.0%) | NS |
| Fever duration prior to admission, days | 3.90 ± 3.06 | 3.97 ± 2.72 | NS |
| Range, days | 1 - 14 | 1-13 | |
| Fever continuation following antibiotic treatment, days | 2.73 ± 1.28 | 3.43 ± 2.05 | NS |
| Range, days | 1 - 7 | 1 - 8 | |
| White blood cell count, (cells/μL) | 19,107 ± 8,772 | 19,600 ± 10,212 | NS |
| Leukocytosis (>15,000 WBC/μL) | 28 (68.3%) | 25 (64.1%) | NS |
| C-reactive protein, (mg/L; normal <5) | 137.7 ± 98.1 | 119.3 ± 74.0 | NS |
| Urine culture | | | |
| *Escherichia coli* | 31 (75.6%) | 28 (71.8%) | NS |
| *E. coli* > $10^5$cfu/mL | 25 (61.0%) | 25 (64.1%) | NS |
| *Klebsiella pneumoniae* | 1 (2.4%) | --- | --- |
| *Pseudomonas aeruginosa* | --- | 1 (2.6%) | --- |
| No isolatable organism | 9 (22.0%) | 10 (25.6%) | NS |
| Blood culture | | | |
| *Escherichia coli* | 1 (2.4%) | 2 (5.1%) | --- |
| *Staphylococcus aureus* | --- | 1 (2.6%) | --- |
| No isolatable organism | 40 (97.6%) | 36 (92.3%) | NS |
| Treatment failure | 7 (17.1%) | 0 (0%) | 0.01 |

NS indicates not significant

Table 3.1. Clinical and laboratory data for 80 children with ALN enrolled for different treatment protocol (Cheng *et al.*, 2006).

None of our patients revealed any evidence of underlying diseases such as diabetes mellitus, immunodeficiency, nor did any feature structural abnormality of the urinary-tract system such as neurogenic bladder, or upper or lower urinary-tract obstruction apart from VUR. Reflux was noted in about 40% of the ALN children in this study, a figure quite comparable to that in several previous studies (Kline *et al.*, 1988; Klar *et al.*, 1996; Uehling *et al.*, 2000). This frequency of VUR among patients with ALN is close to that in children with UTI (Ilyas *et al.*, 2002), thus, VUR may not be a necessary prerequisite for the development of ALN.

Overall, seven treatment failures were noted in this study (8.8%; 95% CI, 2.6%-14.9%), all of which had been managed by a two-week antibiotic course (17.1%; 95% CI, 5.6%-28.6%). Statistical significance was noted in regard to treatment success rate between these two groups (p=0.01). Among these patients with treatment failure, one demonstrated persistent infection during the treatment course, and six others were considered to be relapse by revealing a positive *Escherichia coli* urine culture with the same antibiotic sensitivity profile as had been the case previously.

Table 3.2 lists the clinical characteristics of these seven patients as compared with those successfully treated with the two-week antibiotic course. Proportionally more girls may be noted in the failures group than the non-failures group, but the difference was not statistically significant (p=0.21). The patients failing the two-week antibiotic treatment presented with a more-pronounced fever duration prior to admission (6.00 ± 5.54 vs. 3.47 ± 2.16 days; p=0.04), and they were more likely to be *Escherichia coli* infection positive [>$10^5$ cfu/mL; 100% (7/7) vs. 52.9% (18/34); p=0.03]. The distribution of ALN foci, VCUG characteristics, and other clinical results revealed no difference between the failures and non-failures groups.

For the treatment-failure patients, the antibiotic treatment course was extended/restarted for an additional ten days. Subsequent urine culture and clinical-symptom evaluation at the follow-up exams revealed eventual successful treatment.

| | Failures with two-week treatment protocol (n=7) | Non-failures with two-week treatment protocol (n=34) |
|---|---|---|
| Age, years | 4.07 ± 4.31 | 3.65 ± 4.16 |
| Range | 4 mo - 9 yr | 4 mo - 16 yr |
| Girls | 6 (85.7%) | 18 (52.9%) |
| Fever duration prior to admission, days† | 6.00 ± 5.54 | 3.47 ± 2.16 |
| Range, days | 1 - 14 | 1-10 |
| Fever continuation following antibiotic treatment, days | 2.14 ± 1.21 | 2.85 ± 1.28 |
| Range, days | 1 - 4 | 1-7 |
| White blood cell count, (cells/μL) | 22,257 ± 8,656 | 18,459 ± 8,781 |
| Leukocytosis (>15,000 WBC/μL) | 6 (85.7%) | 22 (64.7%) |
| C-reactive protein, (mg/L; normal <5) | 107.3 ± 113.3 | 143.4 ± 95.9 |
| *Escherichia coli* in urine culture | 7 (100%) | 24 (70.6%) |
| *E. coli* > $10^5$cfu/mL‡ | 7 (100%) | 18 (52.9%) |

†: p=0.04; ‡: p=0.03

Table 3.2. Comparison of demographic data, clinical characteristics and laboratory results between the ALN patients with treatment failure and those with treatment success for the two-week antibiotic therapy protocol (Cheng *et al.*, 2006).

From our results, all ALN patients with the three-week antibiotic course were successfully treated, whereas seven treatment failures (17.1% of treated patients) were noted in the two-week treatment group. This observation suggests that the two-week antibiotic treatment, usually scheduled for APN, may not be appropriate for the treatment of ALN. Patients who failed the two-week treatment modality were more likely to have prolonged fever prior to admission and to reveal positive *Escherichia coli* infection (>$10^5$ cfu/mL). The longer febrile history prior to admission may suggest that these patients may be prone to develop a more severe disease state than their counterparts, and that, by necessity, a longer antibiotic treatment course will be needed for such individuals. Indeed, these treatment failures were all successfully dealt with by an additional ten-day antimicrobial therapy regimen. Whether host factors, or the virulence of *Escherichia coli*, relates to ALN and plays a role leading to treatment failure remains an issue that should be clarified.

## 4. A high incidence of renal scarring is associated with child with acute lobar nephronia

The pathogenesis of renal scarring after a febrile UTI remains unclear. Some risk factors making children with a UTI more vulnerable to renal damage include young age at the time of infection (Winberg *et al.* 1982), delayed treatment (Miller and Phillips 1981; Winberg *et al.* 1982), the presence of vesicoureteral reflux (VUR) (Biggi *et al.* 2001; Chroustova *et al.* 2006; Faust *et al.* 2009), and although mentioned infrequently, the extent of kidney lesions (Biggi *et al.* 2001). ALN is a severe disease entity, with extensive renal parenchymal involvement (Cheng *et al.* 2009). Thus, we performed a prospective study to evaluate renal scar formation after ALN as compared with APN. In this prospective study (Cheng *et al.* 2010a), we also examined nearly all the previously proposed risk factors for renal scarring.

DMSA scintigraphy is a sensitive diagnostic method for renal scarring but does not always distinguish between new and old lesions, or differentiate renal dysplasia from acquired post-infection scars. It is possible that we might have overestimated the occurrence of renal scars that were related to the index infection. Thus, the exclusion of children with history of prior UTI or the development of recurrent UTI before DMSA scintigraphy in current study was designed to keep any overestimation of renal scarring to a minimum.

In this investigation, a total of 218 children with a first documented febrile UTI (109 APN, 109 ALN) who fulfilled our patient selection criteria and completed the final DMSA scintigraphy were analyzed. Patient characteristics were comparable between the two ALN treatment groups (Table 4.1). The frequency of renal scarring at scintigraphy was similar between the 2-week and 3-week successful treatment groups. The demographic and clinical data for the APN (all had received 10-day treatment) and ALN patients are shown in Table 4.2. Acute lobar nephronia was a more severe disease than APN, as judged by higher inflammatory indices and longer fever duration after and/or before treatment. The incidence of renal scarring was much higher in ALN than in APN patients.

Regression analysis of the 218 patients with a first febrile UTI showed that renal scarring was more likely to occur in children with higher inflammatory indices (white blood count: 19802±7652 vs. 15478± 6853; and C-reactive protein: 124.6±89.8 vs. 68.4±69.6; $P < 0.001$), longer duration of fever after ($P < 0.001$) and/or before treatment ($P = 0.001$), and the presence of VUR ($P = 0.044$). However no relationship was found between renal scarring and age at diagnosis or gender.

Higher inflammatory indices and longer fever duration after and/or before treatment were strongly correlated with ALN (Table 4.2), these factors, henceforth, were determined not to be independent predictor variables in a multiple logistic regression analysis on renal scarring. ALN was shown to be the only independent risk factor for renal scarring ($P < 0.001$; Table 4.3)

The duration and route of administration of antibiotics have been shown not to influence the risk for renal scarring in patients with APN (Hoberman and Wald *et al.* 1999; Bouissou *et al.* 2008). Our previous prospective study (Cheng *et al.* 2006) suggested that 3 weeks of antibiotic therapy was the treatment of choice for all radiographically documented ALN patients; a longer duration of antibiotic use resulted in the successful treatment for ALN but did not reduce the risk for renal scarring. In most reported studies, including ours, the outcome in terms of renal scarring seems to be unrelated to the mode and duration of antibiotic treatment.

| Parameter | 2-wk Treatment ALN Group | 3-wk Treatment ALN Group | *P* |
|---|---|---|---|
| Patient number | 54 | 55 | |
| Male/Female | 25/29 | 24/31 | NS |
| Age (years) | 2.62 ± 3.08<br>Median: 1.00<br>Range: (0.25, 15.00) | 3.17 ± 3.01<br>Median: 1.33<br>Range: (0.07, 9.42) | NS |
| WBC count, cells/μl | 21144 ± 7205 | 22014 ± 9608 | NS |
| C-reactive protein, mg/L | 156.1 ± 94.4 | 150.0 ± 85.1 | NS |
| Vesicoureteral reflux | 48.1% (25/52) | 35.9% (19/53) | NS |
| *E. coli* percentage in urine culture[a] | 95.1% (39/41) | 85.7% (36/42) | NS |
| Fever duration before treatment, days | 3.54 ± 2.23 | 4.07 ± 3.37 | NS |
| Fever duration after treatment, days | 3.19 ± 1.76 | 4.02 ± 2.81 | NS |
| Time from ALN to DMSA renal scan, years | 1.27 ± 1.02 | 1.40 ± 1.18 | NS |
| Renal scar formation | 88.9% (48/54) | 89.1% (49/55) | NS |

WBC, white blood cell; DMSA, dimercaptosuccinic acid; NS, not significant. [a] excluding urine cultures showing no growth.

Table 4.1. Demographic and clinical data for 109 patients with ALN (Cheng *et al.* 2010a).

| Parameter | APN | ALN | *P* |
|---|---|---|---|
| Patient number | 109 | 109 | |
| Male/Female | 49/60 | 49/60 | NS |
| Age (years) | 2.80 ± 3.59<br>Median: 1.00<br>Range: (0.16, 15.00) | 2.90 ± 3.04<br>Median: 1.16<br>Range: (0.07, 15.00) | NS |
| WBC count, cells/μl | 14729 ± 4656 | 21583 ± 8475 | < 0.001 |
| C-reactive protein, mg/L | 53.4 ± 46.5 | 153.0 ± 89.5 | < 0.001 |
| Vesicoureteral reflux | 34.6% (36/104) | 41.9% (44/105) | NS |
| *E. coli* percentage in urine culture[a] | 78.8% (82/104) | 90.4% (75/83) | 0.033 |
| Fever duration before treatment, days | 1.90 ± 1.62 | 3.81 ± 2.86 | < 0.001 |
| Fever duration after treatment, days | 1.02 ± 0.75 | 3.61 ± 2.37 | < 0.001 |
| Time from APN or ALN to DMSA renal scan, years | 1.21 ± 1.06 | 1.34 ± 1.10 | NS |
| Renal scar formation | 34.9% (38/109) | 89.0% (97/109) | < 0.001 |

[a] excluding urine cultures showing no growth.

Table 4.2. Demographic and clinical data for patients with APN and patients with ALN (Cheng *et al.* 2010a).

| Variable | aOR | 95% CI | | P |
|---|---|---|---|---|
| | | Lower | Upper | |
| Disease | | | | |
| APN | 1.00 | -- | -- | -- |
| ALN | 13.56 | 6.53 | 28.19 | < 0.001 |
| Gender | | | | |
| Male | 1.00 | -- | -- | -- |
| Female | 0.95 | 0.47 | 1.93 | NS |
| Age | | | | |
| < 1 year | 1.00 | -- | -- | -- |
| 1-5 years | 0.85 | 0.39 | 1.86 | NS |
| > 5 years | 0.91 | 0.35 | 2.33 | NS |
| Vesicoureteral reflux (VUR) | | | | |
| No VUR | 1.00 | -- | -- | -- |
| VUR | 1.83 | 0.90 | 3.74 | 0.096 |

Table 4.3. Multiple logistic regression analysis for scar formation (Cheng *et al.* 2010a).

The severity of APN as evaluated by the extent of renal lesions on acute DMSA scanning has been suggested to be a predictor for renal scarring (Biggi *et al.* 2001; Chiou *et al.* 2001). Our data on higher renal scar odds ratio in ALN, a more severe form of acute renal infection than APN, as well as in higher inflammatory indices and longer fever duration after and/or before treatment strongly support this suggestion.

The role of VUR in the development of renal scars remains controversial (Hoberman and Wald *et al.* 1999; Gordon *et al.* 2003; Hoberman *et al.* 2003; Moorthy *et al.* 2005). Some recent prospective studies (Hoberman *et al.* 2003; Chroustova *et al.* 2006; Polito *et al.* 2006; Bouissou *et al.* 2008) and a cross-sectional meta-analysis (Faust *et al.* 2009) have shown a significant association between the presence of VUR and the risk for renal scarring. However, the presence of VUR was a weak predictor of renal scarring in the present study. The additional effect of VUR above that achieved by including only the presence of ALN (nephromegaly and/or severity of infection) in the multiple logistic regression model was not statistically significant for predicting renal scarring.

In conclusion, our results showed a new finding that ALN is associated with a very high incidence of renal scarring, in comparison to APN, irrespective of the duration of antibiotic treatment.

## 5. Comparison of urovirulence factors and genotypes for bacteria causing acute lobar nephronia and acute pyelonephritis

*Escherichia coli* is the most common cause of various UTIs, including cystitis, prostatitis and pyelonephritis (Johnson and Kuskowski *et al.* 2005). Our early studies showed that *E. coli* was the most common pathogen cultured from the patients with ALN (Cheng *et al.* 2004, 2006), having a higher percentage of pathogens than the first-time UTIs (Hoberman and Wald 1999). This finding has led us to this investigation of the pathogenetic association of the bacterial virulence factors as well as the genotypes of the *E. coli* isolates in pediatric ALN.

Henceforth, we have sought to determine the role of *E. coli* urovirulence factors in the development of ALN as compared to APN in pediatric patients who have no underlying diseases or urinary anatomical anomalies except vesicoureteral reflux (VUR) (Cheng *et al.*, 2007). Through our previous published systematic diagnostic scheme (Cheng *et al.* 2004, 2006), patients who first presented as febrile UTIs and later were diagnosed with positive CT findings of ALN or positive technetium 99m-dimercaptosuccinic acid scintigraphic ($^{99m}$Tc-DMSA) findings of APN were enrolled into this study.

Patients were included for study only if *E. coli* was the sole isolate recovered from their urine specimens. Single colonies of the *E. coli* were randomly selected from the initial culture plate and stored in 20% glycerol at -70°C until used. Urovirulent factors examined included genes associated with various fimbrial and nonfimbrial adhesins (*pap*G I, *pap*G II, *pap*G III, *fimH, sfa, foc, afa*), aerobactin receptor (*iutA*), hemolysin (*hlyA*), and cytotoxic necrotizing factor I (*cnf1*) (Tseng *et al.* 2001, 2002; Johnson 2003; Johnson and Russo 2005). The difference in the prevalence of various *E. coli* urovirulent factors for the pediatric patients with ALN or APN was statistically analyzed. In addition, genotyping of these *E. coli* isolates was also performed to examine the possible clonal differences.

A total of 88 patients who fulfilled enrollment criteria were included for study. Among these, 46 patients were diagnosed with ALN and 42 cases with APN. Seventy-two patients, 42 from the ALN group and 30 from the APN group, underwent VCUG evaluation. Seventeen (40.5%) patients in the ALN group and 12 (40%) in the APN group had VUR. Among the patients with VUR, grade-IV reflux or greater was noted in 3 patients each with APN and ALN. Among patients who underwent VCUG, no difference in the presence of VUR in either frequency or severity was found between the two disease categories.

Among the 88 *E. coli* clinical isolates, *pap*G adhesin genes (including classes I to III) were detected in 44 of the ALN isolates and 32 of the APN ones (95.7% vs. 76.2%, $p<0.05$). The class II allele was more commonly noted in the group of ALN (95.7% vs. 73.9%, $p<0.05$; Table 5.1) (Cheng *et al.*, 2007). In contrast, no significant difference was found for the class III allele between the two groups. None of the isolates had the class I allele. In addition, *pap*G II allele was noted in all ALN patients with normal VCUGs (25/25) while only in 16 of the 18 APN patients with normal VCUGs. The genetic determinant for type 1 fimbriae, *fimH*, was the most common virulence factor (95.5%) found among the isolates; however, no statistically significant difference between the two groups was noted. Similarly, the remaining genetic determinants for other virulence factors did not reveal any significant difference between the two groups. Multivariate logistic regression analysis revealed that *pap*G II allele was significantly associated with ALN ($p<0.005$; odds ratio, 17.16, 95% CI: 2.76-106.70). This association was independent of the presence of VUR.

To cause bacterial infections of the upper urinary tract, the microorganisms need to reach the kidney through ascending or hematogenous routes. Bacterial adherence to the uroepithelial cells by fimbrial or nonfimbrial adhesins is considered to be an important factor in the development of upper urinary tract infection via the ascending route (Tseng *et al.* 2001). Among these adhesins, *pap*G variants, which are located at the tip of P-fimbriae and bind preferentially to different Gal (α 1-4) Gal-containing glycolipids in the human epithelium of proximal and distal tubules and in collecting ducts, have been implicated to be associated with the severity of renal infection (Källenius *et al.* 1981; Johnson 1991; Wang *et al.* 2002; Johnson and Russo 2005). Previous studies have shown that the *pap*G II allele is associated with acute pyelonephritis (APN) (Johanson *et al.* 1993; Otto *et al.* 1993; Jantunen *et al.* 2000), while the *pap*G III allele predominates in less severe genitourinary infections, such as acute cystitis and prostatitis (Johanson *et al.* 1993; Johnson *et al.* 1998; Ruiz *et al.* 2002).

| Virulence factor | ALN group (n=46) | APN group (n=42) | P |
|---|---|---|---|
| *pap*G (P-fimbriae) | | | |
| Class I | 0 (0%) | 0 (0%) | --- |
| Class II | 44 (95.7%) | 31 (73.8%) | 0.01 |
| Class III | 5 (10.9%) | 4 (9.5%) | NS |
| *fimH* (type 1 fimbriae) | 44 (95.7%) | 40 (95.2%) | NS |
| *sfa* (S-fimbriae) | 7 (15.2%) | 4 (9.5%) | NS |
| *foc* (F1C-fimbriae) | 5 (10.9%) | 8 (19.1%) | NS |
| *afa* (afimbrial adhesins) | 3 (6.5%) | 4 (9.5%) | NS |
| *iutA* (aerobactin receptor) | 35 (76.1%) | 32 (76.2%) | NS |
| *hlyA* (hemolysin) | 21 (45.7%) | 23 (54.8%) | NS |
| *Cnf1* (cytotoxic necrotizing factor 1) | 8 (17.4%) | 14 (33.3%) | NS |

NS indicates not significant

Table 5.1. Comparison of virulence factors of *Escherichia coli* isolated from patients with ALN and APN (Cheng *et al.*, 2007).

Results in this study (Cheng *et al.* 2007) also indicated that *pap*G II was significantly more prevalent in pediatric patients with ALN than those with APN. This finding provides further evidence that the *pap*G II allele might play a more important pathogenic role than other adhesins in the development of severe renal infectious diseases. In addition, this finding may offer an insight for the future development of vaccine against such severe renal parenchymal inflammatory diseases.

The *fimH* gene sequence which encodes the type I fimbriae was present uniformly in most of the isolates from either ALN or APN patients. This is in accordance with the fact that type I fimbriae is present in nearly all *E. coli* isolates from patients with various UTIs, ranging from cystitis, prostatitis to APN (Johnson and Stell 2000; Johnson and Russo 2005). This study further extends the proposed mechanism that *fimH* gene (i.e. type I fimbriae) was generally required for renal bacterial infection disease to be occurred, no matter what degree of severity it is. In contrast, other fimbrial and nonfimbrial adhesins (i.e. *sfa*, *foc*, and *afa* genes) were rarely detected among our isolates and their pathogenic roles in ALN and APN are likely of less importance, a finding similar to those reported previously in the less severe renal infection categories (Siitonen *et al.* 1993; Blanco *et al.* 1997; Mitsumori *et al.* 1998).

Host compromise can decrease the requirements for bacterial virulence in causing severe urinary tract infections, and, henceforth, change the distribution of *pap*G pathogenetic determinants among the clinical isolates studied (Jantunen *et al.* 2000; Tseng *et al.* 2001, 2002; Johnson and Russo 2005). In this study, the lack of influence of VUR, the only host compromising factor revealed, on the determination of urovirulence factors could be due to the similar distribution and severity of VUR between these two groups. Such similarities in VUR severity distribution and occurrence frequency were also reported in our earlier studies and many others (Kline *et al.* 1988; Sargent and Stringer 1995; Uehling *et al.* 2000; Cheng *et al.* 2004, 2006). In addition, this frequency of VUR among patients with ALN or APN (~ 40%) is close to that in children with UTI (Ilyas *et al.* 2002). Thus, VUR may not be a necessary prerequisite (i.e. significant predisposing host factor) for the development of ALN.

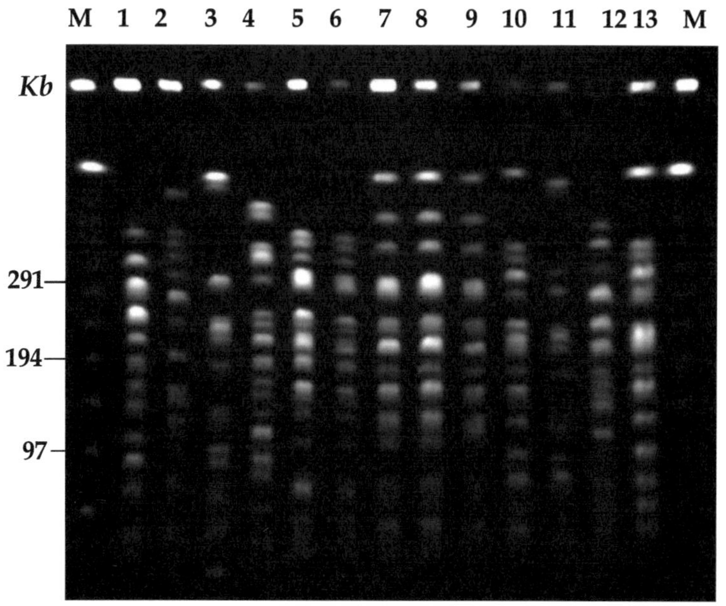


Fig. 5.1. PFGE pattern of representative *Xba*I-digested genomic DNA from *Escherichia coli* isolates. Lane M, lambda DNA concatemer standard; lanes 1-5, 7, and 8, clinical isolates in the APN group; lanes 6, 9-13, clinical isolates in the ALN patients. (Cheng *et al.*, 2007).

A total of 85 genotypes were found among the 88 *E. coli* isolates. Some representative banding patterns are shown in Figure 5.1 (Cheng *et al.*, 2007). These isolates from both ALN and APN patients demonstrated a variety of genotypes. A total of 85 genotypes contained multiple isolates, and 2 genotypes contained isolates from both ALN and APN groups, suggesting that isolates of the same clone could be associated with either entity.

In summary, PFGE analysis indicated that no major genotype was associated with the disease category among these 88 clinical *E. coli* isolates. As to the urovirulence factors examined, the *pap*G class II gene was the most strongly associated pathogenic determinant for the pediatric ALN patients who have no underlying diseases except VUR. Furthermore, even without VUR, patients can still develop clinical symptoms and radiographic characteristics associated with ALN in the presence of *pap*G II gene.

## 6. Comparison of bacterial urovirulence genotypes among patients with urosepsis, acute pyelonephritis, and acute lobar nephronia

Complex pathogen-host interactions determine the patient's susceptibility to bacterial infections (Rushton 1997; Ma and Shortliffe 2004). Various virulence factors have been identified that enhance *E. coli* uropathogenicity, including the facilitation of colonization and invasion of the host, avoidance or disruption of host defense mechanisms, injury to host tissue, and/or stimulation of a noxious host inflammatory responses (Rushton 1997; Johnson and Stell 2000). Furthermore, some virulence factors are more prevalent in specific urinary tract infectious diseases, thus offering insights into future vaccine development (Jantunen *et al.* 2000; Ruiz *et al.* 2002; Tseng *et al.* 2002).

We sought to further elucidate the roles of *E. coli* virulence factors in the development of urosepsis and two other severe renal parenchymal infectious diseases, APN and ALN, in pediatric patients who show no host-compromising factors, except for vesicoureteral reflux (VUR) (Cheng *et al.,* 2010b). Twenty-five virulence factors were analyzed, including genes associated with fimbrial and nonfimbrial adhesins (*pap*AH, *pap*C, *pap*EF, *pap*G I, *pap*G II, *pap*G III, *sfaS*, *focG*, *afa*, *bmaE*, *gafD*, *nfaE*, *fimH*), toxins (*hlyA*, *cnf1*, *cdtB*), siderophores (*fyuA*, *iutA*), capsule synthesis (*kpsMT* II, *kpsMT* III), invasion of brain endothelium (*ibeA*), serum-resistance (*traT*), markers for virulence-associated *E. coli* serogroup O4 (*rfc*) and colcin V plasmids (*cvaC*), and the coding region of PAI from the uropathogenic strain CFT073 (PAI) (Johnson and Stell 2000; Jantunen *et al.* 2000; Tseng *et al.* 2002; Johnson and Kuskowski *et al.* 2005; Cheng *et al.* 2007). Moreover, the prevalence rates of these 25 urovirulence genes for patients with the three invasive UTIs (i.e. APN, ALN, and urosepsis) will also be compared with those for patients diagnosed as cystitis.

The inclusion criteria and diagnostic scheme for patients with documented episodes of ALN or APN were the same as those stated in our earlier publication (Cheng *et al.* 2007). Urosepsis was defined as a patient with bacteremia arising from a urinary tract source (Johnson *et al.* 1988). Cystitis was defined as afebrile pediatric patients with just only localizing symptoms such as dysuria, frequency, urgency, cloudy urine or lower abdominal discomfort. Exclusion criteria included any evidence of underlying diseases such as diabetes or immunodeficiency, or any structural anomalies such as neurogenic bladder, posterior urethral valve, urinary diversion, bladder diverticulum, ureterocele, and urinary tract obstruction apart from VUR.

Among the 123 *E. coli* isolates from APN, ALN and urosepsis, the overall prevalence rate of various virulence factors ranged from 2% (*nfaE*, nonfimbrial adhesin-1) to 97% (*fimH*, Type I fimbriae). In addition, all but one APN clinical isolate presented at least one adhesin. Of the 25 virulence factors examined, 17 showed a statistically significant distribution among these three invasive UTI categories (Table 6.1). ALN isolates differed significantly from other invasive UTI isolates (i.e. APN and urosepsis) due to their lower prevalence of *cdtB* and a medium prevalence of *cvaC*. Moreover, ALN isolates showed a higher prevalence of *pap*AH, *pap*C, *pap*EF, and *pap*G II, compared with APN isolates, and a lower prevalence of *pap*G I, *focG*, *afa*, *bmaE*, *hlyA*, *cnf1*, *iutA*, *kpsMT* III, *rfc*, and *traT* compared with urosepsis isolates. APN isolates were significantly different from other two types of invasive isolates due to a lower prevalence of *cvaC*. Additionally, APN isolates had a lower prevalence of *pap*G I, *focG*, *afa*, *bmaE*, *iutA*, *kpsMT* III, *rfc*, *traT*, and PAI compared with urosepsis isolates. Finally, urosepsis isolates significantly differed from all other two types of invasive UTI isolates due to a higher prevalence of *pap*G I, *focG*, *afa*, *bmaE*, *iutA*, *kpsMT* III, *rfc*, *cvaC*, and *traT* (Table 6.1).

In contrast, among the 24 clinical isolates from cystitis, eight virulence genes were not noted, and in which, six were bacterial adhesins (i.e. *pap*G I, *sfaS*, *afa*, *bmaE*, *gafD*, *nfaE*). However, the highest prevalence rate (100%) was noted in *fimH* adhesin, the virulence gene sequence encoding type I fimbriae. As compared to the combination of three invasive UTI diseases (i.e. APN, ALN and urosepsis), the cystitis isolates had a lower prevalence of *pap*AH, *pap*C, *pap*EF, *pap*G II, *sfaS*, *afa*, *bmaE*, *hlyA*, *cdtB*, *fyuA* and *ibeA* (Table 6.1).

In this investigation, none of the patients presented with any evidence of underlying disease or structural anomalies except VUR, and a similar distribution of severity and frequency of occurrence of VUR was noted among the three different invasive UTI disease groups; APN, ALN, and, urosepsis. Hence, distinct syndrome-specific differences in distribution for certain virulence factors, but conservation across syndromes for others, is likely related to differences in bacterial urovirulence and uropathogenicity among these three invasive bacterial urinary infectious diseases.

| Virulence factor | Cystitis group (n = 24) | APN group (n = 45) | ALN group (n = 48) | Urosepsis group (n = 30) | P[b] | | | |
|---|---|---|---|---|---|---|---|---|
| | | | | | Cystitis vs. (APN+ ALN+ Urosepsis) | APN vs. ALN | ALN vs. Urosepsis | APN vs. Urosepsis |
| Adhesin | | | | | | | | |
| *pap*AH (P-fimbriae) | 8 (33%) | 32 (71%) | 43 (90%) | 24 (80%) | <0.0001 | 0.0242 | --- | --- |
| *pap*C (P-fimbriae) | 6 (25%) | 32 (71%) | 45 (94%) | 25 (83%) | <0.0001 | 0.0038 | --- | --- |
| *pap*EF (P-fimbriae) | 6 (25%) | 34 (76%) | 44 (92%) | 26 (87%) | <0.0001 | 0.0348 | --- | --- |
| *pap*G (P-fimbriae) | | | | | | | | |
| Class I | 0 ( 0%) | 0 ( 0%) | 0 ( 0%) | 13 (43%) | --- | --- | <0.0001 | <0.0001 |
| Class II | 4 (17%) | 33 (73%) | 44 (92%) | 26 (87%) | <0.0001 | 0.0192 | --- | --- |
| Class III | 4 (17%) | 4 ( 9%) | 6 (13%) | 6 (20%) | --- | --- | --- | --- |
| *sfaS* (S-fimbriae) | 0 ( 0%) | 6 (13%) | 7 (15%) | 9 (30%) | 0.0251 | --- | --- | --- |
| *focG* (F1C-fimbriae) | 6 (25%) | 8 (18%) | 5 (10%) | 20 (67%) | --- | --- | <0.0001 | <0.0001 |
| *afa* (afimbrial adhesin) | 0 ( 0%) | 4 ( 9%) | 4 ( 8%) | 27 (90%) | 0.0028 | --- | <0.0001 | <0.0001 |
| *bmaE* (M blood group antigen-specific M fimbriae) | 0 ( 0%) | 1 ( 2%) | 1 ( 2%) | 16 (53%) | 0.0446 | --- | <0.0001 | <0.0001 |
| *gafD* (glucosaminyl-specific G fimbriae) | 0 ( 0%) | 2 ( 4%) | 7 (15%) | 5 (17%) | --- | --- | --- | --- |
| *nfaE* (nonfimbrial adhesion-1) | 0 ( 0%) | 2 ( 4%) | 0 ( 0%) | 0 ( 0%) | --- | --- | --- | --- |
| *fimH* (type 1 fimbriae) | 24 (100%) | 43 (96%) | 46 (96%) | 30 (100%) | --- | --- | --- | --- |
| Toxin | | | | | | | | |
| *hlyA* (hemolysin) | 4 (17%) | 24 (53%) | 22 (46%) | 22 (73%) | 0.0006 | --- | 0.0172 | --- |
| *Cnf1* (cytotoxic necrotizing factor 1) | 4 (17%) | 14 (31%) | 9 (19%) | 16 (53%) | --- | --- | 0.0015 | --- |
| *cdtB* (cytolethal distending toxin) | 0 ( 0%) | 21 (47%) | 4 (8%) | 17 (57%) | 0.0009 | <0.0001 | <0.0001 | --- |

| Virulence factor | Cystitis group (n = 24) | APN group (n = 45) | ALN group (n = 48) | Urosepsis group (n = 30) | $P^b$ | | | |
|---|---|---|---|---|---|---|---|---|
| | | | | | Cystitis vs. (APN+ ALN+ Urosepsis) | APN vs. ALN | ALN vs. Urosepsis | APN vs. Urosepsis |
| Siderophore | | | | | | | | |
| *fyuA* (yersiniabactin receptor) | 14 (58%) | 41 (91%) | 48 (100%) | 29 (97%) | <0.0001 | --- | ---- | --- |
| *iutA* (aerobactin receptor) | 16 (67%) | 35 (78%) | 36 (75%) | 30 (100%) | --- | --- | 0.0024 | 0.0047 |
| Miscellaneous | | | | | | | | |
| *kpsMT* II (capsule synthesis, group II) | 16 (67%) | 38 (84%) | 41 (87%) | 24 (80%) | --- | --- | ---- | --- |
| *kpsMT* III (capsule synthesis, group III) | 0 ( 0%) | 3 (7%) | 3 (6%) | 9 (30%) | --- | --- | 0.0081 | 0.0101 |
| *rfc* (marker for virulence-associated *E. coli* serogroup O4) | 2 ( 8%) | 6 (13%) | 9 (19%) | 16 (53%) | --- | --- | 0.0015 | 0.0002 |
| *ibeA* (invasion of brain endothelium gene) | 14 (58%) | 34 (77%) | 41 (85%) | 28 (93%) | 0.0090 | --- | ---- | --- |
| *cvaC* (marker for ColV, colcin V, plasmids) | 4 (17%) | 4 (9%) | 13 (27%) | 24 (80%) | --- | 0.0233 | <0.0001 | <0.0001 |
| *traT* (serum-resistance associated gene) | 16 (67%) | 30 (67%) | 39 (81%) | 30(100%) | --- | --- | 0.0108 | 0.0004 |
| PAI (coding region of PAI from uropathogenic strain CFT073) | 16 (67%) | 31 (69%) | 39 (81%) | 28 (93%) | --- | --- | --- | 0.0114 |

[a] Data are presented as the number (%) of indicated urovirulence factors.
[b] The *P* values, as determined by $\chi^2$ analysis or 2-sided Fisher's exact tests, as appropriate, are shown only when $P < 0.05$.

Table 6.1. Comparison between virulence factors among 147 *Escherichia coli* isolates from patients with cystitis, acute pyelonephritis (APN), acute lobar nephronia (ALN), or urosepsis. (Cheng *et al.*, 2010b).

The *fimH*, the gene sequence that encodes type I fimbriae, was found in nearly all strains (97%) from these three invasive UTI diseases and did not vary statistically among these three syndromes. This finding further extends the proposed mechanism, namely, that the *fimH* gene is generally required for renal bacterial infectious disease to occur, regardless of level (Johnson and Stell 2000; Tseng *et al.* 2002; Johnson and Russo 2005; Moreno *et al.* 2005; Cheng *et al.* 2007).

An aggregate virulence factor score for each isolate was calculated as the number of unique virulence factors detected, with adjustment for multiple detection of *pap* (P-fimbriae) and *sfa/foc* (S/F1C fimbriae) (Johnson and Kuskowski *et al.* 2005). The median scores were 6.5 (range: 1-12), 9 (range: 2–12), 9 (range: 6–13), and 14 (range: 9–17) for cystitis, APN, ALN, and urosepsis isolates, respectively. A Kruskal-Wallis nonparametric one way ANOVA analysis indicated the aggregate virulence factor score was significantly different among these four disease groups ($p < 0.0001$). *Post hoc* analyses using Dunn method (2-sided) between any two disease categories indicated that urosepsis isolates presented significantly higher aggregate virulence scores than isolates from any other three diseases (urosepsis vs. cystitis, urosepsis vs. APN and urosepsis vs. ALN; $p < 0.0001$). Isolates from cystitis, rather, showed significantly lower aggregate virulence scores than those from any other three invasive UTI diseases (cystitis vs. APN and cystitis vs. ALN; $p < 0.01$; cystitis vs. urosepsis; $p < 0.0001$). However, no significant difference was noted between the APN and ALN isolates ($p = 0.88$).

In summary, for the three invasive urinary infectious diseases, distinct syndrome-specific differences in distribution for certain virulence factors, but conservation across syndromes for others is noted. This likely resulted from the differences in bacterial urovirulence and uropathogenicity. Our findings also suggested that urosepsis isolates carry more virulence factors and are therefore likely more urovirulent compared with cystitis, APN and ALN isolates.

## 7. Genetic polymorphisms and susceptibility for pediatric patients with parenchymal renal infections

Despite of aforementioned efforts on correlating urovirulence factors of uropathogenic *E. coli* with the disease severity, the intra-individual differences in clinical presentations are still noted among UTI patients. This underlies the importance of host factors, such as mechanistic dysfunctions like vesicoureteral reflux (VUR) and genetic variations, in patient's susceptibility to the bacterial invasion and infection (Artifoni *et al.* 2007; Lundstedt and Leijonhufvud *et al.* 2007; Lundstedt and McCarthy *et al.* 2007; Hawn, Scholes and Li *et al.* 2009; Sivick and Mobley 2010).

The inflammatory response caused by the attachment/invasion of uropathogenic *E. coli* into the urinary tract is determined by different molecular interactions between the bacteria and epithelial cells (Artifoni *et al.* 2007; Sivick and Mobley 2010). The initial recognition for bacterial attachment/invasion occurs through the coordination efforts of various toll-like receptors and different Pathogen-Associated Molecular Patterns (PAMPs) such as bacterial flagellin and lipopolysaccharide (Hawn, Scholes and Li *et al.* 2009). Following that, potent chemoattractants secreted by the infected epithelial cells will attract inflammatory cells, and the chemokine receptors will then direct recruited inflammatory cells' interactions with mucosal barrier. Subsequent steps in the inflammatory process will determine the balance between the health and the disease severity (Godaly *et al.* 2001; Artifoni *et al.* 2007). Neutrophil-dependent innate host defense system is considered to be an important antimicrobial process to maintain the sterility of the urinary tract. It starts from signal transmission by cooperative efforts of toll-like receptor 4 (TLR-4) and P fimbriae of uropathogenic *E. coli*, followed by the secretion of main chemoattractant for neutrophils, IL-8. The IL-8 mediates its effects on neutrophil chemotaxis, transepithelial infiltration into the urinary tract, activation and phagocytosis and killing of bacteria through the receptors CXCR1 and CXCR2 (Godaly *et al.* 2001; Lundstedt and Leijonhufvud *et al.* 2007; Lundstedt and McCarthy *et al.* 2007).

Henceforth, we sought to determine the correlations in the polymorphisms for genes regulating the initial recognition of bacterial invasion (i.e. TLR-4, toll-like receptor 4) and subsequent neutrophil infiltration and activation for bacteria clearance (i.e. IL-8, interleukin-8; and CXCR1, CXCR2; receptors for interleukin-8) among the pediatric UTI patients with different clinical severity; namely, acute pyelonephritis (APN) and the clinically more severe UTI disease, acute lobar nephronia (ALN) (Cheng *et al.*, 2011a). In addition, since VUR is a well-known risk factor for severe parenchymal infectious disease as APN (Orellana *et al.* 2004; Artifoni *et al.* 2007), a subgroup of APN and ALN patients without VUR will also be examined to exclude the possible effects caused by VUR.

Statistical analyses using log-additive model has revealed that only IL-8 (rs4073) showed significant difference in genotype frequency between the control group and APN, ALN or combined cases (Table 7.1) for APN vs. control; ALN vs. control and combined vs. control, respectively). In addition, the genotype AA in IL-8 (rs4073) was associated with the severe upper UTIs (i.e. APN and ALN) in comparison to the TT and TA genotypes (Table 7.1) for APN vs. control; ALN vs. control and combined vs. control, respectively). The allele frequency analyses have shown that the minor allele, "A", in IL-8 (rs4073) is more prevalent in the severe upper UTI groups than in the control for APN vs. control; ALN vs. control and combined vs. control, respectively (Table 7.2) (Cheng *et al.* 2011a).

Since vesicoureteral reflux (VUR) has been suggested as the significant host risk factor for upper UTIs (Orellana *et al.* 2004; Artifoni *et al.* 2007), we subsequently evaluated the results of genetic analysis in the subgroup of APN and ALN patients with no VUR. In the no-VUR subgroup of APN and ALN patients, only ALN and APN+ALN group presented a statistically significant difference in IL-8 (rs4073) genotype frequency using log-additive model (OR (95% CI): 1.47 (1.03, 2.10); 1.50 (1.09, 2.06) for ALN vs. control; and combined vs. control, respectively). In comparison to the TT and TA genotypes in IL-8 (rs4073) SNP, a significant higher AA genotype frequency was noted in the no-VUR subgroup of ALN and APN+ALN cases (recessive model, OR (95% CI): 2.31 (1.15, 4.65); 2.15 (1.13, 4.09) for ALN vs. control; and combined vs. control, respectively). These two no-VUR subgroups (i.e. ALN and APN+ALN) also presented a significant higher minor allele (i.e. "A" in IL-8 (rs4073)) frequency than in the control (OR (95%CI): 1.43 (1.02, 2.01); 1.45 (1.07, 1.96) for ALN vs. control and combined vs. control, respectively).

This investigation (Cheng *et al.* 2011a) has indicated that APN and ALN patients have distinctive higher AA genotype frequency and A allele occurrence in IL-8 (rs 4073) as compared to the controls. In contrast, no differences in TLR-4 (rs10759932), CXCR1 (rs16858808) and CXCR2 (rs4674258) were noted among the APN, ALN and control. The polymorphism for IL-8 (rs4073) occurs at -251A>T position in the 5′ promoter region of IL-8.

| SNP | Group | Genotype (%) 00 | 01 | 11 | Log-additive Model OR (95% CI) | P | Dominant Model (01, 11 vs 00) OR (95% CI) | P | Recessive Model (11 vs 00, 01) OR (95% CI) | P |
|---|---|---|---|---|---|---|---|---|---|---|
| | | CC | CT | TT | OR (95% CI) | $P^a$ | OR (95% CI) | $P^a$ | OR (95% CI) | $P^a$ |
| CXCR1 (rs16858808) | Control | 214 (96.4) | 8 (3.6) | 0 (0) | | | | | | |
| | APN | 108 (95.6) | 5 (4.4) | 0 (0) | 1.24 (0.40, 3.88) | | | | | |
| | ALN | 156 (94.0) | 9 (5.4) | 1 (0.6) | 1.79 (0.73, 4.37) | 0.32 | 1.71 (0.66, 4.44) | 0.27 | | 0.43 |
| | Com-bined | 264 (94.6) | 14 (5.0) | 1 (0.4) | 1.57 (0.68, 3.63) | 0.58 | 1.52 (0.63, 3.65) | 0.34 | | |
| | | CC | CT | TT | OR (95% CI) | *P* | OR (95% CI) | *P* | OR (95% CI) | *P* |
| CXCR2 (rs4674258) | Control | 101 (45.7) | 94 (42.5) | 26 (11.8) | | | | | | |
| | APN | 50 (44.2) | 50 (44.2) | 13 (11.6) | 1.03 (0.73, 1.43) | 0.88 | 1.06 (0.67, 1.67) | 0.80 | 0.98 (0.48, 1.98) | 0.94 |
| | ALN | 80 (48.2) | 72 (43.4) | 14 (8.4) | 0.88 (0.64, 1.19) | 0.39 | 0.90 (0.60, 1.35) | 0.63 | 0.69 (0.35, 1.37) | 0.28 |
| | Combi-ned | 130 (46.6) | 122 (43.7) | 27 (9.7) | 0.93 (0.72, 1.22) | 0.62 | 0.96 (0.68, 1.37) | 0.84 | 0.80 (0.45, 1.42) | 0.45 |
| | | TT | TA | AA | OR (95% CI) | *P* | OR (95% CI) | *P* | OR (95% CI) | *P* |
| IL-8 (rs4073) | Control | 94 (42.9) | 107 (48.9) | 18 (8.2) | | | | | | |
| | APN | 40 (35.4) | 54 (47.8) | 19 (16.8) | 1.45 (1.03, 2.06) | **0.03** | 1.37 (0.86, 2.19) | 0.18 | 2.26 (1.13, 4.50) | **0.02** |
| | ALN | 57 (34.3) | 81 (48.8) | 28 (16.9) | 1.49 (1.09, 2.02) | **0.01** | 1.44 (0.95, 2.18) | 0.09 | 2.27 (1.21, 4.26) | **0.01** |
| | Combi-ned | 97 (34.8) | 135 (48.4) | 47 (16.8) | 1.46 (1.12, 1.91) | **0.01** | 1.41 (0.98, 2.03) | 0.06 | 2.26 (1.27, 4.02) | **0.01** |

| SNP | Group | Genotype (%) 00 | 01 | 11 | Log-additive Model | | Dominant Model (01, 11 vs 00) | | Recessive Model (11 vs 00, 01) | |
|---|---|---|---|---|---|---|---|---|---|---|
| | | CC | CT | TT | OR (95% CI) | $P^a$ | OR (95% CI) | $P^a$ | OR (95% CI) | $P^a$ |
| | | TT | TC | CC | OR (95% CI) | $P$ | OR (95% CI) | $P$ | OR (95% CI) | $P$ |
| TLR-4 (rs10759932) | Control | 118 (53.6) | 86 (39.1) | 16 (7.3) | | | | | | |
| | APN | 65 (58.6) | 39 (35.1) | 7 (6.3) | 0.86 (0.59, 1.24) | 0.42 | 0.82 (0.52, 1.30) | 0.40 | 0.86 (0.34, 2.15) | 0.74 |
| | ALN | 87 (52.7) | 68 (41.2) | 10 (6.1) | 0.99 (0.72, 1.37) | 0.96 | 1.04 (0.69, 1.55) | 0.86 | 0.82 (0.36, 1.86) | 0.64 |
| | Comb-ined | 152 (55.1) | 107 (38.8) | 17 (6.1) | 0.94 (0.70, 1.25) | 0.65 | 0.94 (0.66, 1.35) | 0.75 | 0.84 (0.41, 1.70) | 0.62 |

[a] The $P$ values are shown in bold when $P < 0.05$.
[b] Combined: APN+ALN

Table 7.1. Genotypic analysis of single nucleotide polymorphisms (SNPs) (Cheng et al., 2011a).

Hence, current finding is in parallel to an earlier report in which A allele in -251A>T is significantly associated with the presence of dimercapto-succinic acid scan documented APN (Artifoni *et al.* 2007). This has been attributed to the association of A allele with an increase in IL-8 production (Hull *et al.* 2001; Artifoni *et al.* 2007). In addition, AA genotype has been linked to the increased level of fecal IL-8 and the occurrence of enteroaggregative *E. coli*-associated diarrhea (Jiang *et al.* 2003). Therefore, the IL-8 (rs4073) SNP for APN and ALN patients could be related to the up-regulated IL-8 expression that has subsequently resulted in severe clinical inflammatory responses noted clinically. Furthermore, after elimination of VUR, the well-known risk factor for severe UTIs, from analyses, only ALN patients presented SNP in IL-8 (rs4073) while APN did not. Since the inflammatory responses in ALN patients are more sever than in APN ones (e.g. higher CRP value and longer fever duration after antibiotic treatment), this finding further supports the role of polymorphism in IL-8 (rs4073, -251A>T) in IL-8 up-regulation.

In summary, the SNP in the inflammatory chemokine IL-8, a higher frequency in AA genotype and A allele, is involved in the susceptibility and clinical responses in pediatric APN and ALN cases. In addition, after removing VUR, the significant risk factor for parenchymal infection, from statistical analysis, the IL-8 SNP is only noted in the no-VUR subgroup of clinically more severe ALN patients. This suggests IL-8 (rs4073) SNP is correlated to the clinical severity of parenchymal infection, likely due to the up-regulated IL-8 expression by the AA genotype and A allele.

| SNP | Minor allele frequency[a] (%) | | | | APN vs. Control | | ALN vs. Control | | Combined vs. Control | |
|---|---|---|---|---|---|---|---|---|---|---|
| | Control | APN | ALN | Combined[b] | OR (95% CI) | $P^c$ | OR (95% CI) | $P^c$ | OR (95% CI) | $P^c$ |
| CXCR1 (rs16858808) | 1.80 | 2.21 | 3.31 | 2.87 | 1.23 (0.40, 3.81) | 0.72 | 1.87 (0.74, 4.70) | 0.18 | 1.61 (0.68, 3.79) | 0.28 |
| CXCR2 (rs4674258) | 33.03 | 33.63 | 30.12 | 31.54 | 1.03 (0.73, 1.44) | 0.88 | 0.87 (0.64, 1.19) | 0.39 | 0.93 (0.72, 1.22) | 0.62 |
| IL-8 (rs4073) | 32.65 | 40.71 | 41.27 | 41.04 | 1.42 (1.02, 1.97) | **0.04** | 1.45 (1.08, 1.95) | **0.01** | 1.44 (1.11, 1.86) | **0.01** |
| TLR-4 (rs10759932) | 26.82 | 23.87 | 26.67 | 25.54 | 0.86 (0.59, 1.24) | 0.41 | 0.99 (0.72, 1.37) | 0.96 | 0.94 (0.70, 1.24) | 0.65 |

[a] Minor allele: CXCR1, T; CXCR2, T; IL-8, A; TLR-4, C.

[b] Combined: APN+ALN

[c] The $P$ values are shown in bold when $P < 0.05$.

Table 7.2. Allele frequency analysis of single nucleotide polymorphisms (SNPs) by logistic regression model. (Cheng et al., 2011a).

## 8. Conclusion

A new imaging scheme that combines US and CT has been developed for effective ALN diagnosis. In this scheme, patients suspected of suffering from UTI [i.e. who had pyuria (> 5

WBCs/high-power field), fever without focus or any symptoms/signs related to UTI, such as knocking pain, dysuria and frequency] underwent renal US during the 1st-2nd day following their admission to hospital. The CT assessment followed immediately when the initial US findings met either one of these two criteria, evidence of: (1) unilateral or bilateral nephromegaly; and (2) a focal renal mass. For children who presented with borderline nephromegaly ultrasonographically, CT was performed when the patient remained febrile for 72 hours subsequent to antibiotic-treatment commencement. ALN diagnosis was made on the basis of positive CT findings.

Further, with this scheme, we have identified that a three-week antimicrobial therapy protocol, rather than the two-week scheme commonly used for APN treatment, should constitute the treatment of choice for all radiographically documented ALN patients. As for the likelihood in scar formation following the severe parenchymal infections, we have confirmed that pediatric patients with ALN could have higher possibility for scar formation than with APN.

Through the urovirulence factor analyses, we have noted that the *papG* class II gene (gene associated with P-fimbriae of uropathogenic *E. coli*) was the most strongly associated pathogenic determinant for the pediatric ALN patients who have no underlying diseases except VUR. But PFGE analysis indicated that no major genotype was associated with the disease category. Thus the major pathogenic determinants may not be unique to any specific genetic lineage. In addition, using the MDCK epithelial cells model, we have confirmed that the ability to adhere to and produce cytotoxicity against uroepithelial cells appears a prerequisite factor for *E. coli* to cause more severe bacterial kidney infection, such as ALN (Cheng *et al.*, 2011b). Much more, we have confirmed that *E. coli* isolates from urosepsis patients carried more virulence factors as compared to those from patients with cystitis, APN and ALN. This implicated that the number of urovirulent genes found in pathogenic isolates may be correlated with the clinical severity noted in pediatric UTIs.

For the host factors that could influence the patient's susceptibility to the sever parenchymal infections, we have identified SNP in the inflammatory chemokine IL-8, a higher frequency in AA genotype and A allele, is involved in the susceptibility and clinical responses in pediatric APN and ALN cases. Further, among the patients without VUR, this IL-8 SNP is only noted in the ALN patients while not in the APN cases. This finding implicates that this IL-8 SNP could lead to a higher IL-8 secretion level after bacterial infection, and, subsequently, more severe inflammatory responses found in the ALN patients.

Despite of abovementioned findings in the pediatric patients with ALN, we have not explored the host genetic factors for the ALN patient proned to have recurrent UTIs. These patients might have some genetic polymorphisms that increase patient's susceptibility to UTIs. A detailed longitudinal clinical follow-up plan would be needed to further elucidate the likely polymorphisms in these recurrent-UTI-prone ALN patients. In addition, building a proper animal model for ALN study will be attempted in the future study. The IL-8 expression level among the patients diagnosed as cystitis, APN and ALN will also be compared to each other. Since the ALN patients are also likely to have renal scarring according to our previous findings, genetic polymorphisms likely to reduce the renal scars will also be evaluated in the future studies.

## 9. Acknowledgment

Financial support provided by the National Science Council of Taiwan (98-2314-B-182A-007-MY3; 97-2314-B-182A-061; 95-2314-B-182A-111-MY2) and Chang Gung Memorial Hospital

(CMRPG 340351, 470031) are acknowledged. The authors thank Dr. Chee-Jen Chang and his team for their advice and assistance with the statistical analyses. Prof. Lin-Hui Su is acknowledged for her advice in various laboratory works. The excellent technical help from Miss Li-Yun Tseng and editorial assistance from Dr. Jui-Che Lin are also acknowledged. The authors report no conflicts of interest.

## 10. References

Artifoni L, Negrisolo S, Montini G, Zucchetta P, Molinari PP, Cassar W, Destro R, Anglani F, Rigamonti W, Zacchello G, Murer L. (2007) Interleukin-8 and CXCR1 receptor functional polymorphisms and susceptibility to acute pyelonephritis. *J Urol* 177: 1102-1106

Biggi A, Dardanelli L, Cussino P, Pomero G, Noello C, Sernia O, Spada A, Camuzzini G (2001) Prognostic value of the acute DMSA scan in children with first urinary tract infection. *Pediatr Nephrol* 16: 800-804

Blanco M, Blanco JE, Alonso MP, Mora A, Balsalobre C, Muñoa F, Juárez A, Blanco J (1997) Detection of *pap*, *sfa* and *afa* adhesin-encoding operons in uropathogenic *Escherichia coli* strains: relationship with expression of adhesins and production of toxins. *Res Microbiol* 148: 745-755

Boam WD, Miser WF (1995) Acute focal bacterial pyelonephritis. *Am Fam Physician* 52: 919-924

Bouissou F, Munzer C, Decramer S, Roussel B, Novo R, Morin D, Lavocat MP, Guyot C, Taque S, Fischbach M, Ouhayoun E, French Society of Nuclear Medicine and Molecular Imaging, Loirat C, French Society of Pediatric Nephrology (2008) Prospective, randomized trial comparing short and long intravenous antibiotic treatment of acute pyelonephritis in children: dimercaptosuccinic acid scintigraphic evaluation at 9 months. *Pediatrics* 121: e553-e560

Cheng CH, Tsau YK, Hsu SY, Lee TL (2004) Effective ultrasonographic predictor for the diagnosis of acute lobar nephronia. *Pediatr Infect Dis J* 23: 11-14

Cheng CH, Tsau YK, Lin TY (2006) Effective duration of antimicrobial therapy for the treatment of acute lobar nephronia. *Pediatrics* 117: e84-e89

Cheng CH, Tsau YK, Su LH, Lin CL, Lin TY (2007) Comparison of urovirulence factors and genotypes for bacteria causing acute lobar nephronia and acute pyelonephritis. *Pediatr Infect Dis J* 26: 228-232.

Cheng CH, Tsau YK, Chen SY, Lin TY (2009) Clinical courses of children with acute lobar nephronia correlated with computed tomographic patterns. *Pediatr Infect Dis J* 28: 300-303

Cheng CH, Tsau YK, Chang CJ, Chang YC, Kuo CY, Tsai IJ, Hsu YH, Lin TY (2010a) Acute lobar nephronia is associated with a high incidence of renal scarring in childhood urinary tract infections. *Pediatr Infect Dis J* 29: 624-628

Cheng CH, Tsau YK, Kuo CY, Su LH, Lin TY. (2010b) Comparison of extended virulence genotypes for bacteria isolated from pediatric patients with urosepsis, acute pyelonephritis, and acute lobar nephronia. *Pediatr Infect Dis J* 29: 736-740

Cheng CH, Lee YS, Tsau YK, Lin TY. (2011a) Genetic Polymorphisms and Susceptibility for Pediatric Patients with Parenchymal Renal Infections *Pediatr Infect Dis J* 30: 309-314

Cheng CH, Su LH, Tsau YK, Lin TY. (2011b) Comparison of Virulence Variations on MDCK Monolayers by *Escherichia coli* Isolated from Acute Lobar Nephronia and Acute Pyelonephritis. *New Microbiol* 34: 65-72

Chiou YY, Wang ST, Tang MJ, Lee BF, Chiu NT (2001) Renal fibrosis: prediction from acute pyelonephritis focus volume measured at $^{99m}$Tc dimercaptosuccinic acid SPECT. *Radiology* 221: 366-370

Chroustova D, Playzova D, Urbanova I, Kolska M. (2006) Results of a five-year study of 99mTc-DMSA renal scintigraphy in children and adolescents following acute pyelonephritis. *Nucl Med Rev* 9: 46-50

Faust WC, Diaz M, Pohl HG (2009) Incidence of post-pyelonephritic renal scarring: a meta-analysis of the dimercapto-succinic acid literature. *J Urol* 181: 290-298

Godaly G, Bergsten G, Hang L, Fischer H, Frendéus B, Lundstedt AC, Samielsson M, Samuelsson P, Svanborg C. (2001) Neutrophil recruitment, chemokine receptors, and resistance to mucosal infection. *J Leukoc Biol* 69: 899-906

Gordon I, Barkovics M, Pindoria S, Cole TJ, Woolf AS (2003) Primary vesicoureteric reflux as a predictor of renal damage in children hospitalized with urinary tract infection: a systematic review and meta-analysis. *J Am Soc Nephrol* 14: 739-744

Hawn TR, Scholes D, Li SS, Wang H, Yang Y, Robers, PL, Stapleton AE, Janer M, Aderem, A, Stamm, WE, Zhao LP, Hooton TM. (2009) Toll-like receptor polymorphisms and susceptibility to urinary tract infections in adult women. *PLoS ONE* 4: e5990

Hawn TR, Scholes D, Wang H, Li SS, Stapleton AE, Janer M, Anderem A, Stamm WE, Zhao LP, Hooton TM. (2009) Genetic variation of the human urinary tract innate immune response and asymptomatic bacteriuria in women. *PLoS ONE* 4: e8300

Hoberman A, Wald ER (1999) Treatment of urinary tract infections. *Pediatr Infect Dis J* 18: 1020-1021

Hoberman A, Charron M, Hickey RW, Baskin M, Kearney DH, Wald ER (2003) Imaging studies after a first febrile urinary tract infection in young children. *N Engl J Med* 348: 195-202

Hull J, Akerman H, Isles K, Usen S, Pinder M, Thomson A. (2001) Unusual haplotypic structure of IL8, a susceptibility locus for a common respiratory virus. *Am J Hum Genet* 69: 413-419

Ilyas M, Mastin ST, Richard GA (2002) Age-related radiological imaging in children with acute pyelonephritis. *Pediatr Nephrol* 17: 30-34

Jantunen ME, Siitonen A, Koskimies O, Wikström S, Kärkkäinen U, Salo E. Saxén H (2000) Predominance of class II *pap*G allele of *Escherichia coli* in infants with normal urinary tract anatomy. *J Infect Dis* 181: 1822-1824

Jiang ZD, Okhuysen PC, Guo DC, He R, King TM, DuPont HL, Milewicz DM. (2003) Genetic susceptibility to enteroaggregative *Escherichia coli* diarrhea: polymorphism in the interleukin-8 promoter region. *J Infect Dis* 188: 506-11

Johanson IM, Plos K, Marklund BI, Svanborg C. (1993) *Pap*, *pap*G and *prs*G DNA sequences in *Escherichia coli* from the fecal flora and the urinary tract. *Microb Pathog* 15: 121-129

Johnson JR, Moseley SL, Roberts PL, Stamm WE. (1988) Aerobactin and other virulence factor genes among strains of *Escherichia coli* causing urosepsis: association with patient characteristics. *Infect Immun* 56: 405-412

Johnson JR (1991) Virulence factors in *Escherichia coli* urinary tract infection. *Clin Microbiol Rev* 4: 80-128

Johnson JR, Russo TA, Brown JJ, Stapleton A. (1998) *pap*G alleles of *Escherichia coli* strains causing first episode or recurrent acute cystitis in adult women. *J Infect Dis* 177: 97-101

Johnson JR, Stell AL (2000) Extended virulence genotypes of *Escherichia coli* strains from patients with urosepsis in relation to phylogeny and host compromise. *J Infect Dis* 181: 261-272

Johnson JR (2003) Microbial virulence determinants and the pathogenesis of urinary tract infection. *Infect Dis Clin North Am* 17: 261-278

Johnson JR, Kuskowski MA, Gajewski A, Soto S, Horcajada JP, Jimenez de Anta MT, Vila J (2005) Extended virulence genotypes and phylogenetic background of *Escherichia coli* isolates from patients with cystitis, pyelonephritis, or prostatitis. *J Infect Dis* 191: 46-50

Johnson JR, Russo TA (2005) Molecular epidemiology of extraintestinal pathogenic (uropathogenic) *Escherichia coli. Int J Med Microbiol* 295: 383-404

Klar A, Hurvitz H, Berkun Y, Nadjari M, Blinder G, Israeli T, Halamish A, Katz A, Shazberg G, Branski D (1996) Focal bacterial nephritis (lobar nephronia) in children. *J Pediatr* 128: 850-853

Källenius G, Möllby R, Svenson SB, Helin I, Hultberg H, Cedergren B, Winberg J. (1981) Occurrence of p-fimbriated *Escherichia coli* in urinary tract infection. *Lancet* 2: 1369-1372

Kline MW, Kaplan SL, Baker CJ (1988) Acute focal bacterial nephritis: diverse clinical presentations in pediatric patients. *Pediatr Infect Dis J* 7: 346-349

Lee JKT, McClennan BL, Melsen GL, Stanley RJ (1980) Acute focal bacterial nephritis: emphasis on gray scale sonography and computed tomography. *AJR* 135: 87-92

Lundstedt AC, Leijonhufvud I, Ragnarsdottir B, Karpman D, Andersson B, Svanborg C. (2007) Inherited susceptibility to acute pyelonephritis: A family study of urinary tract infection. *J Infect Dis* 195: 1227-1234.

Lundstedt AC, McCarthy S, Gustafsson MCU, Godaly G, Jodal U, Karpman D, Leijonhufvud I, Lindén C, Matinell J, Ragnarsdottir B, Samuelsson M, Truedsson L, Andersson B, Svanborg C. (2007) A genetic basis of susceptibility to acute pyelonephritis. *PLoS ONE* 2: e825

Ma JF, Shortliffe LM. (2004) Urinary tract infection in children: etiology and epidemiology. *Urol Clin N Am* 31: 517-526

Miller T, Phillips S (1981) Pyelonephritis: the relationship between infection, renal scarring, and antimicrobial therapy. *Kidney Int* 19: 654-662

Mitsumori K, Terai A, Yamamkto S, Yoshida O. (1998) Identification of S, F1C and three PapF fimbrial adhesins in uropathogenic *Escherichia coli* by polymerase chain reaction. *FEMS Immunol Med Microbiol* 21: 261-268

Moorthy I, Easty M, McHugh K, Ridout D, Biassoni L, Gordon I (2005) The presence of vesicoureteric reflux does not identify a population at risk for renal scarring following a first urinary tract infection. *Arch Dis Child* 90: 733-736

Moreno E, Planells I, Prats G, Planes AM, Moreno G., Andreu A. (2005) Comparative study of *Escherichia coli* virulence determinants in strains causing urinary tract bacteremia versus strains causing pyelonephritis and other sources of bacteremia. *Diagn Microbiol Infect Dis* 53: 93-99

Nosher JL, Tamminen JL, Amorosa JK, Kallich M (1988) Acute focal bacterial nephritis. *Am J Kidney Dis* 11: 36-42

Orellana P, Baquedano P, Rangarajan V, Zhao JH, Eng ND, Fettich J, Chaiwatanarat T, Sonmezoglu K, Kumar D, Park YH, Samuel AM, Sixt R, Bhatnagar V, Padhy AK. (2004) Relationship between acute pyelonephritis, renal scarring, and vesicoureteral reflux. Results of a coordinated research project. *Pediatr Nephrol* 19: 1122-1126

Otto GS, Sandberg T, Marklund BI, Ulleryd P, Svanborg C. (1993) Virulence factors and pap genotype in *Escherichia coli* isolates form women with acute pyelonephritis, with or without bacteremia. *Clin Infect Dis* 17: 448-456

Polito C, Rambaldi PF, Signoriello G, Mansi L, La Manna A (2006) Permanent renal parenchymal defects after febrile UTI are closely associated with vesicoureteric reflux. *Pediatr Nephrol* 21: 521-526

Rathore NH, Barton LL, Luisiri A (1991) Acute lobar nephronia: a review. *Pediatrics* 87: 728-734

Rosenfield AT, Glickman MG, Taylor KJ, Crade M, Hodson J (1979) Acute focal bacterial nephritis (acute lobar nephronia). *Radiology* 132: 553-561

Riccabona M. (2003) Urinary tract infections in children. *Curr Opin Urol* 13: 59-62

Ruiz J, Simon K, Horcajada JP, Velasco M, Barranco M, Roig G, Moreno-Martínez A, Martínez JA, Jiménez de Anta T, Mensa J, Vila J. (2002) Differences in virulence factors among clinical isolates of *Escherichia coli* causing cystitis and pyelonephritis in women and prostatitis in men. *J Clin Microbiol* 40: 4445-4449

Rushton HG. (1997) Urinary tract infections in children: epidemiology, evaluation, and management. *Pediatr Clin N Am*. 44: 1133-1169

Sargent MA, Stringer DA. (1995) Voiding cystourethrography in children with urinary tract infection: the frequency of vesicoureteric reflux is independent of the specialty of the physician requesting the study. *AJR Am J Roentgenol* 164: 1237-1241

Shimizu M, Katayama K, Kato E, Miyayama S, Sugata T, Ohta K (2005) Evolution of acute focal bacterial nephritis into a renal abscess. *Pediatr Nephrol* 20: 93-95

Siitonen A, Martikainen R, Ikaheimo R, Palmgren J, Makela PH. (1993) Virulence-associated characteristics of *Escherichia coli* in urinary tract infection: a statistical analysis with special attention to type 1C fimbriation. *Microb Pathogen* 15: 65-75

Sivick KE, Mobley HL. (2010) Waging war against uropathogenic *Escherichia coli*: winning back the urinary tract. *Infect Immun* 78: 568-585

Smithson A, Sarrias MR, Barcelo J, Suarez B, Horcajada JP, Soto SM, Soriano A, Vila, J, Martinez JA, Vives J, Mensa J, Lozano F. (2005) Expression of interleukin-8 receptors (CXCR1 and CXCR2) in premenopausal women with recurrent urinary tract infections. Clin *Diagn Lab Immunol* 12:1358-1363

Soulen MC, Fishman EK, Goldman SM, Gatewood OMB (1989) Bacterial renal infection: role of CT. *Radiology* 171: 703-707

Tseng CC, Huang JJ, Ko WC, Yan JJ, Wu JJ (2001) Decreased predominance of *pap*G class II allele in *Escherichia coli* strains isolated from adults with acute pyelonephritis and urinary tract abnormalities. *J Urol* 166: 1643-1646

Tseng CC, Wu JJ, Liu HL, Sung JM, Huang JJ (2002) Roles of host and bacterial virulence factors in the development of upper urinary tract infection caused by *Escherichia coli*. *Am J Kidney Dis* 39: 744-752

Uehling DT, Hahnfeld LE, Scanlan KA (2000) Urinary tract abnormalities in children with acute focal bacterial nephritis. *BJU Int* 85: 885-888.

Wang MC, Tseng CC, Chen CY, Wu JJ, Huang JJ (2002) The role of bacterial virulence and host factors in patients with *Escherichia coli* bacteremia who have acute cholangitis or upper urinary tract infection. *Clin Infect Dis* 35: 1161-1166

Winberg J, Bollgren I, Kallenius G, Mollby R, Svenson SB (1982) Clinical pyelonephritis and focal renal scarring: a selected review of pathogenesis, prevention, and prognosis. *Pediatr Clin North Am* 29: 801-814

Zaontz MR, Pahira JJ, Wolfman M, Gargurevich AJ, Zeman RK (1985) Acute focal bacterial nephritis: a systematic approach to diagnosis and treatment. *J Urol* 133: 752-757